LUNG DISEASE IN THE TROPICS

LUNG BIOLOGY IN HEALTH AND DISEASE

Executive Editor: **Claude Lenfant**

Director, National Heart, Lung, and Blood Institute
National Institutes of Health
Bethesda, Maryland

Volume 1 IMMUNOLOGIC AND INFECTIOUS REACTIONS IN THE LUNG, *edited by Charles H. Kirkpatrick and Herbert Y. Reynolds*

Volume 2 THE BIOCHEMICAL BASIS OF PULMONARY FUNCTION, *edited by Ronald G. Crystal*

Volume 3 BIOENGINEERING ASPECTS OF THE LUNG, *edited by John B. West*

Volume 4 METABOLIC FUNCTIONS OF THE LUNG, *edited by Y. S. Bakhle and John R. Vane*

Volume 5 RESPIRATORY DEFENSE MECHANISMS (in two parts), *edited by Joseph D. Brain, Donald F. Proctor, and Lynne M. Reid*

Volume 6 DEVELOPMENT OF THE LUNG, *edited by W. Alan Hodson*

Volume 7 LUNG WATER AND SOLUTE EXCHANGE, *edited by Norman C. Staub*

Volume 8 EXTRAPULMONARY MANIFESTATIONS OF RESPIRATORY DISEASE, *edited by Eugene Debs Robin*

Volume 9 CHRONIC OBSTRUCTIVE PULMONARY DISEASE, *edited by Thomas L. Petty*

Volume 10 PATHOGENESIS AND THERAPY OF LUNG CANCER, *edited by Curtis C. Harris*

Volume 11 GENETIC DETERMINANTS OF PULMONARY DISEASE, *edited by Stephen D. Litwin*

Volume 12 THE LUNG IN THE TRANSITION BETWEEN HEALTH AND DISEASE, *edited by Peter T. Macklem and Solbert Permutt*

Volume 13 EVOLUTION OF RESPIRATORY PROCESSES: A COMPARATIVE APPROACH, *edited by Stephen C. Wood and Claude Lenfant*

Volume 14 PULMONARY VASCULAR DISEASES, *edited by Kenneth M. Moser*

Volume 15 PHYSIOLOGY AND PHARMACOLOGY OF THE AIRWAYS, *edited by Jay A. Nadel*

Volume 16 DIAGNOSTIC TECHNIQUES IN PULMONARY DISEASE (in two parts), *edited by Marvin A. Sackner*

Volume 17 REGULATION OF BREATHING (in two parts), *edited by Thomas F. Hornbein*

Volume 18 OCCUPATIONAL LUNG DISEASES: RESEARCH APPROACHES AND METHODS, *edited by Hans Weill and Margaret Turner-Warwick*

Volume 19 IMMUNOPHARMACOLOGY OF THE LUNG, *edited by Harold H. Newball*

Volume 20 SARCOIDOSIS AND OTHER GRANULOMATOUS DISEASES OF THE LUNG, *edited by Barry L. Fanburg*

Volume 21 SLEEP AND BREATHING, *edited by Nicholas A. Saunders and Colin E. Sullivan*

Volume 22 *PNEUMOCYSTIS CARINII* PNEUMONIA: PATHOGENESIS, DIAGNOSIS, AND TREATMENT, *edited by Lowell S. Young*

Volume 23 PULMONARY NUCLEAR MEDICINE: TECHNIQUES IN DIAGNOSIS OF LUNG DISEASE, *edited by Harold L. Atkins*

Volume 24 ACUTE RESPIRATORY FAILURE, *edited by Warren M. Zapol and Konrad J. Falke*

Volume 25 GAS MIXING AND DISTRIBUTION IN THE LUNG, *edited by Ludwig A. Engel and Manuel Paiva*

Volume 26 HIGH-FREQUENCY VENTILATION IN INTENSIVE CARE AND DURING SURGERY, *edited by Graziano Carlon and William S. Howland*

Volume 27 PULMONARY DEVELOPMENT: TRANSITION FROM INTRAUTERINE TO EXTRAUTERINE LIFE, *edited by George H. Nelson*

Volume 28 CHRONIC OBSTRUCTIVE PULMONARY DISEASE, second edition, revised and expanded,
edited by Thomas L. Petty

Volume 29 THE THORAX (in two parts),
edited by Charis Roussos and Peter T. Macklem

Volume 30 THE PLEURA IN HEALTH AND DISEASE,
edited by Jacques Chrétien, Jean Bignon, and Albert Hirsch

Volume 31 DRUG THERAPY FOR ASTHMA: RESEARCH AND CLINICAL PRACTICE,
edited by John W. Jenne and Shirley Murphy

Volume 32 PULMONARY ENDOTHELIUM IN HEALTH AND DISEASE,
edited by Una S. Ryan

Volume 33 THE AIRWAYS: NEURAL CONTROL IN HEALTH AND DISEASE,
edited by Michael A. Kaliner and Peter J. Barnes

Volume 34 PATHOPHYSIOLOGY AND TREATMENT OF INHALATION INJURIES,
edited by Jacob Loke

Volume 35 RESPIRATORY FUNCTION OF THE UPPER AIRWAY,
edited by Oommen P. Mathew and Giuseppe Sant'Ambrogio

Volume 36 CHRONIC OBSTRUCTIVE PULMONARY DISEASE: A BEHAVIORAL PERSPECTIVE,
edited by A. John McSweeny and Igor Grant

Volume 37 BIOLOGY OF LUNG CANCER: DIAGNOSIS AND TREATMENT,
edited by Steven T. Rosen, James L. Mulshine, Frank Cuttitta, and Paul G. Abrams

Volume 38 PULMONARY VASCULAR PHYSIOLOGY AND PATHOPHYSIOLOGY,
edited by E. Kenneth Weir and John T. Reeves

Volume 39 COMPARATIVE PULMONARY PHYSIOLOGY: CURRENT CONCEPTS,
edited by Stephen C. Wood

Volume 40 RESPIRATORY PHYSIOLOGY: AN ANALYTICAL APPROACH,
edited by H. K. Chang and Manuel Paiva

Volume 41 LUNG CELL BIOLOGY,
edited by Donald Massaro

Volume 42 HEART-LUNG INTERACTIONS IN HEALTH AND DISEASE,
edited by Steven M. Scharf and Sharon S. Cassidy

Volume 43 CLINICAL EPIDEMIOLOGY OF CHRONIC OBSTRUCTIVE PULMONARY DISEASE
edited by Michael J. Hensley and Nicholas A. Saunders

Volume 44 SURGICAL PATHOLOGY OF LUNG NEOPLASMS
edited by Alberto M. Marchevsky

Volume 45 THE LUNG IN RHEUMATIC DISEASES
edited by Grant W. Cannon and Guy A. Zimmerman

Volume 46 DIAGNOSTIC IMAGING OF THE LUNG
edited by Charles E. Putman

Volume 47 MODELS OF LUNG DISEASE: MICROSCOPY AND STRUCTURAL METHODS
edited by Joan Gil

Volume 48 ELECTRON MICROSCOPY OF THE LUNG
edited by Dean Schraufnagel

Volume 49 ASTHMA: ITS PATHOLOGY AND TREATMENT
edited by Michael A. Kaliner, Peter J. Barnes, and Carl G. A. Persson

Volume 50 ADULT RESPIRATORY DISTRESS SYNDROME
edited by Warren M. Zapol and François Lemaire

Volume 51 LUNG DISEASE IN THE TROPICS
edited by Om P. Sharma

Volume 52 EXERCISE: PULMONARY PHYSIOLOGY AND PATHOPHYSIOLOGY
edited by Brian J. Whipp and Karlman Wasserman

Additional Volumes in Preparation

DEVELOPMENTAL NEUROBIOLOGY OF BREATHING
edited by Gabriel G. Haddad and Jay P. Farber

LUNG DISEASE IN THE TROPICS

Edited by

Om P. Sharma

Department of Medicine
Los Angeles County–University of Southern California
Medical Center

University of Southern California
School of Medicine
Los Angeles, California

MARCEL DEKKER, INC. New York · Basel · Hong Kong

Library of Congress Cataloging--in--Publication Data

Lung disease in the tropics / edited by Om P. Sharma.
p. cm.
Includes bibliographical references and index.
ISBN 0-8247-8398-0
1. Lungs-- --Diseases. 2. Tropical medicine. I. Sharma, Om P.
[DNLM: 1. Lung Diseases. 2. Tropical Medicine. WC 680 L963]
RC732.L84 1990
616.2'4'00193-- --dc20
DNLM/DLC
for Library of Congress 90--14116
CIP

This book is printed on acid-free paper

MARCEL DEKKER, INC.
270 Madison Avenue, New York, New York, 10016

Current printing (last digit):
10 9 8 7 6 5 4 3 2 1

PRINTED IN THE UNITED STATES OF AMERICA

INTRODUCTION

> Sir Edward Parry and his party were going straight towards the pole in one of their arctic expeditions, travelling at the rate of ten miles a day. But the ice over which they travelled was drifting straight towards the equator, at the rate of twelve miles a day, and yet no man among them would have known that he was travelling two miles a day backward unless he had lifted his eyes from the track in which he was plodding. It is not only going backward that the plain practical workman is liable to, if he will not look up and look around; he may go forward to the ends he little dreams of.
>
> *Oliver Wendell Holmes*
> *Massachusetts Medical Society, 1860*

As Dr. Sharma points out in his Preface, "Social, political, and technological developments of the modern era have blurred Nature's boundaries separating tropical, temperate, and arctic land masses." And, thus, today we have many opportunities to "look up and look around"–to observe what medical practices from elsewhere can teach us.

But there is another reason to broaden our view. The practice of medicine in any country is, in part, the result of the culture of that country. In comparison with the rest of the world, America's culture is new. Indeed, medicine has been practiced for thousands of years in many civilizations that preceded ours. From that long experience, principles and precepts have developed; undoubtedly, past experience of these ancient cultures has greatly influenced their practice of modern medicine. We can only benefit from an examination of what is being done elsewhere.

In many ways *Lung Disease in the Tropics* will provide the reader with a panoramic view of the world of medicine. First of all, the purpose of this volume is quite original. It addresses a number of pathological conditions that are common in the tropics, but to some extent rare in the United States. Yet, there is enough migration from the tropics to our country to be concerned about these conditions and to want to learn about them. Next, the contributors to this monograph are recognized experts from the countries and regions of the world where these pulmonary conditions are prevalent and serious public health concerns. They bring to the readers years of experience in recognizing and managing patients affected by these pathologies. Finally, we should acknowledge that much of ancient medicine originated in the areas of the world whence these pulmonary conditions are described. Therefore, the authors are sharing not only their own experience but also ideas and concepts that have evolved from the beginning of medicine.

Few treatises before this one have addressed lung disease in the tropics, but even fewer have assembled contributors from so many countries and regions of the world. This volume truly symbolizes the "blurring of the land masses."

Dr. Sharma and his authors are to be congratulated for such an important contribution. When the series of monographs Lung Biology in Health and Disease was conceived, it was hoped to be an encyclopedia about the lung. As this monograph covers lung diseases from distant parts of the world, it broadens even further the scope of the series. I am grateful to all of the contributors for helping us to "look up and look around."

Claude Lenfant, M.D.
Bethesda, Maryland

PREFACE

> Man, being the servant and interpreter of nature, can do and understand so much and so much only as he has observed in fact or in thought of the course of nature, beyond this he neither knows anything nor can do anything.
>
> Francis Bacon (1561-1626)
> *In Novum Organum, Amphorism i*

Social, political, and technological developments of the modern era have blurred Nature's boundaries separating tropical, subtropical, temperate, and arctic land masses. With increasing travel and intercontinental migration, physicians and other health workers can expect to encounter previously unfamiliar diseases and exotic medical syndromes which once occurred only in tropical and subtropical areas. Several of these diseases manifest primarily in the lungs; whereas others involve the respiratory organs only in conjunction with other tissue systems of the body.

Thus, the modern pulmonologist must learn how to diagnose and treat tropical lung disease and be fully aware of the possibility of an imported illness in every patient he sees, every visitor, immigrant tourist, political refugee, and jet setter he examines.

The authors of the articles on 23 selected topics in this volume, *Lung Disease in the Tropics*, include national and international clinicians who specialize in tropical pulmonary medicine. These elegant essays broaden our vision by exploring interrelationships in medicine and emphasizing the ways of ameliorating human suffering.

In the first article, Lung Immunology in the Tropics, Drs. Zumla and James provide an admirable review of the development of immunology and its clinical application as related to the tropical terrain. They remind us that the host is the battleground between invading antigens whether they are bacteria, viruses, parasites, cancer, or chemicals, The tropical host is a particularly impoverished one who manifests defects of immune deficiency caused by malnutrition.

Pulmonary granulomatous disorders are common in tropical as well as temperate zones. The causes of pulmonary granulomatosis include tuberculosis, fungi, organic antigens, parasites, and chemicals. Drs. Flora and Sharma have given a practical approach to the problem. They admonish us to obtain a thorough history of the residence and recent travels of the patient. A careful history and physical examination enhanced by good quality chest roentgenograms and simple laboratory tests are all that is needed to solve the riddle of lung granulomas.

Drs. Bambery, Jindal, and Kaur from the Postgraduate Institute of Medical Education and Research, Chandigarh, India, paint a dismal picture of the ever-present menace of malaria, a major tropical disorder. About 10 percent of the patients with *Plasmodium falciparum* infection may develop clinical pulmonary disease; pulmonary edema and adult respiratory distress syndrome are the two most serious, potentially lethal, complications. There are many new advances in the treatment of malaria which are succinctly summarized in this review.

Pulmonary melioidosis is endemic in Southeast Asia, particularly Indochina, Hong Kong, Australia, Madagascar, and Guam. Dr. Sumalee Kiatboonsri from Ramathibodi Hospital, Bangkok, Thailand gives us his approach and philosophy of diagnosing and treating this disease. The diagnosis of melioidosis depends on isolation of *Pseudomonas pseudomallei* in tissue fluids; for example, blood, sputum, pus, etc., or a positive serologic test for *Pseudomonas pseudomallei.* However, in endemic areas, patients with negative cultures and serologic tests, but with clinical findings resembling melioidosis, are sometimes treated for melioidosis.

Brucellosis, caused by a Gram-negative bacteria of the germs *Brucella*, was named after Major-General Sir David Bruce, later elected FRS. Medical historians will remember that Bruce also identified the trypanosome causing cattle plague. He also demonstrated that the tse-tse fly was the vector of sleeping sickness. In South Africa, the farmers called him "Bruce of Natal." Drs. Lulu and Araj have distilled their vast experience of brucellosis involving some 400 patients.

In the history of world religions, the Islamic tradition of pilgrimage to Mecca is a unique event. Every year about two million pilgrims from all over the world gather on the Western Coast of the Arabian Peninsula. Dr. El-Kassimi from College of Medicine, King Saud University, Riyadh, Saudi Arabia has made certain unique observations of the effect of heat stroke on the lung. Although William Osler knew about the pulmonary complications of heat stroke, Dr. El-Kassimi was the first to collect hemodynamic data using

Swan-Ganz catheters in patients with adult respiratory distress syndrome due to heat stroke.

Amebiasis has a worldwide distribution and the number of cases seen in some of the large metropolitan county hospitals in this country is impressive. Pleuropulmonary amebiasis should always be included in the differential diagnosis of patients with unexplained pleural effusion or consolidation, particularly in individuals who either live in or have come from an endemic area.

Tropical pulmonary eosinophilia is seen mainly in India, Southeast Asia, and the South Pacific Islands. Although the distribution of the syndrome is similar to Bancroftian and Malayan filariasis, it is far more common in Asia than elsewhere, with Indians comprising a large proportion of the infected population. Professor Deivanayagam tells us that this condition, because of cough, fever, weight loss, and night sweats, may be confused with tuberculosis. In tropical pulmonary eosinophilia, however, serum eosinophil and IgE levels are exceedingly high.

Carlos Chagas, a Brazilian physician who worked at Cruz's Institute in Rio de Janeiro, was the first to describe American trypanosomiasis which is caused by a protozoan, *Trypanosoma cruzi.* The disease has widespread distribution in South and Central Americas. Cases have been reported in the Southern United States as well. In Brazil it is a major health problem, affecting more than six million people. Dr. Newton Bethlem and his colleagues from Rio de Janeiro emphasize that cardiomyopathy is the most important clinical manifestation of Chagas' disease, but the lungs and the airways are also affected.

Although hydatid disease is worldwide in distribution, it is most frequently found in sheep- and cattle-rearing countries because of the close relationship between man, dog, and sheep. The point could be made that it is more a disease of temperate climates than of tropical areas. Drs. Dhar and Wattal from Kashmir, India have amassed significant experience managing pulmonary hydatid disease. Tomaso Casoni, an Italian physician at Ospedale Coloniale Vittorio Emanuele III, Tripoli, first introduced the intradermal test for hydatid disease in 1912. The field of immunology has tremendously widened since; Drs. Dhar and Wattal review the latest development in the diagnosis and treatment of this disease.

In the summer of 1979, an unknown virus capable of decimating the human immune system appeared in our world. The human immunodeficiency virus (HIV) destroys the helper T lymphocytes, the backbone of our cell-mediated immunity. The impaired immune system leaves the victim open to numerous fatal opportunistic infections and tumors. AIDS was first reported among homosexual men and intravenous drug users in North America and Europe. Since then, major outbreaks of the disease have occurred in the Caribbean, Africa, Southeast Asia, and India. AIDS cases have also been reported from Japan. The disease is affecting disadvantaged people all over the world. Drs. Tuchschmidt and Akil remind us that in order to control this global problem, the challenge is not only to develop preventive and curative therapeutic agents, but also to develop means of communication, which will penetrate veins of ignorance.

Worldwide more than 200 million people suffer from ravages of schistosomiasis. In the United States alone there are over 400,000 cases, most of them immigrants from Puerto Rico, the Middle East, the Philippines, and Brazil. There are three major species of *Schistosoma* pathogenic for man; *S. mansoni, S. hematobium,* and *S. japonicum.* Pulmonary disease may occur in the early phase of infection called Katayama fever, or as a chronic event in hepatosplenic schistosomiasis. Drs. Armenio and Isabel Guimarães bring our attention to the fact that pulmonary schistosomiasis should be suspected in anybody with lung disease and associated hepatic or urinary tract disease who is from an endemic area. In schistosomiasis extensive pulmonary involvement and cor pulmonale are rare without marked liver disease. Ova are rarely found in sputum.

Sickle cell anemia and its variants are inherent disorders of hemoglobin structure. The term sickle cell anemia, the homozygous form of the disease (HbSS), has the most severe clinical manifestations. Pulmonary involvement is a common complication with both acute and chronic parenchymal disease causing impairment of lung function and gas exchange. In addition to the microvascular obstruction there is an increased susceptibility to infections; although, the reasons for this pronounced predisposition to infection are not fully understood. Most acute lung infections in sickle cell disease are due to *S. pneumoniae, H. influenza,* and *Mycoplasma pneumoniae.* Dr. Eisenberg outlines the diagnostic difficulties between pulmonary infection and infarction in these patients. The fat embolism syndrome appears to be a common cause of death in sickle cell disease. The occurrence of confusion or mental irritability, thrombocytopenia, hypocalcemia, and hypoxemia in these patients should lead to a search for other evidences of the fat embolism syndrome.

As a medical student, I was taught that paragonimiasis was the most common cause of hemoptysis in the world, although I have never really seen any data validating that opinion. Paragonimiasis is endemic in Korea, Japan, China, and African countries, especially Nigeria, as well as parts of South America and Southeast Asia. This peculiar geographic distribution reflects the presence of appropriate intermediate hosts and substandard sanitation. Clinical features of paragonimiasis resemble those of pulmonary tuberculosis. Hemoptysis is indeed common and is often referred to "endemic hemoptysis" in areas of high prevalence for the disease. Professor C. Nwokolo from Nigeria, provides the perspective of the disease from his vantage point in Enugu, Nigeria.

In tropical and other developing countries, tuberculosis continues to remain the most important of all medical problems. The major task of the tropical physician is to arrive at a correct diagnosis. In the old days when physicians were unduly enamoured with physicial signs, patients who had chronic bronchitis, bronchiectasis, lung abscess, or pneumoconiosis were mistakenly diagnosed to have tuberculosis. Today, the main concern in differential diagnosis is to recognize the unusual pattern of tuberculosis seen particularly in the elderly, in immunosuppressed individuals and in patients with diabetes mellitus or renal failure. This cryptic variety of pulmonary tuberculosis is reviewed by Dr. Yu, who has a vast experience of dealing with difficult patients at Queen Mary Hospital, Hong Kong. Hong Kong antituberculosis drug trials along with Madras and East African studies introduced short-term antituberculosis therapy. In Hong Kong and in other parts of Southeast Asia where the incidence of primary drug resistance is as high as 20 percent or more, the diagnosis of tuberculosis becomes difficult, particularly when the disease occurs in association with immunodeficiency syndromes. Dr. Yu's articles provides guidelines for recognizing and treating obscure manifestations of tuberculosis.

Approximately 10 percent of the world's people are atopic; more than half of these have airway hyperactivity disorders including asthma. The face of asthma is everchanging. In the large metropolitan hospitals in this country, asthma predominantly affects immigrants. Our civilization has introduced asthma, by providing a new set of antigens to virgin tribes in remote parts of the world. The scope and spread of asthma and pulmonary allergic disorders in a country depends on cultural practices, the extent of industrialization and the availability of medical help. Dr. Bovornkitti and his colleagues explore the problem of pulmonary allergic diseases in Southeast Asia where, like Europe, America, and Australia and New Zealand, the incidence of and morbidity due to asthma are on the rise.

Despite a fall in the death rate from chronic bronchitis and emphysema during the last two decades, chronic obstructive lung disease continues to be a major cause of morbidity and mortality. By the time a clinical diagnosis is made, particularly in developing nations, there is often irreversible airway obstruction. While tobacco continues to be the major causative factor, rapid industrialization with little or no regard for human health also plays an important role in the genesis of obstructive airway disease. In the tropics, respiratory tract infections in childhood result in high morbidity and mortality. Some of the survivors develop chronic cough and sputum in later years. Dr. Kamat and his group at Seth G.S. Medical College and K.E.M. Hospital have long been investigating the epidemiology and clinical features of chronic obstructive lung disease. It is possible to separate different types of obstructive airway disease syndromes clinically, but the available therapeutic options in the tropics are limited.

The next three articles provide a Japanese perspective of these pulmonary problems; pneumoconiosis, hypersensitivity pneumonitis, and bronchiolitis. Dr. Hosoda, an international authority on pneumoconiosis, and his colleagues present a basic how-to scheme for diagnosing and assessing the severity of lung damage. Summer-type hypersensitivity pneumonitis is a new addition to the ever-growing list of extrinsic allergic alveolitides. Dr. Ando and his group at the University of Kumamoto have performed pioneering epidemiologic, immunologic, and histopathologic studies which have unraveled the mystery of summer-type hypersensitivity pneumonitis. Dr. Kitaichi and his co-workers have, for many years, been studying the entity of diffuse panbronchiolitis. The clinical picture reminds one of bronchiectasis in its early phase. The article is sure to generate a lot of interest and controversy in countries where bronchiectasis is still a frequent occurrence.

The next essay in the series is from Dr. Adrian Williams, who has condensed the massive literature dealing with pulmonary reactions caused by drugs used for treating tropical diseases. The tropical physician is often seduced in administering pills, capsules, or liquids, no matter their vaunted potency or expected side effects. The crowded dispensaries and hot, humid, dimly lit quarters of underpaid physicians are hardly conducive to scientific medicine. These problems arise from deep-rooted economic sluggishness and educational malaise. Dr. Williams' essay is intended to make the tropical physician think twice before prescribing a potion to a patient.

Finally, Drs. Jindal and Wahi lament the lack of pulmonary function laboratories capable of providing accurate, reliable, and quality controlled data. Their suggestions should be taken seriously by pulmonologists in academic as well as the private practice sector of the developing world.

Of course, this volume is not meant to be a textbook of tropical medicine. It is not comprehensive and contains only selected topics. It is, in a way, unbalanced, for the significance given to various topics does not always reflect their importance. Our aim, however, has been to provide succinct and clear description of those conditions which affect significant numbers of people. We sincerely hope that our efforts will assist those who face practical problems related to tropical medicine, wherever they may be.

Om P. Sharma, M.D.

CONTRIBUTORS

Bisher Akil, M.D. Assistant Professor of Medicine, Divisions of Pulmonary Disease and Critical Care Medicine and Infectious Disease, Los Angeles County-University of Southern California Medical Center, Los Angeles, California

Masayuki Ando, M.D. First Department of Internal Medicine, Kumamoto University Medical School, Kumamoto, Japan

G.F. Araj, Ph.D., ABMM Associate Professor, Department of Microbiology, Mubarak-Al-Kabeer University Hospital, Faculty of Medicine, Kuwait University, Kuwait

P. Bambery, M.D. Associate Professor of Medicine, Department of Internal Medicine, Postgraduate Institute of Medical Education and Research, Chandigarh, India

Newton M. Bethlem, M.D. Emeritus Professor of Pneumology, Servico de Pneumologia-Hospital Universitario de Universidade Federal de Rio de Janeiro, Rio de Janeiro, Brazil

Somchai Bovornkitti, M.D., FRCP Professor, Department of Medicine, Faculty of Medicine, Siriraj Hospital, Mahidol University, Bangkok, Thailand

Suchai Charoenratanakul, M.D., FRCP Department of Medicine Faculty of Medicine, Siriraj Hospital, Mahidol University, Bangkok, Thailand

C.N. Deivanayagam, M.D. Dean, Tamilnadu Arasu Medical Science and Research Institute, Madras, India

Surrender N. Dhar, M.D. Professor, Department of Medicine, Government Medical College, Head of Chest Service, Chest Disease Hospital, Kashmir, India

Harvey Eisenberg, M.D. Chief, Department of Medicine, Lincoln Medical Center, Bronx, New York

Feisal A. El-Kassimi, M.D., MRCP Head, Pulmonary Division, Department of Medicine, King Saud University College of Medicine, Riyadh, Saudi Arabia

Gurdip S. Flora, M.D. Clinical Instructor, Department of Medicine, Los Angeles County-University of Southern California Medical Center, Los Angeles, California

Armenio Guimaraes, M.D., FACP, FACC Professor of Cardiology, Faculty of Medicine, University of Bahia Medical School and Hospital Edgard Santos, Bahia, Brazil

Isabel Guimaraes, M.D. Professor of Cardiology, Faculty of Medicine, University of Bahia Medical School and Hospital Edgard Santos, Bahia, Brazil

Yohmei Hiraga, M.D. JR Sapporo Hospital, Sapporo, Japan

Yutaka Hosada, M.D. Radiation Effects Research Foundation, Hiroshima, Japan

Takateru Izumi, M.D. Professor, Department of Medicine, Chest Disease Research Institute, Kyoto University, Kyoto, Japan

D. Geraint James, M.D., FRCP Adjunct Professor, Department of Medicine, Royal Free Hospital School of Medicine, London, England

Surinder K. Jindal, M.D. Associate Professor of Medicine, Head, Pulmonary Medicine, Department of Chest Diseases, Postgraduate Institute of Medical Education and Research, Chandigarh, India

Sudhakar R. Kamat, M.D. Professor of Medicine, Department of Respiratory Medicine, K.E.M. Hospital, Bombay, India

Upjeet Kaur, M.D., D.M. Associate Professor of Experimental Medicine, Department of Internal Medicine, Postgraduate Institute of Medical Education and Research, Chandigarh, India

Sumalee Kiatboonsri, M.D. Associate Professor, Division of Pulmonary Diseases, Department of Medicine, Ramathibodi Hospital, Bangkok, Thailand

Masanori Kitaichi, M.D. Professor, Department of Medicine, Chest Disease Research Institute, Kyoto University, Kyoto, Japan

Charanjit Lal, M.D. Instructor, Department of Medicine, University of Southern California School of Medicine, Los Angeles, California

W.K. Lam, M.D., FRCP (Edin) Reader, Department of Medicine, University of Hong Kong, Queen Mary Hospital, Hong Kong

Alfred Lemle, M.D. Professor of Medicine and Head, Pulmonary Functions Laboratory, Servico de Pneumologia-Hospital Universitario de Universidade Federal de Rio de Janeiro, Rio de Janeiro, Brazil

A.R. Lulu, M.D., FRCP Professor and Chairman, Department of Medicine, Johra Hospital, Ministry of Public Health, Kuwait

Nanta Maranetra, M.D., MS Professor, Department of Medicine, Faculty of Medicine, Siriraj Hospital, Mahidol University, Bangkok, Thailand

Koichi Nishimura, M.D. Professor, Department of Medicine, Chest Disease Research Institute, Kyoto University, Kyoto, Japan

C. Nwokolo, M.D., FRCP Professor, Department of Medicine, University of Nigeria, Pro-Chancellor and Chairman, Governing Council, Ahmady Bello University, Enugu, Nigeria

Kamlesh Pandya, M.D. Pulmonary Disease Service, Los Angeles County-University of Southern California Medical Center, Los Angeles, California

Rungsun Pushpakom, M.D., MS Professor, Department of Medicine, Faculty of Medicine, Siriraj Hospital, Mahidol University, Bangkok, Thailand

Edson A. Saad, M.D. Professor of Cardiology, Servico de Pneumologia-Hospital Universitario de Universidade Federal de Rio de Janeiro, Rio de Janeiro, Brazil

Om P. Sharma, M.D. Professor, Department of Medicine, University of Southern California School of Medicine, Los Angeles, California

Hisao Shida, M.D. Rosai Hospital for Silicosis, Tochigi, Japan

James Tuchschmidt, M.D. Assistant Professor, Department of Medicine and Director, Medical Intensive Care Unit, Los Angeles County-University of Southern California Medical Center, Los Angeles, California

P.L. Wahi, M.D. Chairman, Department of Cardiology and Director, Postgraduate Institute of Medical Education and Research, Chandigarh, India

Chand Wattal, M.D. Assistant Professor, Department of Microbiology, Sheri Kashmir Institute of Medical Sciences, Kashmir, India

Adrian Williams, M.D. Chief, Pulmonary Disease Service, West Los Angeles Veterans Administration Hospital, Professor, Department of Medicine, University of Southern California School of Medicine, Los Angeles, California

Y.L. Yu, M.D. Senior Lecturer, Department of Medicine, University of Hong Kong, Queen Mary Hospital, Hong Kong

Alimuddin Zumla, MPCP, Ph.D. Lecturer, Departments of Medicine and Immunology, Royal Postgraduate Medical School, Hammersmith Hospital, London, England

CONTENTS

1

Lung Immunology in the Tropics

ALIMUDDIN ZUMLA

Royal Postgraduate Medical School
Hammersmith Hospital
London, England

D. GERAINT JAMES

Royal Free Hospital School of Medicine
London, England

On his deathbed, Louis Pasteur remarked:

> Claude is right
> The organism is nothing
> The terrain is everything.

He was, of course, referring to his friend, guru, and counsellor, Claude Bernard. Here was a bacteriologist, who had spent a lifetime isolating organisms, now switching emphasis to the more important "terrain." A century earlier, John Hunter stressed the importance of the terrain, or soil, by emphasizing the importance of the host's reaction to the disease. This aspect is of particular importance in assessing diseases of the tropics. The host is the battleground between invading antigens, whether they are infections, cancer, or chemicals, and the defenses of the body. At-risk patients are commonplace because of malnutrition, acquired immunodeficiency syndrome (AIDS), cancer, high parasite load, immunosuppressive regimens, cancer chemotherapy, narcotic abuse, hemodialysis, chronic liver and lung diseases, and longer-living diabetics. Many factors impoverish the soil or terrain in what we commonly term the patient with poor terrain.

I. Factors Influencing the Terrain

The antigen deposited in the lung encounters nonspecific immune and nonimmune responses and is also translocated to the lung-associated lymph nodes where a specific immune response is produced. The immune response in lung tissue augments the combination of anatomical barriers, mechanical mechanisms, immunoglobulins, and cellular components (Brain et al., 1977; Table 1). The mucosal surface changes along the airways, with the nares and the oropharynx lined with stratified squamous epithelium. From the nasal turbinates and the upper trachea down to the respiratory bronchioles, a pseudostratified, columnar, ciliated epithelium with mucus-secreting goblet cells exists. In the periphery of the airways, the epithelial layer becomes thinner and less stratified. The cell layer flattens in the terminal air sacs and over the alveolar surface and blends into a single layer of epithelium (type 1 pneumocytes) interspersed with type 2 pneumocytes. Present on the alveolar surface

Table 1 Defenses of the Respiratory Tract

Local	Systemic
Upper respiratory tract	
Nasal filter	Cellular immunity
Tonsils	Humoral immunity
Mucus (IgA)	Phagocytes
Cilia	Complement
Submucosal lymphocytes	HLA system
Lymph nodes (hilar and tracheobronchial)	
Lymph tissue (BALT)	
Lymphatics	
Superficial plexus-pleural	
Deep plexus around bronchioles and blood vessels	
Bronchial macrophages	
Lower respiratory tract	
Alveolar fluid (IgG, surfactant)	
Alveolar macrophages	
Interstitial macrophages	
Mast cells	
Complement	
Neutrophils	
Eosinophils	
Lymphocytes	
Antibody (sIgA and IgG)	

are freely moving phagocytic cells and lymphocytes. Lymphocytes and plasma cells are also distributed in the submucosa and lamina propria. Antigen-specific antibody and immune cells are released into the blood and are recruited into the lung lobes exposed to the antigen (Reynolds, 1986).

A. Cellular and Humoral Immunity

An antigen that manages to penetrate the local defense mechanisms of an individual (skin, cilia, mucous membrane, secretions) will encounter macrophages and two populations of circulating T and B lymphocytes. In the normal lung, lymphocytes make up 10% of all effector cells (Hunninghake et al., 1979). The distribution of lymphocyte subtypes is similar to that in the blood, although there are relatively more T than B cells. They form the cornerstones of an elaborate and powerful defense system (Table 2).

Thymus-mediated T cells, responsible for cellular immunity, recognize antigen presented in association with human leukocyte antigen (HLA) molecules by macrophages, and induce B-cell recruitment (Royer and Reinherz, 1987). Monoclonal antibodies to human T-lymphocyte differentiation antigens have allowed recognition of two distinct subpopulations of T lymphocytes: helper/inducer (T1,T3,T4) and cytotoxic/suppressor cells (T1,T3,T8). The T4 subset signals B cells to proliferate and differentiate into antibody-producing cells, whereas T8 cells exert a cytotoxic function or regulate the immune response. As a result of antigen invasion, macrophages phagocytose and process the antigen, and are activated to produce several cytokines including interleukin-1 (IL-1), which stimulates T cells into activity.

Stimulated T cells produce interleukin-2 (IL-2) and acquire receptors for IL-2, causing clonal expansion of antigen-specific T4 cells. Activated T cells produce a variety of soluble mediator lymphokines to fan the immune response. Apart from the interleukins, these include macrophage chemotactic and migration inhibition factors, α interferon, collagen-stimulating factor, and growth inhibitory and cytotoxic factors. What T cells recognize and the mechanism by which they see it continue to be subjects of intense study (Marx, 1988). T cells are particularly active against organisms that have an intracellular phase during infection, such as viruses, fungi, mycobacteria, *Brucella*, and toxoplasma. The most important cause of depressed T-cell responses in the tropics are protein energy malnutrition (PEM), AIDS, and parasitic diseases.

The B (for bursa of Fabricius) lymphocytes, responsible for humoral immunity, synthesize five major immunoglobulin classes that form the pool of circulating antibodies (reviewed by Bird, 1988). B-cell growth factor (BCGF) (interleukin-4), produced by T4 cells, acts on activated B lymphocytes possessing BCGF receptor and induces their proliferation. Another B-cell-stimulating factor, identical to beta-2 interferon, helps activated B cells to differentiate

Table 2 Comparison of the Properties of T and B Cells

Features	T Cell	B Cell
Site of maturation	Bone marrow Thymus Spleen	(Bursa of Fabricius: chickens) Bone marrow
Immunity	Cellular	Humoral
Life span	Long (months/years)	Short (days/weeks)
Recirculation	Majority	Minority
Percentage of peripheral blood lymphocytes	60-80	8-15
Receptor for antigen	Glycoprotein T-cell receptor (Ti)	Glycoprotein Immunoglobulin
Chemical products	Lymphokines	Immunoglobulins
Assessment methods	In vivo: Delayed hypersensitivity tests: tuberculin In vitro: Fluorescence or proliferation assays	Immunoglobulin levels Autoantibodies Idiotypic expression
Function	Immunity against fungi, viruses, intracellular organisms, and parasites. Cooperation with B cells. Immunosurveillance?	Humoral antibody Defense at portal of entry and in the vascular system
Deficiency-related infections	Viruses, fungi, intracellular bacteria, amoeba, strongyloides, *Pneumocystis*	Pyogenic bacteria
Clinical disorders	AIDS, lepromatous leprosy, Hodgkin's disease, lymphatic leukemia, deficiency syndromes	AIDS, multiple myeloma, macroglobulinemia, infectious mononucleosis, hypogammaglobulinemia
Immunomanipulation	Bone marrow transplant Thymosin Transfer factor	Gamma globulin Plasmapheresis
	Monoclonal antibodies Anti-idiotypes Lymphokines	

into antibody-producing plasma cells. Whereas T4 cells induce B cells to produce IgG, T8 cells suppress or regulate IgG synthesis. Antibodies defend the body in several ways. They may combine with antigen and fix complement, leading to antigen lysis. Antibody may neutralize microorganisms and their products; or opsonization may occur when phagocytosis is enhanced by coating of bacteria with specific antibody. IgG and IgA are present in the mucosa of the respiratory tract, alveolar epithelium, and respiratory secretions (Reynolds, 1988; Reynolds and Newball, 1976). Poor humoral immunity, absolute or functional, is associated with recurrent or chronic pulmonary disease and increased susceptibility to respiratory tract infections (Polmar, 1976).

Defects in cellular and humoral immunity may lead to various pediatric immunodeficiency syndromes (Table 3).

A third class of lymphocyte (non-T, non-B), *natural killer cells* (NK or null cells), can combine with the Fc region of immunoglobulins, cellular antigens, and provoke cell necrosis (Hiserodt et al., 1982; Lotzova and Herberman, 1986). In the tropics, these play a role in early resistance against parasites, serving to limit degree of parasitemia before the development of the necessary T-cell immunity. The role of NK cells in host defense against pulmonary fungal infections remains a controversial issue (Granger and Hobbs, 1988).

B. Phagocytosis

The mobilization of inflammatory cells and phlogistic factors from the intravascular component into the lung is important for effective host defense (Reynolds, 1987). Polymorphonuclear cells are present in few numbers in the normal lung (1% of all cells). Phagocytes (macrophages, monocytes, polymorphonuclear leukocytes) reach the site of invasion by chemotaxis where, with the aid of opsonins and complement, they phagocytose and dispose of foreign particles and organisms. Impairment of function includes poor chemotaxis, intrinsic cellular defects, abnormal opsonization, and neutropenia. The polymorphonuclear neutrophil (PMN) is assumed to be the principal responding cell in the inflammatory focus. Other inflammatory conditions elicit a response of the eosinophils (as in parasitic infections, allergen-induced asthma, or other lung diseases). Several different chemotactic molecules are required for the selective attraction of these cells (Donabedian and Gallin, 1983).

Chemotaxis can be visualized by several in vitro techniques. Poor leukocyte locomotion may be associated with inhibitors, blocking factors, and deficiencies in complement. The role and relative importance of chemotactic factors in pulmonary diseases have been reviewed by Gallin (1976) and Fantone and Ward (1983).

Table 3 Immunodeficiency Disorders

	Infection							Deficiency	
Disorder	Virus	Fungus	Other	Other features	Cause	Treatment	Remarks	Cellular	Humoral B
Thymic hypoplasia (Di George syndrome)	+ (Measles pneumonia)	+	*Pneumocystis*	Hypoplastic parathyroids Neonatal tetany Low-set ears Micrognathia Cardiac defects	Damage to developing anlage during fetal weeks 10-12	Human fetal thymus transplantation	Patients rarely survive to third year without transplant	+	Normal
Severe combined immunodeficiency (SCID)	Respiratory and skin +	+	*Pneumocystis*	Positive family history Chronic diarrhea soon after birth	Inherited X-linked autosomal recessive or sporadic	Gammaglobulin Fresh plasma Bone marrow transplantation Thymic transplant	High infant mortality	+ Also ?defective stem cell	+
Wiskott-Aldrich syndrome	+	+	+	Eczema Thrombocytopenia	Inherited X-linked disorder Postnatal thymic involution	Bone marrow transplants from siblings with preconditioning antilymphocyte globulin	10% develop lymphoreticular malignancy	+	+

Ataxia-telangiectasia	+	+	+	Oculocutaneous telangiectasia (red eyes) Cerebellar ataxia Choreoathetosis Gonadol hypoplasia	Autosomal recessive inheritance	Thymosin Levamisole Fresh plasma Antibiotics	Increased risk of lymphoreticular malignancy Carcinoembryonic antigen and fetoprotein levels may be elevated	+	lLow IgA
Bruton hypogammaglobulinemia			Bacterial only	History of recurrent respiratory and urinary tract bacterial infections	X-linked recessive in males	Weekly I.M. gammaglobulin Antibiotics for recurrent bacterial infection and for prophylaxis		Normal	+
Common variable immunodeficiency (CVI)	+ Warts Molluscum contagiosum Herpes		*Giardia*	Splenomegaly Lymphoid hyperplasia Sprue Protein-losing enteropathy	Develops in teenagers or adults, so difficult to decide whether congenital or acquired	Treatment of infections Gammaglobulin ?Levamisole	Associated with lymphomas and chronic lymphatic leukemia and Epstein-Barr virus infection	+ -	+

Intrinsic cellular defects render phagocytes impotent, as occurs in chronic granulomatous disease of childhood.

Opsonization involves the preparation of bacteria for digestion by phagocytes through the coating of bacterial opsonins such as antibody and the third component of complement C3b. Opsonic activity requires intact receptor sites, and neutrophil attachment to the organism at the Fab site of the opsonizing antibody. Patients with various types of C3b deficiency have poor opsonic activity and are more prone to infections.

C. Immune Opsonins

The role of immune opsonins focuses on the requirements for IgG subclasses to bind to the membrane surface of alveolar macrophages and on specific kinds of antibody contained in the respective subclasses. Alveolar macrophages have cell-surface receptors for IgG and complement. Among the IgG subclasses there are differences in the expression of avidity for Fc gamma receptors.

D. Neutropenia

Neutropenia may be caused by drugs, neoplasia, infections, and hypersplenism. When the neutrophil count in the peripheral blood falls to below 1000/μl, the risk of infection increases. Chronic idiopathic neutropenia is characterized by blood neutrophil counts below 2000/μl for long periods without an obvious cause. It is three times more common in women aged about 30 years than in other persons and its occurrence may be familial. There is a somewhat increased incidence of respiratory tract infections, otitis media, furunculosis, and recurrent oral ulceration. It has a benign course but antibiotics are required for the treatment of severe complicating infections.

E. Eosinophils

Eosinophils represent a minor proportion of alveolar cells, but they play a vital role in immune mechanisms against parasitic diseases, in which eosinophilia is a common finding (Ottessen, 1976; David et al., 1980; Spry, 1988). Produced in the bone marrow, it circulates in the blood before localizing in the tissues. Chemotactic agents for eosinophils include the eosinophil chemotactic factor for anaphylaxis (ECF-A) produced by mast cells, complement activation, lymphokines from sensitized T cells (e.g., eosinophil stimulation promoter, eosinophil chemotactic factor), and hypersensitivity reactions. Their functions include phagocytosis, modification of immediate hypersensitivity reactions by inactivation of mast cell products, parasiticidal effect (by production of oxygen free radicals and enzymes) in the presence of specific antibody, and activation of complement. Mediators released by eosinophils are capable of injuring lung parenchymal cells and matrix. They also release a collagenase capable of cleaving types I and III collagen (Davis et al., 1981). Degranulation of eosinophils into the tissues has adverse effects such as endomyocardial fibrosis, endocarditis, Loeffler's syndrome, and vasculitis.

F. Complement

Factor B and a number of other complement components have been identified in lung lavage fluids. Both the alternative and direct pathways are important in immunity against bacterial and parasitic antigens (Hunninghake et al., 1979; Reynolds et al., 1977).

G. HLA Antigens

This system of antigens lies on the membranes of cells (reviewed by Crumpton, 1987). These tissue antigens are an important constituent of the terrain and there is increasing recognition of an association between particular HLA specificities and respiratory and other disorders (Table 4). The HLA system is a series of closely linked genes that occur on the short arm of the sixth chromosome in the region termed the major histocompatibility complex. The A, B, and C loci code for class I antigens, which are cell surface glycoproteins found on all nucleated cells. Beta 2 microglobulin, which is present as part of the HLA class 1 antigen complex, is found in higher concentrations in pleural fluid than blood in patients with tuberculous and rheumatoid pleurisy compared to exudates of malignancy and lupus erythematosus (Sahn, 1988). The D/DR locus codes for class II cell surface antigens which are expressed on restricted populations of cells, particularly macrophages, B cells, some activated T cells and vascular endothelial cells. Antigen presentation is intimately tied with expression of class II HLA antigens on the surface of monocytes (McDevitt, 1980). It is thought that certain racial groups are more prone to developing tuberculosis due to differences in HLA.

II. Malnutrition and Other Factors

Malnutrition, ischemia, disseminated neoplasia, high parasite load, drugs, and chemotherapy influence the human soil profoundly; these influences on the resistance of the patient are nowhere more striking than the poor, malnourished patients of the tropics (Table 5).

A. Malnutrition

Malnutrition causes depression of cellular immunity and impaired humoral immunity (Chandra, 1988). It may result from poor diet, alcoholism, hepatic cirrhosis, renal disease, drug addiction, or starvation due to wars, flood, and famine, all of which contribute to poor resistance against infection.

Table 4 HLA-Associated Disorders

HLA type	Clinical disorder
B27	Acute anterior uveitis Ankylosing spondylitis Behçet's disease Reiter's disease Psoriatic arthropathy Juvenile rheumatoid arthritis Crohn's arthritis Ulcerative colitis arthritis *Yersinia* and *Salmonella* arthritis Levamisole toxicity
B7	Ankylosing spondylitis in black Americans
B8, DW3	Myasthenia gravis Graves' disease and relapse following carbimazole treatment Sjögren's syndrome Juvenile diabetic retinopathy Thyroiditis Addison's disease Celiac disease Dermatitis herpetiformis Chronic active hepatitis Idiopathic membranous nephropathy
B8, DW2	Systemic lupus erythematosus
B2 and B9	Acute lymphoblastic leukemia (long-term survivors)
B13, B17, CW6	Psoriasis (without arthropathy)
A3, B7, B18, DW2, DW3	Multiple sclerosis
A9	Transitional cell carcinoma of bladder Buerger's disease
B8, BW15, DW2, DW4	Insulin-dependent diabetes mellitus
A3, B14	Hemochromatosis
A1, A11, B5, BW15	Hodgkin's lymphoma
B8	Sarcoid arthritis and uveitis with erythema nodosum Giant cell arteritis Polymyositis and juvenile dermatomyositis Systemic sclerosis Hodgkin's disease (long-term survivors) Hypogonadism Schizophrenia
DR5	Kaposi's sarcoma AIDS
DR2	Narcolepsy, Goodpasture's syndrome
DR3	Adult celiac disease
DR3, DR7	Childhood celiac disease
B40	Chronic myelocytic leukemia

B. Vitamin D

It is becoming increasingly clear that vitamin D_3 metabolites may have immunological functions unrelated to calcium homeostasis (reviewed by Rook, 1988). The hydroxylases that convert the 25(OH) derivative into the active metabolites $1,25(OH)_2D_3$ and $24,25(OH)_2D_3$ occur in several cell types including monocytes and macrophages activated by gamma interferon or endotoxon. In sarcoidosis, activated lung macrophages are the sources of the active hydroxylated D_3 derivatives. The vitamin D-binding protein Gc associates with membranes of lymphocytes and monocytes. On T cells it is associated Fc gamma receptors and on B-cell membranes with immunoglobulins. Gc might be an important signal transducer in these cells. Whether vitamin D3 and its metabolites are relevant to the mechanism that activates macrophages to control the growth of the *Mycobacterium* remains to be elucidated.

C. Ageing

The elderly have become a significantly large group of immunocompromised hosts with impaired resistance against infection, cancer, and an increased risk of such B-cell myeloproliferative disorders. The healthy elderly exhibit impaired cell-mediated immunity, impaired T-cell function, exaggerated but inefficient B-cell function, an increase in circulating immune complexes, and various autoimmune phenomena (Good and Lorenz, 1988). To these immunological alterations may be added atherosclerosis, impaired circulation of the blood, ischemia, a rigid chest wall, inelastic lungs, and dehydration.

D. Antigen Overload

Chronic overstimulation of the immune system by a high antigen load in various chronic infections may interfere with the host's capacity to eliminate infectious agents (Williamson and Greenwood, 1978).

E. Iron

The relationship between infection and iron availability has been a subject of considerable debate (Hershko et al., 1988). The role of iron in host defense may be an important one (Chandra et al., 1977). Reports from tropical countries show an apparent increased incidence and/or severity of infectious diseases after iron treatment.

Table 5 Conditions in Which Impaired Defenses Lead to Infections

Defenses	Diabetes Mellitus	Malnutrition Alcoholism Hepatic Cirrhosis Renal Failure	Drug Addiction	Following Splenectomy
PMNs				
Phagocytosis	±	Leukopenia	Normal	Impaired by underlying disease response for splenectomy
Chemotaxis	Impaired	Impaired		
Cellular immunity	Impaired	T-cell depression, increased null cells	? Impaired	Normal Impaired by any underlying disease, such as Hodgkin's disease
B cells Immunoglobulins Antibodies	Normal	Polyclonal gammopathy when there is underlying liver disease	Polyclonal gammopathy	Impaired primary antibody response Decreased IgM

Miscellaneous				
Opsonins	Normal	Impaired by underlying disease	? Abnormal	Normal
Complement	Normal			Normal
Other contributory factors	Vascular insufficiency Autonomic neuropathy	Vitamin deficiency Alcoholic cirrhosis	Autoinoculation Coma Hypoventilation Pulmonary edema	Hodgkin's disease Sickle cell anemia Thalassemia Congenital spherocytosis Thrombocytopenic purpura
Infection	*Staphylococcus aureus* septicemia and skin infections *Monilia* (*Candida*) *albicans* and other fungi *E. coli* urinary tract Gram-negative cholecystitis	Pneumococcal pneumonia *Klebsiella* pneumonia Anaerobic lung abscess Pulmonary tuberculosis *E. coli* septicemia and peritonitis	*S. aureus* causing pyoderma, cellulitis, endocarditis, osteomyelitis, septic arthritis Pneumococcal pneumonia Tetanus HBSAg hepatitis Pyogenic sacroiliitis	Pneumococcal and streptococcal septicemia Bacterial meningitis There is no increased incidence of viral infections

III. Local Respiratory Tract Factors

Secretory IgA (SIgA) is synthesized by plasma cells in the bronchial mucosa (Hunninghake et al., 1979; Bell et al., 1981). It is a dimer (300,000 daltons) whereas serum IgA is a monomer. Local plasma cells polymerize two 7S monomers of IgA; and a J chain glycoprotein, also made by plasma cells, acts as linkage. Secretory component, made by local epithelial cells, combines with it to form SIgA, which transports more readily across the mucosa into bronchial secretion. It anchors bacteria, neutralizes respiratory viruses, and, with the help of lysozyme and complement, promotes phagocytosis.

Mast cells express membrane receptors for IgE that signal degranulation. They generate and release histamine, leukotrienes, proteases, and eosinophilic chemotactic factors, platelet-activating factors, and prostaglandins (PGD2 and PGF2). These mediators play an important role in bronchial vasoactivity, bronchial asthma, allergic bronchopulmonary aspergillosis, extrinsic allergic alveolitis, and parasitic infections.

Alveolar macrophages are derived from marrow monocytes and also from a local interstitial lung compartment. In the normal lung there are approximately 80 effector cells per alveolus (Crapo et al., 1982). These cells are located within the alveolar interstitium and on the alveolar epithelial surface. More than 90% of these are alveolar macrophages with a life span of months to years. Although macrophages can replicate in the normal lung, most are derived from blood monocytes that migrate through the alveolar walls. Their phagocytic ability is enhanced by the presence of opsonins, but depressed by hypoxia, intoxication with ethanol, and cigarette smoke. Macrophages normally defend the respiratory tract by using surface receptors such as those for the C3b component of complement and the Fc receptor of IgG. In addition, they can phagocytose nonopsonized particles. When activated they release a variety of mediators relevant to inflammatory and immune processes. Activation of the macrophage by immune or nonimmune opsonins or by the complement cascade stimulates them to produce chemotactic factors including protein factors, and leukotrienes such as LTB4, and complement components. These recruit PMNs from the circulating and marginating pools. They generate complement, which amplifies host defenses, and mediates immune mechanisms in the lung. Macrophages play an important role in antigen recognition and presentation to T cells in association with MHC class II products. Together with T and B cells, the cell-to-cell interplay is a crucial pulmonary defense mechanism. And yet, we know very little about the alveolar macrophage. The late Professor Lenzini of Pisa paraphrased Robert Frost as follows:

We all dance around
in a ring
—and suppose
But the macrophage sits
in the middle
—and knows

Alpha-1 antitrypsin (α1AT) is a powerful defender of the lower respiratory tract against proteolytic damage by neutrophil elastase (Reynolds and Newball, 1976). It is a serum glycoprotein produced by mononuclear phagocytes and hepatocytes. It inhibits neutrophil elastase, which is a potent protease. Individuals who inherit genes with a poor protease inhibitor (Pi) type have low serum levels of α1AT and are prone to lung and liver disease. The inadequate inhibition of neutrophil elastase allows progressive destruction of lung parenchyma. The combination of emphysema and hepatic cirrhosis is a late complication that occurs in children and youth.

Cilia form part of the nonimmunological physical mechanisms that make up the mucociliary escalator and the cough reflex (reviewed by Wanner and Ahmed, 1983). They clear particles from the respiratory tract as far as the respiratory bronchioles, where ciliated epithelium gives way to nonciliated epithelium. Over 90% of particles larger than 2.5 μm are cleared by this mechanism, including many fungal and bacterial spores and dust particles. Cilia are vulnerable to disruption by infection and by chemical and physical agents.

In the alveolar lining fluid are several substances such as surfactant (Benson et al., 1983) and fibronectin that act as opsonins. Surfactant has antistaphylococcal and antipneumococcal activity. Palmitoyl lysophosphatidylcholine, which represents a component of surfactant, seems to be the most active fraction. Fibronectin fragments (which originate from plasma, fibroblasts, or macrophages) enhance nonimmune opsonin phagocytosis by macrophages. The fragments are thought to work by interacting with the trypsin-sensitive membrane receptor on the macrophage, which is the putative complement C3b receptor (Proctor, 1987). Fibronectin may serve as a barrier to invasion by parasites such as *Schistosoma* sp., which secrete proteinases during their invasive phase. It may be an important element in the pathogenesis of schistosomal egg granulomas and subsequent tissue fibrosis (Wyler, 1987).

IV. Classification of Immune Reactions

The Coombs-Gell classification of hypersensitivity provides one further dimension in our understanding of tropical lung disease. Immune types, I, II, III, IV, and V depend on the reaction of antigen with antibody, whereas type

Table 6 Types of Immunological Lung Injury

	I: Immediate	II: Cytotoxic	III: Immune complex	IV: Cell-mediated	V: ADCC
Lymphocyte involved	B	B and T	B	T	B and T
Other cells involved	Mast cell Eosinophil	Cytotoxic	PMNs	Macrophages Monocytes Giant epithelioid	Killer cells (NK/Null)
Mechanism	Allergen with IgE degranulates mast cells and basophils	Cross-reactive IgG or IgM with alveolar membrane	Deposited immune complexes and complement evoke inflammation	Antigen, T cells, and macrophages induce chemo and fibroattractants	Antibody-coated antigen/cell induces NK cell-mediated lysis
Respiratory disorders	Hay fever Asthma Leaky hydatid cyst Helminth larvae	Goodpasture's syndrome Chagas disease Transfusion reaction	Sarcoidosis Pulmonary fibrosis Fibrosing alveolitis Migrating larvae Schistosomiasis	Sarcoidosis Nitrofurantoin lung Schistosome ova Lung flukes Helminth larvae	Chagas' disease Trichinosis Filariasis Schistosomiasis Herpes, mumps, Varicella
Pulmonary consequences	Anaphylaxis Loeffler's syndrome Bronchospasm Pulmonary eosinophilia	Hemoptysis Bronchiectasis	Pulmonary eosinophilia Katayama fever Serum sickness	Granulomas Lung fibrosis Vasculitis and pulmonary hypertension	Bronchiectasis Helminthicidal Lysis of infected cell

Table 7 Classification of Lung Granulomas

Infective	Noninfective
Bacterial	Foreign body
Mycobacteria sp.	Snuff/talc
Brucella sp.	Silica/beryllium/asbestos
Pseudomonas pseudomallei	Vascular
Fungal	Wegener's granulomatosis
Hypersensitivity (extrinsic allergic alveolitis)	Polyarteritis
Histoplasma sp.	Tumors
Micropolyspora faeni	*Lymphoma*
Aspergillus sp.	Carcinomatosis
Protozoal	
Toxoplasma gondii	
Leishmania donovani	
Helminths	
Ova *Schistosoma* sp.	
Paragominus sp.	
Opisthorcis sp.	
Migrating helminth larvae	
Rickettsia	
Rickettsia tsutsugamuchi	
Coxiella burnetti	
Arthropods: Pulmonary acariasis	

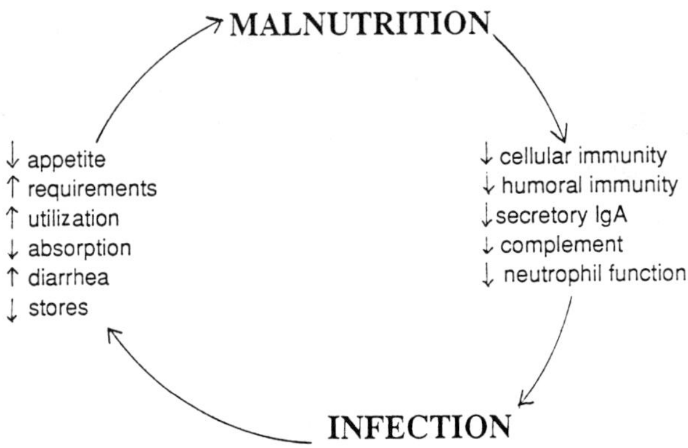

Figure 1 Bugbear of the tropics---the malnutrition-infection cycle.

IV involves mainly T cells (Table 6). The immunopathological appearance of several parasitic diseases can be explained on the basis of these reactions. Granulomatous reactions in the lung causing pathological changes occur in many conditions (Table 7).

V. Disorders with a Poor Terrain

A. Malnutrition

There can be no better example of a poor terrain than the scourge of most developing countries: malnutrition. Protein energy malnutrition (PEM) is the most common cause of T-cell immunodeficiency worldwide (Chandra et al., 1977; Chandra 1983, 1988). The detrimental effect of nutritional defi-

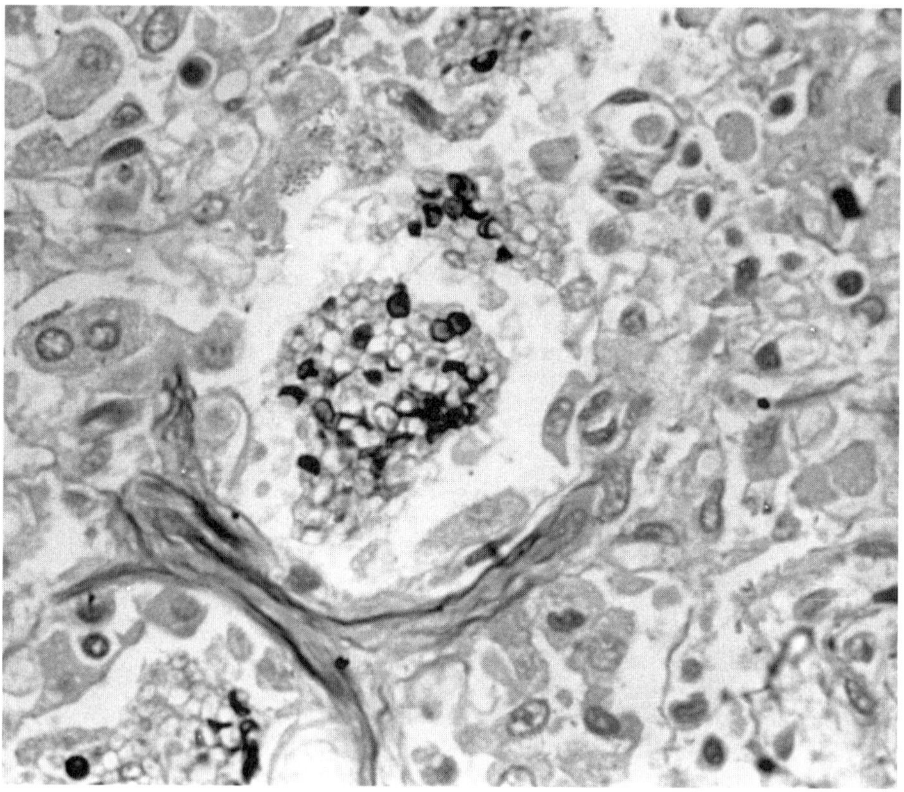

a

Figure 2 a. *Pneumocystis carinii* produces a honeycomb of cystic spaces with cysts in the lung. b. Postmortem lung specimen of an AIDS patient shows extensive consolidation due to *Pneumocystis carinii* pneumonia.

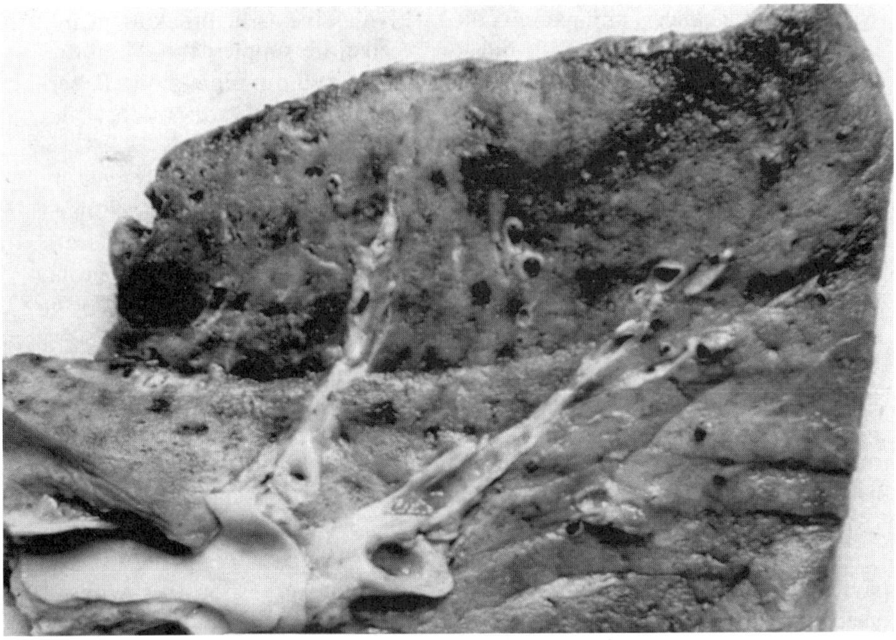

Figure 2b

ciencies on several aspects of immunocompetence has been well documented (Smythe et al., 1971; Chandra et al., 1977; Chandra, 1983, 1988; Keusch et al., 1983; Corman, 1985; Dowd et al., 1986). These include defects in cellular immunity, neutrophil bactericidal effects, complement system, and secretory IgA response. These are accompanied by hypergammaglobulinemia and increased susceptibility to infection. Deficiencies of single nutrients such as zinc, iron, amino acids, pyridoxine, vitamin A, and folic acid can also impair immune responses (Chandra, 1982, 1983; Beisel, 1982). There is a considerable body of evidence to suggest that the malnourished individual is more likely to have a higher incidence or more life-threatening consequence of infection (Chandra, 1972; Mata, 1975; Phillips and Wharton, 1968; Chandra and Newberne, 1977). Epidemiological and clinical studies of children and adults in the tropics have suggested that malnutrition is associated with increased incidence, severity, and/or duration, and higher complications and duration of bacterial, viral, protozoal, and helminthic infections (Fig. 1). A significant relationship has been established between malnutrition and respiratory infections such as tuberculosis, pertussis, measles, *Pneumocystis*, and *Candida*.

Leyton (1946) found a higher incidence of tuberculosis (15-19%) in prisoners of war not receiving protein food supplements compared to those receiving it (1.2%). The tuberculosis was more severe (onset more rapid, worse systemic disturbances, and patients died with massive tissue breakdown and large cavities) in prisoners who did not receive the supplement. Malnutrition is also a significant determinant of response to immunization. Tuberculin conversion after bacillus Calmette-Guirin (BCG) vaccination is decreased in malnourished individuals.

The course and severity of several respiratory diseases are affected by the nutritional status of the subject. Measles is more severe and prolonged (Morley et al., 1966, 1967) and the mortality is increased in children with malnutrition. The respiratory complications of measles—bronchiolitis, croup and interstitial giant cell pneumonia, secondary infection with streptococci, staphylococci, and *Haemophilus*—are also increased.

Several mechanisms have been suggested for malnutrition-associated immunodeficiency (reviewed by Chandra, 1983, 1988). There is thymic atrophy, decrease in lymph node germinal centers, decreased T-cell population in the spleen, and a reduction in circulating T lymphocytes. Decreased chemotaxis and intracellular killing by phagocytes, a depression of cell-mediated immunity related to PEM, and low levels of IgA have been described.

Immune responses to certain vaccines are blunted in the malnourished subject. The antibody response to primary and booster responses to typhoid vaccination is limited (Chandra, 1972). Seroconversion for polio vaccination is low and deficient IgA production against measles vaccination occurs (Chandra, 1975). IgA of the respiratory tract protects the neonate against pertussis but since this does not cross the placenta, and the antibody responses to vaccination are poor, neonates are extremely vulnerable to infection. Whooping cough itself may tip poorly nourished children into frank PEM with a consequent higher mortality. Unexplained geographic differences in the severity of measles in different malnourished communities may be due to differences in strains of the virus or differences in susceptibility due to varying HLA types.

Provision of proper water and sanitary facilities, food supplements, and improved maternal and child health services remain the only means of improving the immune defenses and interrupting the infection-malnutrition cycle.

B. AIDS

Although the AIDS epidemic is well documented in Africa (Biggar, 1986; Berkelman et al., 1989; Fleming, 1989), scientific information is scanty (Lucas et al., 1987) due to political censorship, inadequate medical facilities, and lack of expertise needed for proper investigation and documentation. There are no differences in the pathological manifestations between the two human immunodeficiency viruses (HIV), HIV1 and HIV2, once symptoms and signs develop (Clavell et al., 1987), and thus the features described here will be applicable to both. Several immunological abnormalities, including cellular and humoral defects, have been described in patients with AIDS (reviewed by Koenig and Fauci, 1988). There is a persistent quantitative, irreversible, and functional depression within the T4 lymphocyte subset associated with immunoincompetence. This renders the patient more prone to infection and appearance of neoplasm.

The immunological abnormalities in the lungs of HIV-positive patients have been recently reviewed by Rankin et al. (1988). AIDS-specific cytotoxic T lymphocytes from the lungs of AIDS patients interact with HIV-infected alveolar macrophages (Plata et al., 1988). The functionally defective HIV-infected macrophage serves as a reservoir for virus and also opens the way for bacterial and fungal infections (reviewed by Cook, 1987a). In addition, AIDS may augment the immunosuppressive effects of malnutrition and endemic parasites on the immune system. Published literature on AIDS in Europe and America suggests that the lung is the most common organ involved in patients with AIDS. In one large study, at least 40% of American patients had respiratory manifestatiions (Murray et al., 1984). Lung involvement in AIDS can be due to infection, both opportunistic and nonopportunistic, and noninfectious disorders, such as Kaposi's sarcoma, lymphoid interstitial pneumonitis, and alveolar proteinosis.

C. Opportunistic Lung Infections in AIDS

Infections that take advantage of T-cell and B-cell defects are common in patients with HIV infection (Table 8). *Pneumocystis carinii* pneumonia (PCP) is consequential upon depressed cell mediated immunity and is seen in malnourished or immunosuppressed patients. It causes a chronic interstitial pneumonia and the alveoli become distended with a foamy, amorphous material with few macrophages. The foamy contents consist of a honeycomb of very fine walled cystic spaces in which the parasite may be seen (Fig. 2). The interstitial infiltrate consists of lymphocytes and large number of plasma cells; macrophages and eosinophils are sometimes numerous. In Europe and the United States, PCP is the most common life-threatening opportunistic infection in AIDS patients. This has also been a feature of African AIDS patients treated in Europe (Katlama et al., 1984; Blaser and Cohn, 1986), but PCP appears to be less common in Africa than in Europe and America (Elvin et al., 1989; Mcleod et al., 1989). Since the diagnosis is made with more certainty by transbronchial biopsy, the lack of diagnostic facilities may partly account for some of the difference.

However, several questions arise. Are the differences in geographical variation in incidence of PCP in AIDS patients due to variation in prevalence of the parasite in the environment or are there geographically differing susceptibilities to PCP? A rapid and inexpensive test for detecting *Pneumocystis* antigen in sputum will enable better definition of the problem. Griffin and

Table 8 Pulmonary Manifestations of AIDS

	America/Europe	Africa
Infectious		
Protozoa		
Pneumocystis carinii	Murray et al. (1984)	Lucas (1988)
Toxoplasma gondii	Murray et al. (1984)	Lucas (1988)
Cryptosporidium sp.	Brady et al. (1984)	—
Entamoeba histolytica	—	—
Viruses		
Cytomegalovirus	Macher et al. (1987)	Lucas (1988); Piot (1984)
Herpes simplex	Murray et al. (1987)	—
Severe measles	—	—
Fungi		
Cryptococcus neoformans	Murray et al. (1984)	Lucas and Wamukota (1988)
Candida sp.	Reichart et al. (1983)	Clumeck et al. (1984)
Aspergillus nidulans	Gottlieb (1984)	—
Coccidiodes immitis	Macher et al. (1988)	—
Histoplasma capsulatum	Macher et al. (1988)	Katlama et al. (1984)
Sporothrix schenkii	Macher et al. (1986)	—
Helminths		
Strongyloides stercoralis	Maayan et al. (1987)	—
Other lung parasites	—	—
Bacteria		
Pyogenic organisms		
Staphylococcus aureus	Murray et al. (1987)	
Haemophilus influenza	Murray et al. (1987)	
Streptococcus pneumoniae	Polsky et al. (1986)	
Salmonella sp.	Blaser and Cohn (1986)	Zumla and Luo (1990)
Pseudomonas aeruginosa	Gold (1987)	
Brahmnella sp.	Gold (1987)	

	America/Europe	Africa
Atypical mycobacteria	Murray et al. (1984)	Piot (1984
Mycobacterium tuberculosis	Pitchenik et al. (1984)	Van de Perre et al. (1984)
Nocardia sp.	Holtz et al. (1985)	Van de Perre et al. (1984)
Legionella sp.	Murray et al. (1984)	
Listeria monocytogenes	Real et al. (1984)	—
Noninfectious		
Kaposi's sarcoma	Grieco and Chinoy-Acharya (1985)	Bayley (1988); Piot et al. (1984)
Lymphoid interstitial pneumonitis	Macher et al. (1988)	—
Lymphoid hyperplasia	Macher et al. (1988)	—
Unexplained interstitial pneumonitis	Macher et al. (1988)	Van de Perre et al. (1984)

Lucas (1982), in an experiment designed to determine the presence of *Pneumocystis carinii* in Kenya, exposed immunosuppressed mice to the atmosphere and 5 months later sacrificed them and examined their lungs for histological evidence of PCP. The failure of the mice to contract even light infections suggested a geographical decreased prevalence of the parasite. It is possible that patients with AIDS in the tropics succumb to other more virulent infections before the degree of immunosuppression sufficient needed to permit reactivation of *Pneumocystis* is attained (Blaser and Cohn, 1986).

A "hierarchy of reactivation" of latent infections in AIDS patients may occur (Blaser and Cohn, 1986; Lucas and Wamukota, 1987); a relatively low threshold for reactivation of tuberculosis and toxoplasmosis compared to *Pneumocystis carinii.* As cell-mediated immunity is progressively compromised, more virulent opportunistic or reactivated pathogens proliferate and induce lesions earlier than the less virulent pathogens such as atypical mycobacteria, fungi, and *Pneumocystis.* There may also be differences in susceptibility between persons of black and white origin. PCP occurs in the Caribbean and Brazil with a similar frequency as in the west (Blaser and Cohn, 1986). Results of ongoing *Pneumocystis* research in three areas is anxiously awaited: an inexpensive, simple, and specific diagnostic test; safer and cheaper prophylactic agents; and determination of the underlying mechanisms of the host's lung defenses, wherein lie the answers to prophylaxis and immunotherapy.

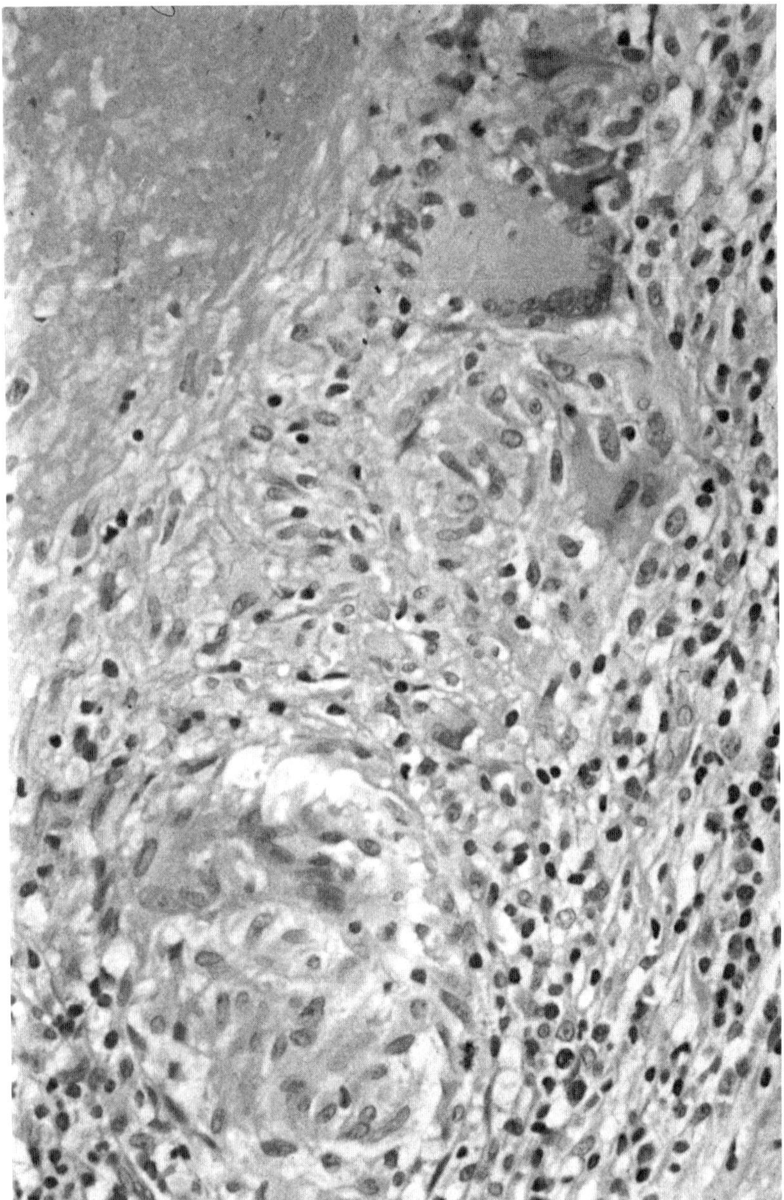

(a)

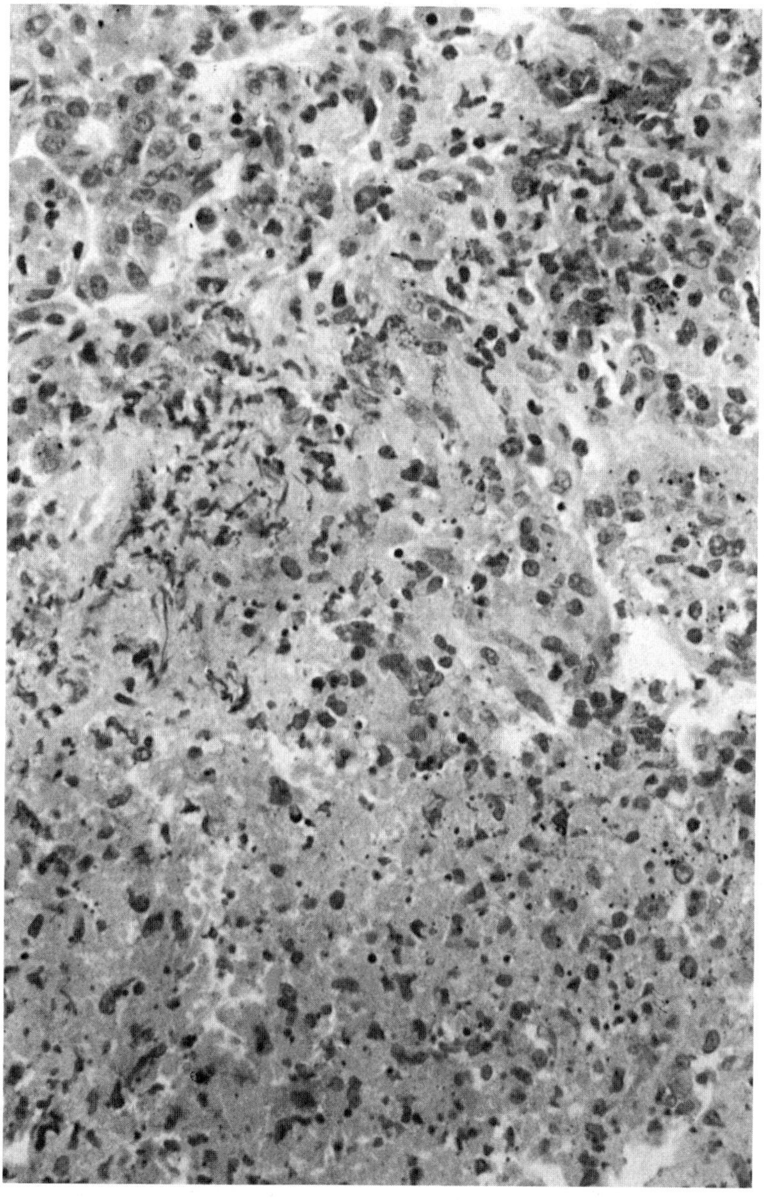

(b)

Figure 3 a. Classic granuloma due to *Mycobacterium tuberculosis*. Note the central area of caseous necrosis with the giant cell and epithelioid cell reaction (courtesy of Dr. Sebastian Lucas, University College and Middlesex Hospitals Medical School, London). b. *Mycobacterium tuberculosis* lung infection in a patient with AIDS shows widespread granular necrosis and a nonreactive "anergic" cellular response. Few lymphocytes and macrophages with no epithelioid cells are present (courtesy of Dr. Sebastian Lucas, University College and Middlesex Hospitals Medical School, London).

Other causes of respiratory disease in African AIDS patients include tuberculosis, cryptococcosis, nocardiosis, pneumococcal pneumonia, *Candida*, cytomegalovirus infection, and Kaposi's sarcoma (Table 8).

D. Mycobacteria and AIDS

Pulmonary tuberculosis due to *Mycobacterium tuberculosis* is one of the most important public health problems in the tropics. The development of tuberculosis may be one trigger for the occurrence of AIDS in the asymptomatic HIV-infected individual. One could predict, on the basis of the decreased cellular responses in AIDS patients, that the overall incidence of tuberculosis would rise and be more common in AIDS patients. Rates of HIV positive reactions have been found to be higher in TB wards than in the general population in Zaire (Mann et al., 1986). Disseminated disease is also more common in AIDS patients (Pitchenik et al., 1984). The most probable mechanism of reactivation or increase in susceptibility to mycobacterial infections is due to HIV infection of T4-positive lymphocytes and macrophages (Bowen et al., 1985; Mann et al., 1986). Quantitative and qualitative defects of these cells lead to impaired granuloma formation (Fig. 3). Observations from Zimbabwe show that HIV-positive patients with pulmonary tuberculosis may manifest miliary reactive histological findings with scanty bacilli or nonreactive histological findings (Lucas et al., 1987). It appears that in African AIDS there appears to be a progression of tuberculosis towards an anergic pathological appearance (Lucas and Wamukota, 1987; Nambuya et al., 1988) as progression of disease occurs. In the United States the clinicopathological pattern of tuberculosis in AIDS also differs from the classic adult-type pulmonary tuberculosis, with less lung fibrocavitary disease and more diseminated visceral disease (Louie et al., 1986; Fig. 4). Lymph node biopsies from African AIDS patients show a range of histopathological findings, with classic caseating granulomas with scanty or no bacilli in 7/16 cases and features of abnormal cell-mediated immunity with abundant necrosis, minimal or no epithelioid cell maturation, and abundant bacilli nonreactive (anergic) tuberculosis in 9 (Nambuya et al., 1988).

Although *Mycobacterium avium-intracellulare* (MAI) is the most common mycobacteria associated with HIV in the west (Hawkins et al., 1986) and the organism is prevalent in most countries, MAI in association with AIDS in Africa appears to be underrepresented (Lucas, 1988). The question of diagnostic facilities may not be the only reason, since MAI was detected in only 3% of Africans receiving care in developed countries compared to 15% in persons native to developed countries (Blaser and Cohn, 1986). Environmental differences in prevalence of the parasite, geographically varying susceptibilities, and the "hierarchy of infection" hypothesis may all contribute to these differences.

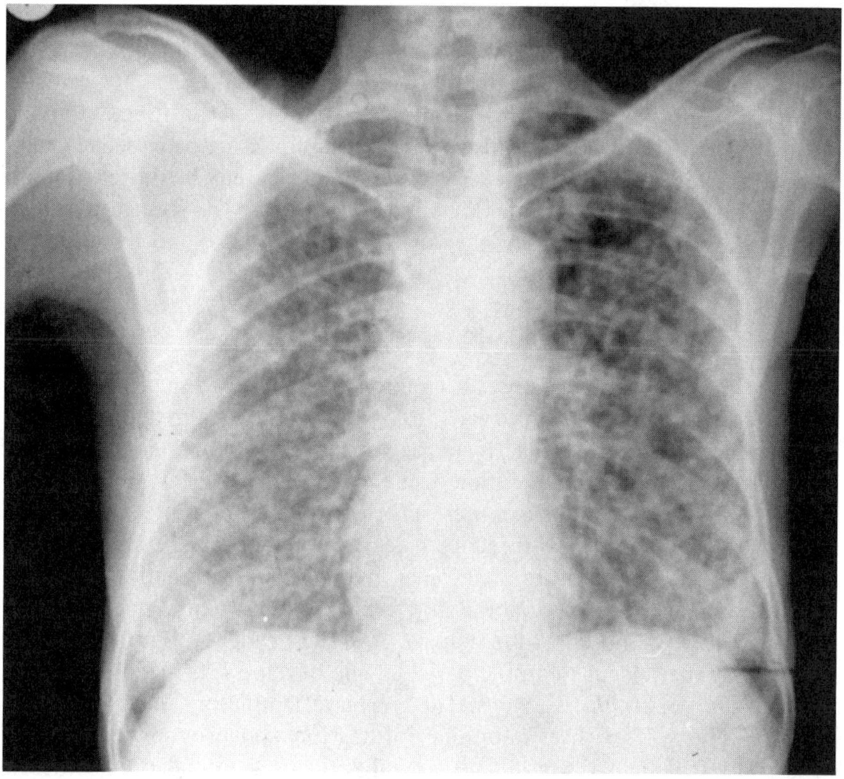

Figure 4 Chest X-ray of an AIDS patient shows extensive miliary tuberculosis (courtesy of Dr. Sebastian Lucas, University College and Middlesex Hospitals Medical School, London).

In the immunocompetent individual, the T lymphocytes in a tuberculous effusion appear to be immunologically committed cells, which, upon exposure to the tubercle bacillus, release lymphokines and activate macrophages necessary for limiting bacterial growth and the formation and maintenance of granulomas (Sahn, 1988). The determination of lymphocyte subpopulations, biochemical markers such as adenosine deaminase, or detection of mycobacterial antigens in pleural fluid using specific monoclonal antibodies as methods for rapid diagnosis have not been exploited as yet and are possible ways of differentiating between mycobacterial and nonmycobacterial pleural infections, and between different mycobacterial species. Furthermore, in light of the immune defects in AIDS patients the response to conventional antituberculous chemotherapy needs urgent study. The infection tends to reactivate after therapy stops and lifelong antituberculous therapy is currently favored. The case for prophylactic antituberculous chemotherapy in AIDS patients can be defined only if baseline data are available.

Pyogenic organisms taking advantage of the B-cell malfunction (Lane et al., 1984) in AIDS patients causing respiratory illness are often seen (Krumholtz et al., 1989) (Table 8). Acute lobar pneumonia may be more common in seropositive African patients (Katlama et al., 1984). The spectrum of bacterial pathogens causing pulmonary disease are similar to those seen in the west (Mcleod et al., 1989).

E. Fungal Infections and AIDS

Cell-mediated immune responses are important in protecting against fungal infections affecting the respiratory tract. Nonspecific local respiratory tract immune mechanisms also inactivate the virulence components of the fungi. In reality, considerable cooperation occurs between leukocytes, complement, and T- and B-cell immune responses. There are several possible outcomes of severe opportunistic fungal infections: recovery following use of antifungal drugs, death, or persistent reinfection. A hypersensitivity reaction may then be triggered, such as aspergilloma in preexisting lung cavities such as those left by treated pulmonary tuberculosis. Allergic bronchopulmonary aspergillosis may then occur in atopic patients who develop IgE-mediated hypersensitivity to *Aspergillus* antigens. There is an inflammatory reaction around the bronchial wall with eosinophilic infiltration and bronchi may be obstructed by fragmented mycelia. If fungal antigens are inhaled by someone with preformed precipitating antibodies the antigen/antibody complexes may form in the respiratory tract, for example, farmers' lung.

In the wake of AIDS, several opportunistic fungal infections have come to light. *Cryptococcus neoformans* causes lung involvement as part of disseminated disease (Fig. 5). In contrast to *Pneumocystis*, it appears to be more common in Africa than in Europe (Blaser and Cohn, 1986). Lucas and Wamukota (1987) found it in 9 of 22 autopsies in Uganda. The reasons for this discrepancy may be similar to those discussed under pneumocystis. Common fungi affecting the lung in the tropics are listed in Table 9 and one can anticipate the emergence of several of these with better definition of the spreading AIDS epidemic.

F. Parasitic Infections in AIDS

Parasitic diseases are endemic in parts of the tropics but there is no convincing evidence that their prevalence or incidence is increasing due to the HIV epidemic. Furthermore, the high prevalence of parasites in the population

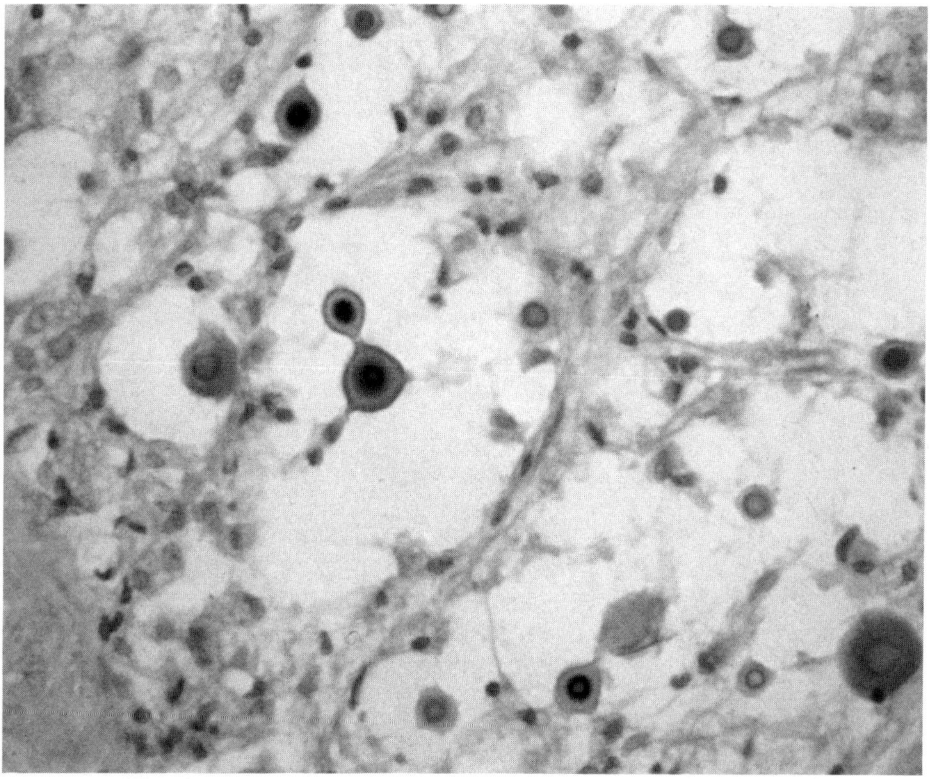

(a)

Figure 5 a. *Cryptococcus neoformans* in the lungs of an AIDS patient (courtesy of Dr. Sebastian Lucas, University College and Middlesex Hospitals Medical School, London). b. Postmortem lung specimen of an African AIDS patient with cryptococcoma (courtesy of Dr. Sebastian Lucas, University College and Middlesex Hospitals Medical School, London).

makes it difficult to know whether an infection is causally related to HIV or not. Potentially invasive parasites that can affect the lung, *Entamoeba histolytica* and *Strongyloides stercoralis*, are closely associated with immunosuppression of cell-mediated immunity. Yet these have not been reported from Africa despite the high prevalence of these two parasites in these populations (Lucas, 1988). This is interesting and paradoxic. In addition, the wide distribution of parasitic infections with known immunosuppressive activity leading to opportunistic infections, and the coexistence of multiple parasites in the same subjects, makes it difficult to identify patients with AIDS.

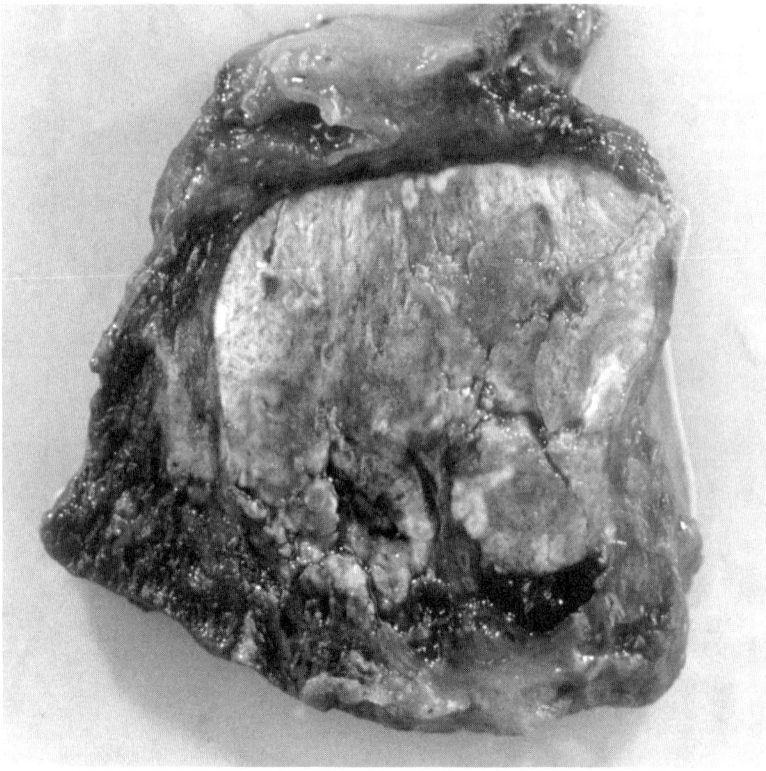

(b)

Figure 5 (continued)

It has been strongly argued that African patients have many reasons, such as malnutrition, to be immunosuppressed without a need to invoke HIV to account for it (Duesberg, 1988). Further observations are required to establish the interaction between HIV and the locally prevalent tropical diseases. Several tropical diseases (e.g., Chagas' disease) cause pathological change by the induction of cross-reactive autoaggressive cytotoxic T lymphocytes. The modification of pathological conditions (perhaps of advantage to the patient) of these due to HIV can be anticipated. That information will be vital for interventional strategies for prophylaxis, diagnosis, treatment, and control. As more information on AIDS becomes available from the tropics it will be interesting to see the physiological mechanisms in the host's terrain that account for reactivation of latent, and increased incidence of other, infections and for the observed geographical variations.

Table 9 Respiratory Mycoses

Fungus	Clinical manifestation	Lung involvement	Immunopathology	Diagnosis	Treatment
Nocardia sp. *Actinomyces* sp.	Actinomycosis	Chronic pneumonia	Granuloma/fibrosis	Microscopy Culture	Minocycline Penicillin
Paracoccidiodes brasiliense	S. American blastomycosis	Bronchopneumonia Pleural effusion Cavitation	Initially: PMN exudate Later: granuloma	Culture Sputa Ag CFT	Amphotericin B 5-FC Sulfadiazine
Coccidioides immitis	Coccidioidomycosis	Bronchopneumonia Cavitation	Chronic granuloma	Culture CFT ELISA	Amphotericin B 5-FC, Miconazole
Cryptococcus neoformans	Cryptococcosis	Pneumonia Infarction Cryptococcoma	Abscess, fibrosis Granuloma	Microscopy Culture	Fluconazole Amphotericin B 5-FC
Candida sp.	Pulmonary moniliasis	Bronchitis Pneumonia	Abscess, necrosis Granuloma	Microscopy Culture	Nystatin Amphotericin B
Sporothrix schenkii	Sporotrichosis	Cavitation	Granuloma	Microscopy Culture	Amphotericin B
Histoplasma capsulatum duboisii	Histoplasmosis	Acute pneumonia Chronic cavitation Histoplasmoma	Granuloma	Microscopy CFT Culture	Amphotericin B Ketoconazole Rifampicin
Aspergillus fumigatus	Aspergillosis	Necrotizing pneumonia	*Aspergillus* Non-suppurative necrotizing granuloma	Microscopy Culture Precipitins	Amphotericin B Itraconazole

G. Kaposi's Sarcoma

The occurrence of Kaposi's sarcoma (KS) in Africa predates the AIDS epidemic (Owor, 1988). The effect of HIV infection on the clinicopathological appearances of KS in central Africa has been the increase in number of cases of atypical aggressive disease (Bayley, 1988). Widespread cutaneous and visceral dissemination including the lungs, in association with a poorer prognosis, occurs. KS may occur in a patient already ill with opportunistic infections or may occur as the only obvious evidence of AIDS. The varying incidence among different ethnic groups has not been adequately explained. In the lungs KS appears grossly as erythematous plaques and nodules (Lucas and Wamukota, 1987; Fig. 6). Serosanguinous pleural effusions may accompany

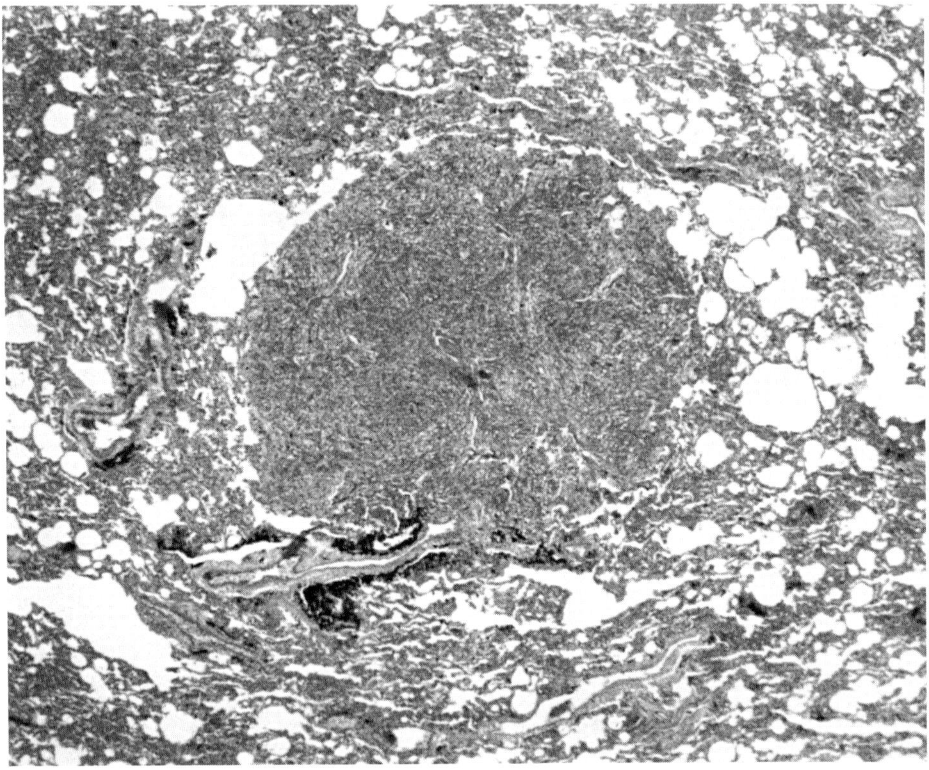

Figure 6 Kaposi's sarcoma nodule in the lung (postmortem specimen) of an AIDS patient (courtesy of Dr. Sebastian Lucas, University College and Middlesex Hospitals Medical School, London).

pleural involvement (Krigel and Friedman-Kien, 1988). It appears that although HIV does not induce the sarcoma, the immunodeficiency may explain the difference and incidence of KS as it presents in AIDS. Kaposi's sarcoma accounts for 3.7% of all de novo malignancies emerging after immunosuppressive chemotherapy for organ transplants. Complete regression or improvement of KS may occur on withdrawal of chemotherapy (Bhoopchand et al., 1986). The immunosurveillance mechanisms that keep KS at bay may ultimately be linked to T-cell function (Downing et al., 1984).

VI. Parasites and the Lung

Parasitic diseases are more important causes of death than cancer or heart disease in the tropics. Pulmonary involvement may be a major feature in some helminthic infections and in others it may be a complication of infection, as the larval stages migrate through the lungs as part of their life cycle in humans. Table 10 lists the range of parasitic diseases affecting the lung in the tropics. Selected examples are discussed here emphasizing the lung immune responses to these parasites.

A. Immune Mechanisms in Pulmonary Parasitic Diseases

The immune response to parasites may have both protective and deleterious effects (Davidson, 1985). The restriction or eradication of infection occurs via several mechanisms. Parasite-specific IgE antibodies play an important role in protection, although the precise mechanism of protection is unknown. IgE antibodies are thought to react with the parasite to form immune complexes that are bound by macrophages via surface receptors for the Fc region of IgE. These activated macrophages then kill the parasite. Eosinophilia is also characteristic of helminthic infections (Spry, 1988). Mobilization of eosinophils may be due to several mechanisms. Activated T cells release lymphokines chemotactic to eosinophils. Mast cells degranulated by bound IgE reacting with parasite antigens release eosinophil chemotactic factor of anaphylaxis. Some parasite material is directly chemotactic to eosinophils. Eosinophils also have an effector function. For example, schistosomes coated with C3 or IgG are killed by eosinophils (Butterworth et al., 1975). The protective role of cell-mediated immune responses to parasites has been difficult to assess. However, the presence of specific delayed hypersensitivity may account for localizing infection. Nonspecific and genetic factors are clearly important in helminthic infections but are not yet clearly defined.

Many parasites generate a prolific humoral immune response much of which is not protective and some harmful. Detection of these IgG and IgM antibodies form the basis of serodiagnosis using the complement fixation test (CFT) and the more specific enzyme-linked immunoassay (ELISA). Sev-

Table 10 Parasites Causing Respiratory Illness

Helminths	Distribution
Nematodes	
Roundworms	
Ascaris lumbricoides	Worldwide
Ascaris suis	
Toxocara canis	
Toxocara cati	
Hookworm	
Necator americanus	S.E. Asia, W. and C. Africa, S. Asia,
Ancylostoma duodenale	S. Europe, N. Africa, India, China, Japan
Ancylostoma caninum	S. USA, Mexico, Africa, Asia, S. America
Necator brasiliense	S. America, Caribbean
Strongyloides stercoralis	Worldwide
Trichinella spiralis	Worldwide
Microfilaria	
Loa loa	W. and C. Africa
Wuchereria bancrofti	Pacific, Asia, Africa, China, Americas
Brugia malayi	S.E. Asia
Brugia pahangi/patei	S.E. Asia, America, S. Africa, Australia
Dirofilaria immitis	S.E. Asia, America, S. Africa, Australia
Gnathostoma spinigerum	India, Philippines, Thailand
Trematodes	
Schistosomes	
Schistosoma mansoni	Africa, S. Arabia, S. America, Caribbean
S. haematobium	Africa, Middle East
S. japonicum	Far East
S. intercalatum	W. and C. Africa
Lung flukes	
Paragonimus westermani	Far East, China, Japan, Philippines
P. africanus/uterobilateralis	Africa
P. caliensis	S. and C. America

Helminths	Distribution
Cestodes	
Hydatid	
Echinococcus granulosus and	Australia, Africa (endemic)
E. multilocularis	Worldwide (sporadic)
Pentastomes	
Linguatula serrata	Worldwide
Armillifus armilata	
Protozoa	
Entamoeba histolytica	Worldwide
Plasmodium falciparum	Africa, S. and C. America, Asia
Pneumocystis carinii	Worldwide
Toxoplasma gondii	Worldwide
Leishmania donovani	Africa, Middle East, S. America, Asia

eral of the clinical features of parasite infection occur due to the host's immune response to parasite antigens (Table 7).

Immediate or type 1 hypersensitivity reactions such as urticaria and angioedema are found in the acute stages of most helminthic infections that have a migratory larval phase of development. Migration through the lungs evokes florid immune responses leading to clinical syndromes such as tropical pulmonary eosinophilia and Loeffler's syndrome. Rupture of a hydatid cyst due to trauma, during surgical removal or even spontaneously, can trigger acute anaphylactic shock.

Cell-mediated immune responses to parasites such as *Schistosoma* sp. and *trypanosoma cruzi* can cause severe tissue damage. Granuloma formation around schistosomal eggs in the lungs can lead to lung fibrosis and pulmonary hypertension. Destruction of autonomic nerves and smooth muscle due to antibody-mediated cell-dependent cytotoxicity occurs in *T. cruzi* infections due to autoaggressive T cells.

B. Pulmonary Eosinophilia

This term is used to describe a heterogeneous group of disorders of the lung interstitium that have three factors in common: respiratory symptoms, peripheral blood eosinophilia, and transient radiographic shadowing on chest x-rays. Loeffler (1932) first described four cases with minimal respiratory symptoms, pulmonary infiltrations on x-ray, and eosinophilia. He believed that this condition was due to a variety of antigens. Muller (1938), having ingested *Ascaris* ova, was able to reproduce what had come to be known as

Loeffler's syndrome and attributed the syndrome to the pulmonary phase of ascariasis. However, the syndrome has been reproduced with a number of causative agents (Table 11). In contradistinction to tropical pulmonary eosinophilia, which is a distinct entity, the eosinophilia is seldom above 20% of the total polymorphonuclear leukocyte count, which itself is only rarely elevated.

C. Tropical Pulmonary Eosinophilia

Weingarten (1943), working as a principal medical officer in India first described a new disease entity under the title "tropical eosinophilia." This was characterized by spasmodic bronchitis, leukocytosis, and a very high eosinophilia. Van der Sar and Hartz (1945) suggested a link between filariasis and tropical eosinophilia. The Indian subcontinent is the most important focus of infection, although cases occur in Africa, South America, Middle East, Indochina, and Australia. Tropical pulmonary eosinophilia (TPE) is now regarded as a specific clinical entity due to a hypersensitivity reaction to migrating animal microfilariae, such as *Brugia pahangi, Brugia patei, Dirofilaria sp* (Fig. 7) in the abnormal host humans. These microfilaria cannot complete their life cycle in humans.

Five diagnostic criteria are essential to make a diagnosis of TPE.

1. Respiratory symptoms
2. Peripheral blood eosinophilia

Table 11 Causes of Pulmonary Eosinophilia

Due to known causes	
Fungi	Allergic bronchopulmonary mycoses
Drugs	Para-amino salicylic acid (PAS), streptomycin, penicillin, tetracycline, sulfonamides, nitrofurantoin, busulfan, chlorpropamide, imipramine, gold
Helminth larvae	Ascaris, hookworm, strongyloides, *Microfilaria, Gnathostoma, Trichinella*
Toxins	Epoxy resins, toxic oils
Due to unknown causes	
Cryptogenic pulmonary eosinophilia	
Vasculitides	Polyarteritis nodosa Churg-Strauss syndrome

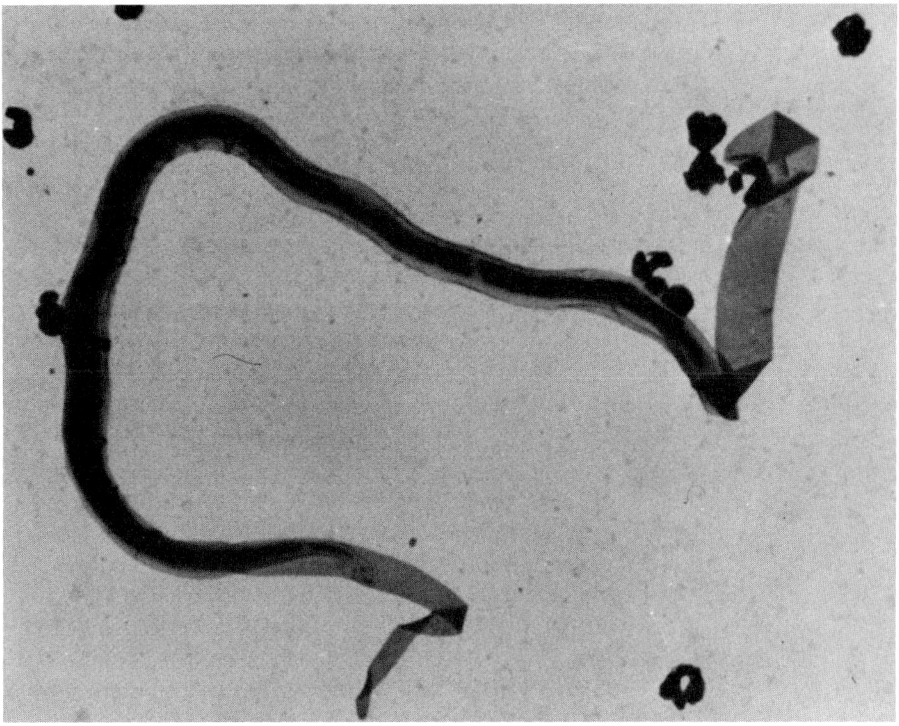

(a)

Figure 7 a. Microfilaria of *Brugia pahangi* (causative agent of TPE). b. Microfilaria of *Dirofilaria immitis* (causative agent of TPE).

3. Transient shadowing on chest x-ray
4. Positive filarial complement fixation test (using a 1% alcoholic extract of *Dirofilaria immitis* as antigen)
5. A clinical and radiological response to treatment with diethylcarbamazine (DEC)

Lung pathological examination shows scattered pneumonic areas with granulomatous changes, numerous focal collection of eosinophils, a few giant cells, and neutrophils. The clinicopathological features are thought to be due to interplay of types I and III hypersensitivity reactions to microfilarial antigens. TPE is more likely where infections are intermittently acquired; the condition is seldom seen in populations who are continuously exposed.

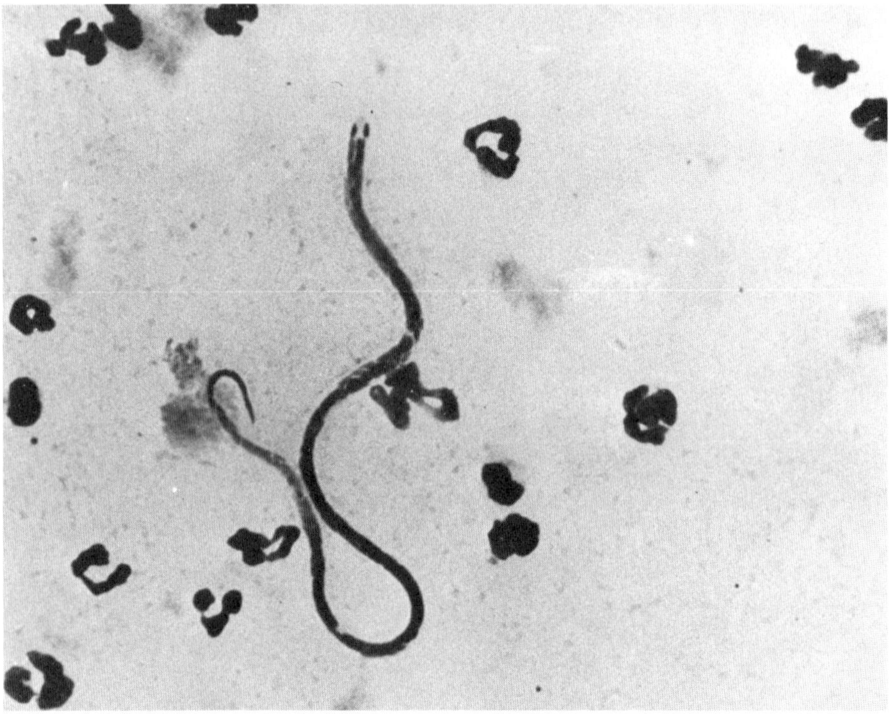

(b)

Figure 7 (continued)

VII. Trematodes and the Lung

A. Schistosomiasis

Schistosomiasis is a disease that is still spreading in association with water and agricultural development projects in the tropics. It is endemic in 74 countries, over 600 million people are exposed to the risk of infection, and an estimated 200 million are infected (WHO, 1985). There are four types of schistosome worms infective to humans. Three of them, *Schistosoma mansoni, S. japonicum,* and *S. intercalatum,* cause intestinal schistosomiasis while *S. haematobium* causes genitourinary schistosomiasis. The organism's life cycle is complex (Manson-Bahr and Bell, 1987a) and a multitude of antigens are present at each stage. The major disease symptoms and pathological findings are due to immune responses to these antigens. As more information on the immune mechanisms against these antigens becomes available, it is becoming increasingly clear that the parasite has outplayed the terrain at every stage in its life cycle in humans, making it one of the most successful parasites of humans (Chen and Mott, 1988a, b). The mechanisms of protective immunity to schistosomiasis remain unsolved despite intense research (Smithers and Doenhoff, 1982; Boros, 1989).

Pulmonary involvement occurs during the initial migratory phase and subsequently due to ectopic deposition of ova and, rarely, adult flukes in the lung. About one-third of all cases of schistosomiasis in Egypt showed some degree of lung involvement (Shaw and Ghareeb;1938). Pulmonary hypertension has been reported to occur in 13% (19/141) of patients with *S. mansoni* infections in Brazil (Guimaraes, 1982). The varying incidence and differences in pathological findings caused by the same parasite may be due to differences in host HLA (Chen and Mott, 1988a).

Pulmonary Eosinophilia and Katayama Fever

After cercarial penetration of the skin, the schistosomula from the primary infection cause few perturbances when passing through the lungs on their way to the portal blood system. Secondary and subsequent migrations through the lung elicit cellular reactions that are markedly earlier and more florid (see discussion of pulmonary eosinophilia). Not all patients develop these symptoms and in many they may go unnoticed. Previous exposure and immune status, together with host HLA types, may account for this variation. Acute schistosomiasis (Katayama fever), characterized by fever, urticaria, hepatosplenomegaly, lymphadenopathy, abdominal pain, nausea, diarrhea, respiratory symptoms, and eosinophilia, occurs within 2-11 weeks of infection. This is thought to coincide with arrival of mature schistosome worms at their destination in the portal or urogenital venous system and commencement of ovideposition.

Immunopathological Mechanisms in Schistosomiasis

Pulmonary inflammatory reactions may cause direct cytotoxic damage to migrating schistosomula (von Lichtenberg et al., 1985; Crabtree and Coulson, 1986). Leukocytosis with eosinophilia is common and serum IgG, IgM, and IgE levels are elevated. There is ample evidence for the eosinophil as an effector cell in schistosome immunity. Eosinophils are the principal cells involved in antibody-dependent cell mediated damage (Butterworth et al., 1974). Eosinophils can adhere to schistosomules and degranulate onto the surface of the worm larva releasing the contents onto the worm. Killing is associated with the major basic protein of the granules causing progressive damage and disruption of the integument of the larva. Adherence of neutrophils and eosinophils to the surface of the larva mediated by antibody and complement is a first step in killing the parasite. Some of the worms are killed by hydrogen peroxide and other oxygen metabolites released from the PMN during the respiratory burst that follows membrane perturbation resulting from contact between PMN and larva. The alternative pathway of complement activation may kill the schistosomula in the absence of antibody (Santoro, 1982). Capron et al. (1975) have demonstrated the important role of parasiticidal IgE antibodies. Other schistosomulae are walled off by granulomas. Warren (1972) suggests that the symptoms of Katayama fever are compatible with those of serum sickness or immune complex disease.

Vascular and Parenchymatous Lung Lesions

Schistosome ova (*S. mansoni* and *S. haematobium* more frequently than *S. japonicum*) may reach the pulmonary circulation as emboli, obstruct small blood vessels, pass through their walls, and come to lie immediately outside them. These are at first surrounded by neutrophil and eosinophil leukocytes and later lymphocytes, multinucleated giant cells, and fibroblasts appear. Some ova are killed by eosinophils (James and Colley, 1976). The macrophages produce fibroblast chemoattractants such as fibronectin (Wyler and Postlewaithe, 1983). Experimental formation of the granuloma can be abrogated by techniques that eliminate cell-mediated immunity (CMI) responses and the ova-specific CMI can be transferred by cells but not serum (Warren et al., 1967). The ova trapped in tissue cause the development of the typical schistosomal granuloma: an end product of hypersensitivity reactions involving type I, III, and IV reactions (Table 6). The cell populations within the granuloma differ according to the duration of the infection and immune status of the individual. The granuloma is induced by release of soluble egg antigens (SEA), is T cell dependent, is independent of humoral effector mechanisms, and can modulate with time. Two types of pathological lesions develop in the lung (Chen and Mott, 1988a, b) as direct and indirect consequences of egg granuloma formation: extensive parenchymatous lesions or Periarteritis, fibrosis, and a diffuse endarteritis obliterans of the pulmonary arterioles (Fig. 8). The clinical consequences of these can be classified into two types: bronchopulmonary schistosomiasis with bronchitis, bronchiectasis, or asthma due to airways obstruction; and cor pulmonale secondary to widespread arteritis and vessel obstruction.

No specific symptoms have been attributed to the presence of ova in the lung until pulmonary hypertension develops. Perivascular fibrous cuffs scattered throughout the lung may give rise to miliary stippling on x-ray studies. If adult flukes embolize to the lung they cause little reaction while they remain alive within the pulmonary arterioles. Severe toxic reactions ensue upon death, including thrombosis of the arteriole, necrosis of surrounding lung tissue, with an eosinophilic and giant cell reaction resulting in fibrosis

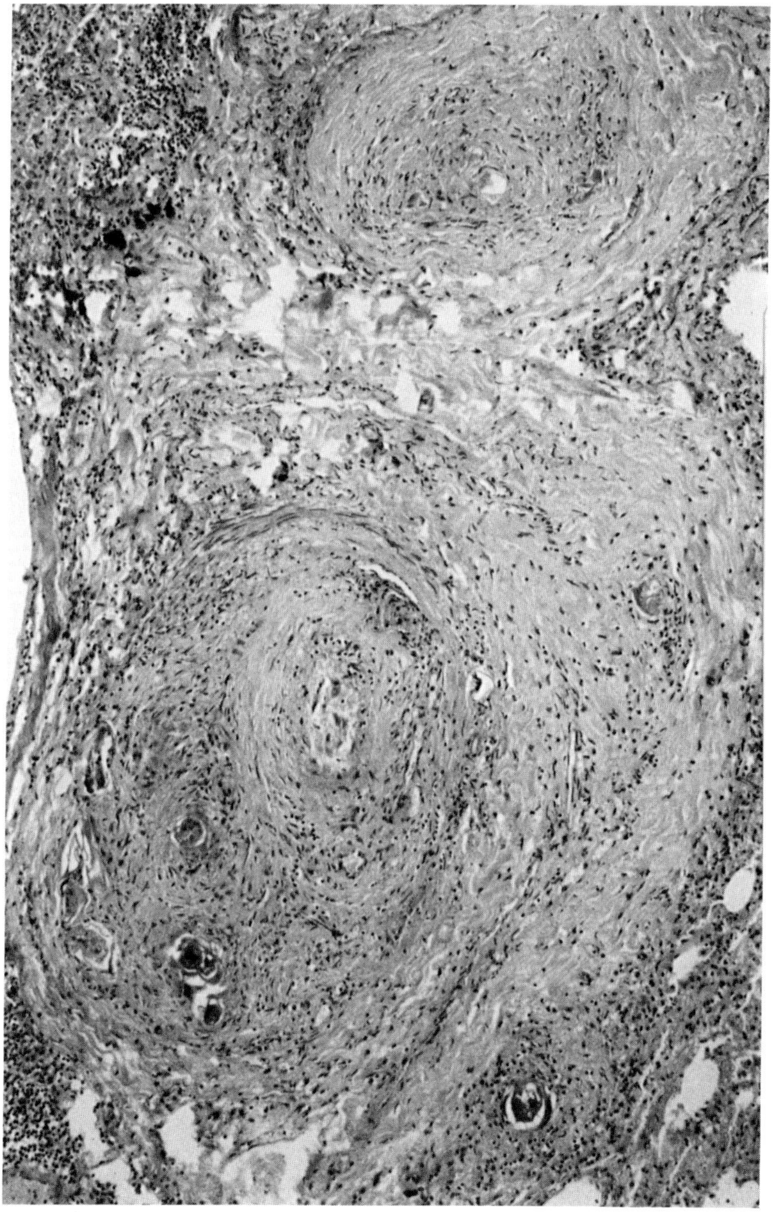

Figure 8 Severe periarteritis and arteritis obliterans with fibrosis in human lung tissue as host's response to ova of *Schistosoma mansoni* (courtesy of Dr. Sebastian Lucas, University College and Middlesex Hospitals Medical School, London).

that may calcify. Pulmonary hypertension is irreversible. Further progression of pathological damage can be arrested by treatment with appropriate antischistosomal drugs (reviewed by Davis, 1986). Praziquantel is currently the treatment of choice for all three species. Oxamniquine remains in favor with some physicians for treatment of *S. mansoni* infections. Posttreatment pneumonia (Davidson et al., 1986) or a Loeffler-like syndrome may occur 24-72 h after treatment with oxamniquine.

B. Paragonimiasis

Paragominus westermani is one of several species of lung flukes endemic in areas where fresh water crab, crayfish, or shrimp is eaten raw or semicooked. The clinical manifestations are similar to those of pulmonary tuberculosis. The flukes can live in humans for many years and persist long after the individual has left an endemic area (Yokogawa, 1965). Once the seafood flesh containing encysted metacercaria is ingested by humans, the larval forms excyst, penetrate the bowel, and migrate through the liver, diaphragm, and pleura into the lung where they pair up and mature into adult flukes (Fig. 8). Although they are hermaphrodite, they cross-fertilize and produce operculated ova that are present in sputum.

Immunopathological features include:

1. Stage of infiltration: hemorrhage and exudative inflammation
2. Encysted stage
3. Nonsuppurative chronic granulomatous reaction containing numerous ova
4. Suppurative lesions
5. Nonhealing chronic lesions.

Secondary infection may intervene at any stage. Eosinophils and polymorphonuclear neutrophils infiltrate around the parasites. Absorption of the worm with collapse of the cyst wall with fibrosis, nodule formation, and calcification may occur. Ova may pass into the interstitial tissue where they evoke a macrophage and giant cell reaction. Pleural thickening or effusions are common findings (Johnson and Johnson, 1983). These vary from small to massive yellow, brown, or white exudates and may occur without parenchymal infiltrates. The leukocyte count in the fluid is generally less than 2000/μl and eosinophilia may be present. Pleural biopsy shows chronic inflammation occasionally with plasma cell and eosinophil infiltration without granulomas (Sahn, 1987). Ova are not usually seen in the pleural fluid. High pleural fluid IgE levels are reported. The diagnosis is made on epidemiological evidence, a positive CFT (usually greater than 1:64), presence of ova in sputum

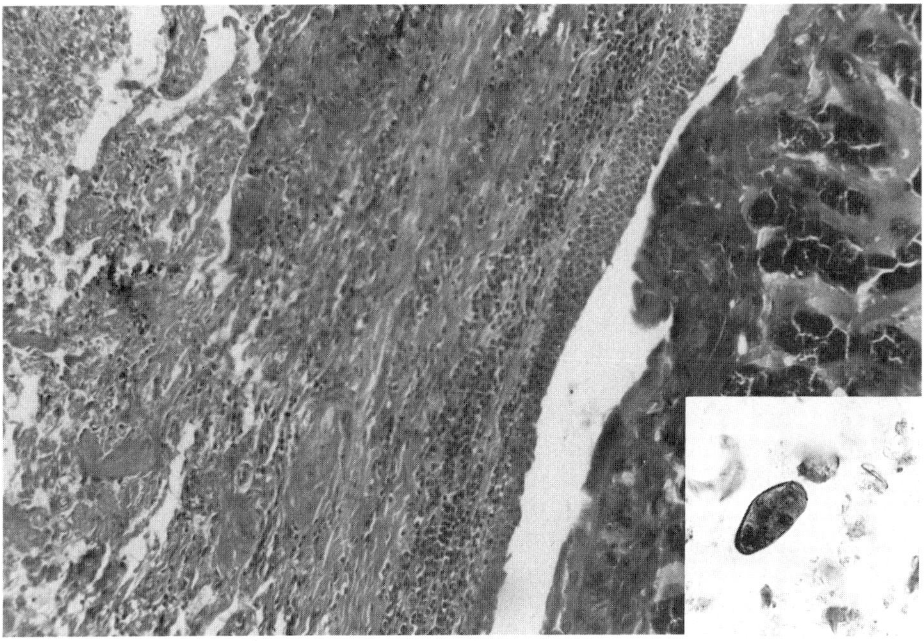

Figure 9 Adult lung fluke *Paragonimus westermani* in the lung. Section shows a chronic fibrous reaction around a part of the parasite. Insert shows an operculated ovum that can be recovered from sputum or feces.

or feces (Fig. 9), and a clinical and serological response to treatment. Recommended treatment is bithional, although some failures do occur. Promising results with praziquantel therapy are being reported.

VIII. Cestodes and the Lung: Pulmonary Hydatid Disease

Echinococcosis is caused by the tapeworms *Echinococcus granulosis* or *E. multilocularis.* It is most commonly seen in sheep- and cattle-raising communities. When humans ingests food contaminated with dog feces containing ova, the shell dissolves in the stomach and upper ileum releasing the embryo (onchosphere), which penetrates the intestinal wall, enters the portal circulation, and is conveyed to the liver, lung, and other tissues where, in a susceptible person, it develops into a hydatid cyst. This consists of a thick laminated layer (ectocyst) and a germinal layer (endocyst) with cyst fluid. Outside the laminated layer lies the fibrous layer formed by the host (pericyst). There is minimal chronic inflammatory cell reaction around the cyst where no leaks or rupture occurs. Brood capsules develop from the germinal layer and these give rise to daughter cysts with scolices, which may be set free if the cyst bursts. The multilocularis or alveolar hydatid lacks the ectocyst and spreads like an infiltrating neoplasm, evoking a granulomatous reaction by the lung.

Rupture of the hydatid cyst, either spontaneously or due to trauma, may result in sudden death due to anaphylactic shock (Werczberger et al., 1979). Scattering of hooklets from the daughter cysts evokes a foreign body giant cell reaction and acute inflammation. The expansion of the cyst may cause rupture of arterioles with hemorrhage. The rate of growth of the cyst is extremely slow and may be dependent on host immune response to it. The cysts may be latent for 10-20 years before the resulting symptoms, which depend on site, type, and rate of growth of the cystic lesion, occur (Dew, 1928). Where lung cysts develop, rupture may be caused by coughing, infection, or muscular strain and produces cough, chest pain, and hemoptyses. The scolices may be present in the sputum. Pneumo- and hemothorax are other recorded complications. Rupture of liver or pulmonary cysts may occur into the mediastinum and pleural cavity (Xanthakis et al., 1972).

Immune responses to the *Echinococcus* include parasite-specific antibodies (Pinon et al., 1979), eosinophils, type 1, and delayed hypersensitivity reactions. Intact T-cell function is a prerequisite for containment of metastasizing protoscolices of *E. multilocularis* (Baron and Tanner, 1976). Survival of the hydatid cysts is relative to the permeability of the cyst to immunoglobulins. Kassis and Tanner (1976) have shown that IgG and IgM occur in the cysts of the two species of *Echinococcus* and hypothesize that insufficient quantities of these cytotoxic antibodies reach the parasite under natural conditions to effect a cytotoxic response. Where pleural effusion develops, thoracentesis reveals turbid yellow fluid with PMN and eosinophil predominance. The diagnosis is established by finding scolices bearing hooklets in sputum or pleural fluid stained by toluidine blue and on the basis of the Weinberg complement fixation test (CFT). The Casoni skin test is out of favor now due to its low sensitivity and potentially dangerous side effects.

Medical therapy with mebendazole for smaller cysts may be successful. Treatment for larger cysts is surgical removal of the cysts and closure of the bronchopleural fistula, and thoracotomy where indicated (Novick et al., 1987).

IX. Nematodes Affecting the Lung

A. Strongyloidiasis

This infection is endemic in the tropics and subtropics. The parasite has a unique life cycle that has enabled it to cause overwhelming and often fatal syndrome of hyperinfection years after the infected individual leaves endemic areas (reviewed by Cook, 1987b; Longworth and Weller, 1986). Infection by *Strongyloides stercoralis* in humans occurs by invasive filariform larvae that penetrate the skin and gain access to the venous system via the lymphatics. These larvae pass through the right side of the heart into the lungs and break out of the capillaries into the alveoli (hemorrhage and edema are common), ascend up the tracheobronchial tree, and are swallowed. The larvae then develop into mature adult worms in the distal duodenum and proximal jejunum. Fertilization can occur by parthenogenesis and ova are laid that hatch immediately into rhabditiform larvae (ovoviviparous) that are excreted in the stool. The rhabditiform larvae may mature into adult worms in the soil or, alternatively, form the infective filariform larvae that penetrate the skin (Manson-Bahr and Bell, 1987b).

During the pulmonary migratory phase, the larvae sometimes develop into adults within the lung, although the accompanying pneumonitis is minimal. Uncomplicated infections with *Strongyloides* are usually minimally symptomatic in the majority of individuals. *Strongyloides* is able to perpetuate itself within a host for years following initial infection (Grove, 1980). This occurs through a process of internal or external autoinfection by which the noninfectious rhabditiform larvae destined to be excreted in feces transform within the colon (internal autoinfection) or perianal skin (external autoinfection) into filariform larvae that then invade the tissues to complete its cycle through the lungs to the small intestine. In the immunocompetent individual this process occurs at a slow rate and is kept in check presumably by the cell-mediated immune response. Persistence of *Strongyloides* in patients who migrated from endemic to nonendemic zones can occur for up to 50 years following initial acquisition of infection in endemic areas (Pelletier, 1984). In certain situations accelerated autoinfection and extremely heavy parasite burdens may develop, giving rise to hyperinfection and disseminated strongyloidiasis, with migration of larvae into organs not normally involved in the parasite's life cycle.

Pulmonary symptoms in uncomplicated strongyloidiasis consist of cough, dyspnea, and wheezing, which occurs as part of the pulmonary eosinophilia caused by the migrating larvae. The precise immunological mechanisms enabling the host to contain infection in uncomplicated strongyloidiasis are unclear (Genta, 1984). The relative importance of cellular and humoral mechanisms is controversial. Serum-modulating factors that suppress the cellular immune response to specific somatic larval antigens have been identified, although their significance remains unclear. Lower eosinophil counts and serum levels of IgG, IgA, and IgM occur in cases of severe strongyloidiasis (Carvalho et al., 1983), which implies that these responses may be important in limiting the disease.

Aberrant localization of ovipositing adult worms in the lungs with a strong eosinophil response has been described as complicating asthma treated with steroids (Higenbottam and Heard, 1976). Hyperinfection and dissemination appear to be phenomena of the immunocompromised host (Ingra-Seigman et al., 1981). It occurs when autoinfection increases in magnitude, which cause large numbers of filariform larvae to penetrate the intestinal mucosa and lodge in the pulmonary circulation. The presence of larvae in tissues may provoke no reaction or a mixed inflammatory infiltrate, while some may be walled off by granulomas. Extensive pneumonic changes may occur in the lung (Fig. 10).

Malnutrition, malignancies, chronic renal disease, chronic infections such as leprosy, tuberculosis, and syphilis, hypogammaglobulinemia, pancytopenia, autoimmune diseases, asthma, inflammatory bowel disease, and alcoholism can cause disseminated disease. While there have been isolated

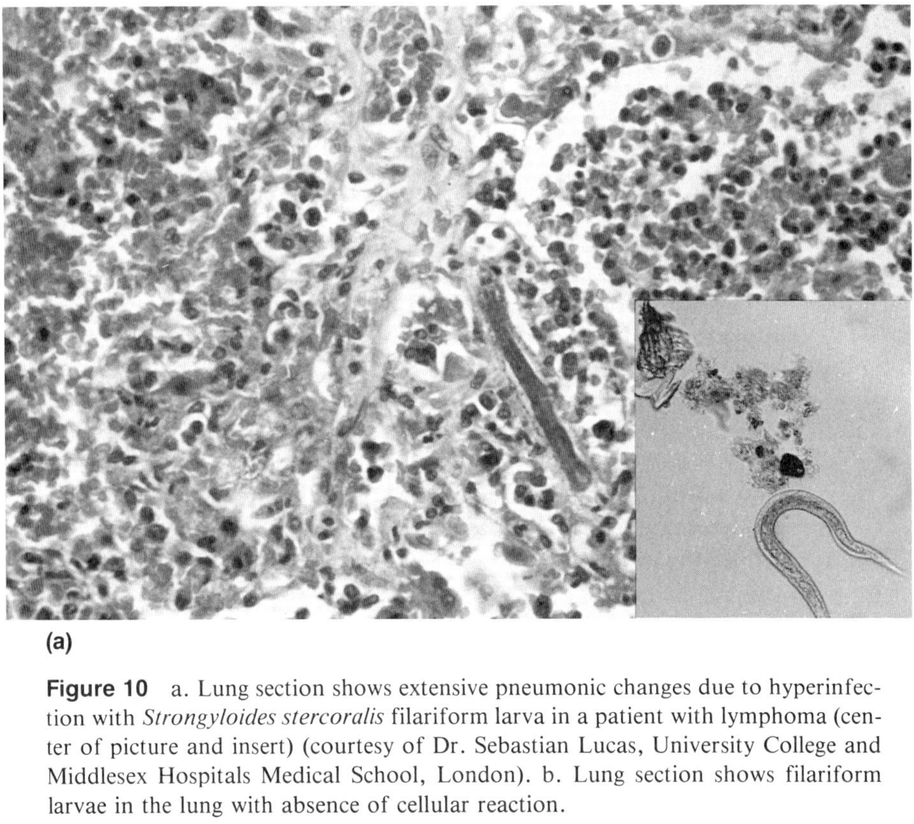

(a)

Figure 10 a. Lung section shows extensive pneumonic changes due to hyperinfection with *Strongyloides stercoralis* filariform larva in a patient with lymphoma (center of picture and insert) (courtesy of Dr. Sebastian Lucas, University College and Middlesex Hospitals Medical School, London). b. Lung section shows filariform larvae in the lung with absence of cellular reaction.

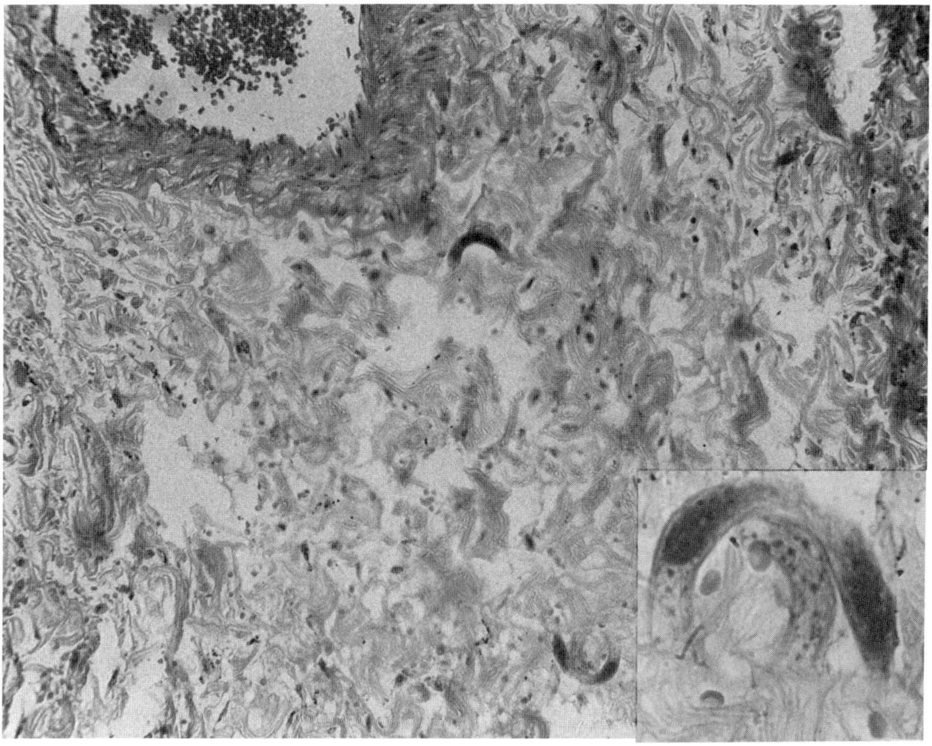

(b)

case reports of strongyloides hyperinfection in AIDS patients in Europe (Vieyra-Herrera et al., 1988; Maayan et al., 1988), there have been no reports of disseminated strongyloidiasis from Africa in the wake of the AIDS epidemic. In the hyperinfection syndrome, gastrointestinal and respiratory symptoms predominate (Longworth and Weller, 1986). Pulmonary manifestations include cough, sputum production, hemoptyses, dyspnea, bronchospasm, and respiratory insufficiency. Radiographic findings include diffuse pulmonary infiltrates, lobar consolidation, and, rarely, lung abscess. Gram-negative septicaemias frequently complicate the course of the hyperinfection syndrome (Ingra-Seigman et al., 1981). Disruption of the mucosal integrity by penetrating filariform larvae may facilitate the entry of gram-negative enteric bacteria. These may also be carried on the integument of the larvae or may be present in the feces of the larvae. Helminths with a migratory larval phase in general can act as vehicles and synergists of other microbial infections in man (Woodruff, 1968). Bronchopneumonia is probably the consequence of the tissue damage inflicted by the invading larvae and the associated sepsis.

Consideration of the diagnosis is vital since most of the clinical features are nonspecific. Physicians in the tropics should actively seek cases of hyperinfection, while in temperate areas a history of past residence or travel to endemic areas together with an eosinophilia of >5% should alert the physician to the possibility of the hyperinfection syndrome. Definitive diagnosis depends on identifying the larvae in stools, jejunal aspirates, sputum, bronchial washings, or transbronchial biopsies. Serological tests such as ELISAs to detect IgG to filariform larval antigen (Neva and Burke, 1981) have not found widespread application in the tropics as yet. In light of AIDS, there is an urgent need for cheaper and more sensitive tests for detection of *Strongyloides* infection in immunosuppressed patients.

A number of chemotherapeutic compounds are available for the treatment of *Strongyloides* infection (Taylor and Denham, 1988). Thiabendazole is the treatment of choice (Grove, 1982). In disseminated infections, low-dose, long term interrupted courses have to be given. Mebendazole, albendazole, and levamisole are alternatives (reviewed by Cook, 1987b). Gram-negative septicemias associated with invasive strongyloidiasis do not respond to antimicrobial therapy unless therapy for strongyloides is promptly initiated concomitantly. The case for prophylactic thiabendazole in immunosuppressed patients in the tropics is stong on theoretical grounds. Further observations are needed to define the magnitude of the problem.

B. Ascariasis

The adult worms live in the small intestine and the parasite has gained the reputation of "wanderlust worms," occasionally being found in organs other than the gut including the liver, brain, and trachea. The eggs are passed in the feces and in a suitable environment a larva develops within the eggs and becomes infective. Eggs containing the infective larva are swallowed by humans and the larva hatch in the small intestine. They begin their migration through the wall of the intestine into the portal system of the liver. They are then carried by the bloodstream to the right heart and lungs, where they remain for several days. The larvae may cause hemorrhage due to capillary damage and pulmonary edema, and evoke a neutrophil and eosinophil reaction before migrating up the bronchus and trachea to the pharynx. They are then swallowed and reenter the small intestine where they become sexually mature within 2 months. The migratory phase of larval development in the liver and lungs requires 8-15 days and is associated with fever, allergic dermatitis, eosinophilia, and pneumonitis or, rarely, pneumonia. A focal granulomatous reaction may occur around dead or dying larvae. A vivid illustration of the clinical features of this phase of the parasite's life cycle is given by Woodruff's description of ingestion of 2,000 viable *Ascaris* ova by Koino (Koino, 1922). Within a week he developed fever, dyspnea, severe cough, cyanosis, and frothy blood-stained sputum lasting over 7 days. Many larvae were recovered from the sputum. *Ascaris* pneumonia may occur 4-16 days after infection and larvae may be found in the sputum. The combination of fever, cough, expectoration, eosinophilia and pulmonary infiltration on x-ray constitutes "Loeffler's syndrome." Portions of larvae have been noted in bronchioles, with a marked patchy infiltrate of polymorphonuclear and eosinophil leukocytes with scattered Charcot Leyden crystals. Sputum may show larvae, eosinophils and Charcot Leyden crystals. A number of antihelminthic drugs (piperazine citrate, biphenium hydroxynapthoate, levamisole, and mebendazole) are active against the adult worm but none are successful in killing migrating larvae.

C. Toxocariasis

Toxocara canis and *Toxocara catis* are roundworms of dogs and cats and in the unusual host (humans) cause visceral larva migrans. The migrating larvae may reach any organ in the body (Ehrhard and Kernbaum, 1979). Pulmonary symptoms are usual and Loeffler's syndrome is simulated. In the lung, initial isolated lesions are composed of fibrinoid material, lymphocytes, and eosinophils. Later an eosinophilic granuloma forms with a fibrous capsule that eventually encloses the larva (Mok, 1968). The parasite reaches an end stage in its life cycle in humans. Children with visceral larva migrans have been shown to have defects in neutrophil function, probably secondary to high levels of IgE.

D. Human Gnathostomiasis

The parasite *Gnathostoma spinigerum* is found throughout Southeast Asia, Africa, America, and the Middle East. Humans become infected by the third-stage larva by eating raw or semicooked the intermeidate hosts of the parasite: fish, snakes, frogs, and chicken. The definitive hosts of the parasite are dogs and cats (Daensuang, 1980). After ingestion, the larvae leave the gut and migrate through the liver, muscles, and subcutaneous tissues. Since humans are not the definitive host, the life cycle is an end stage infection. The disease presents clinically as migratory cutaneous swellings and, more rarely, pneumonitis, pleurisy, and meningoencephalitis. Spontaneous pneumothorax, hemoptyses, and hematuria have all been recorded. Specific diagnosis can be made by ELISA (Dharmkrong et al., 1986). There is no effective chemotherapy. Mebendazole, thiabendazole, and levamisole have all been tried (Janssens, 1985). Spontaneous improvement with resolution usually occurs.

X. Protozoal Lung Infections

A. Amebiasis

An infection caused by the protozoon *Entamoeba histolytica* usually results in dysentery and sometimes involves other viscera. Hepatic abscess is the most common extraintestinal complication. This may, if untreated or inadequately treated, result in rupture into the lung or pleural space and an amebic pleural effusion may occur as a result, leading to empyema (pleuropulmonary amebiasis). *E. histolytica* may reach the lung by way of the lymphatics or, rarely, by the bloodstream (Adams and Macleod, 1977).

Amebic pneumonitis is said to occur in 0.1% of all cases. Although high levels of specific antibody are present, the cell-mediated immune responses are thought to be protective (Sepulveda and Martinez-Palamo, 1982; Ravdin, 1989). Differences in parasite strains (zymodeme differences) or host HLA might account for the invasiveness of the amebae. Amebic lung abscesses are preceded by colliquative necrosis and later multiple hemorrhages and areas of necrosis occur (Brandt and Tamayo, 1970). The hallmark of tissue necrosis is the lack of inflammatory reactions to invading trophozoites. Early changes are accompanied by PMN leukocytosis. The abscess consists of a necrotic center of partly living eosinophils, neutrophils, lymphocytes, macrophages, and cellular debris, and an encircling wall of chronic inflammatory tissue. The trophozoites may be found in the boundary between the two zones. Surrounding the abscess is edematous tissue with collapsed alveoli. Anchovy-sauce-like material may be coughed up and the residual abscess cavity may become secondarily infected. About one-third of patients will have concomitant bacterial infection.

Radiological features include elevation of the right dome of the diaphragm, pleural effusions, pulmonary collapse, and lung abscess. Thoracocentesis shows brown or anchovy-colored fluid from which the trophozoites usually cannot be demonstrated. Computed tomography (CT) and ultrasound will show effusion and liver abscess. Rupture of the abscess into the lung results in respiratory distress and the patient may cough up its contents in sputum. Radiological features include elevation of the right dome of the diaphragm, pleural effusion, pulmonary collapse, and lung abscess. Serological tests (CFT and ELISA) are usually positive. Treatment consists of metronidazole and, in the cases of pleuropneumonic amebiasis, early large tube thoracostomy to drain the thick fluid.

B. Toxoplasmosis and the Lung

Seroprevalence rates of toxoplasmosis in Africa are relatively high (Griffin and Williams, 1983; DeClercq and Lokombe, 1986). *Toxoplasma gondii* is increasingly becoming responsible for a wide range of clinical syndromes in immunocompromised individuals. Although central nervous system involvement is the most common finding (Wong, 1984), lung pathology does occur. Nonspecific bronchopneumonic changes may be found an interstitial pneumonitis with proliferation of alveolar lining cells, many containing parasites. A gelatinous exudate in the alveoli may be diagnostic if observed. Study of monocyte-derived macrophages from patients with AIDS show a decreased ability to kill *T. gondii* (Eales et al., 1989). The mechanism of reactivation of the latent intracellular bradyzoites remains to be elucidated.

C. Malaria and the Lungs

Clinical bronchitis and its complications are common in children with malaria. In the acute stages, the smaller vessels are packed with parasitized erythrocytes (Fig. 11) and small hemorrhages may be present. Hyaline membranes and areas of alveolar hemorrhages have been recorded. Pneumonitis and

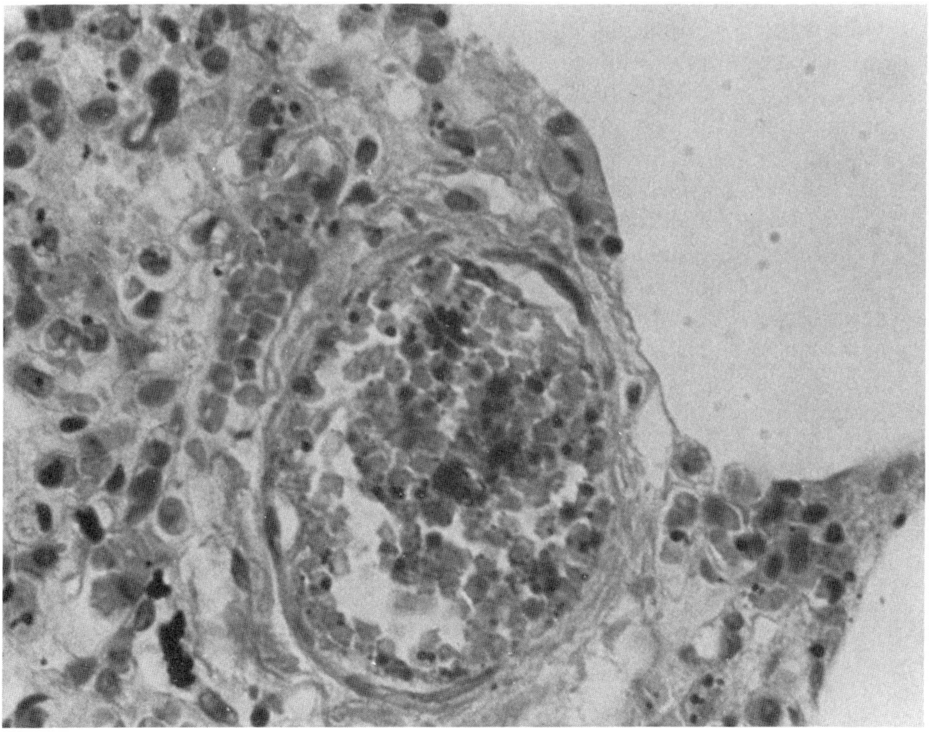

Figure 11 Lung section shows parasitized red blood cells and macrophages with pigment of *Plasmodium falciparum*.

bronchopneumonia are frequent concomitant findings and indicate the general immunosuppression that is a feature of falciparum malaria. Pathological changes in the lung attributable purely to malaria remain a matter of debate.

D. Leishmaniasis and the Lung (Pulmonary Kala Azar)

Coughing as a symptom of visceral leishmaniasis has been well documented (Rees et al., 1983; Marsden and Jones, 1985). It appears early in the disease, persisting throughout the course of the disease and disappears with cure. However, there is scanty information about histopathological lung involvement. Interstitial pneumonitis has been demonstrated in humans with visceral leishmaniasis (Duarte et al., 1989) and also in hamster models of the disease (Duarte and Corbett, 1984). Cells of the reticuloendothelial system present in the lung can become infected with the flagellate *Leishmania donovani.* Following the bite of an infected sandfly, *Phlebotomus* (*Lutzomia*), the infective amastigotes are taken up by mononuclear phagocytes where they multiply happily in their protected site (Russell and Talamas-Rohana, 1989) within macrophages which include lung alveolar cells. Cell-mediated immune responses are thought to be responsible for keeping the infection at bay (Liew, 1989). A nonspecific depression of T lymphocytes may occur during infection which returns to normal after treatment and recovery. The striking feature of the pneumonitis found in visceral leishmaniasis is the marked absence of leishmania amastigotes in lung tissue of humans (Duarte et al., 1989). In addition, interstitial pulmonary involvement by the parasite is thought to facilitate bacterial growth leading to bronchopneumonia.

It is becoming apparent that visceral leishmaniasis is a frequently missed parasitic infection in AIDS patients. Several reports of visceral and cutaneous leishmaniasis occurring as opportunist infections in AIDS patients have been published recently (Zumla, 1989). These have described several difficulties that can arise in diagnosis and management of this condition. Most of the cases were diagnosed incidentally on bone marrow smears or liver biopsy during investigation of pyrexia of unknown origin. Leishmania serology was often negative, response to therapy poor and the mortality high. The high HIV seropositivity rates found in the Tropics (Fleming, 1989) should alert physicians to actively seek for cases of leishmaniasis, many of which could present atypically and be easily overlooked.

E. Pulmonary Chagas

Antibody-dependent cell-mediated cytotoxicity directed towards intracellular *Trypanosoma cruzi* leads to deleterious effects on host tissue. Destruction of the autonomic nerves and smooth muscle leads to the "Mega" organ syn-

Table 12 Zoonoses Affecting the Lung

Zoonosis	Organism	Transmission	Pulmonary features	Serodiagnosis	Diagnosis	Treatment
Q fever	*Coxiella burnetti*	Milk ingestion Tick bite	Atypical pneumonia	CFT, IFAT, ELISA	Sputum, urine, blood culture	Tetracycline
Scrub typhus	*Rickettsia tsutsugamushi*	Mite bite	Atypical pneumonia	CFT, Weil Felix	Sputum, urine, blood culture	Tetracycline Chloramphenicol
Psittacosis	*Chlamydia psittacii*	Bird droppings	Atypical pneumonia	CFT, IFAT, ELISA	Sputum culture	Chlortetracycline Rifampicin
Leptospirosis	*Leptospira* sp.	Rat, pig, and dog urine	Pneumonia Lung abscess	CFT, IFAT, ELISA	Blood, urine, sputum culture	Penicillin
Brucellosis	*Brucella abortus* *mellitensis* *suis*	Milk and meat products	Pneumonia, effusions, pleurisy	CFT, RIA, ELISA Agglutination tests	Blood, marrow, tissue culture	Tetracycline Streptomycin Rifampicin
Plague	*Yersinia pestis*	Flea bite or infective aerosol	Pneumonia	CFT, RIA, ELISA	Sputum smear, blood and sputum culture	Streptomycin Tetracycline Chloramphenicol
Anthrax	*Bacillus anthracis*	Spore inhalation	Hemorrhagic mediastinitis and pneumonia	IFAT	Sputum smear Sputum culture	Penicillin
Melioidosis	*Pseudomonas pseudomalliei*	Soil contamination of skin abrasions	Pneumonia Abscesses	Agglutination CFT	Urine, blood, sputum culture	Tetracycline Chloramphenicol
Tularemia	*Francisella tularensis*	Arthropod bite Waterborne	Pneumonia Abscess	Agglutination	Sputum culture	Streptomycin
DF-2	*Dysgonic fermenter* type-2	Animal bite	Pneumonia	None	Blood culture	Penicillin

IFAT, indirect fluorescent antibody test; RIA, radioimmunoassay; CFT, complement fixation test; ELISA, enzyme-linked immunosorbant assay.

dromes. Rarely, the lung may become involved and bronchiectasis has been documented as a complication of Chagas' disease.

XI. Zoonoses Affecting the Lung

Table 12 lists the characteristics of zoonoses that can affect the lung in the tropics. Of interest is the emerging zoonosis caused by the fastidious gram-negative pleomorphic bacillus, dysgonic fermenter-type 2 (DF-2) (reviewed by Zumla et al., 1988). Most of the 52 reported cases are from Europe or the United States but the first case report from Australia (Waters et al., 1986) indicates that the organism is probably worldwide in distribution. Infection with DF-2 is acquired through contact with domestic animals and presents as a severe community-acquired septicemia. The lung is involved in the pathogenesis in two ways. Ten of the 52 cases (19%) had pneumonia on admission. Persons with chronic respiratory diseases, the immunosuppressed, those without a spleen, and alcoholics appear most susceptible although the healthy are also prone to infection. Of 52 cases reported so far worldwide (Zumla et al., 1988), 8 had chronic respiratory disease as a predisposing factor (4 had chronic obstructive airways disease, 2 fibronodular lung disease, 1 pulmonary tuberculosis, and 1 pulmonary fibrosis). Predisposition to infection by DF-2, an organism of low virulence, of patients with respiratory disease suggests an important role of the lung as an immunological filter. The organism is difficult to grow; despite the paucity of cases, the infection may be more common. Very little is known about its immunology. With the present AIDS epidemic, infection with this "new" organism should be actively sought.

References

Adams, F. B., and Macleod, I. N. (1977). Invasive amoebiasis. *Medicine* **56**: 315-323.

Baron, R. W., and Tanner, C. E. (1976). The effect of immunosuppression on secondary *Echinococcus multilocularis* infection in mice. *Int. J. Parasitol.* **6**:31-33.

Bayley, A. C. (19088). Atypical aggressive Kaposi's sarcoma in Africa. In: *Kaposi's Sarcoma: A Text and Atlas.* Edited by Gottlieb, G. J., and Ackerman, A. B. Philadelphia, Lea & Febiger.

Beisel, W. R. (1982). Single nutrients and Immunity. *Am. J. Clin. Nutr.* **35**: 417-468.

Bell, D. Y., Haseman, J. A., Spock, A., Mclennan, G., and Hook, G. E. R. (1981). Plasma proteins of the bronchalveolar surface of lungs of smokers and non-smokers. *Am. Rev. Respir. Dis.* **124**:72-79.

Benson, B. J., Dobbs, L. G., and Ansfield, M. J. (1983). Immunopharmacology of lung surfactant. In: *Immunopharmacology of the Lung: Lung Biology in Health and Disease* series. Edited by H. H. Newball. New York, Marcel Dekker Inc.

Berkelman, R. L., Heyward, W. L., Stehr-Green, J. K., and Curran, J. W. (1989). Epidemiology of the human immunodeficiency virus infection and acquired immunodeficiency syndrome. *Am. J. Med.* **86**:761-770.

Bhoopchand, A., Cooper, D. K. C., Novitzky, D., Rose, A. G., and Reichart, B. (1986). Regression of Kaposi's sarcoma after reduction of immunosuppressive therapy in a heart transplant patient. *J. Heart Transplant.* **5**:461-564.

Biggar, R. J. (1986). The clinical features of HIV infection in Africa. *Lancet* **2**:1453-1454.

Bird, P. (1988). Structure and function of antibody molecules. In: *B Lymphocytes in Human Disease.* Edited by G. Bird and J. Calvert. Oxford, Oxford Medical Publishers.

Blaser, M. J., and Cohn, D. L. (1986). Opportunistic infections in patients with AIDS; clues to the epidemiology of AIDS and the relative virulence of pathogens. *Rev. Infect. Dis.* **8**:21-30.

Boros, D. L. (1989). Immunopathology of *Schistosoma mansoni* infection. *Clin. Microbiol. Rev.* **2**:3:250-269.

Bowen, D. L., Lane, H. C., and Fauci, A. S. (1985). Immunopathogenesis of the acquired immunodeficiency syndrome. *Ann. Intern. Med.* **103**: 704-709.

Brady, E. M., Margolis, M. L., and Korzeniowski, O. M. (1984). Pulmonary cryptosporidiosis in the acquired immunodeficiency syndrome. *J.A.M.A.* **252**:89-90.

Brain, J. D., Proctor, D. F., and Lynne, M. R. (1977). Respiratory defense mechanisms. In *Lung Biology in Health and Disease*, Vols. 1 and 2. Edited by J. B. Brain, D. F. Proctor, and L. M. Reid. New York, Marcel Dekker Inc.

Brandt, H., and Tamayo, R. P. (1970). Pathology of human amebiasis. *Hum. Pathol.* **1**:351-385.

Butterworth, A. E., Sturrock, R. F., Houba, V., et al. (1974). Antibody-dependent cell-mediated damage to schistosomula in vitro. *Nature* **252**: 503-505.

Butterworth, A. E., Sturrock, R. F., Houba, V. F., Mahmoud, A. F., Sher, A., and Rees, P. H. (1975). Eosinophils as mediators of antibody dependent damage to schistosomula. *Nature* (Lond.) **256**:727-729.

Capron, A., Bazin, H., Dessaint, J. P., and Capron, M. (1975). Specific IgE antibodies in immune adherence of mouse macrophages to schistosoma mansoni schistosomules. *Nature* **253**:474-475.

Carvalho, E. M., Andrade, T. M., Andrade, J. A., and Rocha, H. (1983). Immunologic features in different forms of strongyloidiasis. *Trans. R. Soc. Trop. Med. Hyg.* **77**:3:346-349.

Chandra, R. K. (1972). Immunocompetence in undernutrition. *J. Paediatr.* **81**:1184-1190.

Chandra, R. K. (1975). Reduced serum and secretory antibody responses to live attenuated measles and polio virus vaccines in malnourished children. *Br. Med. J.* **2**:583-585.

Chandra, R. K. (1982). Trace element regulation of immunity and infection. *Nutr. Res.* **2**:721-733.

Chandra, R. K. (1983). Nutrition, Immunity, and infection: present knowledge and future directions. *Lancet* **1**:688-692.

Chandra, R. K. (ed.) (1988). *Contemporary Issues in Clinical Nutrition* II. *Nutrition and Immunology.* New York, Alan Liss.

Chandra, R. K., Au, B., Woodford, G., and Hyam, P. (1977). Iron status, immunocompetence and susceptibility to infection. *Ciba Found. Symp.* **51**:249-268.

Chen, M. G., and Mott, K. E. (1988a). Progress in assessment of morbidity due to *Schistosoma japonicum* infection. *Trop. Dis. Bull.* **85**:6:R2-45.

Chen, M. G., and Mott, K. E. (1988b). Progress in assessment of morbidity due to *Schistosoma mansoni* infection. *Trop. Dis. Bull.* **85**:10:R2-56.

Clavell, F., Mansinho, K., Chamaret, S., et al. (1987). Human immunodeficiency virus type-2 infection associated with AIDS in West Africa. *N. Engl. J. Med.* **316**:1180-1185.

Clumeck, N., Sonnet, J., Taelman, H., Mascart-Lemone, F., et al. (1984). Acquired Immunodeficiency syndrome in African patients. *N. Engl. J. Med.* **310**:492-497.

Cook, G. C. (1987a). Opportunistic parasitic infections associated with the acquired immunodeficiency syndrome (AIDS): parasitology, clinical presentation, diagnosis and management. *Q. J. Med.* **65**:(248):967-983.

Cook, G. C. (1987b). *Strongyloides stercoralis* hyperinfection syndrome: how often is it missed? *Q. J. Med.* **64**:625-629.

Corman, L. C. (1985). The relationship between nutrition, infection and immunity. *Med. Clin. North Am.* **69**:3:519-527.

Crabtree, J. E., and Coulson, P. S. (1986). The rôle of pulmonary cellular reaction in the resistance of vaccinated mice to *Schistosoma mansoni. Parasite. Immunol.* **8**:265-286.

Crapo, J. D., Barry, B. E., Gehr, P., Bachofen, M., and Weibel, E. R. (1982). Cell number and cell characteristics of the normal human lung. *Am. Rev. Respir. Dis.* **126**:332-337.

Crumpton, M. J. (1987). HLA in medicine. *Br. Med. Bull.* **43**:1.

Daensuang, S. A. (1980). A monograph of the genus Gnathostoma and gnathostomiasis in Thailand. Tokyo, SEAMIC/IMFJ.16.

David, J. R., Vadas, M. A., and Butterworth, A. E., et al. (1980). Enhanced helminthotoxic capacity of eosinophils from patients with eosinophilia. *N. Engl. J. Med.* **303**:1147-1152.

Davidson, B. L., El-Kassimi, F., Uz-Zaman, A., and Pillai, D. K. (1986). The lung shift in treated schistosomiasis—bronchoalveolar lavage evidence of eosinophilic pneumonia. *Chest* **89**:455-457.

Davidson, R. A. (1985). Immunology of parasitic infections. *Med. Clin. North Am.* **69**:751-758.

Davis, A. (1986). Recent advances in schistosomiasis. *Q. J. Med.* **58**(226): 95-110.

Davis, W. B., Gadek, J. E., Fells, G. A., and Crystal, R. G. (1981). Role of eosinophils in connective tissue destruction. *Am. Rev. Respir. Dis.* **123**: (4: Part 2):55 (abstract).

DeClercq, D., Henry, M. C., and Lokombe, B. (1986). Serological observations on toxoplasmosis in Zairian AIDS patients. *Trans. Roy. Soc. Trop. Med. Hyg.* **80**:613-614.

Dew, H. R. (1928). *Hydatid Disease: Its Pathology, Diagnosis and Treatment.* Sydney, Australia, Australian Medical Publishing Co.

Dharmkrong, A. T., Migasena, S., Suntharasamai, P., et al. (1986). Enzyme-linked immunosorbant assay for detection of antibody to gnathostoma antigen in patients with intermittent cutaneous migratory swelling. *J. Clin. Microbiol.* **23**:847-851.

Donabedian, H., and Gallin, J. I. (1983). Neutrophil dysfunction and lung disease. In *Immunopharmacology of the Lung.* Edited by H. H. Newball. New York, Marcel Dekker Inc.

Dowd, P. S., Kelleher, J., Walker, B. E., and Guillou, P. J. (1986). Nutrition and cellular immunity in hospital patients. *Br. J. Nutr.* **55**:515-527.

Downing, R. G., Elgin, R. P., and Bayley, A. C. (1984). African Kaposi's sarcoma and AIDS. *Lancet* **1**:478-480.

Duarte, M. I. S. and Corbett, C. E. P. (1984). Histopathological and ultrastructural aspects of interstitial pneumonitis of experimental visceral leishmaniasis. *Trans. Roy. Soc. Trop. Med. Hyg.* **78**:683-688.

Duarte, M. I. S., Matta, V. L. R., Corbett, C. E. P., Laurenti, M. D., Chebabo, R., and Goto, H. (1989). Interstitial pneumonitis in human visceral leishmaniasis. *Trans. Roy. Soc. Trop. Med. Hyg.* **83**:73-76.

Duesberg, P. (1988). The cause of AIDS (letter). *Science* **242**:997-998.

Eales, L-J., Moshtael, O., and Pinching, A. J. (1987). Microbicidal activity of monocyte derived macrophages in AIDS and related disorders. *Clin. Exp. Immunol.* **67**:227-235.

Ehrhard, T., and Kernbaum, S. (1979). Toxocara canis et toxocarose humaine. *Bull. Inst. Pasteur.* **77**:225-235.

Elvin, K. M., Lumbwe, C. M., Luo, N. P., Bjorkman, A., Kallenius, G., and Linder, E. (1989). *Pneumocystis carinii* is not a major cause of pneumonia in HIV infected patients in Lusaka, Zambia. *Trans. Roy. Soc. Trop. Med. Hyg.* **83**:4:553-559.

Fantone, J. C., and Ward, P. A. (1983). Chemotactic mechanisms in the lung. In *Immunopharmacology of the Lung*. Edited by H. H. Newman. New York, Lenfant. Marcel Dekker, pp. 243-272.

Fleming, A. F. (1988). AIDS in Africa—an update. *AIDS* **3**:116-138.

Gallin, J. I. (1976). The role of chemotaxis in the inflammatory immune response of the lung. In *Immunologic and Infectious Reactions in the Lung*. Edited by C. H. Kirkpatrick and H. Y. Reynolds. New York, Marcel Dekker Inc.

Genta, R. M. (1984). Immunobiology of strongyloidiasis. *Trop. Geogr. Med.* **36**:223-229.

Gold, J. W. M. (1987). Infectious complications of the acquired immune deficiency syndrome. In *Advanced Medicine*. Edited by R. E. Pounder and P. L. Chiodini. London, Balliere Tindall, pp. 91-101.

Good, R. A., and Lorenz, E. (1988). Nutrition, immunity, aging and cancer. *Nutr. Rev.* **46**:2:62-67.

Gottlieb, M. S. (1984). Pulmonary disease in the acquired immunodeficiency syndrome. *Chest* **112**:357-382.

Granger, D. L., and Hobbs, M. M. (1988). Do natural killer cells help protect us from disease caused by fungi? *Am. Rev. Respir. Dis.* **138**:510-511.

Grieco, M. H., and Chinoy-Acharya, P. (1985). Lymphocytic interstitial pneumonia associated with the acquired immunodeficiency syndrome. *Am. Rev. Respir. Dis.* **131**:952-955.

Griffin, L., and Lucas, S. B. (1982). Does *Pneumocystis carinii* exist in Kenya? *Trans. R. Soc. Trop. Med. Hyg.* **76**:198-199.

Griffin, L. and Williams, K. A. (1983). Serological and parasitological survey of blood donors in Kenya for toxoplasmosis. *Trans. Roy. Soc. Trop. Med. Hyg.* **80**:613-614.

Grove, D. I. (1980). Strongyloidiasis in ex-prisoners of war in Southeast Asia. *Br. Med. J.* [Clin. Res.] **28**:598-601.

Grove, D. I. (1982). Treatment of strongyloidiasis with thiabendazole. an analysis of toxicity and effectiveness. *Trans. R. Soc. Med. Hyg.* **76**: 114-118.

Guimaraes, A. C. (1982). Situaco atual dos conheci mentos sobre o envoluimento cardiopulmonar na esquistossomose mansonica. *Arq. Bras. Cardiol.* **38**:301-319.

Hawkins, C. H., Gold, J. W. M., Whimbey, E., et al. (1986). *Mycobacterium avium* complex infections in patients with the acquired immunodeficiency syndrome. *Ann. Intern. Med.* **105**:184-188.

Hershko, C., Peto, T. E. A., and Weatherall, D. J. (1988). Iron and Infection. *Br. Med. J.* **296**:660-664.

Higenbottam, T. W., and Heard, B. E. (1976). Opportunistic pulmonary strongyloidiasis complicating asthma treated with steroids. *Thorax* **31**(2): 226-233.

Hiserodt, J. C., Britvan, L. J., and Targan, S. R. (1982). Characterisation of the cytolytic mechanism of human natural killer cells (NK) lymphocyte: resolution into binding, programming and killer cell-independent steps. *J. Immunol.* **129**:1782-1787.

Holtz, H. A., Lavery, D. P., and Kapila, R. (1985). Actinomycetales infection in the acquired immunodeficiency syndrome. *Ann. Intern. Med.* **102**:203-205.

Hunninghake, G. W., Gadek, J. E., Kawanami, O., Ferrans, V. J., and Crystal, R. G. (1979). Inflammatory and immune processes in the human lung in health and disease: evaluation by bronchoalveolar lavage. *Am. J. Pathol.* **97**:149-206.

Ingra-Siegman, Y., Kapila, R., Sen, P., Kaminiski, Z. C., and Louria, D. B. (1981). Syndrome of hyperinfection with *Strongyloides stercoralis. Rev. Infect. Dis.* **3**:397-407.

James, S. L. and Colley, D. G. (1976). Eosinophil mediated destruction of *Schistosoma mansoni* eggs. *J. Reticuloendothel. Soc.* **20**(5):359-374.

Janssens, P. G. (1985). Chemotherapy of gastrointestinal nematodiasis in man. In *Chemotherapy of Gastrointestinal Helminths.* Edited by H. Vanden Bossche, D. Thienpont, and P. G. Janssens. Berlin, Springer-Verlag, pp. 183-368.

Johnson, R. J., and Johnson, J. R. (1983). Paragonimiasis in Indochinese refugees. *Am. Rev. Respir. Dis.* **128**:534-538.

Kassis, A. I., and Tanner, C. E. (1976). The role of complement in hydatid disease: *in vitro* studies. *Int. J. Parasitol.* **6**:25-29.

Katlama, C., Leport, C., Brun-Vezinet, F., Rouziouz, C., et al. (1984). Acquired immunodeficiency syndrome (AIDS) in Africans. *Ann. Soc. Belge. Med. Trop.* **64**:379-389.

Keusch, G. T., Wilson, C. S., and Waksal, S. D. (1983). Nutrition, host defenses and the lymphoid system. In *Advances in Host Defense Mechanisms*, vol. 2. Edited by J. I. Gallin and A. S. Fauci. New York, Raven Press. pp. 275-359.

Koenig, S., and Fauci, A. S. (1988). AIDS: immunopathogenesis and immune response to the human immunodeficiency virus. In *AIDS: Etiology, Diagnosis, Treatment and Prevention*, 2nd ed. Edited by V. T. DeVita, Jr., S. Hellman, and S. A. Rosenberg. Philadelphia, J.B. Lippincott.

Koino, R. (1922). *Jpn. Med. World* **2**:317 (quoted in: Medicine in the Tropics. Edited by A. W. Woodruff. Churchill-Livingstone, 1984).

Krigel, R. L., and Friedman-Kien, A. E. (1988). Kaposi's sarcoma in AIDS. In *AIDS: Etiology, Diagnosis, Treatment and Prevention*, 2nd ed. Edited by V. T. DeVita, Jr., S. Hellman, and S. A. Rosenberg. Philadelphia, J.B. Lippincott.

Lane, H. C., Masur, H., Edgar, L. C., Whallen, G., Rook, A., and Fauci, A. (1984). Abnormalities of B cell activation and immunoregulation in patients with the acquired immunodeficiency syndrome. *N. Engl. J. Med.* **309**:453-458.

Leyton, E. (1946). Effects of slow starvation. *Lancet* **2**:73-79.

Liew, F. Y. (1989). Functional heterogeneity of CD4+ cells in leishmaniasis. *Immunol. Today* **10**:40-45.

Loeffler, W. (1932). Zur differential diagnose der lungennin-filtrierungen: 11. Ueber fluchtige succendan-infiltrate (mit eosinophile). *Beitr. J. Klin. Tuberk.* **79**:368-371.

Longworth, D. L., and Weller, P. F. (1986). Hyperinfection syndrome with strongyloidiasis. In *Current Clinical Topics in Infectious Diseases.* Edited by J. S. Remington and M. N. Swartz, New York, McGraw-Hill, pp. 27-50.

Lotzova, E., and Heberman, R. B. (eds.) (1986). *Immunobiology of Natural Killer Cells*, vols. I and II. Boca Raton, FL, CRC Press.

Louie, E., Rice, L. B., and Holzman, R. S. (1986). Tuberculosis in non-Haitian patients with the acquired immunodeficiency syndrome. *Chest* **90**:542-545.

Lucas, S. (1988). AIDS in Africa—clinicopathological aspects. *Trans. R. Soc. Med.* **82**:801-802.

Lucas, S., and Wamukota, W. (1987). HIV and the local African population. In *Advanced Medicine.* Edited by R. E. Pounder and P. L. Chiodini. London, Balliere-Tindall, pp. 102-111.

Lucas, S., Sewankumbo, N., Nambuya, A., Nsubuga, P., Goodgame, R., Mugerwa, J., and Carswell, J. W. (1987). The morbid anatomy of African AIDS. In *AIDS and Associated Cancers in Africa.* International Symposium, Naples. Basel, Karger, 1988, pp. 124-133.

Maayan, S., Wormser, G. P., Widerhorn, J., Sy, E. R., Kin, Y. E. H.,, and Ernst, J. A. (1987). *Strongyloides stercoralis* hyperinfection in a patient with the Acquired Immune deficiency syndrome. *Am. J. Med.* **83**:945-948.

Macher, A. M., De Vinatea, M. L., Angritt, P., Tuur, S. M., and Reichart, C. M. (1988). Pathologic features of patients infected with the human immunodeficiency virus. In *AIDS: Etiology, Diagnosis, Treatment and Prevention*, 2nd ed. Edited by V. T. DeVita, Jr., S. Hellman, and S. A. Rosenberg. Philadelphia, J.B. Lippincott.

Manson-Bahr, P. E. C., and Bell, D. R. (1987a). Trematode infections: Schistosomiasis. In *Manson's Tropical Diseases*, 19th ed. London, Balliere-Tindall.

Manson-Bahr, P. E. C., and Bell, D. R. (1987b). Soil transmitted helminths: strongyloidiasis. In *Manson's Tropical Diseases*, 19th ed. London, Balliere-Tindall.

Mann, P., Snider, D. E., Francis, H., et al. (1986). Association between HTLV-III/LAV infection and tuberculosis in Zaire. *J.A.M.A.* **256**:346 (letter).

Marsden, P. D. and Jones, T. C. (1985). Clinical manifestations, diagnosis and treatment of leishmaniasis. In *Leishmaniasis.* Edited by K. P. Chang and R. S. Bray. Amsterdam, Elsevier Science Publishers.

Marx, J. I. (1988). What T cells see and how they see it. *Science 242*:863-865.

Mata, L. J. (1975). Malnutrition-infection interactions in the tropics. *Am. J. Trop. Med. Hyg.* **24**(4):564-574.

McDevitt, H. O. (1980). Regulation of the immune response by the major histocompatibility system. *N. Engl. J. Med.* **303**:514-517.

Mcleod, D. T., Neill, P., Robertson, V. J., Latif, A. S., Emmanuel, J. C., Els, J. E., Gwanzura, L. K. Z., Trijssenaar, F. E. J., Nziramasanga, P., Nkanza, N., and Lucas, S. B. (1989). Pulmonary diseases in patients infected with the human immunodeficiency virus in Zimbabwe, Central Africa. *Trans. Roy. Soc. Trop. Med. Hyg.* **83**:694-697.

Mok, C. H. (1968). Visceral larva migrans—a discussion and a review of literature. *Clin. Paediatr.* **7**:565-580.

Morley, D. C., Martin, W. J., and Allen, I. (1966). Measles in West Africa. *W. Afr. Med. J.* **16**:24.

Morley, D. C., Martin, W. J., and Allen, I. (1967). Measles in East and Central Africa. *E. Afr. Med. J.* **44**:12.

Muller, R. W. (1938). Zur pathogenese der fluchtigen eosinophilia lungenin filtrate. *Dtsch. Med. Wochenschr.* **64**:1286-1288.

Murray, J. F., Felton, C. P., Goray, S. M., Gottleib, M. S., Hopewell, P. C., Stover, D. E., and Teirstein, A. S. (1984). Pulmonary complications of the acquired immunodeficiency syndrome: a report of a National Heart, Lung and Blood Institute workshop. *N. Engl. J. Med.* **310**:1682-1685.

Murray, J. F., Garray, S. M., Hopewell, P. C., Mills, J., et al. (1987). Pulmonary complications of the acquired immunodeficiency syndrome. An update. *Am. Rev. Respir. Dis.* **135**:504-509.

Nambuya, A., Sewankambo, N., Mugerwa, J., Goodgame, R., and Lucas, S. (1988). Tuberculous lymphadenitis associated with human immunodeficiency virus infection in Uganda. *J. Clin. Pathol.* **41**:93-96.

Neva, F. A., and Burke, J. (1981). Comparison of larval antigens in an enzyme-linked immunosorbant assay for strongyloidiasis in humans. *J. Infect. Dis.* **144**:427-432.

Novick, R. J., Tchervenkov, C. I., Wilson, J. A., Munro, D. D., and Mulder, D. S. (1987). Surgery for thoracic hydatid disease: a North American experience. *Ann. Thorac. Surg.* **43**:681-686.

Ottesen, E. A. (1976). Eosinophilia and the lung. In *Immunologic and Infectious Reactions in the Lung.* Edited by C. H. Kirkpatrick and H. Y. Reynolds. New York, Marcel Dekker Inc.

Owor, R. (1988). Conventional Kaposi's sarcoma. In *Kaposi's Sarcoma: A Test and Atlas.* Edited by G. Gottlieb and A. B. Ackerman. Philadelphia, Lea & Febiger.

Pelletier, L. L. (1984). Chronic strongyloidiasis in World War II Far East ex-prisoners of war. *Am. J. Trop. Med. Hyg.* **33**:55-61.

Phillips, I., and Wharton, B. A. (1968). Acute bacterial infection in kwashiorkor and marasmus. *Br. Med. J.* **1**:407.

Pinon, J. M., Sulahian, A., Remy, G., and Dropsy, G. (1979). Immunological study of hydatidosis. *Am. J. Trop. Med. Hyg.* **28**:318-324.

Piot, P., Quinn, T. C., Taelman, H., Feinsod, F. M., et al. (1984). Acquired immunodeficiency syndrome in a heterosexual population in Zaire. *Lancet* **2**:65-69.

Pitchenik, A., Cole, C., Russell, B., Fische, M. A., Spira, T. J., and Snider, D. E. (1984). Tuberculosis, atypical mycobacteriosis, and the acquired immunodeficiency syndrome among Haitian and non-haitian patients in south Florida. *Ann. Intern. Med.* **101**:641-645.

Plata, F., Autran, B., Martins, L. P., Wain-Hobson, S., et al., (1988). AIDS virus specific T lymphocytes in lung disorders. *Nature* **328**:348-351.

Polmar, S. H. (1976). Immunodeficiency and pulmonary disease. In *Immunologic and Infectious Reactions in the Lung.* Edited by C. H. Kirkpatrick and H. Y. Reynolds. New York, Marcel Dekker Inc.

Polsky, B., Gold, J. W. M., Whimbey, E., et al. (1986). Bacterial pneumonia in patients with the acquired immunodeficiency syndrome. *Ann. Intern. Med.* **404**:38-41.

Proctor, R. A. (ed.) (1987). Fibronectin and the pathogenesis of infections. *Rev. Infect. Dis.* **9**(Suppl. 4):S317-S430.

Rankin, J. A., Collman, R., and Daniele, R. P. (1988). Acquired immune deficiency syndrome and the lung. *Chest* 94(1):155-164.

Ravdin, J. L. (1989). *Entamoeba histolytica*: from adherence to enteropathy. *J. Infect. Dis.* **159**:3:420-429.

Real, F. X., Gold, J. W. M., Krown, S. E., and Armstrong, D. (1984). *Listeria monocytogenes* bacteraemia in the acquired immunodeficiency syndrome (letter). *Ann. Intern. Med.* **102**:203-205.

Rees, P. H., Krager, P. A., and Bwibo, N. O. (1983). Clinical aspects and treatment of visceral leishmaniasis in Kenya: a retrospective study of 71 patients. In: *Clinical Aspects of Kala Azar in Kenya.* Edited by Krager, P. A., and Rees, P. H. Dordrecht, Netherlands, I.C.G. Printing.

Reichart, C. M., O'Leary, T. J., Levens, D. L., Simrell, C. R., and Macher, A. M. (1983). Autopsy pathology in the acquired immunodeficiency syndrome. *Am. J. Pathol.* **112**:357-382.

Reynolds, H. Y. (1986). Lung immunology and its contribution to the immunopathogenesis of certain respiratory diseases. *J. Allergy. Clin. Immunol.* **78**:5:833-847.

Reynolds, H. Y. (1987). Lung inflammation: normal host defense or a complication of some diseases? *Annu. Rev. Med.* **38**:295-323.
Reynolds, H. Y. (1988). Subject review: immunoglobulin G and its function in the human respiratory Tract. *Mayo. Clin. Proc.* **63**:161-174.
Reynolds, H. Y., and Newball, H. H. (1976). Fluid and cellular millieu of the human respiratory tract. In *Immunologic and Infectious Reactions in the Lung*. Edited by C. H. Kirkpatrick and H. Y. Reynolds. New York, Marcel Dekker, Inc.
Reynolds, H. Y., Fulmer, J. D., Kazmeirowski, J. A., Roberts, W. C., Frank, M. M., and Crystal, R. G. (1977). Analysis of cellular and protein content of broncho-alveolar lavage fluid from patients with idiopathic pulmonary fibrosis and chronic hypersensitivity pneumonitis.
Rook, G. A. W. (1988). The role of vitamin D in tuberculosis. *Am. Rev. Respir. Dis.* **138**:768-770.
Royer, H. D., and Reinherz, E. L. (1987). T Lymphocytes: ontogeny, function and relevance to clinical disorders. *N. Engl. J. Med.* **317**(8):1136-1142.
Russell, D. G., and Talamas-Rohana, P. (1989). Leishmania and the macrophage: a marriage of inconvenience. *Immunol. Today* **10**(10):328-332.
Sahn, S. A. (1988). State of the art: the pleura. *Am. Rev. Respir. Dis.* **138**: 184-234.
Santoro, F. (1982). Interaction of complement with parasite surfaces. (1982). *Clin. Immunol. Allergy* **2**:639-654.
Shaw, A. F. B., and Ghareeb, A. A. (1938). The pathogenesis of pulmonary schistosomiasis in Egypt with special reference to Ayersa's disease. *J. Pathol. Bacteriol.* **46**:401-424.
Smithers, S. R., and Doenhoff, M. J. (1982). Schistosomiasis. In *Immunology of Parasitic Infections.* Edited by S. Cohen and K. S. Warren. London, Blackwell Scientific.
Smythe, P. M., Schonland, D. M., Brereton-Stiles, G. C., et al. (1971). thymolymphatic deficiency and depression of cell-mediated immunity in protein-calorie malnutrition. *Lancet* **2**:939-944.
Spry, C. J. F. (1988). Parasitic diseases. In *Eosiniphils—A Comprehensive Review and Guide to the Scientific and Medical Literature.* Oxford/ New York, Oxford University Press.
Sepulveda, B., and Martinez-Palamo, A. (1982). Immunology of amoebiasis by *Entamoeba histolytica.* In *Immunology of Parasitic Infections*, 2nd ed. Edited by S. Cohen and K. S. Warren. Oxford, Blackwell Scientific.
Taylor, A. E. R., and Denham, D. A. (1988). Intestinal nematode infections of man. *Trop. Dis. Bull.* **35**(4):R21.
Van de Perre, P., Rouvroy, D., Lepage, P., et al. (1984). Acquired Immunodeficiency Syndrome in Rwanda. *Lancet* **2**(8394):62-65.
Van der Sar, A., and Hartz, P. (1945). The syndrome tropical eosinophilia and microfilaria. *Am. J. Trop. Med.* **25**:83-87.

Vieyra-Herrera, G., Becerril-Carmana, G., and Padua-Gabriel, A. (1988). *Strongyloides stercoralis* hyperinfection in a patient with the acquired immune deficiency syndrome. *Acta. Cytol.* **10**:277-279.

von Lichtenberg, F., Correa-Olivecira, R., and Sher, A. (1985). The fate of challenge schistosomula in murine anti-schistosome vaccine model. *Am. J. Trop. Med. Hyg.* **34**:96-106.

Wanner, A., and Ahmed, T. (1983). Immunopharmacology of the mucociliary system. In *Immunopharmacology of the Lung*. Edited by H. H. Newball. New York, Marcel Dekker, Inc.

Warren, K. S. (1972). Immunopathogenesis of schistosomiasis: a multidisciplinary approach. *Trans. R. Soc. Trop. Med. Hyg.* **66**:417-434.

Warren, K. S., Domingo, E. O., and Cowan, R. B. T. (1967). Granuloma formation around schistosome eggs as a manifestation of delayed hypersensitivity. *Am. J. Pathol.* **51**:735-756.

Waters, M. J., Stern, L., and Andrew, J. H. (1986). Dysgonic fermenter-2 septicaemia. *Pathology* **18**(1):162-164.

Weingarten, R. G. (1943). Tropical eosinophilia. *Lancet* **1**:103.

Werczberger, A., et al. (1979). Disseminated echinococcosis with repeated anaphylactic shock treated with mebendazole. *Chest* **76**:482.

WHO (1985). Tropical diseases research (TDR). Seventh Programme Report. Schistosomiasis. 3/1. Geneva, World Health Organization.

Williamson, W. A., and Greenwood, B. M. (1978). Impairment of the immune response to vaccination after acute malaria. *Lancet* **1**:1328-1329.

Woodruff, A. W. (1968). Helminths as vehicles and synergists of microbial infections. *Trans. R. Soc. Trop. Med.* **62**(3):446-452.

Wong, B. (1984). Parasitic diseases in immunocompromised hosts. *Am. J. Med.* **76**:479-486.

Wyler, D. J. (1987). Fibronectin in parasitic diseases. *Rev. Infect. Dis.* **9** (suppl. 4):S391-399.

Wyler, D. J., and Postlethwaite, W. E. (1983). Fibroblast stimulation in schistosomiasis. IV. Isolated egg granulomas elaborate a fibroblast chemoattractant in vitro. *J. Immunol.* **130**:1371-1375.

Xanthakis, D., Efthimiadis, M., Papadakis, G., et al. (1972). Hydatid disease of the chest. Report of 91 surgically treated cases. *Thorax* **27**:517-534.

Yokogawa, M. (1965). Paragonimus and paragonimiasis. *Adv. Parasitol.* **3**:99-158.

Zumla, A., Lipscomb, G., Corbett, M., and McCarthy, M. (1988). Dysgonic fermenter type-2: an emerging zoonosis. Report of 2 cases and review. *Q. J. Med.* **68**(257):741-752.

Zumla, A. (1989). Emergence of Leishmaniasis in the wake of AIDS (letter). *South Afr. Med. J.* **76**(6):285.

Zumla, A., and Luo, N. P. (1990). Salmonella and surgery (letter). *Br. Med. J.* **300**:1342.

2

Granulomatous Lung Diseases in the Tropics

OM P. SHARMA and GURDIP S. FLORA

Los Angeles County-University of Southern California Medical Center
Los Angeles, California

A granuloma is a focal chronic inflammatory reaction characterized by the presence of mononuclear cells, macrophages, epithelioid, and giant cells along with a number of lymphocytes, plasma cells, and fibroblasts (Williams and Jones-Williams, 1983). Granulomatous reactions may be classified functionally into two major categories (Myrvik, 1982). The first category is composed of lesions characterized by a delayed-type hypersensitivity, antigen-specific immunological response. These have a high rate of cell turnover, are very active lesions, and are seen in tuberculosis, sarcoidosis, hypersensitivity pneumonitis, and schistosomiasis. The second type is a foreign body granuloma that lacks an antigen-specific response and often is an inactive, minimally destructive lesion. These low-turnover granulomas are seen in berylliosis, where the offending agent is inanimate and inert. The composition of the evoking irritant and its degradability and immunogenicity are decisive factors in the development of the lesion (Boros, 1978). Rapid advances in immunology and histopathology have enabled researchers to analyze the fundamental mechanism of granuloma formation but much remains unknown.

I. Morphology of Granulomas

Granulomas are dynamic entities going through evolutionary and involutionary phases of cell proliferation and death that are probably regulated by localized cell-cell interactions. The mature granuloma is caused by the influx of hematogenous mononuclear phagocytes and their local multiplication, maturation, and activation (Ando et al., 1972).

A. Epithelioid Cells

These are derived from macrophages, and are large mononuclear cells about 20 μm in diameter. The maturation of macrophages is influenced by many stimuli such as immune complexes, phagocytic burden, membrane perturbants such as phorbol esters, arachidonate metabolites, and specific activators such as lymphokines, chemotactic factors, and interferon (Adams and Hamilton, 1984). Epithelioid cells are round or oval in shape and may be of two morphological types: one with abundant granular endoplasmic reticulum and mitochondria, the other predominantly with vacuoles containing pale fibrillar material (Jones-Williams et al., 1970). They are poorly phagocytic but actively pinocytic, with strong microbicidal activity (Papadimitriou and Spector, 1971). They also possess avid secretory properties that have been confirmed by immunocytochemical localization of products such as angiotensin converting enzyme (ACE) and 1,25-dihydroxy vitamin D3 (Pertschuk et al., 1981; Adams et al., 1986).

B. Giant Cells

These are formed by the fusion of macrophages or epithelioid cells and may be up to 300 μm in diameter and contain as many as 30 nuclei (Fig. 1) (Postlethwaite, 1982). Fusion takes place either as a result of secretion of specific lymphokines or of membrane events associated with attempts by mononuclear cells to phagocytose large particles. The two mechanisms may act synergistically. Fusion initially results in a heterokaryon with randomly scattered nuclei that later redistribute by a microtubule-dependent mechanism to form a peripheral ring (Chambers, 1978). Foreign body and Langhans' giant cells thus seem to be different maturational stages of the same cell. Giant cells are poorly phagocytic and their function is uncertain (Boros, 1978).

C. Inclusion Bodies

Both epithelioid cells and giant cells may contain curious, calcium-rich, star-shaped, or conchoid inclusion bodies—Schaumann, asteroid, and residual bodies—all of which are nonspecific and nondiagnostic. They represent the

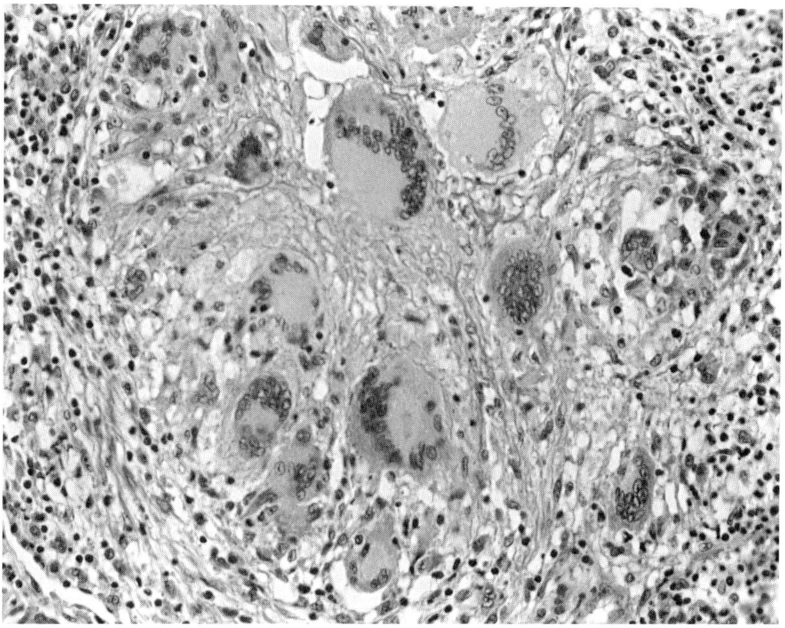

Figure 1 A typical noncaseating granuloma with many giant cells and inclusion bodies (hematoxylin and eosin, ×200).

end products of active metabolism and secretion. Inclusion bodies are found in tuberculosis, syphilis, sarcoidosis, chronic beryllium lung disease, Crohn's disease, and extrinsic allergic alveolitis (Jones-Williams, 1960; Sharma, 1984).

D. Lymphocytes

Granulomas often contain lymphocytes of both T and B types. T lymphocytes usually form a peripheral rim, whereas B cells are found within the granuloma and can be identified by immunofluorescence tests. Immunoperoxidase techniques to analyze lymphocytes and identify various patterns of T-helper and T-suppressor cell arrangements have been used (Van Voorhis et al., 1982). Granulomas from an effective cell-mediated response, as in tuberculoid leprosy, sarcoidosis, and tuberculosis, demonstrate a high number of helper cells within epitheloid cell aggregates in gramulomas, surrounded by a rim of suppressor cells. Granulomas from a poor cell-mediated response, as in lepromatous leprosy, granuloma annulare, and rhinoscleroma, show a near equal number of helper and suppressor phenotypes evenly distributed throughout the granuloma (Modlin et al., 1983; Gupta et al., 1982). In general,

T-helper cells are involved in the maintenance of a granuloma (Narayanan et al., 1983). Cyclosporin A, a potent T-cell suppressor, can completely inhibit granuloma formation (Semenzato et al., 1982).

II. Function of Granulomas

The basic function of a granuloma is to keep the offending agent subdued and, eventually, to destroy it. In doing so, the granuloma disturbs the traffic of circulating immune reactor cells within lymphoid organs and other tissues. This could contribute to the peripheral depression of delayed-type hypersensitivity commonly observed in granulomatous disorders (Bullock et al., 1976). Macrophages, which are not very phagocytic, are highly active secretory cells capable of releasing a variety of potent enzymes including lysozyme, ACE, plasminogen activator, collagenase, elastase, and 1,25-dihydroxy D3 (Adams et al., 1983; Gordon, 1976; Weinstock, 1986). Many of these enzymes are capable of lysing extracellular fibrin, collagen, and elastin. Plasmin can activate enzymatic cascades generating mediators of inflammation (Ryan and Majno, 1977).

III. Immunologic Events at the Site of Granuloma

Granuloma formation is the expression of a series of complex inflammatory events. Most studies analyzing the immunopathogenesis of granuloma formation have been performed in patients with sarcoidosis and hypersensitivity pneumonitis.

Evidence has accumulated in recent years to suggest that cytokines, such as interleukin-1 (IL-1), migration inhibition factor, and chemotactic factors, may play important roles in the initiation and maintenance of hypersensitivity granuloma formation (Masih et al., 1979; Yoshida, 1980; Kobayashi et al., 1985). In both hypersensitivity and foreign body granuloma models, IL-1, but not IL-2, activity was detected in the granuloma extracts in association with activity and size of granulomas. Kasahara and associates (1988) provided direct evidence for the granuloma-inducing activity of IL-1 by inducing experimental pulmonary granuloma formation in mice by IL-1-coupled beads. Natural killer (NK) cell cytolytic activity is known to be suppressed in active pulmonary granulomatous inflammation (Remick et al., 1988b).

Gallium (^{67}Ga) lung scans during active granuloma formation have demonstrated the presence of a large number of activated alveolar macrophages in the lung parenchyma. These activated macrophages process and present antigen in a manner three times more active than normal. They produce IL-1, a protein that serves as a maturational signal and augments T-cell proliferation (Dinarello, 1984; Hunninghake, 1984). The helper T-cells release IL-2, which is non-antigen-specific. Under its influence, the responding T cell acquires IL-2 receptors, proliferates, and differentiates into an effector T-cell (Hunninghake, 1983). Lymphocytes from the lung also produce gamma-interferon, a chemotactic factor for circulating monocytes and other lymphokines, including migration inhibition factor (MIF). These chemical mediators provide cells for the continuing maintenance of granulomas (Yoshida, 1980).

IV. Causes of Lung Granulomas

There are numerous causes of pulmonary granulomatosis. Some of these are well known, others are only partially identified, and still others are barely understood and difficult to identify. Certain granulomatous lung diseases are limited to the tropics or are more common there than in temperate regions because of the tremendous variations in the epidemiological factors that determine the distribution, prevalence, incidence, and endemic nature of diseases, especially those with infectious causes. Some of these are frequently seen in this country in immigrants from tropical regions, visitors, and returning travelers. The causative agents range from live replicating intracellular organisms (bacteria, mycobacteria, viruses, fungi) to nonreplicating metazoans (helminths) to inanimate substances (metals, chemical agents) and organic antigens (Table 1).

V. Differential Diagnosis

A careful history and physical examination are mandatory. The points discussed below should be emphasized.

A. Location and Travels

In India, the most common cause of pulmonary granuloma is tuberculosis, whereas in Egypt and North Africa schistosomiasis should be included in the differential diagnosis. Granulomas in association with visceral leishmaniasis should be considered in inhabitants of eastern India and the Mediterranean littorals, while those in association with helminthic infestations should be considered in residents of almost every developing country. In sharp contrast to the tropics, coccidioidomycosis and sarcoidosis head the list in California, whereas histoplasmosis is the frequent culprit in the midwestern United States. Thus, it is absolutely essential to obtain a thorough history of the patient's residence and recent travels.

Table 1 Classification of Pulmonary Granulomas

Infection	
Bacteria	Mycobacteria
Brucella	*M. tuberculosis*
Francisella	*M. kansasii*
Propioni	*M. avium*
Yersinia	*M. leprae*
	M. marinum
Spirochetes	Protozoa
T. pallidum	*Toxoplasma*
T. carateum	*Leishmania*
Metazoa	Fungi
Toxocara	*Histoplasma*
Schistosoma	*Coccidioidomyces*
Extrinsic allergic alveolitis	
Farmer's lung	Bird fancier's lung
Parakeet lung	Mushroom worker's lung
Suberosis (cork)	Bagassosis (sugarcane)
Chemicals	
Beryllium	Zirconium
Silicon	
Neoplasia	
Lymphoma	
Carcinoma	
Idiopathic	
Sarcoidosis	
Lymphomatoid granulomatosis	
Necrotizing sarcoidal granulomatosis	
Wegener's granulomatosis	

B. Occupational History

Brucellosis is an occupational hazard of veterinary surgeons, laboratory personnel, and abbatoir workers. In Kuwait, brucellosis is a major health hazard among sheep and camel herders, most of whom drink raw milk and have close contact with animals. Farmer's lung disease is caused by antigenic products of thermophilic actinomyces (*Micropolyspora faeni*). The causative agent is not histologically detectable but a positive history of exposure is of diagnostic value, since it might lead one to estimate levels of circulating precipitins against the antigen. Chronic beryllium disease, although rare, continues to be a hazard because the metal is being used increasingly in a variety of industries, especially ceramics and metallurgy. The diagnosis of berylliosis is based on a history of exposure, compatible radiological features, and presence of granulomas.

C. Hobbies

Pigeon breeder's disease, parakeet lung, talc granulomatosis, mushroom picker's lung, and many others are acquired while the individual indulges in an apparently harmless pursuit of pleasure. Intravenous drug abuse involving injection of talc-containing drugs intended for oral use is known to cause granulomatous inflammation in the lung. This habit is usually the result of a shortage of available heroin. Granulomas due to *Coccidioides* may occur in individuals indulging in such activities as unearthing Indian relics and rock hunting. A careful social history including hobbies and habits may, therefore, provide invaluable clues to determining the causes of some pulmonary granulomatous diseases.

D. Family History

If more than one member of the family is ill, the answer might lie in the home environment. The incidence of tuberculosis diminishes as social and economic conditions improve. Poor housing with associated overcrowding increases the risk of massive infection or reinfection if one of the occupants has infectious tuberculosis. Leprosy has long been considered to occur only after exposure to a human case, the most important mode of spread of *Mycobacterium leprae* being by droplets from the sneezes of lepromatous patients with heavily infected nasal mucosa. However, evidence has been accumulating that this conventional view is wrong and that an environmental nonhuman source is critical to some *Mycobacterium leprae* infections. Recent observations with monoclonal antibodies have shown that phenolic glycolipid I antigen, which is unique to the *M. leprae* cell wall, is found in soil (Blake et al., 1987; Reich, 1987).

E. Physical Examination

Sarcoidosis and tuberculosis are multisystem disorders. The patient should be examined carefully for ocular lesions, dermatological changes, joint involvement, peripheral lymphadenopathy, splenomegaly, and neurological involvement (Table 2). Remittent fever, splenomegaly, and hepatomegaly in a chronically ill patient may suggest visceral leishmaniasis.

Table 2 Differences Between Sarcoidosis and Tuberculosis

Features	Sarcoidosis	Tuberculosis
Clinical		
Age of incidence (years)	20-50	20-50
Sex	Commonly affects women	Commonly affects men
Fever, chills	Unusual	Usual
Anorexia, weight loss	Uncommon	Common
Erythema nodosum	Common	Uncommon
Skin lesions	Lupus pernio, rash, papules	Lupus vulgaris, draining sinuses
Parotid enlargement	Common	Rare
Peritonitis, pericarditis, meningitis	Rare	Common
Radiological		
Chest x-ray		
Hilar lymphadenopathy	Bilateral	Unilateral
Pulmonary cavitation	Rare	Common
Pleural effusion	Rare	Common
Bone lesions	Common	Rare
Histological		
Granuloma	Noncaseating	Caseating
Acid-fast bacilli	Absent	Present
Immunological		
Delayed-type hypersensitivity	Depressed	Normal
Kveim test	Positive	Negative
Hyperglobulinemia	Present	May be present
Therapeutic		
Antituberculous drugs	Unhelpful	Treatment of choice
Corticosteroids	Helpful	May be helpful in some cases
Chloroquine	May be helpful	Not indicated
Immunosuppressive drugs	May be helpful	Not indicated

F. Chest Radiograph

In pulmonary tuberculosis, the chest roentgenogram may show unilateral hilar adenopathy, miliary infiltration, and an upper lobe infiltrate with or without a cavity (Fig. 2a). In sarcoidosis, bilateral hilar adenopathy occurs in more than 50% of the patients (Fig. 2b). In lymphoma or Hodgkin's disease, mediastinal adenopathy is the rule (Fig. 2c). The x-ray findings in beryllium lung disease are nonspecific. In the early stages, there is a general haziness, or ground glass appearance throughout both lungs. As the disease progresses, however, bronchovascular and hilar shadows increase (Fig. 2d). Reticulation may be observed in some cases, primarily in the upper lung regions, with emphysematous changes at the bases. Thus, an ability to recognize a few radiographic patterns goes a long way in evaluating a patient with a lung granuloma (Table 3).

G. Histopathological Findings

Recognition of typical features of a granuloma, special stains (AFB, fungi), culture of tissue, and examination of tissue under a polarizing light microscope considerably narrow the diagnostic possibilities (Table 4). Caseation is characteristic of the *Mycobacterium*-induced granulomas (Fig. 3), whereas the sarcoid or beryllium-induced granulomas practically never undergo caseation. The histological picture of hypersensitivity granulomas, however, is seldom specific and cannot be independently used as a diagnostic tool for the identification of specific diseases.

H. Skin Tests

The Kveim-Siltzbach skin test is most helpful in differentiating sarcoidosis from all other granulomatous disorders. However, not only is the antigen not generally available but there is also a lack of standardized preparations. Tuberculin, histoplasmin, and coccidioidin skin tests have minor but important roles. There are no skin tests for hypersensitivity pneumonitis.

I. Laboratory Tests

A determination of the serum and bronchoalveolar lavage fluid (BALF) ACE may be useful in establishing the diagnosis of sarcoidosis. The serum level of ACE (SACE) is thought to reflect the granulomatous load in the body, and is elevated in up to 80% of patients with sarcoidosis. SACE levels fall with resolution of granulomata and can prove useful in monitoring the course of the disease. SACE levels are nonspecific, however, and may be elevated in many diseases (Table 5). Even so, elevated SACE levels associated with hypercalcemia strongly suggests sarcoidosis. This combination, however,

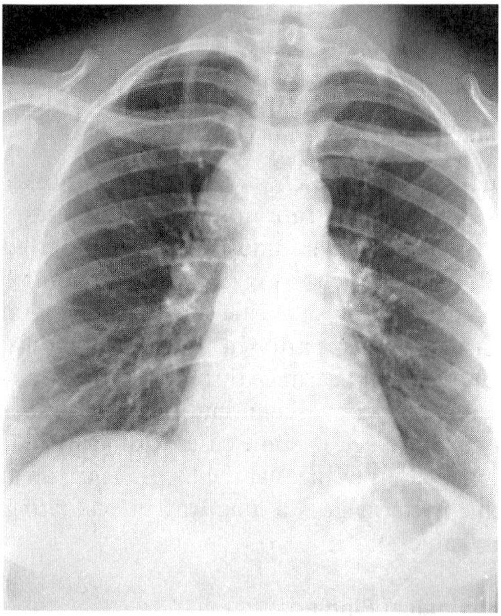

a

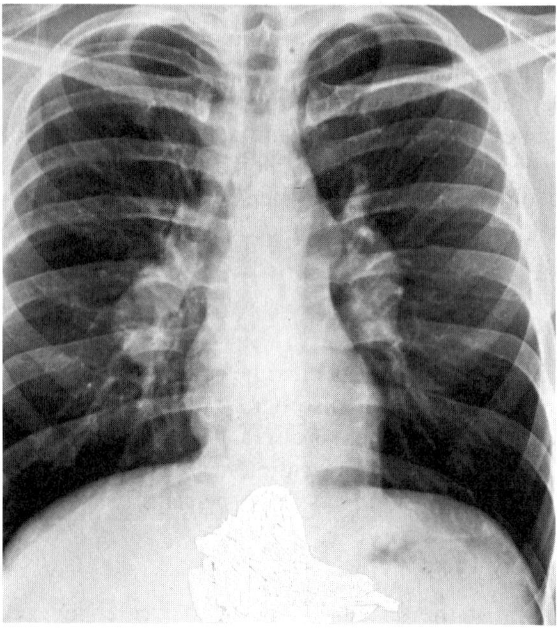

b

Figure 2 Typical pulmonary presentations in some of the granulomatous reactions. a. Right hilar and paratracheal adenopathy in a young man with tuberculosis. b. Bilateral hilar adenopathy in a 20-year-old man from Calcutta, India, who showed noncaseating granuloma consistent with sarcoidosis. c. Left hilar adenopathy in a patient with Hodgkin's disease. d. Diffuse interstitial infiltrate in a patient with chronic beryllium exposure.

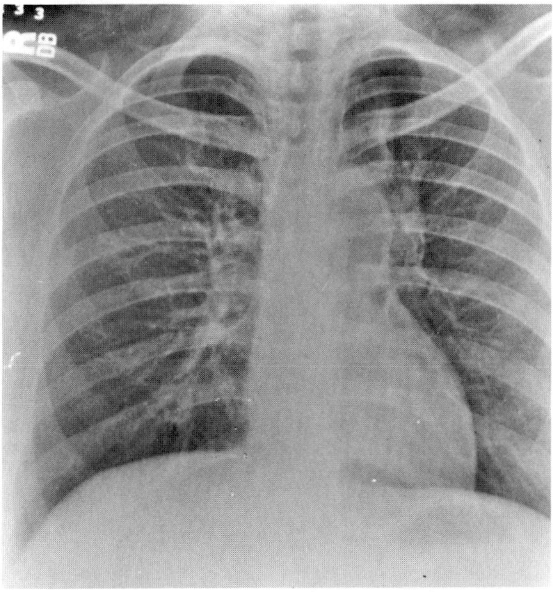

c

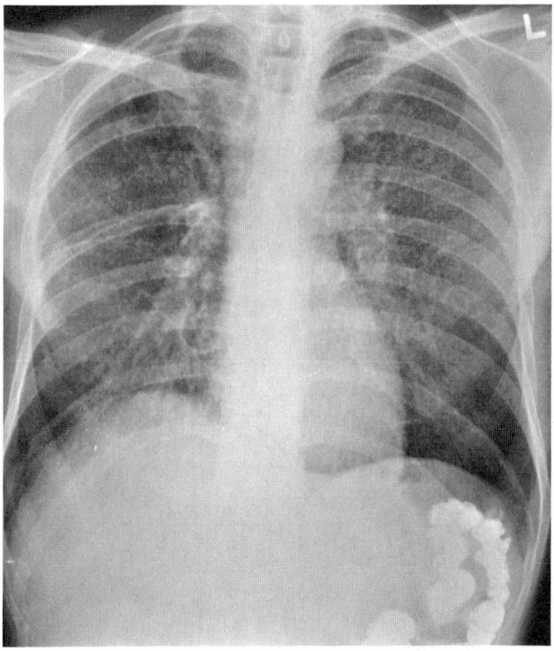

d

Figure 2 Continued

Table 3 Common Chest Radiographic Patterns

Features	TB	Sarcoidosis	EAA	CBD	WG	Hodgkin's disease
Hilar adenopathy	Unilateral	Bilateral	Absent	Rare	Absent	Unilateral
Parenchymal infiltrate	May be miliary	More in lower and mid fields	Diffuse	Diffuse	Rare	Uncommon
Cavity formation	Common	Rare	Rare	Rare	Common	Rare
Mediastinal adenopathy	May occur	Uncommon	Absent	Absent	Absent	Common
Pleural effusion	Common	Rare	Absent	Absent	Rare	May occur
Large nodules	May occur	May occur	Absent	Absent	Common	Common

TB, tuberculosis; EAA, extrinsic allergic alveolitis; CBD, chronic beryllium disease; WG, Wegener's granulomatosis.

Table 4 Histological Appearance of Common Pulmonary Granulomas

Features	TB	Sarcoidosis	EAA	Fungi	Leprosy	Brucellosis	WG	CBD
Granuloma	Present	Present	Present	Present	Present	Present	Rare	Present
Caseation	Present	Absent	Rare	Absent	Present	Absent	Absent	Rare
Necrosis	Present	Absent	Rare	Present	Present	May be present	Common	Rare
Inclusion bodies	Rare	Present (70%)	Rare	Rare	Rare	Rare	Absent	Present (80%)
Alveolitis	Minimal	Present	Prominent	Absent	Absent	Absent	Present	Prominent
Vasculitis	Rare	Present	Absent	Absent	Absent	Absent	Present	Rare
Bronchiolitis	Rare	Rare	Present	Absent	Absent	Absent	Absent	Rare

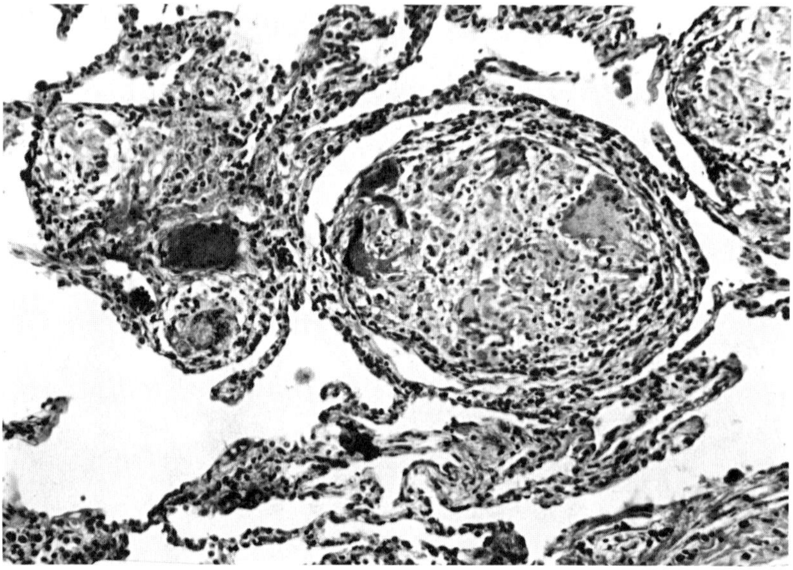

a

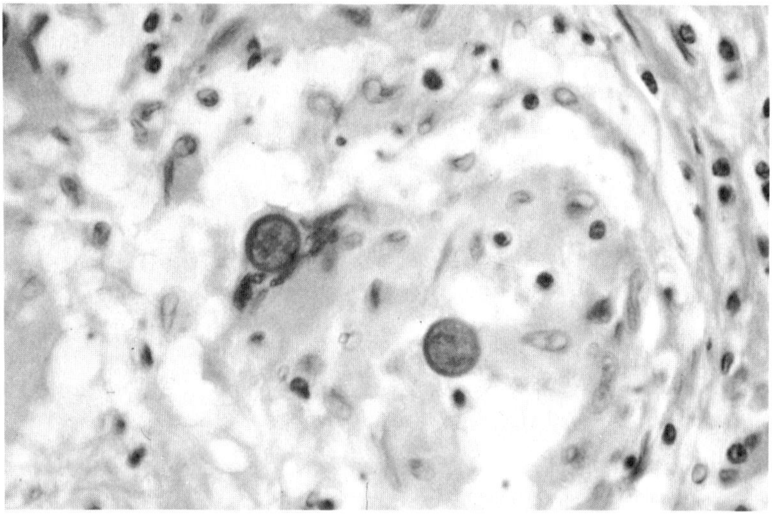

b

Figure 3 Various granulomatous reactions involving the lungs. a. Typical sarcoidosis granuloma consists of a compact collection of epithelioid cells, a few giant cells, and a layer or two of lymphocytes. b. Typical granuloma due to coccidioidomycosis shows cocci spherules. c. Brucellosis granulomas are poorly formed structure with no organisms or foreign body reaction. d. A poorly formed talc granuloma is usually packed with birefringent foreign body particles.

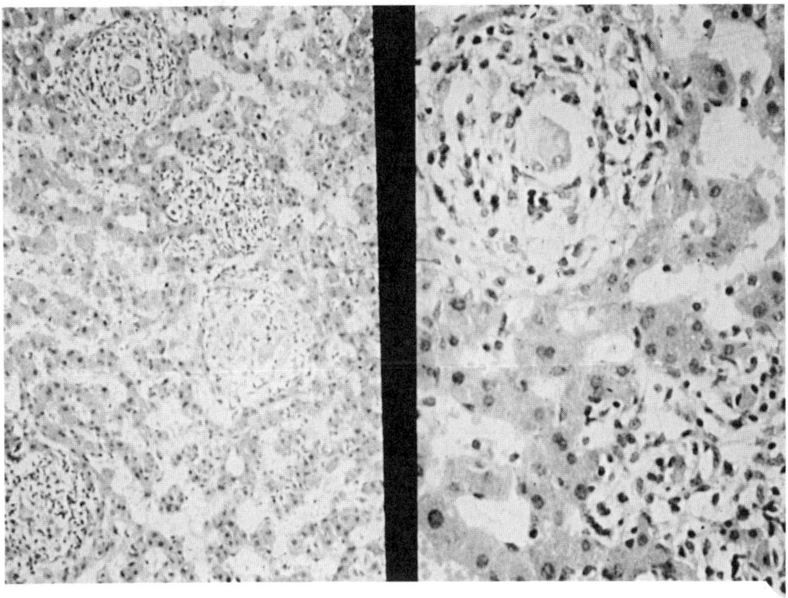

c

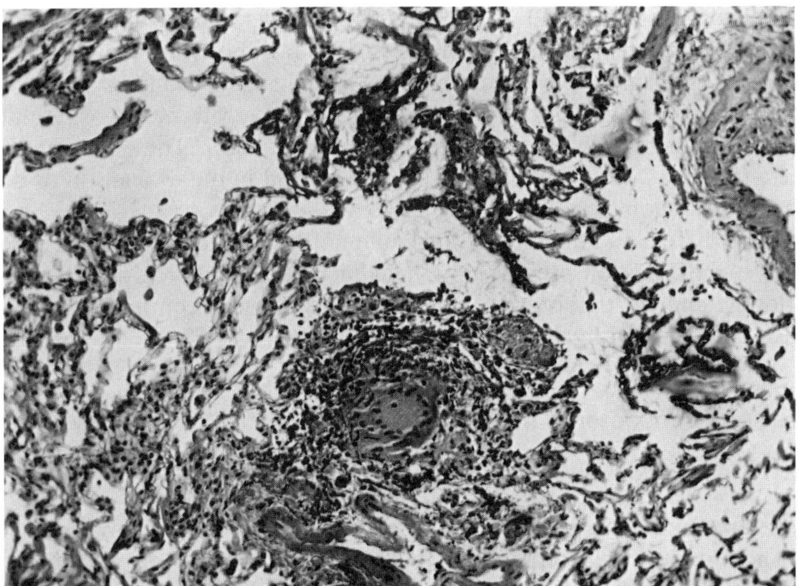

d

Table 5 Conditions Associated with Elevated Serum ACE Level

Likely to be confused with sarcoidosis	Unlikely to be confused with sarcoidosis
Asbestosis	Coccidioidomycosis
Berylliosis	Diabetes mellitus
Granulomatous hepatitis	Gaucher's disease
Hypersensitivity pneumonitis	Idiopathic respiratory disease syndrome
Lymphoma	Inflammatory bowel disease
Miliary tuberculosis	Pulmonary neoplasm
Primary biliary cirrhosis	Leprosy
Silicosis	Liver cirrhosis

may also occur in Hodgkin's disease and miliary tuberculosis. Both agglutinating and complement-fixing antibody titers may be used in the diagnosis of brucellosis. Titers may persist at low levels for months or years, especially in patients with chronic infection. There is a problem of cross-reaction with *Francisella tularensis, Yersinia enterolitica,* and other organisms, however (Mittal and Tizzard, 1979). Serological titers are very important in the diagnosis of brucellosis, because the organisms are fastidious and require special media for optimal recovery from blood. The only abnormal laboratory findings in chronic infections with *Schistosoma* may be peripheral eosinophilia and a mild increase of serum globulins, especially IgG. The sedimentation rate and C-reactive proteins levels are not helpful in the evaluation of pulmonary granulomas.

The differential diagnosis of granulomatous disorders demands a synthesis of information provided by the clinician, the radiologist, the microbiologist, and the pathologist. Some of the conditions commonly encountered are discussed in the next sections.

VI. Mycobacterial Infections

A. Tuberculosis

There are more documented tuberculosis cases in the world today than have ever been recorded before, and with many Third World countries documenting high resistance rates to single and multiple drugs, it has become a major health problem worldwide (Sbarbaro, 1989). The tuberculous granulomas are usually characterized by central caseous necrosis, but in miliary tuberculosis noncaseating granulomas are more common. The granulomas usually tend to be multiple without a dominant lesion, and are generally surrounded by fibroblastic fibrosis, and extensive vasculitis (Ulbright and Katzenstein, 1980). Hypercalcemia and elevated SACE levels may occur in miliary tuberculosis. Acid-fast stains and culture of body fluids or biopsied tissues are needed to confirm the diagnosis. Many laboratories use a fluorochrome staining procedure with auramine O as the stain. This requires a fluorescent microscope for examination but is much faster because the slide can be scanned at a lower magnification. Assessment of pulmonary functions in patients treated for pulmonary tuberculosis has revealed evidence of chronic obstructive airways disease (Willcox and Ferguson, 1989).

B. Leprosy

This chronic infectious disease is caused by *Mycobacterium leprae*, an organism with suspected high infectivity but low pathogenicity and with a preference for growth in cool areas of the body (Woodruff and Wright, 1987). The disease is endemic in most of the tropical and warm, temperate countries of the world including S.E. Asia, Africa, and South America. Incidence and prevalence figures are inaccurate because of the limited resources for health care in the areas most affected, and the stigma attached to the diagnosis. The conventional view regarding the mode of spread of *M. leprae*, including prolonged close contact and transmission by nasal droplet, is being strongly challenged (Reich, 1987; Blake et al., 1987). The granulomas in tuberculoid leprosy have little or no caseation (Narayanan, 1988). *M. leprae* bacilli are scant or altogether absent and cannot be cultured or transmitted to usual laboratory animals (Reich, 1987). Systemic infections develop in thymectomized or irradiated mice, in nude mice, and in about 50% of normal nine-banded armadillos. The latter are the main source of leprosy bacilli used for research. Elevated SACE levels may be noted in patients with leprosy patients (Lieberman and Rea, 1977). Leprosy may mimic other diseases involving the skin and peripheral nerves. The diagnosis is established by clinical evidence of the disease and biopsy. The lepromin test is usually positive in tuberculoid leprosy (TT) and negative in lepromatous leprosy (LL) polar types (Woodruff and Wright, 1987). Recent studies based on detection of *M. leprae*-specific phenolic glycolipid I give rise to the possibility of a serodiagnostic test for leprosy in the future (Blake et al., 1987). In terms of pulmonary function in leprosy, there is evidence of universal hyporesponsiveness in lepromatous leprosy, which is attributed to autonomic system involvement (Jindal et al., 1989).

VII. Fungal Diseases: Histoplasmosis

This granulomatous infection is acquired by inhalation. It has been reported from over 50 countries, including Africa, Southeast Asia, Mexico, and South America, with the first case being recognized in Panama in 1905. In the United States, the midwestern portion of the country is the area of highest endemicity. Histoplasmosis may resemble sarcoidosis clinically as well as pathologically and radiologically (Goodwin and Des prez, 1978). Histoplasma granulomas tend to be round, are often microscopically solitary, and, if multiple, usually contain one dominant lesion (Ulbright and Katzenstein, 1980). They are generally surrounded by sclerosing fibrosis and often contain calcium. Since the standard hematoxylin and eosin stain is inadequate, special stains such as silver and periodic acid-Schiff (PAS) may be necessary to visualize the organism in tissue sections. Although important in epidemiological studies, the histoplasmin skin test is not often helpful diagnostically and has the disadvantage of occasionally boosting a subsequent complement fixation titer. Serum complement fixation, immunodiffusion, and radioimmunoassay may be needed for accurate diagnosis (Goodwin and Des Prez, 1978).

VIII. Parasitic Diseases

A. Protozoa: Leishmaniasis

Visceral leishmaniasis (kala azar) is a disease characterized by a long incubation period and a chronic course, remittent fever, leukopenia, anemia, and enlargement of the spleen and liver (Woodruff and Wright, 1987). The Mediterranean type is prevalent in the Mediterranean and Red Sea littorals, Sudan, Asian Russia, and Arabia, whereas the Indian type is prevalent in parts of India and Burma bordering the Bay of Bengal (Manson-Bahr and Apted, 1982). The parasites, known as Leishman-Donovan bodies, are found in the cytoplasm of reticuloendothelial cells or free in the blood plasma. Transmission is either by the bite of the female sandfly, *Phlebotomus* spp. or transfusion of infected blood. Pulmonary involvement is usually characterized by signs and symptoms of bronchitis or bronchopneumonia. There is usually an increase in gammaglobulins, mainly IgG. The diagnosis depends on appropriate history, clinical evidence of splenomegaly, hepatomegaly, progressive granulocytopenia, and profound anemia (Wyler and Marsden, 1984). With the increase in incidence of human immunodeficiency virus (HIV) infections in Africa and other tropical countries, kala azar is emerging as an important opportunistic infection in patients with the acquired immunodeficiency syndrome (AIDS) (Berenguer et al., 1989). A serodiagnostic assay for visceral leishmaniasis using monoclonal antibodies has been recently developed (Jaffe and McMahon-Pratt, 1987).

B. Metazoa

Nematodes

Parasitic helminths are common in almost all developing countries due to the prevailing sanitary conditions. Migration of a helminth through the lung may induce a foreign-body type cellular reaction with subsequent granuloma formation. Metazoan tissue parasites such as *Trichinella spiralis* larva and others are too large to be phagocytosed, but can secrete various antigens that are probably ingested by pinocytosis by the surrounding macrophages. The slow degradability of metazoans and the continuous antigenic stimuli emanating from them ensure that conditions for granuloma formation are fulfilled (Boros and Warren, 1970). Refractile structures representing fragments of the helminth may be seen in the center of the granuloma on lung biopsy (Ulbright and Katzenstein, 1980). Patients may present with a visceral larva migrans syndrome, asthmatic symptoms, and eosinophilia (Aftandelians et al., 1977). The nematodes causing pulmonary granulomas include *Ascaris lumbricoides, Toxocara canis, Capillaria aerophila,* and others. Eosinophilia may be absent at the onset of respiratory symptoms. Compounding the diagnostic dilemma, stool samples may be negative for ova and parasites.

Tropical Pulmonary Eosinophilia

This disease is found mostly in India, Southeast Asia, and the South Pacific islands, and should be considered in all patients with eosinophilia and miliary pulmonary infiltrates who give the appropriate history. It is thought to be caused by infection due to human filarial species, *Wuchereria bancrofti* and *Brugia malayi*, but microfilariae are virtually never located in the blood and are rarely found in tissue biopsy specimens. The discovery of elevated microfilarial antibody titers, the demonstration of microfilaria in foci of inflammation, and the dramatic clinical response to diethylcarbamazine in suspected pulmonary eosinophilia have almost certainly implicated microfilaria as the causative agent. Tropical eosinophilia is hypothesized to represent a host hypersensitivity response to microfilariae (Ottesen et al., 1979). Not all individuals infected with microfilariae develop a hypersensitivity reaction and the reason for this idiosyncrasy is not known. The IgG4 subclass of IgG antibodies, which rises in response to filariasis, may function as a blocking antibody and a higher IgG4 response may be associated with protection against developing pulmonary eosinophilia (Hussain and Ottesen, 1986).

Clinical manifestations include low-grade fever, weight loss, and fatigue together with cough and wheeze, which are usually worse at night. In addition to the lungs, the lymph nodes, pericardium, the central nervous system may be involved (Spry and Kumaraswami, 1982). The chest radiograph may be normal or may reveal a reticulonodular pattern, focal areas of consolidation, hilar adenopathy, or pleural effusions. Lung functions reveal mixed obstructive-restrictive defects (Chhabra and Gaur, 1988; Fig. 4).

Diagnosis is confirmed by marked eosinophilia, elevated IgE levels, and elevated microfilarial titers. Histopathological studies show early histiocytic infiltration followed by eosinophilic bronchopneumonia. Chronic disease state may reveal a mixed cellular infiltrate of histiocytes, lymphocytes, and eosinophils with increased fibrosis (Neva and Ottesen, 1978).

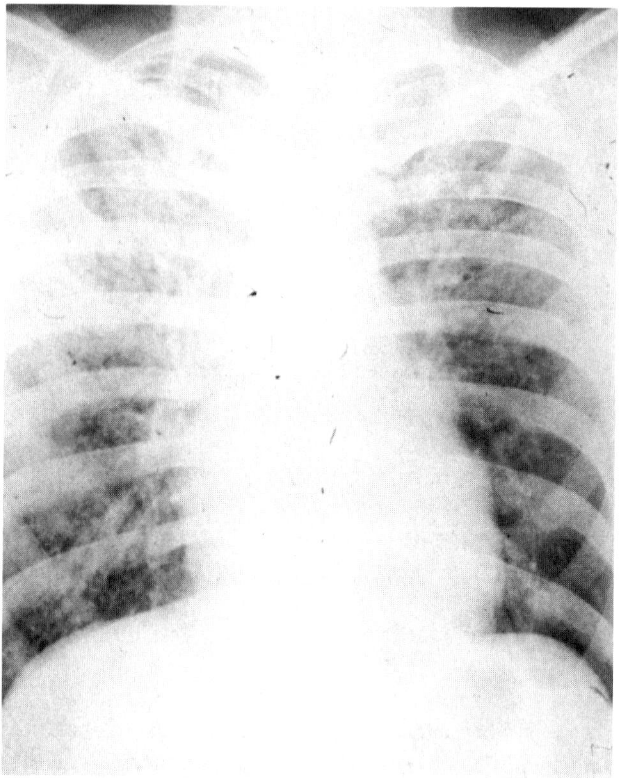

Figure 4 Posteroanterior view of the chest shows a diffuse nodular infiltrate in a man with tropical eosinophilia (reproduced with kind permission of *Chest,* 1989).

C. Trematodes: Schistosomiasis

Schistosoma mansoni has a wide geographical distribution including Africa, the eastern Mediterranean, South America, and the West Indies. The disease is mainly due to eggs deposited in host tissue by the adult female worms, which induce inflammatory and fibrotic lesions in the host organs, including the intestines, liver, and lungs. Pulmonary hypertension and cor pulmonale induced by pulmonary arteritis as a result of *S. mansoni* egg deposition have been well documented in the literature (Andrade and Andrade, 1970; Irusta, 1978; Nash et al., 1982). Such pathological effects are due to collateral circulation in patients with liver fibrosis and portal hypertension, which provide direct access of eggs to the lungs (Adams, 1980). The *S. mansoni* egg granuloma is a T-cell-mediated, delayed-type hypersensitivity granuloma (Remick et al., 1988a). Pulmonary hypertension and cor pulmonale are less common with *S. japonicum* or *S. hematobium* infection (Watt et al., 1986). A solitary pulmonary bilharzioma measuring 5 cm was reported several years ago (Thompson et al., 1979). Diagnosis and assessment of morbidity are based on clinical features, stool egg count, and other laboratory findings (Nash et al., 1982).

IX. Bacterial Diseases

A. Brucellosis

This zoonotic infection is caused by bacteria of the genus *Brucella.* It is an acute or chronic illness manifested principally by chills, relapses of fever, weakness, and vague aches and pains. In the United States, brucellosis is rare and is largely an occupational hazard of slaughterhouse workers and veterinarians. It is common in the Far East, Kuwait and other Gulf countries, South America, Mexico, and the Mediterranean region. The disease can be caused by any of the four species, each usually confined to its major animal host: *B. melitensis* (goat), *B. suis* (hogs), *B. abortus* (cattle), and *B. canis* (dogs) (Charters, 1980). After uptake by macrophages, the organisms are broken down rapidly, but a residual 20% remains undegraded. Low solubility and poor degradability of the residual antigen ensure the prolonged antigenic stimulus necessary for maintenance of the chronic granulomatous reaction (Boros, 1988). Granulomas are small and poorly defined (Jordans and Bruin, 1980). Involvement of the pleura in the form of brucellar pleuritis may occur (Sirera Jimenez et al., 1987). The diagnosis depends on occupational history, clinical features, and serologic evidence. A single titer of 1:160 or higher, or a fourfold or greater rise in titer of specimens drawn 1-4 weeks apart, indicates recent infection (Moyer et al., 1987; Young, 1983).

B. Tularemia

Francisella (*Pasturella*) *tularensis* is a small gram-negative coccobacillus spread by contact with infected animals or by insect vectors such as ticks (Woodruff and Wright, 1987). Tularemia is an occupational hazard of sheep herders, trappers, and butchers. Tularemia may present in different ways depending upon the site of inoculation, but the most common clinical features are local ulcer formation and regional lymphadenopathy in association with symptoms of systemic febrile illness (Woodruff and Wright, 1987). Host defense mechanisms are not fully understood. However, immunity is associated with the appearance of delayed hypersensitivity to tularemia skin antigen (Buchanan et al., 1971). Septicemic tularemia usually causes miliary microabscesses in the liver, spleen, and lungs (Dienst, 1963). With healing, these abscesses organize and granulomas may occur. There are many pathological similarities between tularemia and tuberculosis. On microscopic examination, mononuclear cells are prominent in the lesions and some may undergo caseous necrosis (Lillie and Francis, 1936). Various degrees of organization, occasionally with giant cells present, occur with healing (Lillie and Francis, 1936). Granulomatous pleuritis may be confused with tuberculous pleuritis (Schmid et al., 1983). Because the organism is fastidious and highly infective, serological responses are usually used for diagnosis (Bevanger et al., 1988).

X. Granulomatous Diseases of Unknown Cause

These are a group of chronic granulomatous lung diseases in which no causative agents have been found.

A. Sarcoidosis

This granulomatous disorder of unknown cause has a worldwide distribution. Although it is much less frequent in tropical Africa, India, and Southeast Asia, the frequency of sarcoidosis in the central mountainous district of Japan is high (Sharma, 1984; Gupta, 1989). It most commonly affects young adults and presents most frequently with bilateral hilar adenopathy, pulmonary infiltration, and skin or eye lesions. It can involve almost any organ system in various combinations, giving rise to many clinical syndromes embracing all branches of medicine. Immunological features include depression of delayed-type hypersensitivity, suggesting impaired cell-mediated immunity, and elevated or abnormal immunoglobulins. Alveolar macrophages from sarcoidosis patients are HLA-DR/DS+, can present a variety of antigens to autologous blood T cells, can spontaneously secrete IL-1 immune interferon and fibronectin, and display C3b and Fc membrane receptors

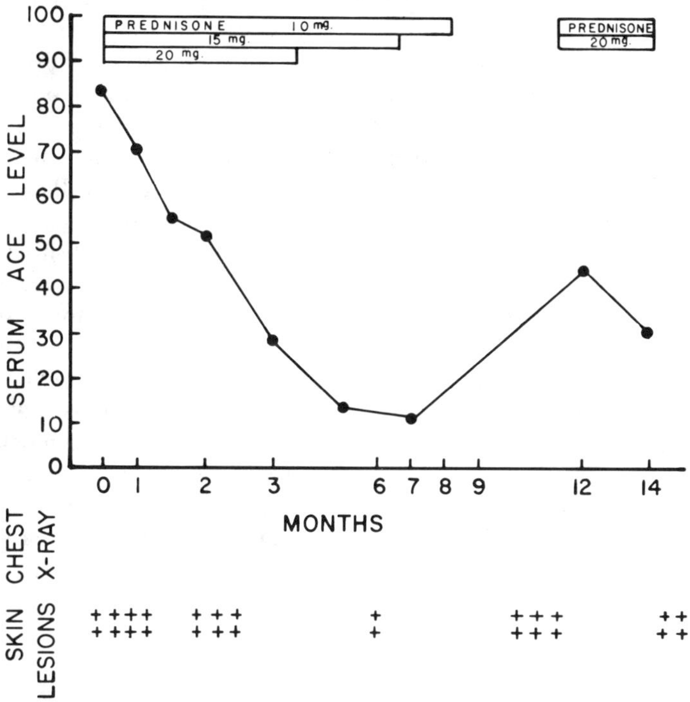

Figure 5 Course of ACE and serum calcium levels in a patient with sarcoidosis. Note that elevated ACE and calcium levels may also occur in patients with tuberculosis.

(Hunninghake, 1983, 1984). The diagnosis depends on the evidence of multisystem involvement, typical chest roentgenographic findings, and the presence of noncaseating granulomata in a tissue biopsy specimen. Elevated SACE and calcium levels are helpful (Sharma, 1984; Fig. 5).

B. Wegener's Granulomatosis

This disease, first described in the 1930s, is an organ-specific necrotizing granulomatous vasculitis involving principally the lungs, upper respiratory tract, and kidneys. The presentation may be generalized, with involvement of the nose, lungs, and kidneys, or limited to only the lungs (Liebow, 1973; Liebow et al., 1972; Israel and Patchefsky, 1971). Common presenting symptoms include nasal crusting and bleeding. A long history of sinusitis or rhinitis may precede discovery of lung or renal involvement. Pulmonary symptoms include cough, hemoptysis, and chest pain. Renal symptoms, when present, usually occur after the onset of respiratory symptoms. Constitutional symptoms such as low-grade fever, weight loss, and malaise are more common in the presence of respiratory symptoms. The skin may be involved with maculopapular or ulcerative lesions. Neurological involvement may be present in up to 25% of patients with systemic Wegener's granulomatosis (Fauci and Wolff, 1973). Other organ systems are rarely involved in the absence of the classic triad of upper respiratory tract, lungs, and kidneys (Bambry et al., 1987). Based on the granulomatous histopathological findings, the disease is presumed to be a manifestation of the delayed hypersensitivity response to an as yet unidentified antigen. Because patients with Wegener's granulomatosis sometimes respond to treatment with trimethoprim-sulfamethoxazole, it is possible that the causative agent for the disease may be an as yet unidentified infectious agent (West et al., 1987). The predilection of the granulomatous inflammations to occur in the vessel wall has not been explained. The detection of circulating immune complexes in certain patients could indicate that the granulogenic agents are the large complexes that lodge in the vessel walls and are ingested by macrophages initiating the granulomatous process. However, complex formation may be secondary to the delayed hypersensitivity response induced by a granulogenic agent (Fauci et al., 1978).

C. Pulmonary Allergic Granulomatosis

Churg and Strauss described in 1951 a series of patients with asthma, eosinophilia, and vascular lesions similar to the type seen in polyarteritis nodosa. It remains a relatively rarely diagnosed syndrome. The disease may be organized into three distinct phases (Lanham et al., 1984). The prodromal or allergic phase is characterized by asthma with or without associated allergic rhinitis. Peripheral blood eosinophilia and eosinophilic tissue infiltrates mimicking Loeffler's syndrome, chronic eosinophilic pneumonia, or eosinophilic gastroenteritis characterize the second phase. Systemic vasculitis characterizes the third phase. The chest radiographic pattern is nonspecific, typically revealing transient patchy infiltrates, massive bilateral nodular infiltrates without evidence of cavitation, or an interstitial pattern (Chumbley et al., 1977). The cause of the illness is unknown. Diagnosis is made by a history of asthma, eosinophilia, elevated IgE levels, and histological features of necritizing vasculitis, tissue infiltration by eosinophils, and extravascular granulomas.

D. Lymphomatoid Granulomatosis

This disease was first described in 1972 as an entity distinct from lymphomas, to which it bears histological similarities, and from limited Wegener's granulomatosis, to which it bears both clinical and histological similarities (Liebow et al., 1972). It is characterized by pulmonary lymphoreticular infiltrates that are angiocentric and angiodestructive. Pulmonary symptoms are common and include cough, dyspnea, and chest pain. Constitutional symptoms are frequent. Dermatological and neurological involvement is also quite common. Chest radiographs usually reveal bilateral nodular infiltrates that are frequently peripheral and may be mistaken for metastatic tumors. Other possible radiological features include cavitation, indistinct lesions resembling pneumonias, and lesions that change in configuration and size. Unilateral disease is rare. Hilar adenopathy is uncommon and when present suggests lymphoma or other disease process (Katzenstein et al., 1979). Approximately 10% of pulmonary disease that is initially diagnosed as lymphomatoid granulomatosis eventually is manifested as malignant lymphomas (Katzenstein et al., 1979; Cohen et al., 1979). Pulmonary involvement is the major cause of death, although a significant number of patients die from central nervous system involvement.

E. Bronchocentric Granulomatosis

This is a necrotizing granulomatous disease of the lungs centered principally around bronchi and bronchioles. Clinical manifestations include fever, cough, chest pain, and malaise. Most patients (50%) have a history of chronic asthma. Some patients have multiple allergies. Positive skin tests and serum precipitins to *Aspergillus* and isolation of *Aspergillus* from sputum cultures from several patients have been observed (Katzenstein et al., 1975; Hanson et al., 1977). Chest radiographic studies may reveal involvement of a single lobe or multiple lobes, with unilateral or bilateral involvement. Other radiological manifestations include multiple small or large nodules, consolidation, infarction patterns, and collapse (mucus plugging). Bronchograms may reveal segmental obstruction. The pathogenesis of bronchocentric granulomatosis in asthmatic patients is likely to be related to hypersensitivity against *Aspergillus* antigens. The cause in nonasthmatic patients is not known.

XI. Hypersensitivity Pneumonitides

This group of pulmonary disorders includes several diseases such as farmer's lung, mushroom worker's lung, maltworker's lung, maple bark disease, bird fancier's lung, and others. They are initiated in nonatopic subjects by inhalation of organic dust leading to chronic alveolar inflammation, interstitial infiltration, granuloma formation, and fibrosis. Spores of thermophilic actinomycetes, avian serum proteins in bird droppings, or powdered pituitary hormones inhaled by patients with diabetes insipidus can serve as offending agents. Repeated inhalation of the agents induces sensitization in a certain percentage of exposed individuals. Histopathological changes of the lung, during the acute stage, are characterized by infiltration of lymphocytes, macrophages, and plasma cells into the walls of the alveoli and the alveolar space, thickening of the alveolar septae, and appearance of noncaseating granulomas with epithelioid and giant cells. In the chronic stage, lymphocytic infiltration persists and interstitial fibrosis is pronounced. Although an immune cause has been implicated in the disease, the types of hypersensitivity reactions participating in the reactions are not clearly known.

The presence of high levels of precipitins in persons exposed to *Micropolyspora faeni*, the organism causing farmer's lung, was thought to indicate that antigen-antibody complexes may be responsible, but no correlation has been found between the presence or absence of precipitins and symptoms of the disease (Fink et al., 1972). The presence of epithelioid-cell-containing granulomas is indicative of a delayed type hypersensitivity reaction. Examination of BALF from chronically ill patients revealed that the number of T lymphocytes was considerably elevated over that found in the circulation (Reynolds et al., 1977). There appears to be no difference in the ratio of T4/T8 in asymptomatic or symptomatic pigeon breeders (Leatherman et al., 1984). It is interesting that T8 lymphocytes are the predominant phenotype of T cells in either group. Hypersensitivity pneumonitis should be suspected when a person regularly exposed to a heavy concentration of organic dusts complains, a few hours after reexposure to the same dust, of general malaise, dry cough, and dyspnea without wheeze. If not detected early, and further exposure to the dust hazard is permitted, the symptoms continue and become very severe in some cases. At this stage, the patient may be febrile, cyanosed, and dyspneic at rest. A chest radiograph may show diffuse micronodular shadowing (Hargreave et al., 1972). Spirometry usually reveals a restrictive ventilatory defect without airflow obstruction, but a mixed restrictive-obstructive picture may be present (Allen et al., 1976). Diagnosis is confirmed serologically by a positive precipitin test and, if necessary, by a positive provocation test. Inhalation of the relevant aerosolized antigen is followed 3-6 h later by fever, and a drop in FVC, often with recurrence of symptoms.

XII. Berylliosis

The inhalation of beryllium dusts, salts, or fumes is associated with two types of pulmonary disease: an acute chemical pneumonitis caused by short exposures to high concentrations, and a chronic interstitial granulomatous lung disease caused by lower levels of exposure over a prolonged period (Kriebel et la., 1988). The natural source for beryllium, beryl ore, is mined in India, the Soviet Union, parts of Europe, and the United States. Modern uses for beryllium are found in the nuclear, electronics, and aerospace industry. Because of the widespread use of beryllium and its salt in industry, the incidence of chronic, dermal, and pulmonary berylliosis has sharply increased. The major organ affected by beryllium is the lung.

The acute pneumonitis is probably caused by direct injury of the lung by beryllium, whereas the chronic pulmonary disease is associated with an alveolitis characterized by a diffuse accumulation of lymphocytes and mononuclear phagocytes in the alveolar structures and the formation of noncaseating granulomas, features suggestive of a chronic, delayed-type hypersensitivity reaction (Cullen et al., 1987; Rossman et al., 1988). Beryllium is thought to act as a class II restricted antigen, stimulating local proliferation and accumulation in the lung of beryllium-specific CD4+ (helper/inducer) cells (Saltini et al., 1989). The onset of symptoms may appear long after the initial exposure. These include progressive dyspnea, chronic nonproductive cough, weight loss, fatigue, and other symptoms. The chest x-ray may show a mottled appearance in both lungs with hilar adenopathy (Weber et al., 1965; Klech, 1986). On histological examination, chronic interstitial pneumonitis and noncaseating granulomas are present with epithelioid and giant cells (Langerhans type), making it difficult to differentiate from sarcoid granulomas. At the later stage, fibrosis may be pronounced, with development of cor pulmonale. A mild exposure to beryllium may result in reversion of inflammation and healing without much residual disease, but higher intensities of exposure may cause permanent, severe disease (Sprince et al., 1978). The diagnosis depends on a history of exposure, the presence of beryllium in tissues and body fluids, and pathological findings.

XIII. Drug-Induced Pulmonary Granulomas

The drugs that are known to be associated with the production or induction of pulmonary granulomas are mineral oil, disodium cromoglycate, magnesium trisilicate (talc), methotrexate, and bacillus Calmette-Guerin (BCG). Aspirated oil is the most common cause of drug-induced granulomas. Abnormalities range from an asymptomatic solitary pulmonary nodule to diffuse disease. On aspiration, the oils are emulsified and engulfed by macrophages. Eventually a fibrosis or a granulomatous reaction, which is usually a localized reaction, occurs. Pulmonary granulomas due to inhalation of cromolyn sodium in powder form are rare. There is only one case report of a postulated, tissue-proven cromolyn-induced diffuse pulmonary granulomatous reaction (Burgher et al., 1974). Magnesium trisilicate, which is used as an excipient or bonding agent in the manufacture of methadone, methylphenidate, dextropropoxyphene, and amphetamine pills, may incite a granulomatous reaction in the pulmonary interstitium, arteries, and arterioles

(Waller et al., 1980). Intravenous injection of talc-containing drugs intended for oral use may incite granulomatous inflammation and fibrosis surrounding the talc particles in the pulmonary interstitium in addition to causing emphysema (Peter Pare et al., 1989). BCG, which is used extensively in developing countries as a vaccination against *Mycobacterium tuberculosis* infection, and more recently as a stimulant of the body's immune system to treat or prevent various metastatic malignant diseases, has also been described to cause pulmonary granulomas (Gormsen, 1955; Au et al., 1978). Methotrexate (MTX) is widely used for the treatment of a variety of tumors as well as for nonneoplastic conditions. Pneumonitis associated with this drug is well described, although the mechanism of lung injury is not known (Cooper et al., 1986). The clinical presentation with fever and eosinophilia, the occasional findings of granuloma and multinucleated giant cells in pathological specimens, and the dramatic improvement in some patients following corticosteroid therapy suggest an immunological pathogenesis (White et al., 1984). The presence of increased BALF phenotypic helper/suppressor T cells in patients with MTX pneumonitis suggests an immunologically mediated injury rather than a direct toxic effect of this drug (White et al., 1989) (Fig. 6).

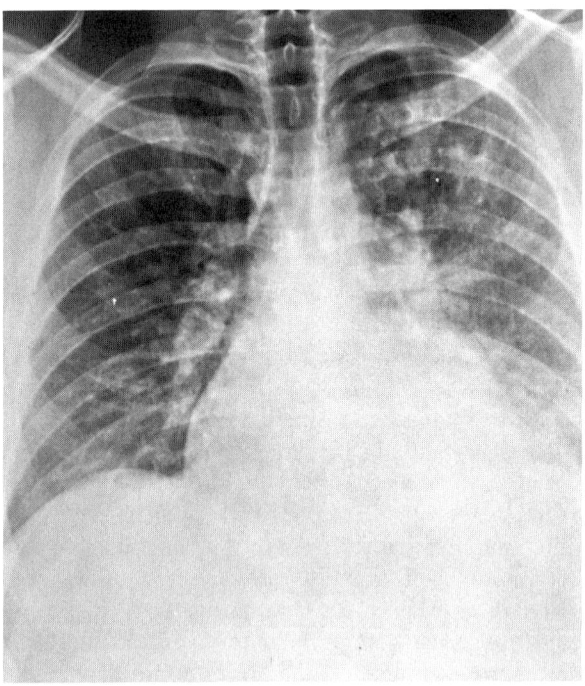

Figure 6 Diffuse pulmonary infiltration in a patient with methotrexate lung reaction.

XIV. Conclusion

International travel, student exchanges, and changing immigration patterns are steadily transforming tuberculosis and other granulomatous lung diseases in the United States and other developed countries. It is imperative that the clinician be aware of the increasing prevalence of illnesses previously regarded as "exotic." The definitive diagnosis of the cause of pulmonary granulomas is important. Mycobacterial, fungal, parasitic, and other infections must be differentiated distinguished from a variety of noninfectious granulomatous lesions since therapy is significantly different and, if inappropriate, may not only be ineffective but also, in many cases, deleterious.

References

Adams, A. R. D. (1980). Schistosomiasis. In *Clinical Tropical Disease*, 7th ed. London, Blackwell Scientific Publications, pp. 370-393.

Adams, D. O., and Hamilton, T. A. (1984). The cell biology of macrophage activation. *Annu. Rev. Immunol.* **2**:283-318.

Adams, J. S., Sharma, O. P., Gacad, M. A., et al. (1983). Metabolism of 25-hydroxy-vitamin D3 by cultured pulmonary alveolar macrophages in sarcoidosis. *J. Clin. Invest.* **72**:1856-1860.

Adams, J. S., Gacad, M., Singer, F. R., and Sharma, O. P. (1986). Production of 1,25-dihydroxyvitamin D3 by pulmonary alveolar macrophages from patients with sarcoidosis. *Ann. N.Y. Acad. Sci.* **465**:587-594.

Aftandelians, R., Raafat, F., Taffazoli, M., and Beaver, P. C. (1977). Pulmonary capillariasis in a child in Iran. *Am. J. Trop. Med. Hyg.* **26**:64-71.

Allen, D. H., Williams, G. V., and Woolcock, A. J. (1976). Bird breeder's hypersensitivity pneumonitis. Progress studies of lung function after cessation of exposure to the provoking antigen. *Am. Rev. Respir. Dis.* **114**:555-566.

Ando, M., Dannenberg, A. M., and Shima, K. (1972). Macrophage accumulation, division, maturation, and digestive and microbicidal capacities in tuberculous lesions. II. Rate at which mononuclear cells enter and divide in primary BCG lesions and those of re-infection. *J. Immunol.* **109**:8-19.

Andrade, Z. A., and Andrade, S. G. (1970). Pathogenesis of schistosomal pulmonary arteritis. *Am. J. Trop. Med. Hyg.* **19**:305-310.

Au, F. C., Webber, B., and Rosenberg, S. A. (1978). Pulmonary granulomas induced by BCG. *Cancer* **41**:2209-2214.

Bambry, P., Gupta, A., Sakhuja, V., Kaur, U., Gangwar, D. N., Jain, I. S., and Deodhar, S. D. (1987). Ocular manifestations of Wegener's granulomatosis in North India. *Sarcoidosis* **5**:132-135.

Berenguer, J., Cercenado, M. S., Bernaldo De Quiros, J. C. L., et al. (1989). Visceral leishmaniasis in patients with human immunodeficiency virus (HIV) infection. *Ann. Intern. Med.* **111**:129-132.

Bevanger, L., Maeland, J. A., and Naess, A. I. (1988). Agglutinins and antibodies to *Francisella tularensis* outer membrane antigens in the early diagnosis of disease during an outbreak of tularemia. *J. Clin. Microbiol.* **26**:433-437.

Blake, L. A., West, B. C., Lary, C. H., and Todd, J. R. (1987). Environmental nonhuman sources of leprosy. *Rev. Infect. Dis.* **9**(3):562-577.

Boros, D. L. (1978). Granulomatous inflammation. *Prog. Allergy* **24**:184-243.

Boros, D. L. (1988). Hypersensitivity granulomas. In *Allergy Principles and Practice*, 3rd ed. St. Louis, CV Mosby, pp. 275-294.

Boros, D. L., and Warren, K. S. (1970). Delayed hypersensitivity-type granuloma formation and dermal reaction induced and elicited by a soluble factor isolated from *Schistosoma mansoni* eggs. *J. Exp. Med.* **132**:488-507.

Buchanan, T. M., Brooks, G. F., and Brachman, P. S. (1971). The tularemia skin test. 325 skin tests in 210 persons: serologic correlation and review of the literature. *Ann. Intern. Med.* **74**:336-343.

Bullock, W. E., Evans, P. E., Wyatt, C., et al. (1976). Disturbance of lymphocyte circulation and mobilization in granulomatous disorders of the lymphoid system. *Ann. N.Y. Acad. Sci.* **276**:19-28.

Burgher, L. W., Kass, I., and Schenken, J. R. (1984). Pulmonary allergic granulomatosis: a possible drug reaction in a patient receiving cromolyn sodium. *Chest* **66**:84-86.

Chambers, T. J. (1978). Multinucleate giant cells. *J. Pathol.* **126**:125-148.

Charters, A. D. (1980). Brucellosis. *Aust. Fam. Physician* **9**(10):707-712.

Chhabra, S. K., and Gaur, S. N. (1988). Airway hyperreactivity in tropical pulmonary eosinophilia. *Chest* **93**:1105-1106.

Chumbley, L. C., Harrison, E. G., Jr., and DeRemee, R. A. (1977). Allergic granulomatosis and angiitis (Churg-Strauss syndrome). Report and analysis of 30 cases. *Mayo Clin. Proc.* **52**:477-484.

Churg, S., and Strauss, L. (1951). Allergic granulomatosis, allergic angiitis and periarteritis nodosa. *Am. J. Pathol.* **27**:277-301.

Cohen, M. L., Dawkins, R. L., Henderson, D. W., Sterrett, G. F., and Papadimitriou, J. M. (1979). Pulmonary lymphomatoid granulomatosis with immunodeficiency terminating as malignant lymphoma. *Pathology* **11**:537-550.

Cooper, J. A. D., White, D. A., and Matthay, R. A. (1986). Drug-induced pulmonary disease. Part I: cytotoxic drugs. *Am. Rev. Respir. Dis.* **133**:321-340.

Cullen, M. R., Kominsky, J. R., Rossman, M. D., et al. (1987). Chronic beryllium disease in a precious metal refinery. *Am. Rev. Respir. Dis.* **135**:201-208.

Dienst, F. T., Jr. (1963). Tularemia. A perusal of three hundred thirty-nine cases. *J. Louisiana State Med. Soc.* **115**:114-127.

Dinarello, C. A. (1984). Interleukin-1. *Rev. Infect. Dis.* **6**:51-95.

Fauci, A. S., and Wolff, S. M. (1973). Wegener's granulomatosis: studies in eighteen patients and a review of the literature. *Medicine* (*Baltimore*) **52**:535-561.

Fauci, A. S., Haynes, B. F., and Katz, P. (1978). The spectrum of vasculitis: clinical, pathologic, immunologic, and therapeutic considerations. *Ann. Intern. Med.* **89**:660-676.

Fink, J. N., Schleuter, D., and Sosman, A. (1972). Clinical survey of pigeon breeders. *Chest* **62**:277-281.

Goodwin, R. A., Jr., and Des Prez, R. M. (1978). State of the art: histoplasmosis. *Am. Rev. Respir. Dis.* **117**:929-956.

Gordon, S. (1976). Macrophage neutral proteinases and chronic inflammation. *Ann. N.Y. Acad. Sci.* **278**:176-189.

Gormsen, H. (1955). On the occurrence of epitheloid cell granulomas in the organs of BCG-vaccinated human beings. *Acta Pathol. Microbiol. Scand.* **111** (suppl):117-120.

Gupta, S. (1989). Treatment of sarcoidosis by steroid aerosol: a ten year prospective study from Eastern India. *Sarcoidosis* **5**:51-54.

Gupta, S. K., Bhutani, L. K., and Nath, I. (1982). The in situ characteristics of mononuclear cell infiltrates in dermal lesions of leprosy. *Int. J. Leprosy* **50**:297-305.

Hanson, G., Flod, N., Wells, I., Novey, H., and Galant, S. (1977). Bronchocentric granulomatosis: a complication of allergic bronchopulmonary aspergillosis. *J. Allergy Clin. Immunol.* **59**:83-90.

Hargreave, F., Hinson, K. F., Reid, L., Simon, G., and McCarthy, D. S. (1972). The radiologic appearance of allergic alveolitis due to bird sensitivity (bird fancier's lung). *Clin. Radiol.* **23**:1-10.

Hunninghake, G. W. (1983). Role of interleukin-2 release by lung T-cells in active pulmonary sarcoidosis. *Am. Rev. Resp. Dis.* **128**: 634-640.

Hunninghake, G. W. (1984). Correlation of interleukin-1 release by alveolar macrophages with disease active in pulmonary sarcoidosis. *Am. Rev. Respir. Dis.* **129**:569-574.

Hussain, R., and Ottesen, E. A. (1986). IgE responses in human filariasis. IV. Parallel antigen recongition by IgE and IgG4 subclass antibodies. *J. Immunol.* **135**:1859-1863.

Irusta, V. R. C. (1978). Contribuicao ao estudo da patologia pulmonar esquistossomotica experimental. *Revista de patologia tropical* **7**:203-242.

Israel, H. L., and Patchefsky, A. S. (1971). Wegener's granulomatosis of the lung. Diagnosis and treatment experience with 12 cases. *Ann. Intern. Med.* **74**:881-891.

Jaffe, C. L., and McMahon-Pratt, D. (1987). Serodiagnostic assay for visceral leishmaniasis employing monoclonal antibodies. Transactions of the Royal Society of Tropical Medicine and Hygiene; **81**(4):587-594.

Jindal, S. K., Dattatreya, R., Kumar, B., and Kaur, S. (1989). Airway hyporesponsiveness in leprosy—a clinical model of chronic pulmonary denervation, antithetic to asthma (abstract). *Chest* **92**:249S.

Jones-Williams, W. (1960). The nature and origin of Schaumann bodies. *J. Pathol. Bacteriol.* **79**:193-201.

Jones-Williams, W., Erasmus, D. A., James, V. E. M., and Davies, T. (1970). The fine structure of sarcoid and tuberculous granulomas. *Postgrad. Med.* **46**:496-500.

Jordans, H. G., and Debruin, K. D. (1980). Granulomas in *Brucella melitensis* infection (letter). *Ann. Intern. Med.* **92**:264-265.

Kasahara, K., Kobayashi, K., Shikama, Y., Yoneya, I., Soezima, K., Ide, H., and Takahashi, T. (1988). Direct evidence for granuloma-inducing activity of interleukin-1: induction of experimental pulmonary granuloma formation in mice by interleukin-1-coupled beads. *Am. J. Pathol.* **130**:;629-638.

Katzenstein, A. A., Liebow, A. A., and Friedman, P. J. (1975). Bronchocentric granulomatosis, mucoid impaction and hypersensitivity to fungi. *Am. Rev. Respir. Dis.* **111**:497-537.

Katzenstein, A. A., Carrington, C. B., and Liebow, A. A. (1979). Lymphomatoid granulomatosis. A clinicopathologic study of 152 cases. *Cancer* **43**:360-373.

Klech, H. (1986). Sarcoidosis: differential diagnosis. *Semin. Respir. Med.* **8**:72-94.

Kobayashi, K., Allred, C., Cohen, S., and Yoshida, T. (1985). Role of interleukin 1 in experimental pulmonary granuloma in mice. *J. Immunol.* **134**:358-364.

Kriebel, D., Brain, J. D., Sprince, N. L., and Kazemi, H. (1988). The pulmonary toxicity of beryllium. *Am. Rev. Respir. Dis.* **137**:;464-473.

Lanham, J. G., Elkon, K. B., Pusey, C. D., and Hughes, G. R. (1984). Systemic vasculitis with asthma and eosinophilia: a clinical approach to the Churg-Strauss syndrome. *Medicine* (*Baltimore*) **63**(2):65-81.

Leatherman, J. W., Michael, A. F., Schwartz, B. A., and Hoidal, J. R. (1984). Lung T cells in hypersensitivity pneumonitis. *Ann. Intern. Med.* **100**:390-392.

Lieberman, J., and Rea, T. H. (1977). Serum angiotensin-converting enzyme in leprosy and coccidiomycosis. *Ann. Intern. Med.* **87**:423-425.

Liebow, A. (1973). The J. Burns Anderson Lecture: Pulmonary angiitis and granulomatosis. *Am. Rev. Respir. Dis.* **108**:1-18.

Liebow, A., Carrington, C. B., and Friedman, P. J. (1972). Lymphomatoid granulomatosis. *Hum. Pathol.* **3**:457-558.

Lillie, R. D., and Francis, E. (1936). The pathology of tularemia in man (*Homo sapiens*). In *The Pathology of Tularemia.* National Institute of Health Bulletin 167. Washington, D.C., Public Health Service, pp. 1-82.

Manson-Bahr, P. E. C., and Apted, F. I. C. (1982). Leishmaniasis. In *Manson's Tropical Diseases*, 18th ed. London, Balliere Tindall, pp. 93-104.

Masih, N., Majeska, J., and Yoshida, T. (1979). Studies on experimental pulmonary granulomas: I. Detection of lymphokines in granulomatous lesions. *Am. J. Pathol.* **95**:391-406.

Mittal, K. R., and Tizzard, I. R. (1979). Experimental studies on the serologic relationships between *Yersinia enterocolitica* and *Brucella abortus. Res. Vet. Sci.* **27**:354-360.

Modlin, R. L., Hofman, F. M., Meyers, R. P., Sharma, O. P., Taylor, C. R., and Rea, T. H. (1983). In situ demonstration of T lymphocyte subsets in granulomatous inflammation: leprosy, rhinoscleroma, and sarcoidosis. *Clin. Exp. Immunol.* **51**:430-438.

Moyer, N. P., Evins, G. M., Pigott, N. E., Hudson, J. D., Farshy, C. E., et al. (1987). Comparison of serologic screening tests for brucellosis. *J. Clin. Microbiol.* **25**(10):1969-1972.

Myrvik, Q. N. (1982). Immunopathology of pulmonary granulomas. *Adv. Exp. Med. Biol.* **155**:649-657.

Narayanan, R. B. (1988). Immunopathology of leprosy granulomas—current status: a review. *Lepr. Rev.* **59**:75-82.

Narayanan, R. B., Bhutani, L. K., Sharma, A. K., and Nath, I. (1983). T-cell subsets in leprosy lesions; in situ characterization using monoclonal antibodies. *Clin. Exp. Immunol.* **51**:421-429.

Nash, T. E., Cheever, A. W., Ottesen, E. A., and Cook, J. A. (1982). Schistosome infections in humans: perspectives and recent findings. *Ann. Intern. Med.* **97**:740-754.

Neva, F. A., and Ottesen, E. A. (1978). Tropical (filarial) eosinophilia. *N. Engl. J. Med.* **298**:1129-1131.

Ottesen, E. A., Neva, F. A., Paranjape, R. S., Tripathy, S. P., Thiruvengadam, K. V., and Beaven, M. A. (1979). Specific allergic sensitisation to filarial antigens in tropical eosinophilia syndrome. *Lancet* **1**:1158-1161.

Papadimitriou, J. M., and Spector, W. G. (1971). The origin, properties and fate of epitheloid cells. *J. Pathol.* **105**:187-203.

Pertschuk, L. P., Silverstein, E., and Friedland, J. (1981). Immunohistologic diagnosis of sarcoidosis. Detection of angiotensin converting enzyme in sarcoid granulomas. *Am. J. Clin. Pathol.* **75**:350-361.

Peter Pare, J., Cote, G., and Fraser, R. S. (1989). Long-term follow-up of drug abusers with intravenous talcosis. *Am. Rev. Respir. Dis.* **139**:233-241.

Postlethwaite, A. E., Jackson, B. K., Beachey, E. H., and Kang, A. H. (1982). Formation of multinucleate giant cells from human monocyte precursors. Mediation by a soluble protein from antigen and mitogen stimulated lymphocytes. *J. Exp. Med.* **155**:168-178.

Reich, C. V. (1987). Leprosy: cause, transmission, and a new theory of pathogenesis. *Rev. Infect. Dis.* **9**(3):590-594.

Remick, D. G., Chensue, S. W., Hiserodt, J. C., Higashi, G. I., and Kunkel, S. L. (1988a). Flow-cytometric evaluation of lymphocyte subpopulations in synchronously developed *Schistosoma mansoni* egg and sephadex bead pulmonary granulomas. *Am. J. Pathol.* **131**:298-307.

Remick, D. G., Kunkel, S. L., Higashi, G. I., and Hiserodt, J. C. (1988b). Suppression of natural killer cytolytic activity in mice undergoing pulmonary granulomatous inflammation. *J. Immunol.* **140**:2225-2230.

Reynolds, H. Y., Fulmer, J. D., Kazierowski, J. A., et al. (1977). Analysis of cellular and protein content of bronchoalveolar lavage fluid from patients with idiopathic pulmonary fibrosis and chronic hypersensitivity pneumonitis. *J. Clin. Invest.* **59**:165-175.

Rossman, M. D., Kern, J. A., and Elias, J. A. (1988). Proliferative response of bronchoalveolar lymphocytes to beryllium. *Ann. Intern. Med.* **108**: 687-693.

Ryan, G. B., and Majno, G. (1977). Acute inflammation: a review. *Am. J. Pathol.* **86**:183-276.

Saltini, C., Winestock, K., Kirby, M., Pinkston, P., and Crystal, R. (1989). Maintenance of alveolitis in patients with chronic beryllium disease by beryllium-specific helper T cells. *N. Engl. J. Med.* **320**:1103-1109.

Sbarbaro, J. (1989). To treat or not to treat, that was the question (editorial). *Am. Rev. Respir. Dis.* **139**:865-866.

Schmid, G. P., Catino, D., Suffin, S. C., Martone, W. J., and Kaufmann, A. F. (1983). Granulomatous pleuritis caused by *Francisella tularensis*: possible confusion with tuberculous pleuritis. *Am. Rev. Respir. Dis.* **128**:314-316.

Semenzato, G., Pezzutto, A., Chiloso, M., and Pizzolo, G. (1982). Redistribution of T-lymphocytes in the lymph nodes of patients with sarcoidosis. *N. Engl. J. Med.* **306**:48-49.

Sharma, O. P. (1984). *Sarcoidosis: Clinical Management.* London, Butterworths.

Sirera Jimenez, G., et al. (1987). Brucellar pleuritis with a positive culture (letter). *Med. Clin. (Barc.)* **89**(16):708-709.

Sprince, N. L., Kanarek, D. J., Weber, A. L., Chamberlin, R. I., and Kazemi, H. (1978). Reversible respiratory disease in beryllium workers. *Am. Rev. Respir. Dis.* **117**:1011-1017.

Spry, C. J. F., and Kumaraswami, V. (1982). Tropical eosinophilia. *Semin. Hematol.* **19**:107-115.

Thompson, H. T., Pettigrew, R., and Johnson, E. A. (1979). Solitary pulmonary bilharzioma. *Thorax* **34**:401-403.

Ulbright, T. M., and Katzenstein, A. A. (1980). Solitary necrotizing granulomas of the lung. Differentiating features and etiology. *Am. J. Surg. Pathol.* **4**:13-28.

Van Voorhis, W. C., Kaplan, G., Sarno, E. N., Horwitz, M. A., et al. (1982). The cutaneous infiltrates of leprosy: cellular characteristics and predominant T cell phenotypes. *N. Engl. J. Med.* **307**:1593-1597.

Waller, B. F., Browmlee, W. J., and Roberts, W. C. (1980). Self-induced pulmonary granulomatosis. A consequence of intravenous injection of drugs intended for oral use. *Chest* **78**:90-94.

Watt, G., Long, G. W., Calubaquib, C., and Ranoa, C. P. (1986). Cardiopulmonary involvement rare in severe *Schistosoma japonicum. Trop. Geogr. Med.* **38**:233-239.

Weber, A. L., Stoeckle, J. D., and Hardy, H. L. (1965). Roentgenologic patterns in long-standing beryllium disease: report of 8 cases. *Am. J. Roentgenol.* **93**:879-890.

Weinstock, J. V. (1986). The significance of angiotensin 1 converting enzyme in granulomatous inflammation: function of ACE in granulomas. *Sarcoidosis* **3**:19-26.

West, B. C., Todd, J. R., and King, J. W. (1987). Wegener granulomatosis and trimethoprim-sulfamethoxazole. Complete remission after a twenty-year course. *Ann. Intern. Med.* **106**:840-842.

White, D. A., Orenstein, M., Godwin, T. A., and Stover, D. E. (1984). Chemotherapy-associated pulmonary toxic reactions during treatment for breast cancer. *Arch. Intern. Med.* **144**:953-956.

White, D. A., Rankin, J. A., Stover, D. E., Gellene, R. A., and Gupta, S. (1989). Methotrexate pneumonitis. Bronchoalveolar lavage findings suggest an immunologic disorder. *Am. Rev. Respir. Dis.* **139**:18-21.

Willcox, P. A., and Ferguson, A. D. (1989). Chronic obstructive airways disease following treated pulmonary tuberculosis. *Respir. Med.* **83**: 195-198.

Williams, G. T., and Jones-Williams, W. (1983). Granulomatous inflammation: a review. *J. Clin. Pathol.* **36**:723-730.

Woodruff, A. W., and Wright, S. G. (1987). *A Synopsis of Infectious and Tropical Diseases*, 3rd ed. Bristol, Wright.

Wyler, D. J., and Mardsen, P. D. (1984). Leishmaniasis. In *Tropical and Geographic Medicine.* Edited by K. S. Warren and A. A. F. Mahmoud. New York, McGraw-Hill, pp. 270-280.

Yoshida, T. (1980). Role of lymphokines in the induction and maintenance of the granuloma. In *Basic and Clinical Aspects of Granulomatous Diseases.* Edited by D. L. Boros and T. Yoshida. New York, Elsevier North Holland, pp. 81-94.

Young, E. J. (1983). Brucellosis. *Rev. Infect. Dis.* **5**(5):821-842.

3

Pulmonary Complications of Malaria

PRADEEP BAMBERY, SURINDER K. JINDAL, and UPJEET KAUR

Postgraduate Institute of Medical Education and Research
Chandigarh, India

I. Malaria: The Problem

Malaria continues to ravage large tracts of the tropics relentlessly. Although it is a major tropical disorder, the rise in world travel has rendered it an almost global phenomenon. Thus medical personnel far removed from the tropics must also be informed of the protean manifestations and devastating complications of this potentially curable infection (Miller et al., 1989).

Despite impressive progress in understanding the biology of the malarial parasite and its interactions with cells of the human body, we are still far from finding a solution to the problem of malaria eradication (Neva, 1967; Wernsdorfer, 1980). The heady optimism regarding malaria eradication in India during the 1950s and 1960s has now been replaced by a more cautious and pragmatic program of control. Eradication has been thwarted by a conglomeration of factors, which include vector resistance to pesticides, parasite resistance to drugs, alterations in the ecology, and the movement of populations. Given the prevailing conditions in most parts of the malarious world, these problems are likely to increase in magnitude. It is also well established that most nations, in which malaria severely curtails national productivity, lack the financial resources to launch effective control programs (Wernsdorfer, 1980). In addition, the territories where drug-resistant malaria is frequent now cover large tracts of Southeast Asia, the Pacific, Africa, South and Central America (Neva, 1967; Cook, 1986). In the 1950s, drug resistance was confined to much smaller pockets. It is estimated that 150 million persons are affected by malaria in Asia, Africa, and South America and that 1 million die as a consequence each year (Quinn and Plorde, 1981). Excluding the incidence in sub-Saharan Africa, 6 million new cases are notified annually (Cook, 1986).

II. Historical Perspective

Human malaria has been known since the earliest of times. The first recognizable references were found in ancient Egyptian papyri (Boyd, 1949; Wernsdorfer, 1980). Hippocrates described the fever accurately (Boyd, 1949). Effective therapy became available almost 200 years before the cause was identified. The alkaloid quinine was purified in the early years of the last century. The causative parasite, its life cycle, and transmission to humans by the vector were detailed towards the turn of the century (Ross, 1902; Boyd, 1949; Wernsdorfer, 1980). The greatest stimulus to the development of malariology was, however, provided by its adverse effects on military operations during the wars of the last 100 years. Ross (1902) commented on the serious impact of malaria on the fitness, morale, and battle-worthiness of the British Army in India. The Gallipoli campaign in World War I, the Far East and Pacific actions during World War II, and the experience in Vietnam have served to sustain and further reinforce this contention (Boyd, 1949; Blount, 1964, 1969; Neva, 1967; Wernsdorfer, 1980). So great was the need of the military that most of the antimalarial drugs in use today had their origins in military research programs (Peters, 1980).

The pulmonary complications of malaria had been recognized towards the end of the 1800s (Marchiafava and Bignami, 1900; Ross, 1902; Watson, 1905). Pneumonitis (Applebaum and Shrager, 1944) was initially considered the major problem; however, detailed pathological studies later demonstrated pulmonary edema, pleural effusion, and bacterial pneumonia (Spitz, 1946). Clinical recognition of noncardiogenic pulmonary edema was made in the 1960s (Sheehy and Reba, 1967; Brooks et al., 1968). Pulmonary abnormalities occur only in infections with *Plasmodium falciparum* or in mixed infections with both *P. vivax* and *P. falciparum* (WHO Malaria Action Programme 1986; Warrell, 1987).

III. Life Cycle of the Malaria Parasite

Human malaria is caused by four species belonging to the genus *Plasmodium* (*Plasmodium vivax, P. falciparum, P. ovale,* and *P. malariae*). The parasite is transmitted to humans following the bite of an infected female anopheline mosquito. The sporozoites injected enter the bloodstream briefly and then enter the host liver cells, probably guided by a chemotactic stimulus and aided by reticuloendothelial cells (Wernsdorfer, 1980). Exoerythrocytic schizogony ensues and after 12-16 nuclear divisions 2000-30,000 merozoites are liberated by rupture of the schizont. The apical ends of the merozoites contain rhoptries and micronemes that facilitate attachment to and invagination into the red cell (Aikawa and Seed, 1980). Erythrocytic schizogony entails formation and growth of a trophozoite that ingests homoglobin. Three to five divisions later erythrocytic merozoites are formed and liberated by schizont rupture. These merozoites either continue the process of erythrocytic schizogony or undergo gametogony. The gametes fuse in the lumen of the mosquito stomach after an infected blood meal and form an ookinete that penetrates the gut epithelium to become an oocyst. Motile sporozoites are released into the hemolymph by oocyst rupture and move to the salivary glands (Ross, 1902; Wernsdorfer, 1980).

Plasmodium falciparum, by virtue of its capacity to infect red cells of all ages, produces very high levels of parasitemia (Field, 1949; Neva et al., 1970) and is thus the only parasite associated with the development of severe complicated malaria. (WHO Malaria Action Programme, 1986). *Plasmodium vivax* infection can occasionally result in severe malaria also, but invariably in a mixed infection with *P. falciparum*.

IV. Host Defenses

The ability to resist the development of malaria has a genetic and immunological basis (Warrell, 1987). In addition, the nutritional status of an individual may adversely affect the maturation of the parasite. Undernourished children have less severe malaria and epidemics of malaria are less devastating when there is a coexistent famine (Garnham, 1980). Conflicting reports are available regarding the protective role of riboflavin deficiency (Cook, 1986; Das et al., 1988).

A. Genetic Defenses

Genetic mechanisms prevent merozoite attachment to the red cell membrane and also inhibit the intracellular development of the parasite (Perrin et al., 1982; Warrell, 1987; Plorde and White, 1987). Duffy blood-group-negative red cells are naturally resistant to the attachment and entry of *Plasmodium knowlesi* and *P. vivax* merozoites. Surface treatment with chymotrypsin also confers this property to Duffy-positive cells (Barnwell et al., 1989). This suggests that the Duffy material on the cell membrane is a specific receptor. No such absolute phenomena have been described in *P. falciparum* malaria.

The intracellular development of *P. falciparum* is, however, adversely affected by the presence of fetal hemoglobin (HbF), sickle cell anemia (HbS), glucose-6-phosphate dehydrogenase (G-6 PD) deficiency, and the thalassemia syndromes (Neva et al., 1970; Perrin et al., 1982). In HbS disease, normal parasite development is possible in the presence of normal oxygen tension. However, in vivo trapping of infected red cells in deep visceral circulation where oxygenation is poor results in parasite death.

B. Immunological Defenses

From observations in highly endemic areas it is clear that acquired immunity prevents severe *P. falciparum* malaria (Warrell, 1987). In such areas, children constitute the most susceptible population. Severe *P. falciparum* malaria develops in the indigenous adult population in these areas consequent to immune suppression. These conditions include pregnancy (Editorial, 1983), steroid and cytotoxic drug therapy, splenectomy (Eling, 1980; Garnham, 1980), and a prolonged stay away from the area, in a low or nonendemic zone. The exact humoral factor responsible is, as yet, unidentified.

V. Pathophysiology of Severe Malaria: Pulmonary Edema

Pulmonary edema is a dreaded, highly fatal complication of severe *P. falciparum* malaria (Brooks et al., 1967; Punyagupta et al., 1974; Barrett-Connor, 1982; James, 1985; WHO Malaria Action Programme, 1986; Plorde and White, 1987; Warrell, 1987). There is paucity of information on its development in human disease. However, a frequently coexisting complication, cerebral malaria, has been extensively studied. Elegant animal experiments have revealed several other pathogenetic mechanisms that have been postulated to operate in humans. This extrapolation is fraught with difficulties since concrete evidence is as yet unavailable. These studies have, however, served to highlight the myriad factors that may contribute to pulmonary edema (Robin et al., 1973; Ingram, 1987). The possible interplay of these factors is summarized in Figure 1.

A. Alterations in Infected Red Blood Cells

Infection of red blood cells (RBC) by merozoites of *P. falciparum* result in many structural and functional changes.

Anemia

Severe anemia is a well documented feature of *P. falciparum* malaria (Abdalla et al., 1980; Perrin et al., 1982). Schizont rupture and hemolysis, increased

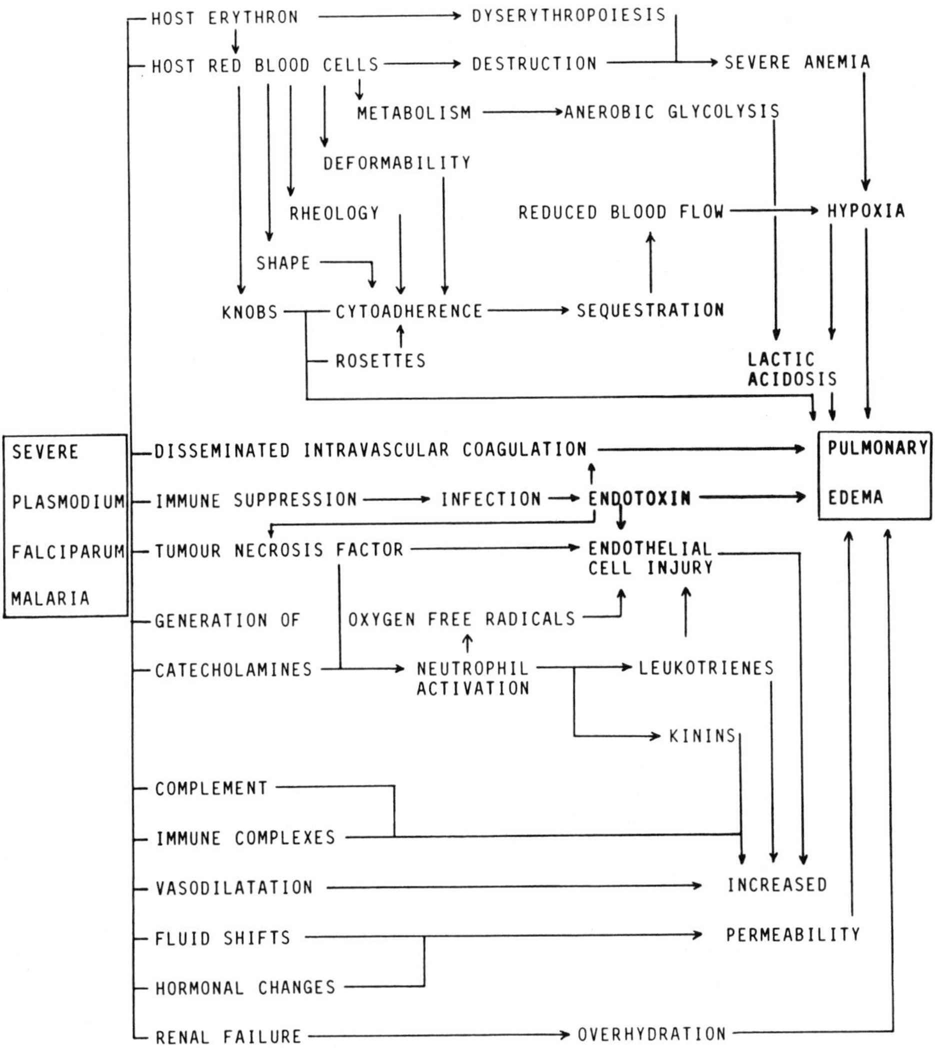

Figure 1 Schematic representation of the possible pathogenesis of malarial pulmonary edema.

phagocytosis of the infected cells, immune-mediated hemolysis, and dyserythropoiesis are the mechanisms involved. A Coombs-positive hemolytic anemia supports the immunological basis (Holmes, 1987).

Altered RBC Metabolism

These changes result in increasing anerobic glycolysis (Warrell, 1987).

Altered RBC Deformability

Parasitized RBC are less deformable than normal cells (Miller et al., 1972) and the degree increases with parasite maturity (Cranston et al., 1984). As a consequence, it would be expected that these cells would fail to negotiate the narrowest portions of the capillaries, but this was not demonstrated on a careful human ultrastructural study (MacPherson et al., 1985).

Changes in the RBC Membrane

Infected cells show extensive pitting and undergo a gradual change in shape to spherical with increasing maturity of the parasite (Aikawa and Seed, 1980). Alterations in cell surface charge, glycoprotein content, fluidity, and enzyme distribution result in deranged rheological properties and enhanced sequestration (Warrell, 1987).

Development of Surface Knobs

These projections are formed and increase in number with the maturity of the parasite. They facilitate adherence to endothelial cells (Udeinya et al., 1981; Perrin et al., 1982) and amelanotic melanoma cells (Sherman and Valdez, 1989) by binding to receptors. A parasite-related protein, rich in histidine, is found to underlie the knobs. The process of binding involves the projection of strain-specific, potent malarial antigenic protein (adhesin) through the knob into close proximity of an endothelial ligand identical to thrombospondin (Lawler, 1986). Binding is inhibited by antibodies to thrombospondin. Intact splenic function facilitates binding (David et al., 1983) while splenectomy prevents or reduces it considerably (Garnham, 1980). Recent evidence suggests that infected RBC induce spontaneous rosette formation by noninfected cells, thereby aiding adherence (David et al., 1988; Udomsangpetch et al., 1989). This is inhibited by immune serum and heparin. Knobs have also been implicated in respiratory distress (Corbett et al., 1989).

B. Mediators and Mechanisms of Injury

A large number of substances have been implicated in the development of increased vascular permeability, which has been postulated as a major pathogenetic mechanism in pulmonary edema observed in severe malaria. Although increased permeability has not been demonstrated to play a part in human cerebral malaria, and Warrell (1987) insists that experiments have refuted any possible role in cerebral disease, pulmonary edema is a complication at considerable variance from the others encountered during the course of severe complicated malaria (WHO Malaria Action Programme, 1986). The pathological appearance of malarial pulmonary edema suggests that increased permeability does indeed play a major role in its development. The mediators and mechanisms are discussed in the sections below.

Histamine

High circulating levels were found in animal and human subjects (Maegraith and Onabanjo, 1970) but the use of specific H_1 and H_2 receptor blockers in further studies eliminated any major role (Martins et al., 1986).

Kinins

These were initially suggested as mediators of vasodilatation and increased permeability via a catecholamine-induced neutrophil injury (Onabanjo and Maegraith 1970a,b; Janoff et al., 1988). Elevated levels of kallikrein (Onabanjo and Maegraith, 1970a) and bradykinin (Cordiero et al., 1983) have been observed to correlate with increased permeability in animal studies.

Reduced Serum Albumin

Reduced synthesis consequent to subclinical hepatic injury was proposed (Hall, 1977) but later refuted by results of detailed studies (Cordiero et al., 1983; Warrell, 1987).

Oxygen Free Radicals

Generation of these radicals during the respiratory burst of neutrophils adherent to endothelial cells is a final common mechanism in cellular injury (Warrell, 1987; Ingram, 1987; Arias and Walter, 1988) and has been implicated in the damage to endothelial cells. This phenomenon is also operative in endotoxin-induced RBC injury and hemolysis (Clark and Hunt, 1983). Neutrophil injury also releases other mediators—leukotrienes and products of the arachidonic acid system (Ingram, 1987)—both of which are mediators of cellular injury.

Tumor Necrosis Factor

Experimental studies (Clark et al., 1987) showed that this substance induced several pathological processes documented in malaria. It resulted in endothelial cell damage, neutrophil activation, hemolysis, dyserythropoiesis, and possibly abortions in pregnant animals (Clark and Chaudhri, 1988). Elevated levels have also been observed in human disease.

Immunological Mechanisms

Complement activation and immune complex formation are well-described causes of vascular injury and consequent increased permeability. Conflicting observations on the role of complement are available (Neva et al., 1970; Warrell, 1987) but its depletion in human disease has been confirmed (Warrel, 1987). Immune complexes have been demonstrated in human malaria but no vasculitis is seen (MacPherson et al., 1985). In a mouse *Plasmodium berghei* experimental model, Weiss and Kubat (1983) convincingly demonstrated immune complexes comprised of IgM, C_3, C_4, and malarial antigen in the kidneys and the lungs. Their clinical observations on these animals also revealed several similarities to human pulmonary edema. The recently observed phenomenon of spontaneous rosetting of uninfected RBC around an infected RBC substantiates the immunological basis of injury (David et al., 1988; Udomsangpetch et al., 1989).

Current evidence suggests that human immune competence is also compromised in severe malaria (Marsh and Greenwood, 1986) and that there is an increased susceptibility to secondary infections and septicemia (Bygbjerg and Lanng, 1982).

Endotoxin

Elevated levels of endotoxin have been demonstrated in human malaria due to *P. falciparum* (Tubbs, 1980; WHO Malaria Action Programme, 1986) but the parasite itself does not contain it (Warrell, 1987). The elevation is ascribed to coexistent bacterial infection. Endotoxin has been implicated in hemolysis-related vascular injury, release of tumor necrosis factor, and disseminated intravascular coagulation (DIC) (Clark and Hunt, 1983).

DIC

Punyagupta et al. (1974) reported a high incidence of DIC in their patients with pulmonary edema and suggested that heparin be used as treatment. Their findings could also be ascribed to other complications observed in their group of patients (Warrell, 1987). Renal failure, heparin and corticosteroid therapy, and low-molecular-weight dextran infusion could have significantly contributed to the bleeding observed in their patients.

Vasodilation and Fluid Shifts

These were documented in human disease (Brooks et al., 1967; Malloy et al., 1967) and could contribute to pulmonary edema.

Overhydration and Cardiac Dysfunction

Uncontrolled fluid administration to patients who have renal failure has resulted in pulmonary edema (Brooks et al., 1968; James, 1985). However, in the majority of patients, the central venous pressure was low (James, 1985) and there was no convincing evidence of significant cardiac dysfunction in malaria (Sprague, 1946).

Reduced Oxygen Uptake

This was demonstrated in volunteer experiments with *Plasmodium vivax* (Henschel et al., 1950).

It must be stressed that the development of pulmonary edema is a dynamic event of great complexity. The factors mentioned may all play major parts at different times during the pathogenesis and are, hence, either ignored or overemphasized depending upon the timing of the studies. It is expected that once the pathogenesis is clearly elucidated, newer modes of therapy may emerge based on specific inhibitors of major mediators of injury.

VI. Pulmonary Syndromes in Malaria

Symptoms and signs of pulmonary disease occur in 3-10% of patients with *Plasmodium falciparum* malaria (Brooks et al., 1968). The clinical picture is varied and ranges from mild upper respiratory problems to severe and rapidly fatal pulmonary edema (Sheehy and Reba, 1967; Brooks et al., 1968). The major pulmonary complications of malaria in humans are pulmonary edema and the adult respiratory distress syndrome (ARDS). Pneumonitis, pleural effusion, and secondary bacterial pneumonias also occur. Functional impairment, in the absence of clinical symptoms or signs of pulmonary involvement (Tong et al., 1972a), has been described.

Pulmonary edema was observed in only 3 of 3,300 patients (Sheehy and Reba, 1967) in Vietnam, but was not encountered in another series of over 2,000 patients from the same area (Blount, 1969). In Brazil, 4% of 200 patients with *P. falciparum* malaria required mechanical ventilation (Duarte et al., 1985) while in India 5 of 425 patients developed this complication (Mehta et al., 1989). It is thus an uncommon problem (Barrett-Connor, 1982) but carries the highest mortality (80%) associated with any complication of severe malaria (Plorde and White, 1987). Pneumonia was recorded in 3.7% of patients with malaria in the Panama Canal Zone (Applebaum and Shrager, 1944), but this included an equal number of patients with *P. falciparum* and *P. vivax* malaria. Pleural effusions are a frequent autopsy finding but a clinically significant effusion has been described in only one patient (Al-Ibrahim and Holzman, 1975). The clinical features, pathological appearance, an illustrative case report, and the experimental models useful in the study of pulmonary edema are described below.

A. Pulmonary Edema and ARDS

The first clinical description was made by Watson (1905), but it was not accorded significance (Kitchen, 1949) until several decades later when it was seen in several patients during the Vietnam War (Sheehy and Reba, 1967; Brooks et al., 1968; Deaton, 1970; Neva et al., 1970; Tong et al., 1972a). The pathological lesion had, however, been recognized much earlier (Marchiafava and Bignami, 1900; Spitz, 1946; Clark and Tomlinson, 1949).

In many respects, pulmonary edema is an unusual complication of *P. falciparum* malaria. Unlike cerebral malaria, anemia, and renal failure, it occurs late in the course of the disease, often several days after antimalarial drug therapy has been instituted (Deaton, 1970; Neva et al., 1970; Punyagupta et al., 1974; James, 1985; WHO Malaria Action Programme, 1986). There may be little or no evidence of heavy parasitemia at the time of development, unlike cerebral malaria. It carried the highest mortality among the pernicious malaria complications and apparently has different pathophysiological influences operative in its genesis compared to cerebral malaria (WHO Malaria Action Programme, 1986; Warrell, 1987). The prime determinant of the outcome of such patients was not only the adequacy of the antimalarial therapy but also the intensive management of hypoxia (James, 1985). As with other malarial complications, recovery, if it occurred, was remarkable and complete (Punyagupta et al., 1974; Marks et al., 1977; Fein et al., 1978; Martell et al., 1979; James, 1985; WHO Malaria Action Programme, 1986). Pregnant women (Editorial, 1983; WHO Malaria Action Programme, 1986), immunocompromised patients, nonimmune adults, and very young children developed this complication frequently.

In its most severe form, pulmonary edema is preceded by a sense of tightening of the chest, a dry cough, and an entirely normal chest examination. This is followed within hours by the catastrophic development of rapidly progressive restlessness and agitation, dyspnea, orthopnea, cyanosis, productive cough, and pink frothy sputum. The lungs then show the characterstic signs of pulmonary edema that are easily confirmed radiologically (Punyagupta et al., 1974). Such patients often had coexisting cerebral, renal, hemostatic, and hematological complications of malaria (WHO Malaria Action Programme, 1986).

In highly endemic areas, such a constellation was easily recognized as a potentially lethal consequence of malaria and treatment was usually started immediately. However, it must be differentiated from aspiration pneumonia, overhydration in the presence of renal failure, and other causes of ARDS. This group of clinical features is nonspecific and in nontropical areas may lead to a markedly delayed diagnosis (Neva et al., 1970; Barrett-Connor, 1982) and high mortality. Milder forms of pulmonary interstitial edema that cleared quickly and did not necessitate mechanical ventilation have also been described occasionally (Cayea et al., 1981; Godard and Hansen, 1971). It is not clear at this time why certain individuals developed severe and others developed mild pulmonary edema. It may be related to the virulence of the parasite (Schmidt, 1978; Warrell, 1987) or the immune response of the host. In patients who survived severe pulmonary edema, the radiological clearing commenced by day 3 and was usually completed in another 2-5 days (Punyagupta et al., 1974; James, 1985).

Hemodynamic monitoring of these patients excluded significant cardiac dysfunction. The findings were low central venous pressure, reduced pulmonary artery wedge pressure (except in coexistent renal insufficiency where these may be high), and a normal cardiac index (Fein et al., 1978; Martell et al., 1979). The response of fully developed pulmonary edema to therapy with diurectics, digitalis, nasal oxygen, corticosteroids, heparin, tourniquets, and low-molecular-weight dextran infusion has been uniformly poor (Punyagupta et al., 1974). Only the prompt correction of hypoxia by mechanical ventilation has helped to save some patients (James, 1985).

Controversy exists regarding the role of DIC in the genesis of pulmonary edema. Punyagupta et al. (1974) observed DIC in 10 of their 12 patients with pulmonary edema, but these observations have not been substantiated by others. Warrell (1987) ascribed DIC to the administration of heparin and low-molecular-weight dextran infusion in patients with secondary infections, renal failure, and cerebral malaria.

B. Malarial Pneumonitis

In the clinical setting of severe complicated malaria, the development of pneumonitis can be attributed to several factors other than the malarial parasite (Applebaum and Shrager, 1944; Kitchen, 1949; Tong et al., 1972b; WHO Malaria Action Programme, 1986). Pneumonitis in patients with malaria was classified as viral or atypical, secondary bacterial, and true malarial based on the response to therapy. The first group did not respond at all, the second responded to sulfonamides, and the third to antimalarials (Applebaum and Shrager, 1944). Response was judged clinically and by radiological disappearance of opacities in the lungs. Today we know that sulfonamides have an antimalarial effect also. Nearly 4% of malaria patients in the Panama Canal Zone developed pneumonitis, with equal numbers being due to *Plasmodium falciparum* and *P. vivax* infections. There was only 1 death among 125 patients. If malarial pneumonia genuinely exists, it is a minor cause of mortality.

Cough, expectoration, chest pain, rales, bronchial breathing, and dullness to percussion were the clinical features, in decreasing order of frequency. Hemoptysis and pleural rub were rare. At radiological examination lobular consolidation was seen in all patients, except in 7% who had lobar pneumonia (Applebaum and Shrager, 1944). Since the publication of this series, there has been no major work on this phenomenon except for a small study during the Vietnam war (Tong et al., 1972b). There has been no convincing demonstration of parasites in the sputum, nor has there been any conclusive elimination of other pathogens as causative factors. However, the response of consolidation to antimalarial therapy alone does support the existence of such entities.

C. Pleural Effusion

A clinically significant effusion necessitating drainage has been described in only one patient with *P. falciparum* malaria (Al-Ibrahim and Holzman, 1975) and this patient also had histoplasmosis. Applebaum and Shrager (1944) reported an overall incidence of 2.5% in their patients with pneumonitis, but did not specify the responsible parasite/organism.

Pleural effusions are frequently found at autopsy in patients dying of pulmonary edema. Punyagupta et al. (1974) observed effusions varying from 70 to 560 ml in eight of nine autopsied patients; Brooks et al. (1968) likewise reported them in four of five patients. Excess pleural fluid at necropsy was also noted by others (Deaton, 1970; Neva et al., 1970; Tong et al., 1972b). These effusions probably have little if any clinical significance, since they are never large enough to compromise respiratory function seriously. Some of the experimental models of malaria in mammals also showed pleural effusions at autopsy (MacCallum, 1968; Schmidt, 1978).

D. Secondary Bacterial Pneumonia

Cerebral symptoms, coma, convulsions, vomiting, aspiration, renal failure, corticosteroid administration, and innate immune suppression are all part of the syndrome of severe complicated malaria (WHO Malaria Action Programme, 1986), and contribute to the frequent development of bacterial (gram-negative bacillary) pneumonia in such patients (Warrell, 1987). These infections also contribute significantly to morbidity and mortality. Ross (1902) alluded to pneumonia being a common mode of death in patients who were severely debilitated by malaria.

Septicemia and its associated complications must be avidly sought and either excluded or energetically treated to minimize the high mortality rate.

E. Pulmonary Function Abnormalities

Arterial hypoxemia was observed during the course of malarial infection several years ago (Meldolesi, 1931). However, to date there has only been one well-documented study of functional abnormalities in patients with *P. falciparum* malaria (Tong et al., 1972a). Results were compared with normal subjects and two groups of patients were identified on the basis of presence or absence of respiratory complaints. Even those patients who had no pulmonary symptoms had reduced $PaCO_2$, increased blood pH, increased work of breathing, and tachypnea compared to normals. Those with pulmonary edema had hypoxia, reduced compliance, increased shunting, alkalosis, and marked tachypnea. This study convincingly demonstrated that functional impairment preceded radiological evidence of pulmonary involvement and also confirmed an earlier study in demonstrating an increase in the work of breathing (Henschel et al., 1950). James (1985) observed hypoxia in 7 of 10 nonimmune white patients with malaria but in only 3 of 20 native black patients, thus reinforcing the contention that indigenous immune populations are less susceptible to severe complications.

F. Pulmonary Pathological Findings

On gross examination the lungs have a slaty grey pigmented appearance and are overweight (Spitz, 1946; Clark and Tomlinson, 1949; Punyagupta et al., 1974; Aikawa et al., 1980). The combined weight of the lungs may be in excess of 2000 g. Spitz (1946) demonstrated pulmonary edema in all of 50 autopsied patients. Twenty-five of them also had pneumonitis. Subpleural petichiae and pulmonary hemorrhages were also documented.

On light microscopic examination the predominant features observed were alveolar, septal, and interstitial edema; cogestion of blood vessels; hyaline membrane formation; alveolar hemorrhage; and occasionally fibrin deposition. These findings are quite nonspecific and a definite diagnosis of malaria-related pulmonary edema must be based on the demonstration of parasitized RBC in the dilated and packed vascular channels. Malarial pigment-laden macrophages must also be visible. Goodall (1973) described giant nuclear masses in the peripheral blood and lungs of two patients who died of pulmonary edema of malarial origin. This finding has not yet been substantiated even with electron microsopic examination (Duarte et al., 1985). In severe human *P. falciparum* malaria, parasitized RBCs are observed in the largest numbers in the cerebral vessels followed by the cardiac, hepatic, pulmonary, and renal vasculature (MacPherson et al., 1985).

Ultrastructural study of the lungs in a patient who died of *P. falciparum* malaria-related pulmonary edema revealed alveolar septal edema and dissociation of the normally close association between the matrix and fibrils of the alveolar septa. The capillary lumen was compromised due to the swelling of endothelial cells that contained mildly distorted rough endoplasmic reticulum and mitochondria. There were no major changes in the type I and type II pneumocytes (Duarte et al., 1985). A more recent study has suggested the close association between the surface knobs of the parasitized RBC and the genesis of pulmonary edema. Cytoadherent knob-bearing RBC were demonstrated in both patients who died of pulmonary edema and were conspicuous by their absence in the third patient who did not have edema (Corbett et al., 1989). There was no evidence of dilated lymphatics, as had been demonstrated in the hamster *Plasmodium berghei* model (MacCallum, 1968).

G. Case Report

A 30-year-old pregnant woman in the 37th week of gestation was referred in deep coma, with a history of intermittent, high-grade fever accompanied by chills and rigors and altered sensorium for the preceding 4 days. At another hospital, a diagnosis of cerebral malaria has been considered and established by the demonstration of ring and gamete forms of *Plasmodium falciparum*. She had received parenteral dexamethasone and oral pyrimethamine 25 mg plus sulfalene 500 mg with no improvement over 3 days. She was already in the second stage of labor at the time of admission and soon delivered a stillborn boy. The third stage of labor and the early puerperal period were not complicated by excessive bleeding. At the time of admission she was deeply comatose and unresponsive. Reflexes were exaggerated and the plantar response was extensor. Although she was tachypneic (rate 40/min) the lungs were clinically clear. She had severe anemia (hemoglobin 4 g/dl) and leukocytosis (initial leukocyte count 15,000/mm^3 and later 34,000/mm^3) with 80-92% polymorphonuclear leukocytes. Ring forms and gametes of *Plasmodium falciparum* were seen. She also had renal insufficiency (serum creatinine level 3.0 mg/dl).

Under strict monitoring, fluids and blood were infused along with parenteral quinine 600 mg in a drip every 8 h. Penicillin, metronidazole, and gentamicin were administered for treatment of possible secondary infection. On the second day the blood findings of malarial parasites became negative yet on the third day she experienced seizures and refractory pulmonary edema. Blood gas analysis revealed PaO_2 70 mmHg, $PaCO_2$ 20 mmHg, pH 7.54, and HCO_3 16 mEq/L. Coagulation parameters were abnormal, with a prothrombin index of 60% and a 27 s prolongation in the partial thromboplastin time, but there was no bleeding diathesis. She died a day later.

The placenta was heavily parasitized. At necropsy the typical gross and microscopic features of cerebral malaria were present. The lungs were congested and edamatous (Fig. 2a). Thickened alveolar septa and hyaline membrane formation were seen (Fig. 2b). Blood vessels were packed with cells and macrophages were laden with malarial pigment (Fig. 2c). Patchy consolidation, presumably bacterial, was seen (Fig. 2d) along with parasitized RBCs in the dilated septal vessels (Fig. 2e).

This patient demonstrated several clinically important aspects of severe *P. falciparum* malaria (WHO Malaria Action Programme, 1986). Increased

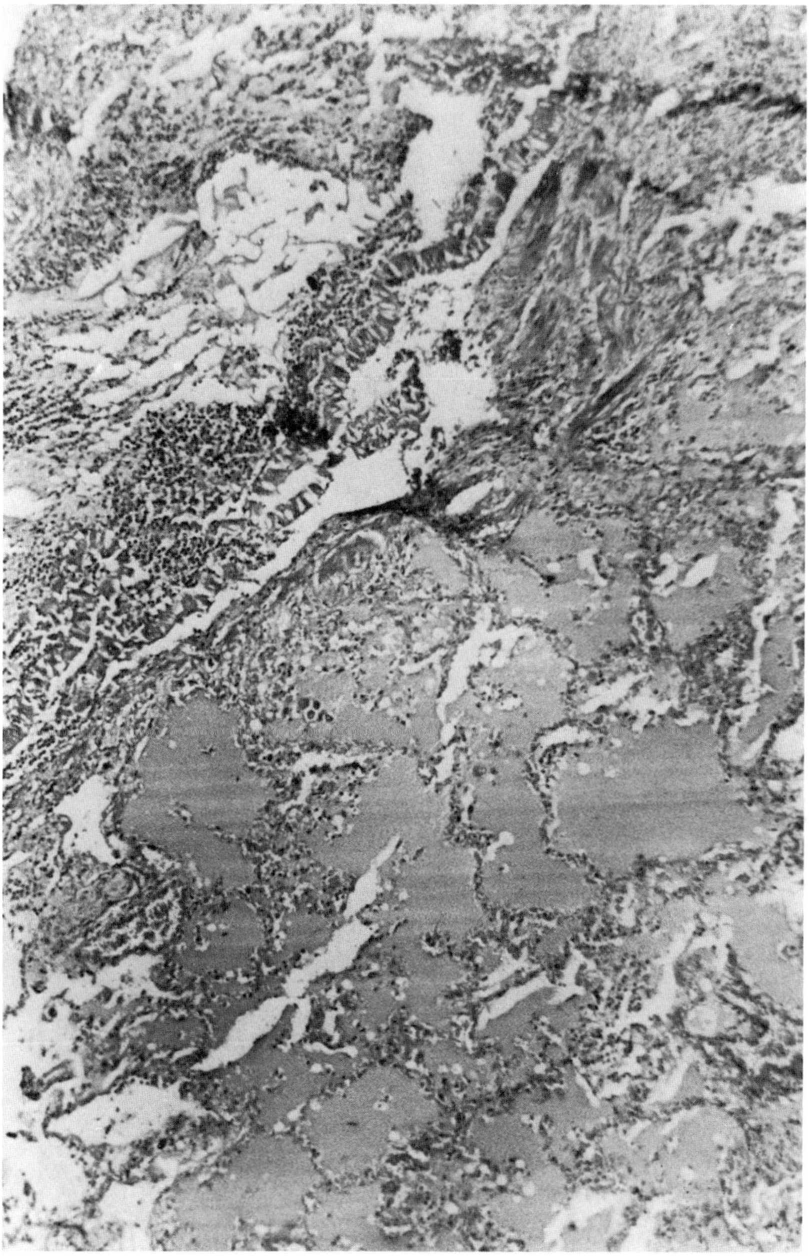

Figure 2 Histological appearance of the lung at autopsy. **a**. Extensive pulmonary edema (hematoxylin and eosin × 120).

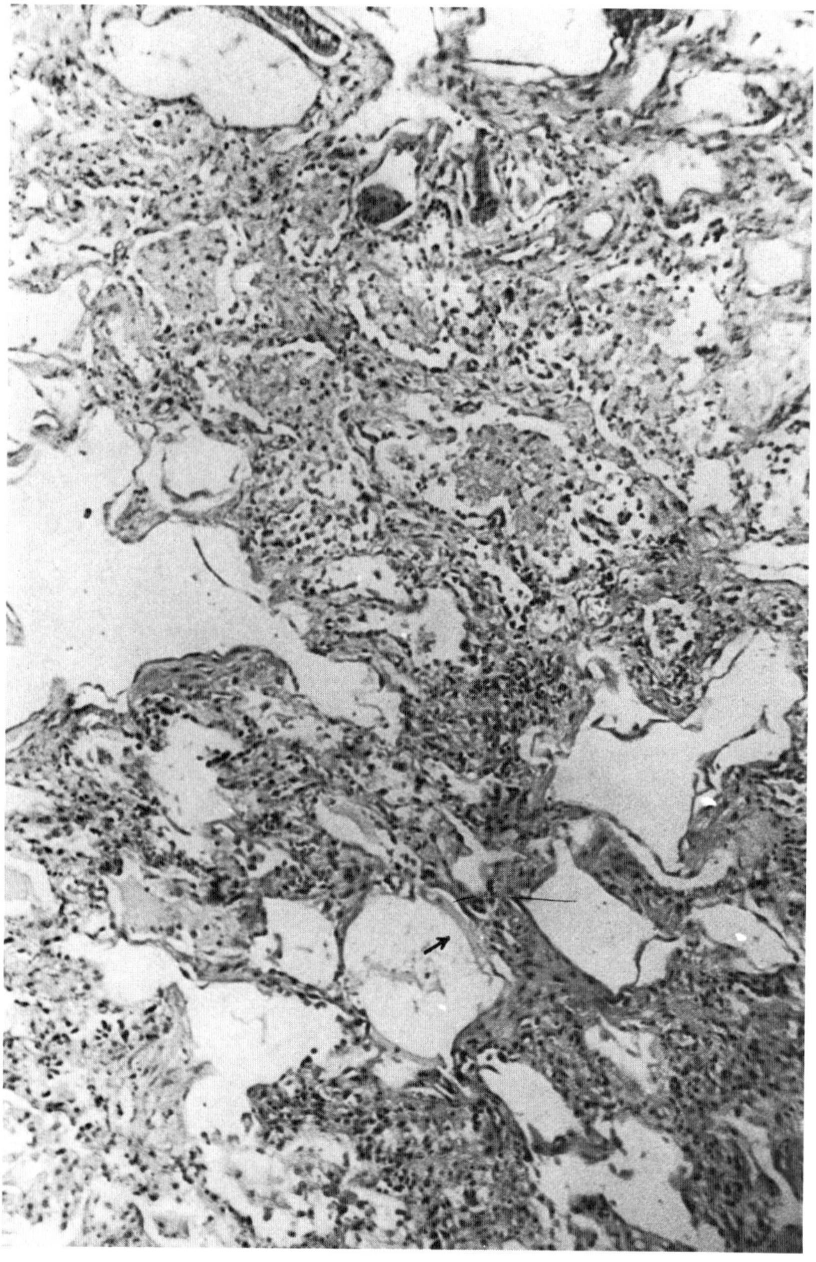

Figure 2b Markedly thickened alveolar septa and hyaline membrane formation (→); (hematoxylin and eosin × 120).

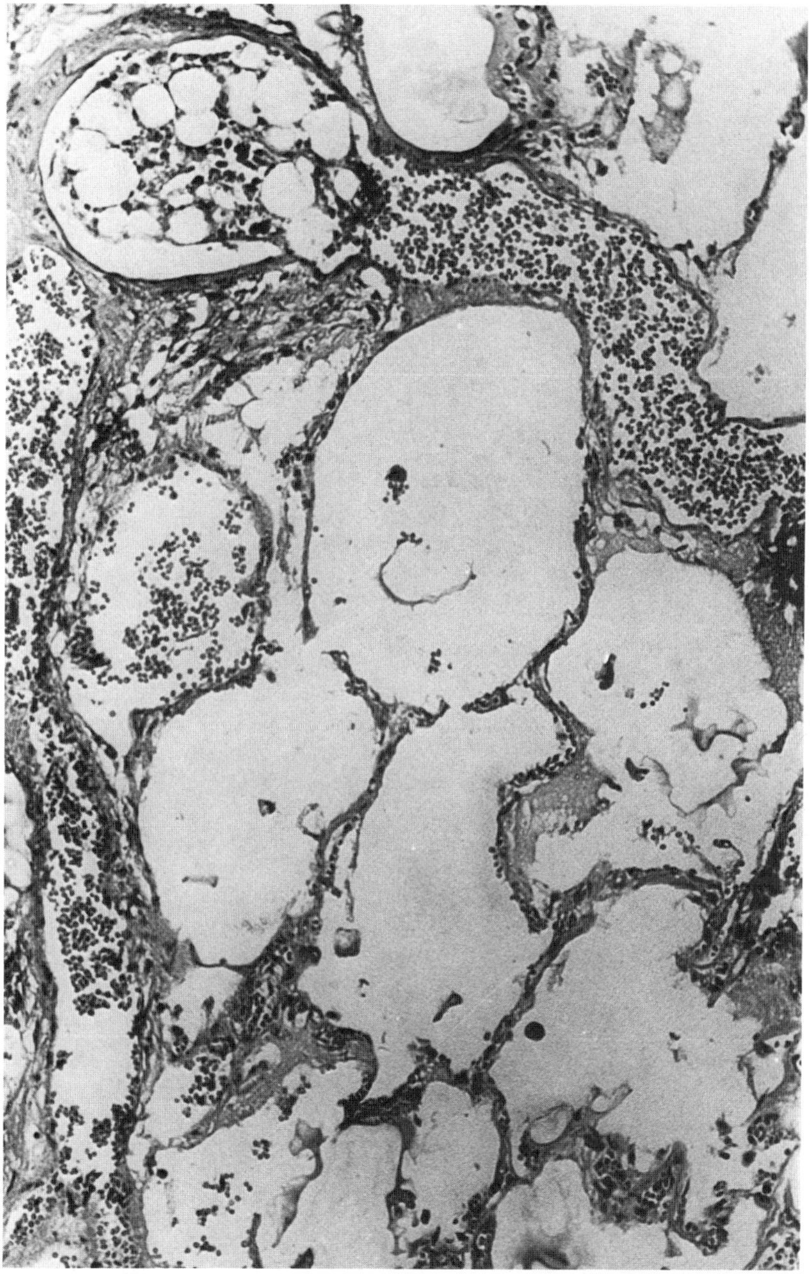

Figure 2c Marked vascular congestion and an incidental bone marrow embolus (hematoxylin and eosin × 120).

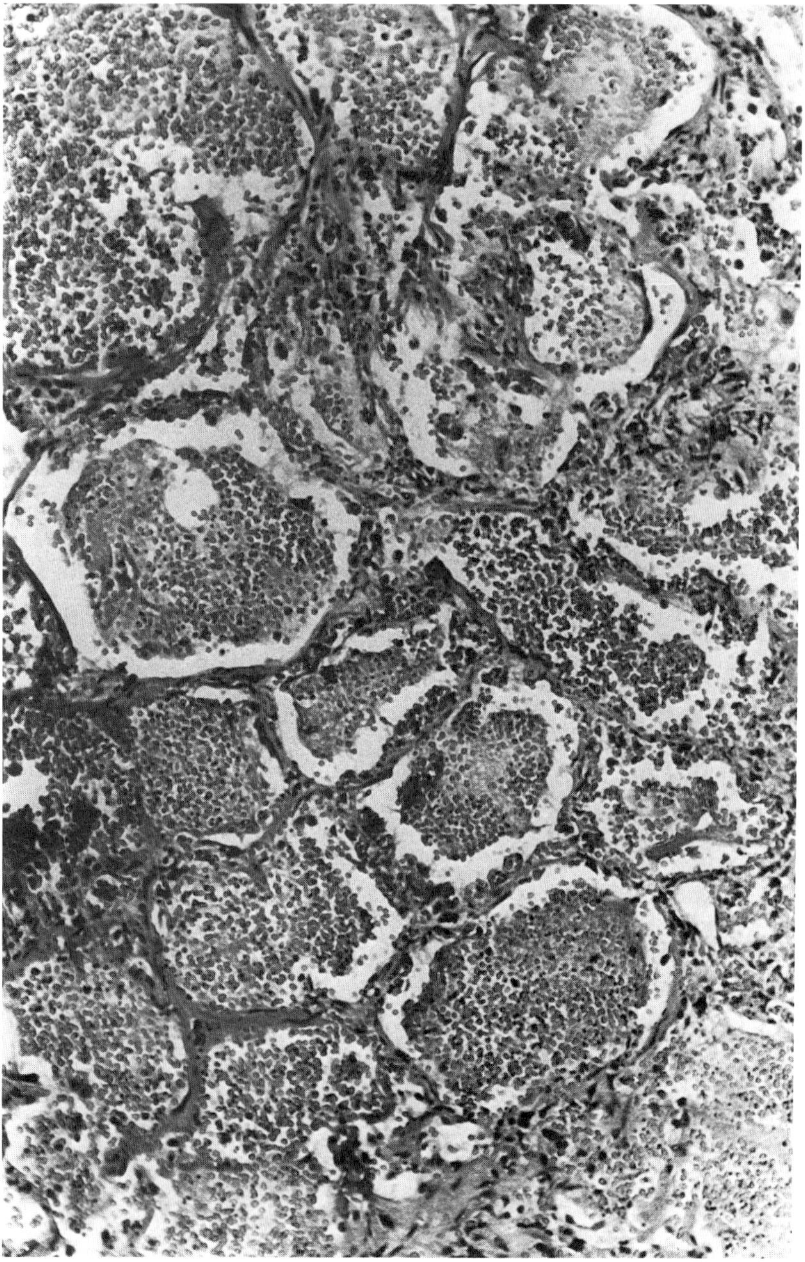

Figure 2d Coexistent bacterial pneumonia (hematoxylin and eosin × 120).

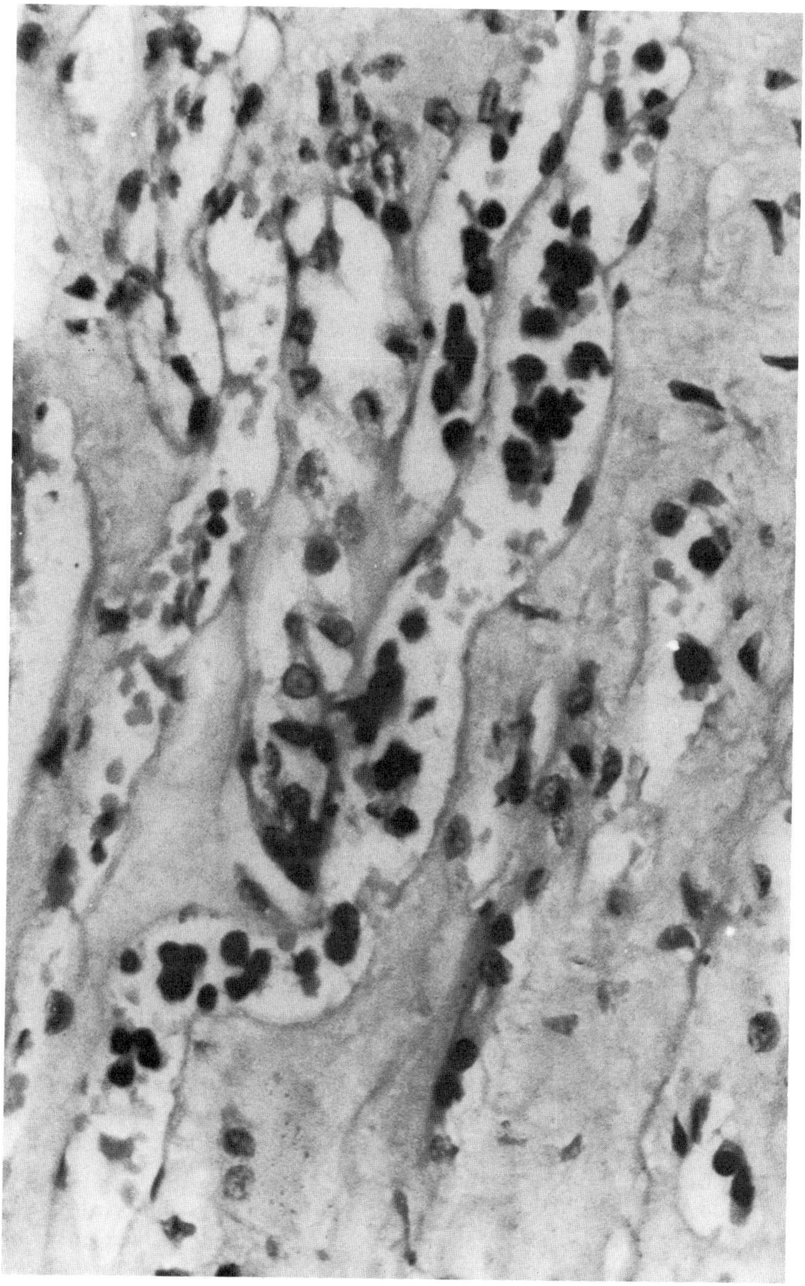

Figure 2e Higher-power photomicrograph shows parasitized red cells in septal capillaries (hematoxylin and eosin × 1080).

fetal loss, abortion, or premature labor and an increased susceptibility to infection and other pernicious complications of malaria are well-recognized problems of malaria in pregnancy (Editorial, 1983). Delay in diagnosis and inadequate and inappropriate treatment are major management problems in malaria (WHO Malaria Action Programme, 1986). The temporal profile of cerebral malaria followed by severe anemia, renal insufficiency, coagulation abnormalities without bleeding, leukocytosis, and finally pulmonary edema suggests that factors other than mere sequestration are operational in causing pulmonary edema. It may be a cascade phenomenon.

H. Animals Models of Pulmonary Edema in Malaria

Animal models of severe complicated malaria do not exactly reproduce human *P. falciparum* malaria. There is, for instance, no entirely satisfactory model for cerebral malaria (Yoeli, 1976; Warrell, 1987). Pulmonary abnormalities are demonstrated in several species during experimental malaria (MacCallum, 1968), including canaries, ducks, chickens, mice, rats, hamsters, and several species of monkeys. There are, however, three good experimental models for studies on malarial pulmonary edema.

The Panamanian owl monkey (*Aotus trivirigatus*) was infected with human material-based *Plasmodium falciparum* (Schmidt, 1978). These animals showed two distinct patterns at necropsy. The animals who survived less than 15 days from the establishment of patency demonstrated hyperacute changes in the lungs that included edema, alveolar hemorrhage and pleural effusion. Those that survived longer than 20 days do not show these changes.

Hamsters (*Mesocricetus auratus*) infected with *Plasmodium berghei* and sequentially sacrificed (MacCallum, 1968) revealed progressive increase in the number of pigment-laden macrophages and parasitized RBCs followed by adherence to venular endothelial cells by the macrophages, blockage of the vascular channels, lymphatic dilatation, and, finally, pulmonary edema. Lymphatic dilatation is not observed in human *P. falciparum* malaria (Duarte et al., 1985; Corbett et al., 1989). Host modification, including neonatal thymectomy and splenectomy (Wright, 1968; Eling, 1980), prevented these developments thereby strongly supporting the role of immunity in their evolution.

The clinical and pathological profile of male Swiss C3H/Z mice infected with *Plasmodium berghei* (Weiss and Kubat, 1983) showed several remarkable similarities to complicated human *P. falciparum* malaria. A sudden fall in hematocrit around the seventh day of patency was followed by severe pulmonary edema and sudden death. The lung and kidneys showed immune complexes of IgM, C_3, C_4 and malarial antigen. The lungs of three surviving mice were clear. There was no obstruction to blood flow due to pigment-laden macrophages as observed in the hamster model.

The development of pulmonary edema was recently observed in a *Macaca mulatta Plasmodium knowlesi* model (M. Tatke and G. Bazaz-Mallik personal communication, February 1989; Fig. 3). These authors believed that the marked septal damage by parasitized cells led to the pulmonary edema.

The high levels of parasitemia achieved in these models are seldom observed in human disease. Nevertheless, these models reflect the problems in human *P. falciparum* malaria and offer a unique opportunity to study malaria-related pulmonary edema. Weiss and Kubat (1983) observed that the genesis of malarial lung in their model suggested an anaphylactoid reaction, possibly due to the sudden release of large amounts of antigen. This can occur in a highly synchronized human *P. falciparum* infection (WHO Malaria Action Programme, 1986).

VII. Diagnosis of Malaria

Careful examination of well-stained thick and thin smears of the peripheral blood by an experienced observer is the most easily available and reliable method for the diagnosis of malarial infection. If results of the examination are negative, it must be repeated several times since the parasites may not be demonstrated at all times. If maturation is highly synchronized, the para-

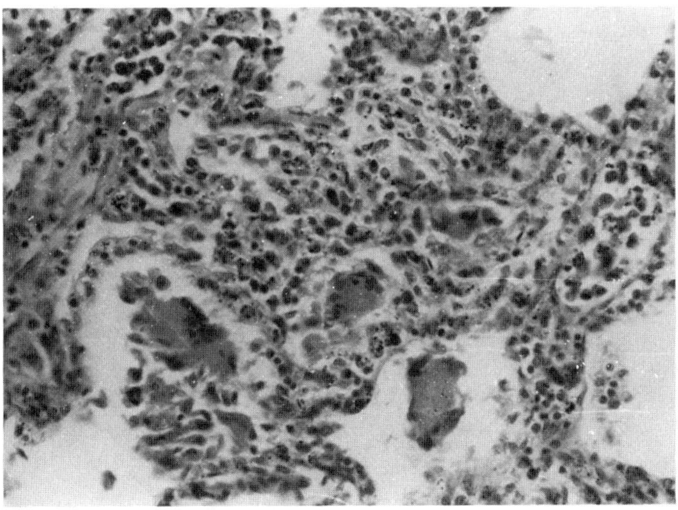

Figure 3 Experimental malaria in *Macaca mulatta* infected with *Plasmodium knowlesi*. Photomicrograph of the lung shows thickened septa and heavy parasitemia of sequestered RBC (courtesy of Drs. M. Tatke and G. Bazaz-Mallik).

site withdraws into the deeper circulation for the development of the schizont (WHO Malaria Action Programme, 1986). A new diagnostic method for the demonstration of parasitized RBCs, based on the reduced density of infected cells compared to normal RBC and hence placement just below the buffy coat in special acridin-orange-containing centrifugation tubes (QBC) viewed under ultraviolet light, has been shown to be better and about eight times more sensitive (Speilman et al., 1988) than blood smear examination.

Estimation of the extent of parasitemia is also important, since it is clearly established that higher values correlate directly with subsequent mortality (Field, 1949). A detailed analysis of the immunological methods of diagnosis is beyond the scope of this chapter. These methods (Mahajan et al., 1981; Lim, 1988) are of great epidemiological significance and are also helpful in identifying totally nonimmune groups at special risk of developing severe malaria (Cook, 1986).

VIII. Management

Pulmonary edema and pneumonia are the major management problems posed by malarial infection. Such patients should be admitted to intensive care units fully equipped to monitor and, when required, ventilate them mechanically.Unfortunately, such facilities are usually not available in the areas where malaria is rampant (WHO Malaria Action Programme, 1986). The management of such patients will be considered below.

A. General Measures

Since many of these patients have other complications of severe malaria, the extent and severity of the coexistent problems must be assessed. Patency and adequacy of the airway must be established. If necessary, intubation with a cuffed endotracheal tube may be required. Intravenous access must be obtained and the stomach emptied to prevent aspiration. Drugs must be administered parenterally as far as possible and in the appropriate dosage based on the patient's body weight. Urinary output should be used as a guide to fluid therapy. If renal failure is present, the need for dialysis should be ascertained. Severe anemia necessitates whole blood transfusion, while seizures and secondary infection must be treated with anticonvulsants and antibiotics, respectively (WHO Malaria Action Programme, 1986; Cook, 1986).

B. Specific Drug Therapy

It is perhaps a quirk of nature that *P. falciparum*, which is invariably responsible for severe, complicated malaria, is also the only parasite that can be easily treated with curative intent because it lacks a tissue phase that serves to sustain other malarial infections. The curability is, however, dependent on drug sensitivity. Various stages of erythrocytic schizogony—the ring, trophozoite, and schizont—have been demonstrated to be variably sensitive to different drugs. Ammonium chloride destroyed the ring stage selectively while amodiaquin, mefloquin, quinine, chloroquin, qinghaosu, halofantrine, rifampicin, cyclohexamide, actinomycin D, and antimycin A are active schizonticides. Tetracyclines, clindamycin, and halofuginone act on all the three stages (Geary et al., 1989). The use of these agents in severe malaria complicated by pulmonary edema and infection is discussed below. The detailed pharmacology, kinetics, and toxicity are beyond the scope of this chapter. Excellent reviews of the subject are available (Peters, 1980; Cook, 1986; WHO Malaria Action Programme, 1986).

Chloroquin

Chloroquin is an excellent schizonticidal agent but its wide use as a chemoprophylactic agent and over-the-counter febrifuge has rendered several strains of *P. falciparum* resistant to it. However, even in areas where there is a high incidence of resistance, intravenous chloroquin has been of demonstrated usefulness (WHO Malaria Action Programme, 1986; Cook, 1986). The recommended dosage is 10 mg base/kg diluted in 500 ml and infused over 4 h followed by 5 mg/kg infusion every 12 h for 3 doses.

Quinine

Quinine is the drug of first choice in the management of severe malarial infection because there is widespread resistance to chloroquin in several areas. Extensive use has removed doubts regarding serious toxicity, which was maximally observed when large bolus injections were administered. Such drug delivery resulted in serious cardiovascular complications and severe hypoglycemia (WHO Malaria Action Programme, 1986). A slow, steady infusion of 10-20 mg/kg at 8 h intervals results in sustained therapeutic drug levels. Administration must be continued for at least 72 h after the asexual forms of the parasite have disappeared from the peripheral blood.

Quinidine

Quinidine is as potent as quinine as a schizonticide. In areas of emerging quinine resistance it may be more effective (WHO Malaria Action Programme, 1986). Presently, its use is recommended in the management of severe malaria in countries where quinine is not freely available. The results have been very satisfying (WHO Malaria Action Programme, 1986; Miller et al., 1989).

The dosage is 10-15 mg/kg as a loading dose followed by 7-10 mg/kg every 8 h. The slow infusion minimizes the risk of cardiovascular and hypoglycemic complications.

Mefloquin

Mefloquin is not available for parenteral use but can be given by nasogastric tube after administration of an antiemetic. This drug is useful in the treatment of multiple drug-resistant *P. falciparum* malaria. A single 1500 mg dose is used usually after a course of quinine therapy.

Qinghaosu

Qinghaosu is a traditional Chinese remedy for malaria and has been shown to be highly effective in complicated *P. falciparum* malaria (PeThan Myint and Tin Shwe, 1987). The drug is administered intravenously as an infusion of 1000 mg and repeated 24 h later. The parasite clearance and clinical response occur earlier than with quinine treatment.

Amodiaquin

Amodiaquin sensitivity may be preserved even in the face of chloroquin resistance. (WHO Malaria Action Programme, 1986).

Tetracycline

Tetracycline 5-6 mg/kg every 6 h for 7-10 days and clindamycin 10 mg/kg every 12 h for 5 days have been effective in the treatment of severe malaria as adjuncts to quinine administration (Cook, 1986).

Pyrimethamine/Sulfonamide

Pyrimethamine and sulfonamide combinations are poor drugs for the treatment of malaria because of emerging resistance consequent to their widespread prophylactic and ill-advised therapeutic use. These drugs may be useful after a course of quinine (WHO Malaria Action Programme, 1986).

Phenanthrene Methanols

Phenanthrene methanols are not readily available. Halofantrine has excellent potential in the treatment of severe multiple drug-resistant *P. falciparum* malaria (Cook, 1986).

C. Exchange Transfusion

This modality has been demonstrated to rapidly reduce the levels of parasitemia. Patients exhibiting greater than 5% parasitized RBCs should receive this treatment (Miller et al., 1989). Excellent results have been obtained when exchange was used in conjunction with quinine (WHO Malaria Action Programme, 1986; Cook, 1986) and quinidine (Miller et al., 1989). Use of mechanical and automatic devices has yielded similar results.

D. Oxygenation

This is the most vital need in the management of pulmonary edema. Once the airway has been established, frequent suction must be used to maintain its patency. Nasal catheters, prongs, or masks may be used initially but if oxygenation cannot be maintained in the face of severe pulmonary edema, mechanical ventilation should be instituted early. The principles of ventilatory management in malarial pulmonary edema are the same as for any other cause of ARDS (Ingram, 1987). The results have been very encouraging (James, 1985). The FiO_2 should be kept at the lowest level that maintains oxygenation.

E. Other Measures

Severe hyperpyrexia and convulsions adversely effect the outcome of a pateint who is also hypoxic (WHO Malaria Action Programme, 1986). Fever must be reduced by sponging, fanning, or other methods of cooling and the administration of paracetamol (acetaminophen). Diazepam, phenytoin, or paraldehyde may be used to control seizures. Hypoglycemia must be corrected. For complicating bacterial infections usually due to gram-negative bacilli, antibiotics of the aminoglycoside group can be used, but care must be taken to adjust the dosages according to the patient's renal function.

F. Controversial Measures

One of the greatest controversies in the management of severe malaria surrounds the use of corticosteroids. Based on the increased permeability hypothesis, this form of treatment was shown to be harmful rather than helpful in the management of cerebral malaria (Warrell et al., 1982). Since the role of steroids in pulmonary edema is also not firmly established (Ingram, 1987), the use of these agents should be avoided. Heparin and low-molecular-weight dextrans can confound an already complicated situation by inducing bleeding. They do not have any prophylactic role in the prevention of DIC. (WHO Malaria Action Programme, 1986).

G. Newer Trends in Therapy

The sweeping advance of drug-resistant malaria has prompted the search for newer drugs and delivery systems. In the last few years published information has suggested possible therapeutic potential for the agents listed below:

1. Trimethoprim—sulfamethoxazole was used successfully in Japan (Yoshida et al., 1987).
2. Analogs of riboflavin were used to induce deficiency of riboflavin, which is believed to be protective. Experimental studies confirm this (Cowden et al., 1987).
3. Ciprofloxacin and Norfloxacin were used successfully (Krishna et al., 1988; Sharma, 1989)
4. In vitro studies confirmed the effectiveness of pyronaridine against *P. falciparum* (Childs et al., 1988).
5. Orally active iron chelators (alpha-keto hydroxypyridines), devoid of the problems of desferroxamine administration, were shown to be active against *P. falciparum*. This group of drugs offers a unique new concept in the treatment of malaria (Heppner et al., 1988).
6. The concomitant use of verapamil abolished chloroquin resistance in *P. falciparum* malaria. (Jacobs et al., 1988).
7. Experimental malaria was treated successfully using a liposome drug delivery system that allows selective drug targeting and reduces systemic drug toxicity (Peeters et al., 1989).

IX. Prevention of Malaria

Malaria can be prevented if the mosquito is not allowed to bite. *Plasmodium-falciparum*-bearing mosquitoes are nocturnal and bite between dusk and dawn (Cook, 1986). Mosquito nets, screening of rooms with a wire mesh, and application of mosquito repellants have gained added significance since it was established that chemoprophylaxis only suppressed infection and did not eradicate it, while it prompted the emergence of drug resistance. Chemoprophylaxis is advised only to special nonimmune groups at great risk of developing malaria:

1. Pregnant women or those contemplating conception during a stay in an endemic area
2. Very young children residing in highly endemic zones
3. Patients receiving immunosuppressive drug therapy in highly endemic areas
4. Travellers from malaria-free areas visiting highly endemic zones
5. Persons returning to such areas after prolonged absence (Cook, 1986)

The choice of drugs depends on the parasite behavior in the area.

The development of an effective malaria vaccine remains a dream (Bruce-Chwatt, 1987), but the quest has stimulated searches into the molecular biology of one of the oldest scourges of mankind (Kabilan et al., 1988) and success in the near future appears more of a reality.

Acknowledgments

We are grateful to Dr. (Mrs.) C.K. Bannerjee, Additional Professor of Pathology, for her help with the case description. We would like to dedicate this work to the memory of the late Dr. S.K. Malik who taught us to think pulmonary. Mr. Brij Raj deserves special mention for the expeditious typing of the manuscript.

References

Abdalla, S., Weatherall, D. J., Wickramasinghe, S. N., and Hughes, M. (1980). The anemia of *Plasmodium falciparum* malaria. *Br. J. Haematol.* **46**:171-183.

Aikawa, M., and Seed, T. M. (1980). Morphology of plasmodia. In *Malaria* Vol. 1. Edited by J. P. Kreier. New York, Academic Press, pp. 285-346.

Aikawa, M., Suzuki, M., and Gutierrez, Y. (1980). Pathology of malaria. In *Malaria* Vol. 2. Edited by J. P. Kreier. New York, Academic Press, pp. 47-102.

Al-Ibrahim, M. S., Holzman, R. S. (1975). Bilateral pleural effusions with *Plasmodium falciparum* infection. *Am. J. Trop. Med. Hyg.* **24**:910-912.

Applebaum, I. L., and Shrager, J. (1944). Pneumonitis associated with malaria. *Arch. Intern. Med.* **74**:155-162.

Arias, A. E., and Walter, R. D. (1988). *Plasmodium falciparum*: association with erythrocyte superoxide dismutase. *J. Protozool.* **35**:348-351.

Barnwell, J. W., Nichols, M. E., and Rubenstein, P. (1989). In vitro evaluation of the role of the Duffy blood group in erythrocyte invasion by *Plasmodium vivax*. *J. Exp. Med.* **169**:1795-1802.

Barrett-Connor, E. (1982). Parasitic pulmonary disease. *Am. Rev. Respir. Dis.* **126**:558-563.

Blount, R. E. (1964). Malaria: an unsolved military medical problem. *Am. J. Med. Sci.* **247**:407-411.

Blount, R. E. (1969). Acute falciparum malaria: field experience with quinine/pyrimethamine combined therapy. *Ann. Intern. Med.* **70**:142-147.

Boyd, M. F. (1949). Historical review. In *Malariology* Vol. 1. Edited by M. F. Boyd. Philadelphia, W. B. Saunders, pp. 3-28.

Brooks, M. H., Malloy, J. P., Bartelloni, P. J., Tigertt, W. D., Sheehy, T. W., and Barry, K. G. (1967). Pathophysiology of acute Falciparum malaria. I. Correlation of clinical and biochemical abnormalities. *Am. J. Med.* **43**:735-744.

Brooks, M. H., Kiel, F. W., Sheehy, T. W., and Barry, K. G. (1968). Acute pulmonary edema in falciparum malaria. *N. Engl. J. Med.* **279**:732-737.

Bruce-Chwatt, L. J. (1987). The challenge of malaria vaccine: trials and tribulations. *Lancet* **1**:371-373.

Bygbjerg, I. C., and Lanng, C. (1982). Septicemia as a complication of falciparum malaria. *Trans. R. Soc. Trop. Med. Hyg.* **73**:705.

Cayea, P. D., Robin, E., and Teixidor, H. S. (1981). Atypical pulmonary malaria. *AJR* **137**:51-55.

Childs, G. E., Hausler, B., Milhous, N., Chen, C., Wimonwattrawatte, T., Pooyindee, N., and Boudreau, E. F. (1988). In vitro activity of pyronaridine against field isolates and reference clones of *Plasmodium falciparum. Am. J. Trop. Med. Hyg.* **38**:24-29.

Clark, I. A., and Chaudhri, G. (1988). Tumor necrosis factor in malaria induced abortion. *Am. J. Trop. Med. Hyg.* **39**:246-249.

Clark, I. A., and Hunt, N. H. (1983). Evidence for reactive oxygen intermediates causing haemolysis and parasite death in malaria. *Infect. Immun.* **39**:1-6.

Clark, H. C., and Tomlinson, W. J. (1949). The pathologic anatomy of malaria. In *Malariology* Vol. 2. Edited by M. F. Boyd. Philadelphia, W. B. Saunders, pp. 874-903.

Clark, I. A., Cowden, W. B., Butcher, G. A., and Hunt, N. H. (1987). Possible roles of tumor necrosis factor in the pathology of malaria. *Am. J. Pathol.* **129**:192-199.

Cook, G. C. (1986). *Plasmodium falciparum* infection: problems in prophylaxis and treatment in 1986. *Q. J. Med.* **61**:1091-1115.

Corbett, C. E. P., Duarte, M. I. S., Lancellotti, C. L. P., Silva, M. A. L. G., and Andrade, H. F. (1989). Cytoadherence in human falciparum malaria as a cause of respiratory distress. *J. Trop. Med. Hyg.* **92**:112-120.

Cordeiro, R. S. B., Cunha, F. Q., Filho, J. A., Flores, C. A., Vasconcelos, H. N., and Martins, M. A. (1983). *Plasmodium berghei*: pathophysiological changes during infections in mice. *Ann. Trop. Med. Parasitol.* **77**:455-465.

Cowden, W. B., Butcher, G. A., Hunt, N. H., Clark, I. A., and Yoneda, F. (1987). Antimalarial activity of a riboflavin analog against *Plasmodium vinckei* in vivo and *Plasmodium falciparum* in vitro. *Am. J. Trop. Med. Hyg.* **37**:495-500.

Cranston, H. A., Boylan, C. W., and Carroll, G. L. (1984). *Plasmodium falciparum* maturation abolishes physiological red cell deformability. *Science* **223**:400-402.

Das, B. S., Das, D. B., Satpathy, R. N., Patnaik, J. K., and Bose, T. K. (1988). Riboflavin deficiency and severity of malaria. *Eur. J. Clin. Nutr.* **42**:277-283.

David, P. H., Hommel, M., Miller, L. H., Udeinya, I. J., and Oligino, L. D. (1983). Parasite sequestration in *Plasmodium falciparum* malaria: spleen and antibody modulation of cytoadherence of infected erythrocytes. *Proc. Natl. Acad. Sci. U.S.A.* **80**:5075-5079.

David, P. H., Handunnetti, S. M., Leech, J. H., Gamage, P., and Mendis, K. N. (1988). Rosetting: a new cytoadherence property of malaria infected erythrocytes. *Am. J. Trop. Med. Hyg.* **38**:289-297.

Deaton, J. G. (1970). Fatal pulmonary edema as a complication of acute falciparum malaria. *Am. J. Trop. Med. Hyg.* **19**:196-201.

Duarte, M. I. S., Corbett, C. E. P., Boulos, M., and Neto, V. A. (1985). Ultrastructure of the lung in falciparum malaria. *Am. J. Trop. Med. Hyg.* **34**:31-35.

Editorial (1983). Malaria in pregnancy. *Lancet* **2**:84-85.

Eling, W. M. C. (1980). Role of spleen in morbidity and mortality of *Plasmodium berghei* infection in mice. *Infect. Immun.* **30**:635-641.

Fein, I. A., Rackow, E. C., and Shapiro, L. (1978). Pulmonary edema in *Plasmodium falciparum* malaria. *Am. Rev. Respir. Dis.* **118**:425-428.

Field, J. W. (1949). Blood examination and prognosis in acute falciparum malaria. *Trans. R. Soc. Trop. Med. Hyg.* **43**:33-48.

Garnham, P. C. C. (1980). Malaria in its various vertebrate hosts. In *Malaria* Vol. 1. Edited by J. P. Kreier. New York, Academic Press, pp. 95-144.

Geary, T. G., Divo, A. A., and Jensen, J. B. (1989). Stage specific actions of antimalarial drugs on *Plasmodium falciparum* in culture. *Am. J. Trop. Med. Hyg.* **40**:240-244.

Godard, J. E., and Hansen, R. A. (1971). Interstitial pulmonary edema in acute malaria. *Radiology* **101**:523-524.

Goodall, H. B. (1973). Giant nuclear masses in the lungs and blood in malignant malaria. *Lancet* **2**:1124-1126.

Hall, A. P. (1977). The treatment of severe falciparum malaria. *Trans. R. Soc. Trop. Med. Hyg.* **71**:367-378.

Henschel, A., Taylor, H. L., and Keys, A. (1950). Experimental malaria in man. I. Physical deterioration and recovery. *J. Clin. Invest.* **29**:52-59.

Heppner, D. G., Hallaway, P. E., Kontoghiorghes, G. J., and Eaton, J. W. (1988). Antimalarial properties of orally active iron chelators. *Blood* **72**:358-361.

Holmes, P. H. (1987). Pathophysiology of parasitic infections. *Parasitology (Suppl.)* **94**:S29-S51.

Ingram, R. H. (1987). Adult respiratory distress syndrome. In *Harrison's Principles of Internal Medicine*, 11th ed., vol. 2. Edited by E. Braunwald, K. J. Isselbacher, R. G. Petersdorf, J. D. Wilson, J. B. Martin, and A. S. Fauci. New York, McGraw Hill, pp. 1134-1137.

Jacobs, G. H., Oduola, A. M. J., Kyle, D. E., Milhous, W. K., Martin, S. K., and Aikawa, M. (1988). Ultrastructural study of the effects of chloroquin and verapamil on *Plasmodium falciparum*. *Am. J. Trop. Med. Hyg.* **39**: 15-20.

James, M. F. M. (1985). Pulmonary damage associated with falciparum malaria: a report of ten cases. *Ann. Trop. Med. Parasitol.* **79**:123-138.

Janoff, A., Roth, W. J., Sinha, S., and Barnwell, J. W. (1988). Degradation of plasmodial antigens by human neutrophil elastase. *J. Immunol.* **141**: 1332-1340.

Kabilan, L., Troye-Blomberg, M., and Perlmann, H. (1988). T-cell epitopes in PF 155/RESA, a major candidate for a *Plasmodium falciparum* malaria vaccine. *Proc. Natl. Acad. Sci. U.S.A.* **85**:5659-5663.

Kitchen, S. F. (1949). Falciparum malaria. In Malariology Vol. 2. Edited by M. F. Boyd. Philadelphia, W. B. Saunders, pp. 995-1016.

Krishna, S., Davis, T. M. E., Chan, P. C. Y., Wells, R. A., and Robson, K. J. H. (1988). Ciprofloxacin in malaria. *Lancet* **1**:1231-1232.

Lawler, J. (1986). The structural and functional properties of thrombospondin. *Blood* **67**:1197-1209.

Lim, T. S. (1988). A sensitive malaria immunoperoxidase assay for the detection of *Plasmodium falciparum* antibody. *Am. J. Trop. Med. Hyg.* **38**: 255-257.

MacCallum, D. K. (1968). Pulmonary changes resulting from experimental malaria infection in hamsters. *Arch. Pathol.* **86**:681-688.

MacPherson, G. G., Warrell, M. J., White, N. J., Looareesuwan, S., and Warrell, D. A. (1985). Human cerebral malaria: a quantitative ultrastructural analysis of parasitized erythrocyte sequestration. *Am. J. Pathol.* **119**:385-401.

Maegraith, B. G., and Onabanjo, A. O. (1970). The effects of histamine in malaria. *Br. J. Pharmacol.* **39**:755-764.

Mahajan, R. C., Ganguly, N. K., Thadani, M., Gill, N., and Chandnani, R. E. (1981). Comparison of ELISA with indirect haemagglutination and indirect fluorescent antibody tests in malaria. *Ind. J. Med. Res.* **73**:874-879.

Malloy, J. P., Brooks, M. H., and Barry, K. G. (1967). Pathophysiology of acute Falciparum malaria. II. Fluid compartmentalization. *Am. J. Med.* **43**:745-750.

Marchiafava, E., and Bignami, A. (1900). Malaria. In *Twentieth Century Practice: An International Encyclopaedia of Modern Medical Science.* Vol. 19. Edited by T. L. Stedman. New York, William Wood, pp. 225-252.

Marks, S. M., Holland, S., and Gelfand, M. (1977). Malarial lung: report of a case from Africa successfully treated with intermittent positive pressure ventilation. *Am. J. Trop. Med. Hyg.* **26**:179-180.

Marsh, K., and Greenwood, B. M. (1986). The immunopathology of malaria. *Clin. Trop. Med. Communic. Dis.* **1**:91-125.

Martell, R. W., Kallenbach, J., and Zwi, S. (1979). Pulmonary edema in falciparum malaria. *Br. Med. J.* **2**:1761-1762.

Martins, M. A. E., Silva, P. M. R., Henriques, M. G. M. O., Cordeiro, R. S. B., and Correa, F. M. A. (1986). *Plasmodium berghei* infected mice: lack of effect of meclizine and cimetidine on the development of pulmonary edema. *Ann. Trop. Med. Parasitol.* **80**:491-499.

Mehta, S. R., Naidu, G., Chandar, V., Singh, I. P., Johri, S., and Ahuja, R. C. (1989). Falciparum malaria-present day problems. An experience with 425 cases. *J. Assoc. Physicians India* **37**:264-267.

Meldolesi, G. (1931). Respiratory disorders in Malaria. *Boll. Atti Accad. Med. Roma.* **57**:310-316.

Miller, K. D., Greenberg, A. E., and Campbell, C. C. (1989). Treatment of severe malaria in the United States with a continuous infusion of quinidine gluconate and exchange transfusion. *N. Engl. J. Med.* **321**:65-70.

Miller, L. H., Chien, S., and Usami, S. (1972). Decreased deformability of *Plasmodium coatneyi* infected red cells and its possible relation to cerebral malaria. *Am. J. Trop. Med. Hyg.* **21**:133-137.

Neva, F. A. (1967). Malaria—recent progress and problems. *N. Engl. J. Med.* **277**:1241-1252.

Neva, F. A., Sheagren, J. N., Shulman, N. R., and Canfield, C. J. (1970). Malaria: host defense mechanisms and complications. *Ann. Intern. Med.* **73**:295-306.

Onabanjo, A. O., and Maegraith, B. G. (1970 a). Inflammatory changes in small blood vessels induced by kallikrein (kininogenase) in the blood of *Macaca mulatta* infected with *Plasmodium knowlesi. Ann. Trop. Med. Parasitol.* **64**:227-236.

Onabanjo, A. O., and Maegraith, B. G. (1970 b). Pathological lesions produced in the brain by kallikrein (kininogenase) in *Macaca mulatta* infected with *Plasmodium knowlesi. Ann. Trop. Med. Parasitol.* **64**:237-242.

Peeters, P. A. M., Huiskamp, C. W. E. N., Eling, W. M. C., and Crommelin, D. J. A. (1989). Chloroquin containing liposomes in the chemotherapy of murine malaria. *Parasitology* **98**:381-386.

Perrin, L. H., Mackey, L. J., and Miescher, P. A. (1982). The hematology of malaria in man. *Semin. Hematol.* **19**:70-82.

Peters, W. (1980). Chemotherapy of malaria. In *Malaria* Vol. 1. Edited by J. P. Kreier. New York, Academic Press, pp. 145-273.

PeThan Myint and Tin Shwe (1987). A controlled clinical trial of artemether (Qinghaosu derivative) versus quinine in complicated severe malaria. *Trans. R. Soc. Trop. Med. Hyg.* **81**:559-561.

Plorde, J. J., and White, N. J. (1987). Malaria. In *Harrison's Principles of Internal Medicine*, 11th ed., Vol. 1. Edited by E. Braunwald, K. J. Isselbacher, R. G. Petersdorf, J. D. Wilson, J. B. Martin, and A. S. Fauci. New York, McGraw Hill, pp. 778-784.

Punyagupta, S., Srichaikul, T., Nitiyanant, P., and Petchalai, B. (1974). Acute pulmonary insufficiency in falciparum malaria: summary of 12 cases with evidence of disseminated intravascular coagulation. *Am. J. Trop. Med. Hyg.* **23**:551-559.

Quinn, T. C., and Plorde, J. J. (1981). The resurgence of malaria: Diagnostic and therapeutic dilemmas. *Arch. Intern. Med.* **141**:1123-1124.

Robin, E. D., Cross, C. E., and Zelis, R. (1973). Pulmonary edema. (Second of two parts). *N. Engl. J. Med.* **288**:292-304.

Ross, R. (1902). Researches on malaria. The Nobel lecture, Dec. 12, 1902. In *Nobel Lectures* (*Medicine and Physiology*) *1901-1921*. Nobel Foundation Stockholm, Sweden. Amsterdam, Elsevier Publishing Co., (1967) pp. 25-116.

Sarma, P. S. (1989). Norfloxacin: a new drug in the treatment of falciparum malaria. *Ann. Intern. Med.* **111**:336-337.

Schmidt, L. H. (1978). *Plasmodium falciparum* and *Plasmodium vivax* infections in the owl monkey (*Aotus trivirgatus*). I. The course of untreated infections. *Am. J. Trop. Med. Hyg.* **27**:671-702.

Sheehy, T. W., and Reba, R. C. (1967). Complications of falciparum malaria and their treatment. *Ann. Intern. Med.* **66**:807-809.

Sherman, I. W., and Valdez, E. (1989). In vitro cytoadherence of *Plasmodium falciparum* infected erythrocytes to melanoma cells: factors affecting adhesion. *Parasitology* **98**:359-369.

Speilman, A., Perrone, J. B., Taklehaimanot, A., Balcha, F., Wardlaw, S. C., and Levine, R. A. (1988). Malaria diagnosis by direct observation of centrifuged samples of blood. *Am. J. Trop. Med. Hyg.* **39**:337-342.

Spitz, S. (1946). The pathology of acute falciparum malaria. *Milit. Surg.* **99**:555-572.

Sprague, H. B. (1946). The effects of malaria on the heart. *Am. Heart. J.* **31**:426-430.

Tong, M. J., Ballantine, T. V. N., and Youel, D. B. (1972a). Pulmonary function studies in *Plasmodium falciparum* malaria. *Am. Rev. Respir. Dis.* **106**:23-29.

Tong, M. J., Youel, D. B., and Cotten, C. L. (1972b). Acute pneumonia in tropical infections. *Am. J. Trop. Med. Hyg.* **21**:50-57.

Tubbs, H. (1980). Endotoxin in human and murine malaria. *Trans. R. Soc. Trop. Med. Hyg.* **74**:121-123.

Udeinya, I. J., Schmidt, J. A., Aikawa, M., Miller, L. H., and Green, I. (1981). Falciparum malaria infected erythrocytes specifically bind to cultured human endothelial cells. *Science* **213**:555-557.

Udomsangpetch, R., Wahlin, B., Carlson, J., Berzino, K., Torii, M., Aikawa, M., Perlmann, P., and Wahlgren, M. (1989). *Plasmodium falciparum*-infected erythrocytes form spontaneous erythrocyte rosettes. *J. Exp. med.* **169**:1835-1840.

Warrell, D. A. (1987). Pathophysiology of severe falciparum malaria in man. *Parasitology* (*Suppl.*) **94**:S29-S51.

Warrell, D. A., Looareesuwan, S., Warrell, M. J., Kasemsarn, P., Intaraprasert, R., Bunnag, D., and Harinasuta, T. (1982). Dexamethasone proves deleterious in cerebral malaria. A double line trial in 100 comatose patients. *N. Engl. J. Med.* **306**:313-319.

Watson, M. (1905). Some clinical features of quartan malaria. *Ind. Med. Gaz.* **40**:49-52.

Weiss, M. L., and Kubat, K. (1983). *Plasmodium berghei*: a mouse model for the "sudden death" and "malarial lung" syndromes. *Exp. Parasitol.* **56**:143-151.

Wernsdorfer, W. H. (1980). The importance of malaria in the world. In *Malaria* Vol. 1. Edited by J. P. Kreier. New York, Academic Press, pp. 1-93.

World Health Organization Malaria Action Programme (1986). Severe and complicated malaria. *Trans. R. Soc. Trop. Med. Hyg.* (*Suppl.*) **80**:3-50.

Wright, D. H. (1968). The effects of neonatal thymectomy on the survival of golden hamsters infected with *Plasmodium berghei*. *Br. J. Exp. Pathol.* **49**:379-384.

Yoeli, M. (1976). Cerebral malaria—the quest for suitable experimental model in parasite disease of man. *Trans. R. Soc. Trop. Med. Hyg.* **70**:24-35.

Yoshida, Y., Matsumoto, Y., and Yamada, M. (1987). Clinical trial of trimethoprim—sulfamethoxazole in treatment of vivax, ovale and falciparum malaria. *Jpn. J. Trop. Med. Hyg.* **15**:105-116.

4

Melioidosis

SUMALEE KIATBOONSRI

Ramathibodi Hospital
Bangkok, Thailand

I. Historical Background

In 1912, Whitmore and Krishnaswami reported an undescribed infective disease among the population of Rangoon. The disease was caused by a gram-negative bacilli, which was later named "*Pseudomonas pseudomallei.*" Its clinical features resembled "glanders" in the animal and the disease was called "melioidosis." Most of the reported cases were from Southeast Asian countries during World War II where attention to the disease was first drawn. Many clinical and laboratory studies were also conducted in the 1960s during the Vietnam war since many American veterans were affected by the disease. Case findings in the last two decades were confined mainly to Southeast Asia, especially Thailand, from which most of the cases were reported (Alexander et al., 1970; Clayton et al., 1973; Nigg, 1963; Pack and Zwanenburg, 1947; Paton et al., 1947; Weber et al., 1969).

II. Epidemiology

Unlike the worldwide diseases caused by other pseudomonads, melioidosis is endemic mainly in the Southeast Asian countries, particularly Indochina (Dhiensiri et al., 1988; Howe et al., 1971; Kiatboonsri and Sathapatayavongs, 1985; Kiatboonsri and Vathesatogkit, 1979; Nachiangmai et al., 1985; So, 1985; Susaengrat et al., 1987). Other endemic areas include Hong Kong, Australia, Madagascar, and Guam. These are tropical and subtropical countries located between latitude 20 degrees north and latitude 20 degrees south. In Thailand, the most endemic area is the northeastern part, where more than 50 new cases were found each year. Cases from other parts of the country were reported not infrequently.

Pseudomonas pseudomallei normally inhabitats the environment of the endemic countries and can be isolated from soil, well and rice field water, rice seeds, and other agricultural instruments. The positive isolation rate varies from 40 to 80%. Human subjects acquire the disease by direct contact with the organisms from the environment. There are two main routes of entry.

A. Abraded Skin or Open Wound

Examples are patients in car accidents with open wounds or abraded skin contaminated by local soil and water; and people, particularly farmers and plantation workers, who work in close contact with soil and water in endemic areas.

B. Aspiration or Inhalation

Examples are patients who survived drowning with aspiration of contaminated water; and Vietnam veterans who inhaled contaminated dusts raised by helicopter propellers.

A few cases of laboratory-acquired melioidosis and a rare occasion of human-to-human sexual transmission have been reported (Green and Tuffnell, 1968; McCormick et al., 1975; Schlech et al., 1981). These are not considered the usual routes of entry.

III. Clinical Manifestations

Reported cases of melioidosis ranges from newborns to men over 70, with more than half of the cases in people of working age, 30-60 years (Achana et al., 1985; Carruthers, 1981; Cooper, 1967; Everett and Nelson, 1975; Jackson et al., 1972; Kiatboonsri and Sathapatayavongs, 1985; Mays and Ricketts, 1975; Piggott and Hochholzer, 1970; Prevatt and Hunt, 1957; Sanford, 1971; Spotnitz et al., 1967; Thin et al., 1970; Thisyakorn, 1986; Weber et al., 1969).

The disease occurs more frequently in men, with a male/female ratio of 2-3:1. As mentioned above, farmers are predisposed to the disease and account for more than 50% of the cases. Thus, it is said that "melioidosis is mostly a disease of active working men who work in close contact to soil and water." Host factors or basic underlying diseases also play important roles in its occurrence and severity. Among the various diseases reported, diabetes mellitus was found to be the most common concurrent condition, occurring in 50-60% of cases. Other less common concurrent diseases included cirrhosis, drug addiction, alcoholism, renal stones, thalassemia, and various forms of malignant diseases.

Melioidosis is an example of disease with a wide range of clinical manifestations. At one extreme, a patient may have the insidious onset of fever for months, with a very low mortality rate. At the other extreme, he or she may be acutely ill with shock, respiratory failure, and extremely high mortality rate despite appropriate antibiotic treatment. These clinical manifestations have been previously classified into acute septicemic melioidosis, chronic melioidosis, and subclinical melioidosis. It was noted later that not all patients with blood-culture-positive, septicemic melioidosis were acutely ill or experienced high mortality rates. Some ran subacute clinical courses, which mimicked chronic melioidosis, with a low fatality rate. Thus the former classification made it impossible to compare the outcome of treatments from different institutes or the efficacy of various antibiotic regimens.

In November, 1985, the National Workshop on Melioidosis was held in Bangkok by the Infectious Disease Association of Thailand. Various aspects of melioidosis from different institutes of the country were discussed. Attention was drawn to the newer, more proper clinical classification so that disease states with different levels of severity and prognosis could be clearly differentiated. The newly classified clinical forms include disseminated septicemic melioidosis, nondisseminated septicemic melioidosis, localized melioidosis, and subclinical melioidosis.

A. Disseminated Septicemic Melioidosis

Patients usually present with acute febrile illness and deteriorate rapidly within 2-3 days. Signs and symptoms are indistinguishable from severe gram-negative sepsis and more than 90% of cases experience septicemic shock. Acute respiratory failure is present in most cases and may progress to adult respiratory distress syndrome (ARDS). Physical examination and laboratory investigation show evidences of multiple organ infections (usually three or more). The most common findings are multiple small superficial skin pustules, bilateral diffuse alveolar infiltrations of bloodborne pneumonia type on chest x-ray, and multiple hepatic and splenic abscesses demonstrated by

Table 1 Clinical Classification of Melioidosis

	Positive Blood Culture	Positive Culture from Other Organs	Positive Serological Results	Septic Shock	Clinical Foci	Foci Clinical Progress	Need for Treatment	Expected Mortality Rate
Disseminated septicemic melioidosis	Yes	3 +	0-2 +	Frequent (80-90%)	Multiple	Rapid	Very urgent	High (70-80%)
Nondisseminated septicemic melioidosis	Yes	1-2 +	0-2 +	Not common	Few	Varied	Urgent	Low
Localized melioidosis	No	0-1 +	0-3 +	Usually no	Few	Slow	Less urgent	Low
Subclinical melioidosis	No	0	Yes	Never	Not detected	None	None	None

computed tomographic scanning or ultrasonography. Postmortem examination commonly shows diffuse abscess formations in the lungs, liver, spleen, intestinal wall, myocardium, and brain. These suggest bloodstream dissemination with simultaneous implantation of organisms in various organs. Primary site of infection as a source of dissemination may or may not be found. Some patients habor localized benign infections for months prior to disease dissemination. Attempts to drain a melioid abscess or corticosteroid therapy without previous proper antibiotic coverage are highly associated with aggravation of dissemination.

Disseminated septicemic melioidosis usually runs a rapid course and most patients die within 2-3 days after disease has disseminated. The mortality rate approaches 70-80% despite early, proper antibiotic treatments. Death is usually attributed to irreversible septic shock and intractable hypoxcmia. Most patients carry one or more concurrent diseases, among which uncontrolled diabetes mellitus was found to be most common (over 50% of cases). Others include hematologic malignancies, rheumatic heart disease, and chronic renal failure.

Case 1

A 45-year-old Thai farmer with uncontrolled diabetes was admitted because of fever with chill for 4 days and progressive dyspnea for 2 days. He was found to be cyanotic, in distress, and markedly dyspneic. His blood pressure was 70/50 mmHg, pulse 130/min, and respiratory rate 40/min. Auscultation revealed medium to fine crepitations over both lungs and a hepatomegaly of 3 inches below the right costal margin was palpated with diffuse tenderness. Small superficial skin pustules 1-2 mm in diameter were distributed on the extremities and trunk. Chest x-ray revealed bilateral patchy, alveolar infiltrations (Figure 1). Liver scan showed multiple hepatic and splenic abscesses, 0.5-1 cm in diameter. Gram's stain of pus from skin pustules showed rare, faint-staining gram-negative rods with a safety pin appearance. The provisional diagnosis of disseminated septicemic melioidosis was made and treatment with cotrimoxazole, kanamycin, and chloramphenicol was initiated. Aggressive resuscitation of shock and assisted ventilation were also started promptly. However, the patient deteriorated rapidly and died 48 h after admission. Cultures from blood, sputum, and urine all grew *Pseudomonas pseudomallei*, which were sensitive to the antibiotics given. Postmortem examination demonstrated diffuse bronchopneumonia in both lungs, and multiple small abscesses in liver, spleen, intestinal wall, and kidneys.

Case 2

A 48-year-old male plant worker with a 5 year history of diabetes had experienced intermittent fever and right upper quadrant pain for 2 months. Physical

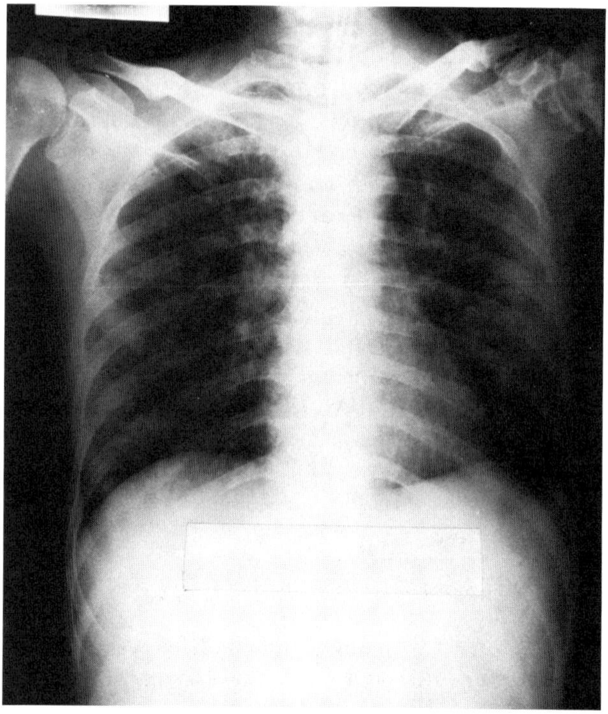

Figure 1 Chest x-ray demonstrates bilateral patchy alveolar infiltrations at time of admission.

examination revealed a middle-aged man who was not in distress with mild jaundice. His temperature was 37.5 °C, pulse rate 84/min, and blood pressure 130/80 mmHg. The rest of the examination was normal except for an enlarged liver measured 4 inches below the right costal margin with mild tenderness. The liver scan showed a 5 × 6 cm^2 space occupying lesion in the superior part of the right lobe. The diagnosis of amebic liver abscess was suspected and metronidazole was given. Direct needle aspiration of the abscess was done on the third hospital day and obtained 3 ml of anchovy-colored pus. Gram's stain of the liver aspirate revealed no organism.

Twelve hours after the procedure, the patient experienced spike of fever (40 °C) and diffuse abdominal tenderness. At 36 h, he became dyspneic, cyanotic, and hypotensive (blood pressure 60/40 mmHg). Chest x-ray showed bilateral alveolar infiltration (Figure 2). The diagnosis of ruptured or leakage of hepatic abscess was made and a laparotomy was performed. No abscess was found in the abdominal cavity; instead, there were small abscesses 2-3 mm

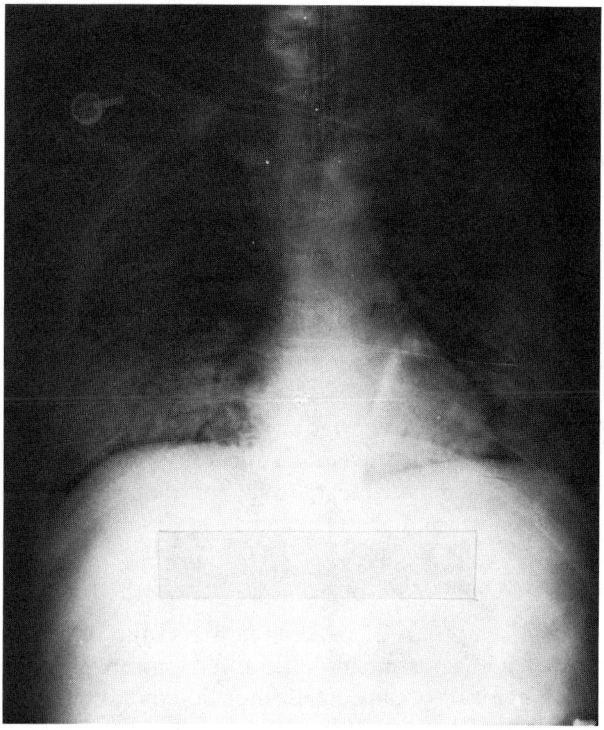

Figure 2 Chest x-ray demonstrates bilateral alveolar infiltrations that appeared 36 h after surgery.

in diameter distributed over the surface of liver, spleen, intestinal wall, and omentum. Postoperatively, he was in profound shock and hypoxemic states despite aggressive resuscitative treatments and died 48 h later. Cultures of pus obtained from liver, intraabdominal abscess, blood, and sputum grew *Pseudomonas pseudomallei* resistant to the antibiotics prescribed.

Comments

Both patients had uncontrolled diabetes mellitus as an underlying disease and experienced rapid fatal deterioration within a few days after their disease disseminated. This happened despite early appropriate antibiotic treatment. Profound shock and severe hypoxemia usually contributed to death before the antibiotics took action. It was surprising that the primary source of infection in the first patient could not be identified. The second patient had carried a silent liver abscess for months. Needle aspiration of the abscess led to rapid spreading of the organisms into the bloodstream to various organs. Thus, in cases of suspected melioidosis, a full range of antibiotic coverage is recommended before any surgical attempt is made.

B. Nondisseminated Septicemic Melioidosis

The usual presenting symptoms of patients with disease in this group are fever of undetermined origin or fever with chronic identified localized infections limited to one or two organs. Despite the positive blood cultures, no evidence of widespread, multiple organ infections or acute septicemia (e.g., hypotension, acute respiratory failure) is detected. Patients usually run benign and uneventful clinical courses, with very low fatality rates. Liver abscesses and pneumonitis are the most common localized infections found and account for 30-60% of cases. Other reported organ infections included prostatitis, arthritis, lymphadenitis, osteomyelitis, pericarditis, and brain abscesses. As in the patients with disseminated septicemia, most habor one or more concurrent diseases, among which diabetes mellitus was found to be most common.

C. Localized Melioidosis

Clinical signs and symptoms of patients in this group resemble those with nondisseminated septicemic melioidosis. Infections are chronic, localized, and limited to one or two organs. Septicemia does not occur and thus blood cultures are negative. The organs involved are similar but higher incidences of urinary tract infection and lymphadenitis are found. Some patients may have concurrent illness but more than half of these patients have been previously healthy. Outcome of treatment is usually good, with a very low fatality rate.

Case 3

A 48-year-old man from the southern part of Thailand had experienced fever and productive cough of yellowish sputum for 2 weeks. Physical examination was unremarkable except for a temperature of 39.7 °C and crepitations over the right upper lung field. Chest x-ray showed alveolar infiltration with multiple cavities involving the entire right upper lobe (Fig. 3). Gram's stain of the sputum revealed mixed gram-positive cocci and gram-negative coccobacilli. Anaerobic pneumonia was initially diagnosed and intravenous penicillin G was given. Since the x-ray findings were unable to exclude tuberculosis, isoniazid, ethambutol, and streptomycin were added on the fourth hospital day despite the acid fast bacilli- (AFB) negative sputum. Admission blood and sputum cultures were negative. On the seventh day of his hospitalization, sputum culture revealed growth of *Pseudomonas pseudomallei*.

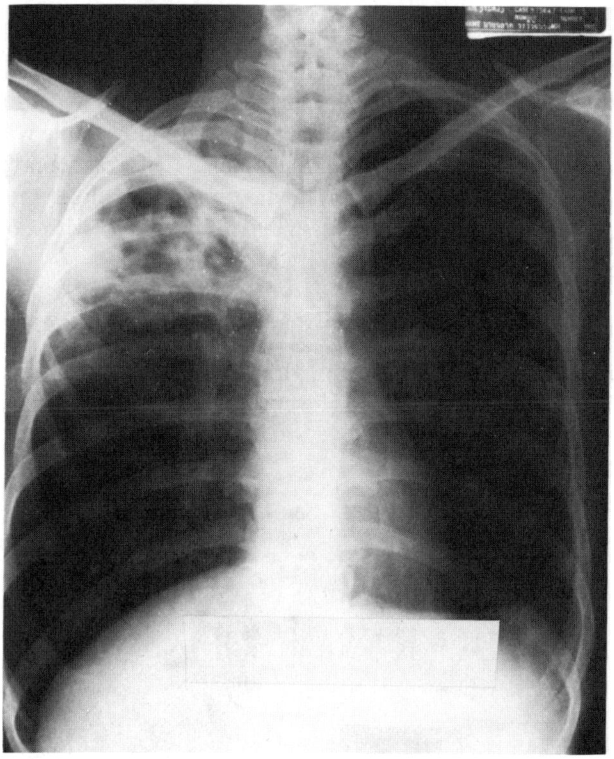

Figure 3 Chest x-ray demonstrates cavitating infiltrations involving the entire right upper lobe.

Penicillin and antituberculous drugs were then replaced by cotrimoxazole and kanamycin. The patient's clinical symptoms improved gradually and he became afebrile after 5 days of treatment. The indirect hemagglutination titer for melioidosis was 1:320 and monotherapy with cotrimoxazole was contined for 6 months.

Case 4

A 17-year-old farmer from the northeastern part of Thailand was admitted because of intermittent fever, cough with scanty sputum, and an abnormal chest x-ray. He was treated in the local hospital with three antituberculous drugs for 3 months without clinical or roentgenographic improvement. Physical examination was unremarkable except for a diminished breath sound over the right lower lung area. Chest x-ray (Fig. 4a) showed cavitary infiltration in the right middle lobe that was unchanged from the film taken 3 months earlier. Repeated blood cultures were negative. Gram's stain of sputum revealed mixed organisms and the culture grew normal flora. Antituberculous drugs were then replaced by clindamycin. Assessment after 3 weeks of treatment showed no improvement. A blood sample was then taken for indirect hemagglutination test for melioidosis. This was found to be strongly positive, with a titer of 1:1280. The diagnosis of melioid pneumonia was finally made and the patient was successfully treated with cotrimoxazole (Fig. 4b,c).

Comments

Cases 3 and 4 demonstrated chronic, localized pulmonary melioidosis with its typical benign clinical course. The chronicity and x-ray appearance made

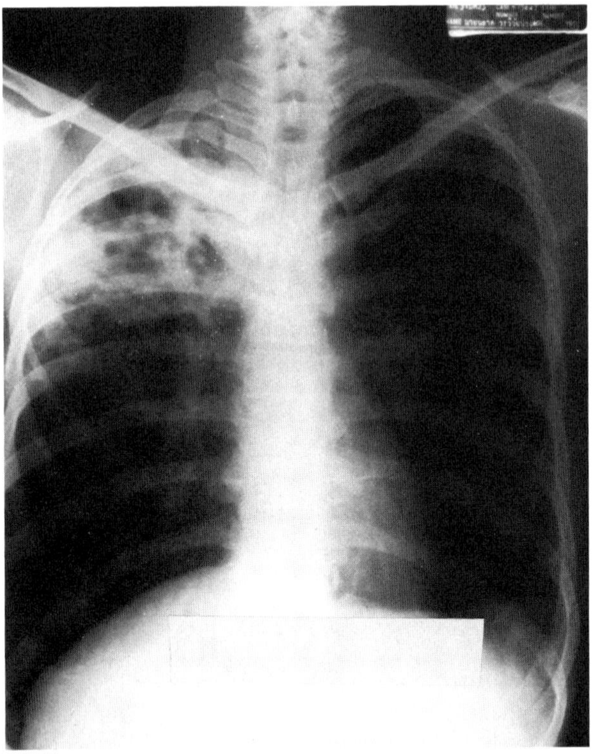

(a)

Figure 4 a. Admission chest x-ray demonstrates cavitating infiltrations in the right middle lobe. b,c. Chest radiographs at 2 and 6 months after treatment.

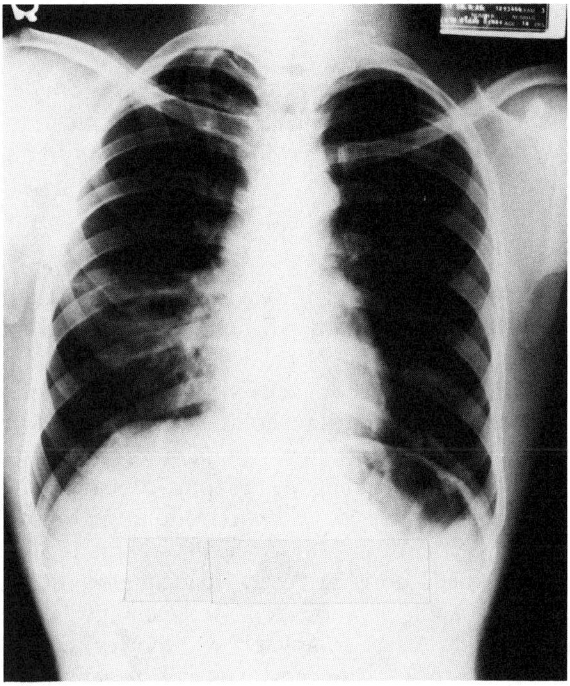

(b)

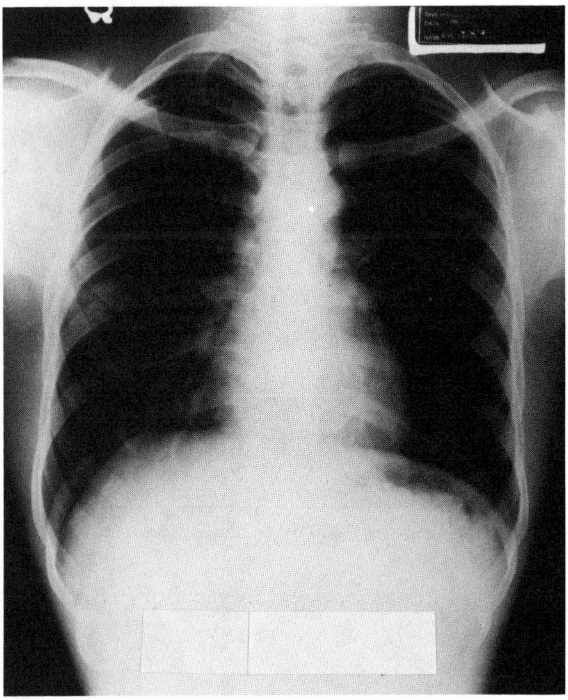

(c)

it difficult to differentiate from tuberculosis. This creates a diagnostic problem, particularly in places where the incidence of tuberculosis is very high. Once the disease is diagnosed, therapy will not be difficult to administer and response is usually good.

D. Subclinical Melioidosis

This is manifest in patients who have a positive serologic test for melioidosis but no evident clinical infection. This may indicate previous infection with development of host immunity.

The course of each form of melioidosis is interrelated (Fig. 5). The benign form of localized or subclinical melioidosis can be transformed to the more malignant form whenever the host's immunity is impaired.

Case 2 involved an example of the transformation of localized hepatic melioidosis to disseminated septicemic melioidosis following breakage of the abscess wall. Patients who survive acute fulminating courses of disseminated septicemic melioidosis but receive inadequate antibiotic treatment will carry infections in some organs as localized melioidosis. If chemotherapy is adequate, they will recover completely with no foci of residual infections. Most of these patients will show positive serological tests for years or indefinately. The condition is termed *subclinical melioidosis* since the presence of antibodies does not prevent the reactivation of disease in the future. Recrudescence is a well-known feature of melioidosis and usually occurs following factors or diseases that impair host defenses: uncontrolled diabetes mellitus,

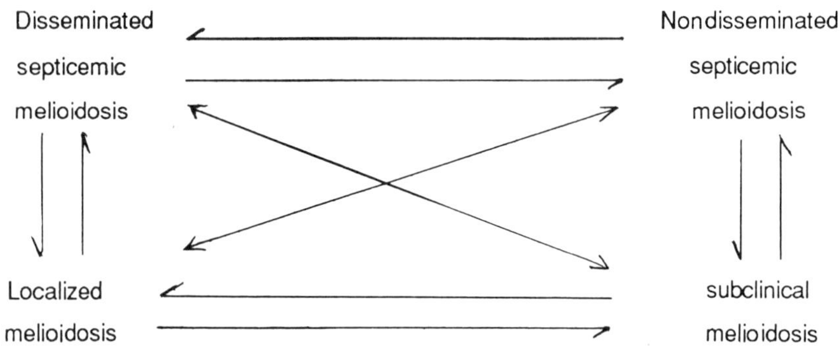

Figure 5 Diagram illustrates interrelationship of each clinical form of melioidosis.

corticosteroid therapy, and emergence of a new malignant tumor. The time interval between each reactivation varies: it may be few months or more than 20 years.

IV. Bacteriological Findings

Pseudomonas pseudomallei is a rapidly motile, non-acid-fast, noncapsulated, gram-negative bacilli with a characteristic safety pin appearance (Bassett, 1971; Cheong et al., 1987; Eickhoff et al., 1970; Everett and Kishimoto, 1973; Hall and Manion, 1973; Howe et al., 1971, Jayanetra et al., 1975). Many synonyms for this organism have been used in the past, including *Loefflerella whitmori, Pfeifferella whitmori, Malleomyces pseudomallei,* and *Actinobacillus pseudomallei.* It grows easily in conventional culture media (e.g., blood agar, eosin-methylene blue agar, and nutrient agar). At 24 h after incubation, the colony is 1 mm, convex, and mucoid. After 72 h, shrinkage occurs, which causes folds radiating from the convex center. This resembles an old yeast colony and often leads to confusion, particularly when it grows together with other bacteria. The colony does not produce soluble pigment but may have different colors due to the nonspecific uptake of dye from the culture media. The characteristic finding that alerts laboratory workers to the early recognition of the organism is its strong musty or earthy odor. This is almost pathognomonic and can be detected very early, soon after the colonies are visible on the culture plate.

The characteristic antibiotic sensitivity pattern makes *Pseudomonas pseudomallei* distinct from other gram-negative bacilli. The organisms are highly sensitive to sulfisoxazole, kanamycin, and novobiocin. As a rule, they are resistant to drugs in the penicillin group, lincomycin, and the first and second generations of cephalosporins. Other antipseudomonal drugs (e.g., polymyxin, carbenicillin, and aminoglycosides other than kanamycin) are also ineffective. Recently, a combination of trimethoprim and sulfamethoxazole or cotrimoxazole was found to have great inhibitory effect in vitro and has been used widely and successfully in clinical treatment during the past 10 years.

New beta-lactam drugs (e.g., ceftazidime, piperacillin, amoxycillin, clavulanic acid, azlocillin, mezlocillin, monobactam, and imipenem) have been found to have very low minimum inhibitory concentrations (MIC), with an MIC_{50} of 0.8-1.6 g/L. However, the time kill effects are not satisfactory and the organisms are not killed completely after 8 h of incubation.

An in vitro synergistic effect has been found in combinations of chloramphenicol and tetracycline, chloramphenicol and cotrimoxazole, tetracycline and cotrimoxazole, cotrimoxazole and kanamycin. Antagonism occurs when tetracycline is combined with kanamycin and chloramphenicol with kanamycin. These are all laboratory data; no well-documented synergism or antagonism has been shown in clinical use.

V. Serological Findings

Pseudomonas pseudomallei infection elicits both cellular and humoral immune responses (Alexander et al., 1970; Ashdown, 1981a,b; Howe et al., 1971; Ismail et al., 1987; Khupulsup and Petchclai, 1986; Nigg, 1963; Nigg and Johnston, 1961). It is unclear which antigen is responsible for each immune response. An antigen called whitmorine or melioidin was once used in the skin test for melioidosis, but was found later to be nonspecific. Humoral immunity studies have been carried out widely; the methods used included direct hemagglutination test, indirect hemagglutination test (IHA), and complement fixation test (CF). The later two tests have proven to be more sensitive and specific. However, IHA has been used most commonly in routine diagnostic tests because of its simplicity and low cost. In general, the levels of antibodies are considered significant are a CF titer over 1:4 and IHA titer over 1:40. In Thailand, where infection is more prevalent, population surveys revealed higher antibody levels in the general population and the IHA titer must exceed 1:80 or 1:160 to be considered positive. False-positive IHA or cross-reactivity is also found in patients infected by *Pseudomonas aeruginosa, Staphylococcus,* and Enterobacteriaceae, but the titers are usually low.

Only 60-80% of patients with clinical melioidosis show a positive IHA test. Those with more chronic and localized form of melioidosis usually exhibit higher incidence of positive IHA with higher titer than those with the acute form. One week after infection, 40% of patients will show a significant IHA titer; the rate will rise to 60-70% by the end of the second week. Thereafter, the antibody level will be persistently high for years regardless of the treatment and clinical response. Transient anergy may occur occasionally in cases of recrudescent disseminated septicemic melioidosis despite previous positive IHA. Thus, IHA is a useful diagnostic test but is of no value in following the response and outcome of treatment. In recent years, new diagnostic serologic tests with higher sensitivity and specificity have been developed. Examples are enzyme-linked immunosorbent assay (ELISA) and indirect fluorescent antibody-IgM (IFA-IgM) techniques. Much attention was drawn to the IFA-IgM, since it is claimed to be useful in differentiating clinical and subclinical melioidosis.

VI. Laboratory Findings

Blood analyses in patients with melioidosis are of little diagnostic aid. Patients may have normal leukocyte count, leukocytosis or leukopenia (Bateson and Webling, 1981; Dhiensiri et al., 1988; Everett and Nelson, 1975; Kiatboonsri and Sathapatayavongs, 1985). Laboratory tests that may be of special use in diagnosing melioidosis are described below.

A. Chest X-Ray

Chest x-ray findings in melioidosis are generally of the two forms discussed here.

Diffuse, Bilateral Patchy Alveolar Infiltration

This type of infiltration is found in 80% of patients with disseminated septicemic melioidosis (Figs. 1,2). The patchy infiltrates distributed bilaterally resemble classic hematogenously spreaded pneumonia. Associated infections in various organs are almost always found. Since the disease process is very acute, most of the infiltrates contain no cavity on first presentation. If patients present late, small cavities may occur. Clearing is mostly complete in patients who survive and recover, with no residual scar on the following chest x-ray.

Localized Infiltration

This form is found in nondisseminated septicemic melioidosis and localized melioidosis. Clinical features and chest x-ray findings closely resemble pulmonary tuberculosis (cases 3,4). Weeks or months of fever and cough with varying amount of sputum are the most frequent presenting symptoms. Accompanying hemoptysis and chest pain are also not uncommonly found. The lesions seen on chest x-ray usually consist of lobar or segmental infiltration of one or two sites. Unilateral or bilateral upper lobe infiltration is the most common finding, occurring in 70-90% of cases. Cavitations occur in 40-70% of the infiltrates, most of which are small (0.5-1 cm in diameter) and multiple (Figs. 3, 4a). It is very unusual to find an abscess larger than 2.5 cm in diameter or an air fluid level in the cavity. Unlike the anaerobic lung abscess, most melioid abscesses do not produce large amount of purulent sputum. After treatment, clearing is mostly incomplete in these cavitating lesions, with some residual fibrotic scar (Fig. 4c).

As mentioned above, tuberculosis cannot be differentiated from localized melioidosis based on clinical and chest x-ray findings. Diagnosis must rely on cultures and serologic studies. However, localized pulmonary melioidosis still shows some characteristics of gram-negative pneumonia that differ from pulmonary tuberculosis. Some of the following points may alert clinicians and lead to earlier recognition of the disease.

Rate of Progression of Pulmonary Lesions

Although localized pulmonary melioidosis may have unchanged or persistent infiltrates for weeks or months, some patients do have clinical and roentgenographic progression within a few days or a week during investigations. This makes pulmonary tuberculosis unlikely, since this needs months for such roentgenographic deterioration.

Rate of Roentgenographic Resolution after Appropriate Medical Treatments

In contrast to the uncertain rate of deterioration, localized pulmonary melioidosis usually responds to treatment well and has apparent roentgenographic improvement within 7-14 days. Such rapid improvement rate is not a feature of pulmonary tuberculosis.

Pleural Effusion

Pleural effusion is found in 5-15% of patients with localized pulmonary melioidosis. This is parapneumonic effusion and thus associated pulmonary infiltrates are almost always found. The amount of fluid is not large; therefore, pressure effect is not a common presenting symptom. This is contrast to tuberculous pleuritis, in which large amount of pleural fluid without underlying pulmonary infiltrates are commonly found.

Other Features

Hilar adenopathy is very uncommon in melioidosis (less than 2-5%). This differs from the more frequent hilar adenopathy found in primary tuberculosis. Although upper lobe infiltrations are commonly found, melioidosis usually does not cause dense calcification, dense fibrosis, or typical upper lobe atelectasis as found in pulmonary tuberculosis. Furthermore, some observers found that apical segment involvement was less common than in tuberculosis.

B. Ultrasonography and Computed Tomography

These procedures are usually used in cases suspected of hepatic or splenic abscess. When such abscesses are present, they are mostly small (0.2-3 cm) and multiple, with central white spots or target appearance. If the abscess is larger than 3 cm, it will usually contain small lucent areas within the cavity. This may represent an aggregate of small abscesses or a true single abscess with multiloculation. These features are not commonly found in amebic liver abscess or pyogenic liver abscess caused by other bacteria.

C. Gram's Stains

Gram's stains of sputum from patients with pulmonary lesions and pus or aspirates from abscesses have their distinctive features that are worth mentioning. The organisms, if present, are characteristically few in number or rarely found with faint staining. These are different from most pyogenic infections in which an early diagnosis can be easily made based on clinical specimen stainings.

VII. Diagnosis

Definitive diagnosis of melioidosis depends on one of the following criteria: isolation of *Pseudomonas pseudomallei* from clinical specimens (e.g., blood, sputum, pus, urine, etc.), or positive serologic test for *Pseudomonas pseudomallei* (e.g., IHA titer greater than 1:80, CF titer greater than 1:4, or fourfold rising titer of either test in the convalescent serum).

In endemic areas, patients whose clinical findings are close to those of melioidosis but with negative cultures and routine results of serologic tests are, in some instances, treated as having melioidosis. If improvement is prompt and dramatic, therapy is continued to the complete course. These patients are labeled as having "probable melioidosis" to alert clinicians about possible future recrudescence.

VIII. Treatment

A. Antibiotics

Antibiotic treatment is still the mainstay of therapy in melioidosis (John, 1976; Kiatboonsri and Vathesatogkit, 1979; Sathapatayavongs and Kiatboonsri, 1985; Zajtchuk et al., 1973). In disseminated septicemic melioidosis, antibiotics should be started immediately when the disease is suspected. At least two or three bactericidal drugs are usually used initially. This is followed by use of one or two drugs until the disease is cured. This can be evident by disappearance of inflammation or localized infections, and improvement of the chest roentgenogram with no further clearing. The total duration of treatment should be more than 4-6 weeks. Usually, it ranges from 2 to 6 months, depending on the response to the treatment. Examples of drug combinations are cotrimoxazole plus chloramphenicol plus ceftazidime followed by cotrimoxazole; tetracycline plus cotrimoxazole plus kanamycin followed by cotrimoxazole or tetracycline. The dosage of each drug should be two to three times normal at initiation. This is gradually reduced when clinical signs and symptoms improve. Monotherapy with a drug with a very low MIC, such as the new beta-lactam derivatives, is not recommended, since in vitro killing is slow and incomplete. Furthermore, clinical studies of some of these drugs showed no definite benefit over the old regimens. They should therefore be used in a combination rather than as a single drug in the treatment of disseminated septicemic melioidosis.

Patients with nondisseminated septicemic melioidosis and localized melioidosis are usually treated initially with one or two organism-sensitive antibiotics until clinical improvement is evident. This is followed by a single drug for the rest of the course. The dosage and duration of treatment are not different from those used in disseminated septicemic melioidosis. Because of the possible transformation of their disease to the disseminated form, patients with nondisseminated septicemic melioidosis and localized melioidosis should receive antibiotic treatment soon after the diagnosis is suspected.

Antibiotic treatment of subclinical melioidosis is not recommended, since there is no indicator for the timing of its clinical transformation. Furthermore, treatment in the symptom-free period may not prevent future recrudescence.

B. Surgical Treatment

This is used as an adjunct to medical treatment. Examples are drainage of pus from various organ abscesses, empyema, and pericardial effusion. Antibiotics should be started prior to any surgical procedure to prevent systemic dissemination and be continued until the disease is cured. Patients who undergo surgical drainage without appropriate antibiotic coverage will experience persistent chronic sinuses, a feature similar to tuberculosis.

C. Supportive Treatment

This includes aggressive management of severe hypoxemia and profound septicemic shock in the acute stage of disseminated septicemic melioidosis. Such treatments outweight antibiotics in the first few days and usually determine the early survival. Patients who survive the acute catastrophic period are often malnourished and need a prolonged hospital stay. Adequate nutritional supplements and prevention of nosocomial infection are thus important and determine the late survival.

In summary, complete cycled treatments are needed in the management of melioidosis. These included appropriate use of antibiotics, good critical care, good chronic supportive care, and awareness of future recrudescence.

References

Achana, V., Silpapojakul, K., Thininta, W., and Kalnaowakul, S. (1985). Acute *Pseudomonas pseudomallei* pneumonia and septicemia following aspiration of contaminated water: a case report. *Southeast Asian J. Trop. Med. Public Health* **16**:500-504.

Alexander, A.D., Huxoll, D. L., Warner, A. R., Shepler, V., and Dorsey, A. (1970). Serological diagnosis of human melioidosis with indirect hemagglutination and complement fixation test. *Appl. Microbiol.* **20**:825-833.

Ashdown, L. R. (1981a). Demonstration of human antibodies to *Pseudomonas pseudomallei* by indirect fluorescent antibody staining. *Pathology* **13**:597-601.

Ashdown, L. R. (1981b). Realtionship and significance of specific immunoglobulin M antibody response in clinical and subclinical melioidosis. *J. Clin. Microbiol.* **14**:361-364.

Bassett, D. C. J. (1971). The sensitivity of *Pseudomonas pseudomallei* to trimethoprim and sulfamethoxazole in vitro. *J. Clin. Pathol.* **24**:798-800.

Bateson, E. M., and Webling, D. D. A. (1981). The radiological appearances of pulmonary melioidosis: a report on twenty three cases. *Australas. Radiol.* **25**:239-245.

Carruthers, M. M. (1981). Recrudescent melioidosis mimicking lung abscess. *Am. Rev. Respir. dis.* **124**:756-758.

Cheong, Y. M., Joseph, P. G., and Koay, A. S. (1987). In vitro susceptibility of *Pseudomonas pseudomallei* isolated in Malaysia to some new cephalosporins and quinoline. *Southeast Asian J. Trop. Med. Publ. Health* **18**:94-96.

Clayton, A. J., Lisella, R. S., and Martin, D. G. (1973). Melioidosis: a serological survey in military personel. *Milit. Med.* **138**:24-26.

Cooper, E. B. (1967). Melioidosis. *J.A.M.A.* **200**:452-453.

Dhiensiri, T., Paupairoj, S., and Susaengrat, W. (1988). Pulmonary melioidosis: clinical-radiologic correlation in 183 cases in Northeastern Thailand. *Radiology* **166**:711-715.

Eickhoff, T. C., Bennett, J. V., Hayes, P. S., and Feeley, J. (1970). *Pseudomonas pseudomallei*: susceptibility to chemotherapeutic agents. *J. Infect. Dis.* **121**:95-101.

Everett, E. D., and Kishimoto, R. A. (1973). In vivo sensitivity of 33 strains of *Pseudomonas pseudomallei* to trimethoprim and sulfamethoxazole. *J. Infect. Dis.* **128** (Suppl):539-542.

Everett, E. D., and Nelson, R. A. (1975). Pulmonary melioidosis: observation in thirty-nine cases. *Am. Rev. Respir. Dis.* **112**:331-340.

Green, R. N., and Tuffnell, P. G. (1968). Laboratory acquired melioidosis. *Am. J. Med.* **44**:599-605.

Hall, W. H., and Manion, R. E. (1973). Antibiotic susceptibility of Pseudomonas pseudomallei. *Antimicrob. Agents. Chemother.* **4**:193-195.

Howe, C., Samphath, A., and Spotnitz, M. (1971). The pseudomallei group: a review. *J. Infect. Dis.* **124**:598-606.

Ismail, G., Noor Embi, M., Omar, O., Allen, C., and Smith, C. J. (1987). A competitive immunosorbent assay for detection of *Pseudomonas pseudomallei* exotoxin. *J. Med. Microbiol.* **23**:353-357.

Jackson, A. E., Moor, W. L., and Sanford, J. P. (1972). Recrudescent melioidosis associated with diabetic ketoacidosis. *Arch. Intern. Med.* **130**: 268-271.

Jayanetra, P., Vorachit, M., and Bhatarakamol, S. (1975). *Pseudomonas pseudomallei*: II. Laboratory and experimental studies in animals. *Southeast Asian. J. Trop. Med. Public Health* **6**:10-17.

John, J. F. (1976). Trimethoprim-sulfamethoxazole therapy of pulmonary melioidosis. *Am. Rev. Respir. Dis.* **114**:1021-1025.

Khupulsup, K., and Petchclai, B. (1986). Application of indirect hemagglutination test and indirect fluorescent antibody test for IgM antibody for diagnosis of melioidosis in Thailand. *Am. J. Trop. Med. Hyg.* **35**: 366-369.

Kiatboonsri, S., and Sathapatayavongs, B. (1985). Non-bacteremic and bacteremic melioidosis: a clinical study. In *Abstracts of the National Workshop on Melioidosis*, Bangkok, Thailand, pp. 46-56.

Kiatboonsri, S., and Vathesatogkit, P. (1979). Melioidosis. *Thai Med. Council Bull.* **6**:593-612.

Mays, E. E., and Ricketts, E. A. (1975). Melioidosis: recrudescence associated with bronchogenic carcinoma twenty six years following initial geographic exposure. *Chest* **68**:261-263.

McCormick, J. B., Sexton, D. J., McMurray, J. G., Carey, E., Hayes, P., and Feldman, R. A. (1975). Human-to-human transmission of *Pseudomonas pseudomallei. Ann. Intern. Med.* **83**:512-513.

Nachiangmai, N., Patamasucon, P., Tipayamonthein, B., Kongpon, A., and Nakaviroj, S. (1985). *Pseudomonas pseudomallei* in southern Thailand. *Southeast Asian J. Trop. Med. Pub. Health* **16**:83-87.

Nigg, C. (1963). Serologic studies on subclinical melioidosis. *J. Immunol.* **91**:18-28.

Nigg, C., and Johnston, M. M. (1961). Complement fixation test in experimental clinical and subclinical melioidosis. *J. Bacteriol.* **82**:159-169.

Pack, C. R., and Zwanenburg, T. (1947). A case of melioidosis presenting as an abscess in the neck. *Br. Med. J.* **1**:337-338.

Paton, J. P. J., Peck, C. R., and Van de Schaaf, A. (1947). Report on a case of melioidosis from Siam. *Br. Med. J.* **1**:336-337.

Piggott, J. A., and Hochholzer, L. (1970). Human melioidosis: a histopathologic study of acute and chronic melioidosis. *Arch. Pathol.* **90**:101-111.

Prevatt, A. L., and Hunt, J. S. (1957). Chronic systematic melioidosis. *Am. J. Med.* **23**:810-823.

Sanford, J. P. (1971). Recrudescent melioidosis: a Southeast Asian legacy. *Am. Rev. Respir. Dis.* **104**:452-453.

Sathapatayavongs, B., and Kiatboonsri, S. (1985). Outcome treatments of melioidosis in Ramathibodi Hospital (1973-1985). In *Abstracts of the National Workshop on Melioidosis.* Bangkok, Thailand, pp. 144-148.

Schlech, W. F., 3d, Turchik, J. B., Westlake, R. E., Jr., Klein, G. C., Band, J. D., and Weaver, R. E. (1981). Laboratory-acquired infection with *Pseudomonas pseudomallei* (melioidosis). *N. Engl. J. Med.* **305**:1133-1135.

So, S. Y. (1985). Melioidosis: an overlooked problem in Hong Kong. *Hong Kong Practitioner* **7**:1111-1114.

Spotnitz, M., Rudnitzky, J., and Rambaud, J. J. (1967). Melioidosis pneumonitis. *J.A.M.A.* **202**:950-954.

Susaengrat, W., Dhiensiri, T., Sinavatana, P., and Sitprija, V. (1987). Renal failure in melioidosis. *Nephron* **46**:167-169.

Thin, R. N. T., Brown, M., Stewart, J. B., and Garrett, C. J. (1970). Melioidosis: a report of ten cases. *Q. J. Med.* **39**:115-127.

Thisyakorn, U. (1986). Melioidosis in children at children's hospital, Bangkok. *Southeast. Asian. J. Trop. Med. Pub. Health* **17**:101-103.

Weber, D. R., Douglass, L. E., Brundage, W. G., and Stallkamp, T. C. (1969). Acute varieties of melioidosis occurring in U.S. soldiers in Vietnam. *Am. J. Med.* **46**:234-244.

Whitmore, A., and Krishnaswami, C. S. (1912). An account of the discovery of a hitherto undescribed infective disease occurring among the population of Rangoon. *Indian. Med. Gaz.* **47**:262-267.

Zajtchuk, R., Guiton, C. R., Sadler, T. R., Heydorn, W. H., and Strevey, T. E. (1973). Surgical treatment of pulmonary melioidosis. *J. Thorac. Cardiovasc. Surg.* **66**:838-840.

5

Pulmonary Complications of Brucellosis

A. R. LULU

Johra Hospital
Kuwait

G. F. ARAJ

Mubarek-Al-Kabeer University Hospital
Kuwait University
Kuwait

I. Introduction

Brucellosis, a zoonotic disease, has a worldwide distribution. It is transmitted to humans from animal reservoirs such as cattle, sheep, goats, camels, and dogs (Hughes, 1897; Spink, 1956; Williams, 1982; Young, 1983). It is caused by aerobic gram-negative bacteria of the genus *Brucella* (named after David Bruce). So far, six species have been identified: *B. melitensis, B. abortus, B. suis, B. canis, B. ovis,* and *B. neotomae,* only the first four are known to cause diseases in humans. The disease has protean manifestations and could affect several body organs or systems (Lulu et al., 1988; Williams, 1982).

Although brucellosis has been controlled in North America, certain European countries, and Japan, it remains a significant public health problem in many countries around the world especially in Latin America, the Mediterranean and the Middle East (Alausa, 1980; Al Kandari et al., 1987; Matyas and Fujikara, 1984; Williams, 1982). In the United States, the reported cases decreased from 6000 in 1949 to 133 in 1985; while in Kuwait it increased from 12 in 1976 to 1168 (69 per 100,000 population) in 1985 (Lulu et al., 1988; Salata, 1988). The World Health Organization still reports over

500,000 cases yearly. In addition, infection in countries that enforced effective control measures is usually occupational: veterinarians, farmers, meat handlers, and laboratory personnel. Although the disease occurs in a wide spectrum of the population, it essentially remains an occupational disorder (Lulu et al., 1988; Gotuzzo et al., 1982; Williams, 1982; Young, 1983; Salata, 1988).

II. Transmission

Brucellosis is acquired by ingestion of contaminated unpasteurized milk or dairy products, contact with an infected animal or its tissues, through abraded skin, via the conjunctiva, or by inhalation of infectious aerosols (Kaufmann et al., 1980; Williams, 1982; Young, 1983). Other routes such as interhuman or blood transfusion are rare (Stanec-Paulinic et al., 1983; Economidow et al., 1976). The relative importance of each route varies with the epidemiological and occupational setting. The majority of cases reported in the literature had a history of ingestion of raw milk or its products (Lulu et al., 1988; Schirger et al., 1960; Sharda and Lubani, 1986). Inhalation of infectious aerosols, as a route of acquiring brucellosis, has been implicated in laboratory, meat packing factory, and abattoir workers and in camping sites soiled by urine or abortion products of infected animals (Kerr et al., 1966; Miller et al., 1987; Hendricks et al., 1962; Buchanan et al., 1974a,b; Feiz et al., 1973; Mousa et al., 1987).

III. Sex and Age Distribution

The ratio of affected males to females ranges from 7:1 in countries where brucella is controlled to 2:1 in endemic areas. It occurs predominantly in those in the 20-40-year age group. Although infection in children was thought to be infrequent, reports from endemic areas show a high incidence of brucellosis in children (Hagebusch and Frei, 1940; Sharda and Lubani, 1986; Young, 1983; Lulu et al., 1988).

IV. Clinical Features

After entry, the microorganisms, engulfed by macrophages and neutrophils, are carried to regional lymph nodes and through the blood to reticuloendothelial tissue and then to other organs. The incubation period is variable, ranging from 10 days to 2 months. The onset may be abrupt but it is mostly insidious. The clinical features are nonspecific and include fever, arthralgia, myalgia, low back pain, arthritis, hepatomegaly, and splenomegaly. Based on the duration of signs and symptoms, brucellosis has been categorized as acute (< 2 months), subacute (2 months to 1 year), and chronic (> 1 year). Complications may occur with variable incidence in various body systems such as the musculoskeletal (30%), genital (8.5%), neurological (7%), psychiatric (6%), cardiovascular (2%), urinary (1.3%), and pulmonary (1%) as reported by us and others (Lulu et al., 1988; Pfischner et al., 1957; Schirger et al., 1960; Sharda and Lubani, 1986; Williams, 1982; Spink, 1956; Young, 1983).

V. Involvement of the Respiratory System

The exact factors involved in the pathogenesis of pulmonary brucellosis remain unclear. Although inhalation is one of the routes of acquiring brucellosis, there is no solid evidence to suggest that this route is associated with pulmonary complications in human brucellosis. It appears that the most likely source of lung disease is hematogenous spread. Experimental studies in guinea pigs have shown that the *Brucella* microorganisms readily invade the lungs by respiratory challenge but do not result in primary pneumonia (De Mello et al., 1967; Elberg and Henderson, 1948). It is suggested, however, that the mode of contracting *Brucella* may influence its clinical presentation (Mousa et al., 1987; Young, 1983; Di Pace et al., 1976).

Respiratory symptoms could occur in 31% of patients with brucellosis but the incidence of serious complications is usually low (≤ 2%). The symptoms are mostly referable to upper respiratory tract and include cough with or without sputum, transient bronchitis, or vague chest pain. These patients usually have normal chest radiographs (Lulu et al., 1988; Mathur, 1960; Pfischner et al., 1957; Robinson, 1938; Mousa et al., 1988).

Pulmonary complications due to brucellosis are rare. The literature (mostly non-English European) on this subject is scarce and mostly reported before 1960. It is probably due to lack of awareness or recognition of the multisystem involvement by *Brucella* microorganisms (Greer, 1956; Herden et al., 1946; Harvey, 1948; Mathur, 1960). There are sporadic case reports of pulmonary brucellosis (Chavez and Veach, 1976; Lafferty and Phillips, 1937; Webb and Thorougham, 1966). In our studies, the incidence of pulmonary complications was 1% of 400 patients in adults and 0.4% of 1100 children with brucellosis. However, higher incidence rates, ranging from 8.7 to 16.4% have been reported by others from this part of the world (Matyas and Fujikura, 1984; Patel et al., 1988).

The epidemiological, demographic, and clinical features of patients with pulmonary complications are generally similar to those with systemic brucellosis, except for the chest findings (Tables 1, 2). For the convenience of this discussion we have categorized pulmonary brucellosis into two clinical types: acute and chronic, depending on whether the duration of the respiratory

Table 1 Clinical Manifestations in Patients with Acute or Chronic Pulmonary Brucellosis

	Percent of patients with signs or symptoms	
	Acute[a] (n = 23)	Chronic[b] (n = 18)
Symptoms		
Fever	100	100
Cough	100	39
Arthralgia	39	67
Sweating	35	67
Chills	30	67
Anorexia	30	50
Weakness	30	100
Myalgia	26	89
Chest pain	17	0
Dyspnea	8	0
Delirium	4	0
Signs/Complications		
Weight loss	30	100
Hepatosplenomegaly	30	27
Arthritis	26	55
Splenomegaly	8	11
Hepatomegaly	8	5
Pericarditis	4	0
Orchitis	4	0

[a]Twelve patients from Kuwait (nine from M. M. Lubani et al. [1989b] and three unpublished before, A. R. Lulu) and 11 from India by T. N. Mathur (1960).
[b]Greer (1956).

Table 2 Chest Radiographic Findings in Patients with Acute Pulmonary Brucellosis from Kuwait, Saudi Arabia, and USA

Findings	Patients Kuwait (n = 12)[a]	Saudi Arabia (n = 27)	USA (n = 10)
Consolidation	5	3	1
Pleural effusion	4	0	1
Hilar or paratracheal lymphadenopathy	3	6	0
Diffuse fluffy coarse infiltrations	2	4	0
Interstitial pneumonitis	1	0	0
Solitary granuloma	1	0	0
Soft miliary mottling	0	10	0
Parenchymal nodules	0	3	0
Pneumothorax	0	1	0
Bronchopneumonia	0	0	8

[a]Three patients had combined lesions each of : consolidation + pleural effusion + hilar lymphadenopathy, effusion + hilar lymphadenopathy, and granuloma + hilar lymphadenopathy.
Data from: Kuwait (nine patients from M. M. Lubani et al. [1989b] and three unpublished before, A. R. Lulu); Saudi Arabia (Patel et al. [1988]); USA (Greer [1956]).

involvement was less or more than 3 months. In both types, a variety of pulmonary lesions have been encountered: bronchitis, bronchopneumonia, pneumonia, pneumonitis, interstitial pneumonitis (Fig. 1), interstitial fibrosis (Fig. 2), miliary infiltrations or calcifications, diffuse perihilar and peribronchial infiltrations, diffuse parynchymal nodulation, solitary pulmonary granuloma (Fig. 3), hilar and paratrachial lymphadenopathy, pleural effusion (Fig. 4), encysted interlobar effusion (Fig. 5), empyema, pneumothorax, pyopneumothorax, abscess, atelectasis, zonal lung fibrosis, and pleural or septal thickening. Table 3 classifies these various clinical and radiographic forms of acute and chronic pulmonary brucellosis as localized or generalized. The most common lesions encountered in the acute form are pneumonia, soft miliary mottling, bronchopneumonia, and hilar and paratracheal lymphadenopathy, while those more common in the chronic form are perihilar

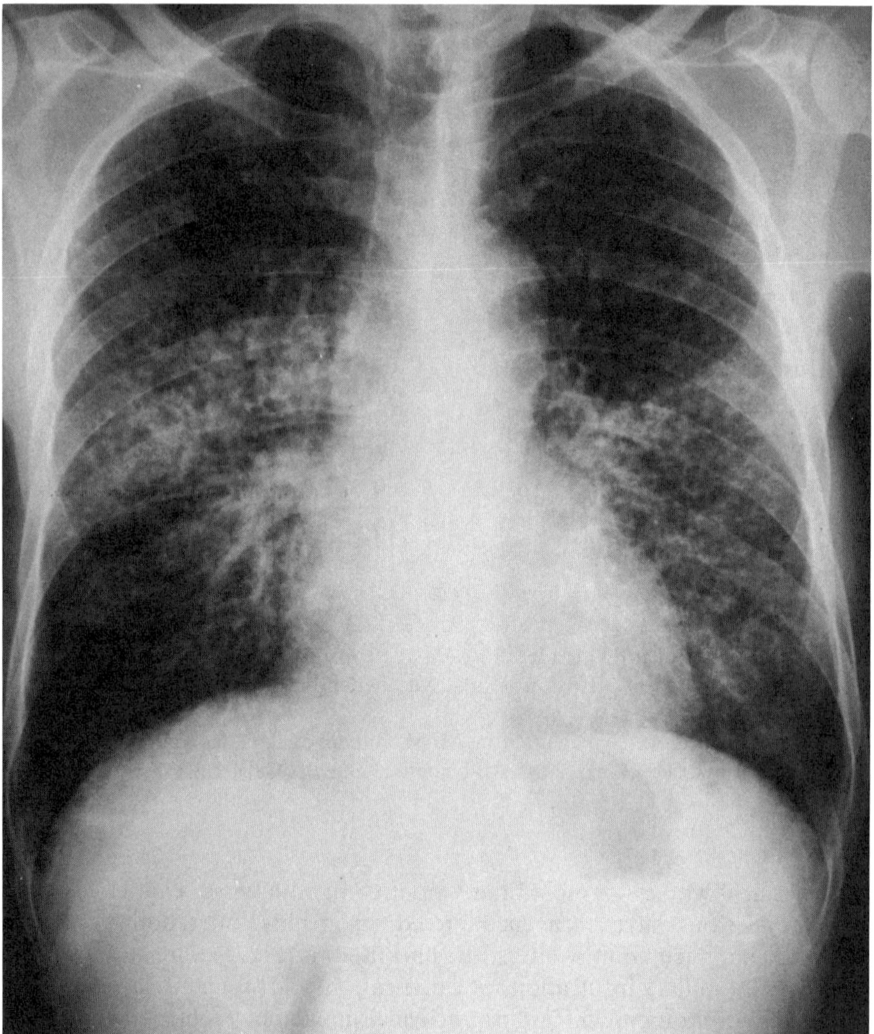

Figure 1 Chest radiograph shows bilateral interstitial pneumonitis.

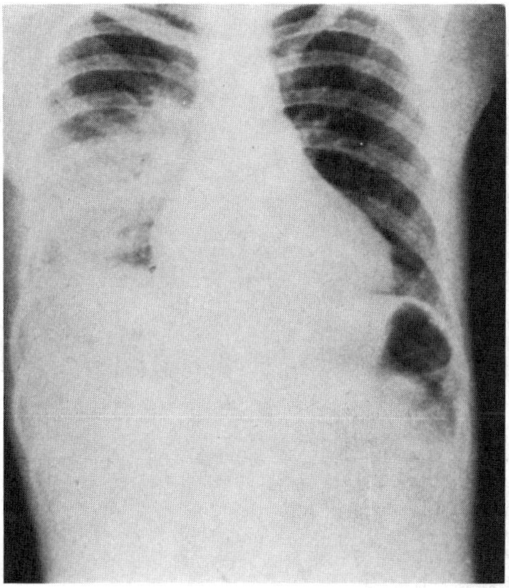

Figure 2 Chest radiograph shows diffuse interstitial fibrosis.

and peribronchial infiltrations, diffuse parynchymal nodulations, and interstitial lung fibrosis (Beatty, 1937; Elson and Ingelfinger, 1942; Greer, 1956; Harvey, 1948; Johnson, 1935; Lubani, 1989a; Mathur, 1960; MacDonald, 1939; Patel et al., 1988; Shipley, 1945; Webb and Thorougham, 1966; Ramah et al., 1959; Bogart, 1936; Weed et al., 1956).

In areas of endemic *Brucella*, acute pulmonary brucellosis occurs as a complication of acute systemic brucellosis, while in nonendemic areas chronic pulmonary complication forms predominate over the acute with a ratio of 3:1. This difference could be due to the high index of suspicion among physicians in endemic areas, resulting in early diagnosis and specific treatment of sufficient duration. In our experience with thousands of cases with brucellosis, we encountered only the acute pulmonary forms.

Acute pulmonary brucellosis usually has an abrupt onset with high fever (101-104°F) and cough, which is mostly mucopurulent. In contrast, chronic pulmonary brucellosis has an insidious onset. It usually occurs in the setting

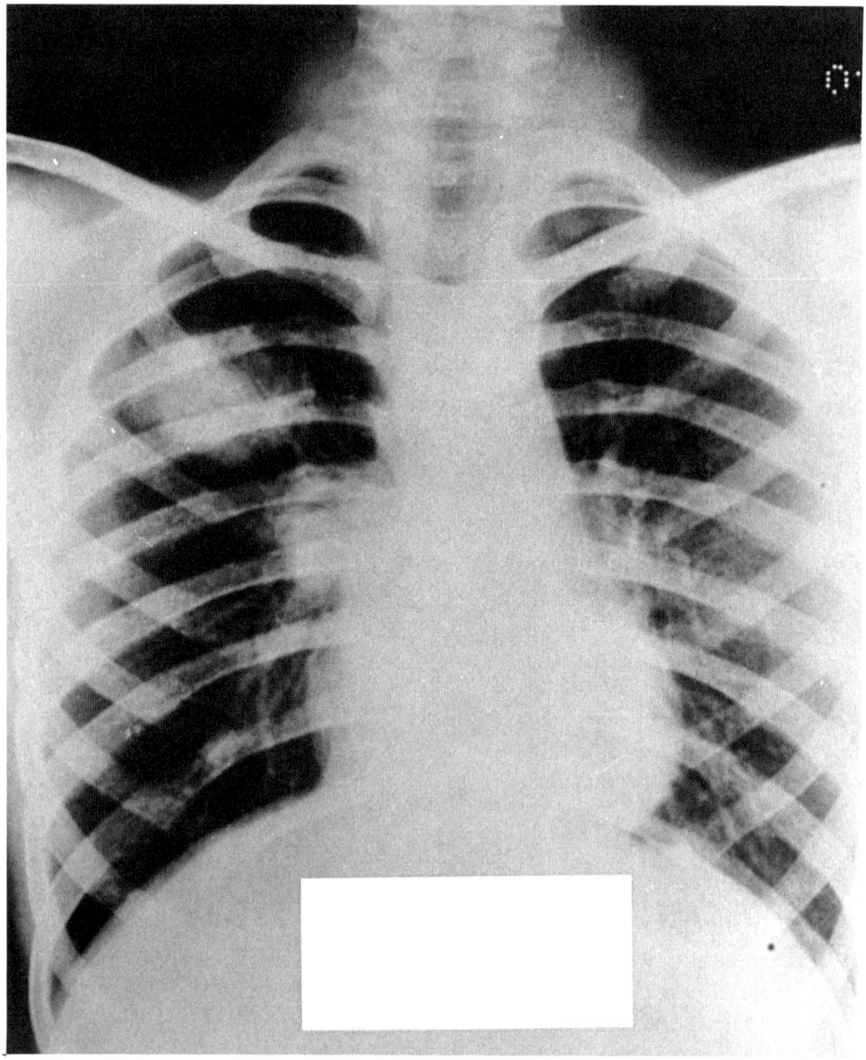

Figure 3 Chest radiographs shows right upper zone solitary pulmonary nodule (granuloma) and right hilar lymphadenopathy.

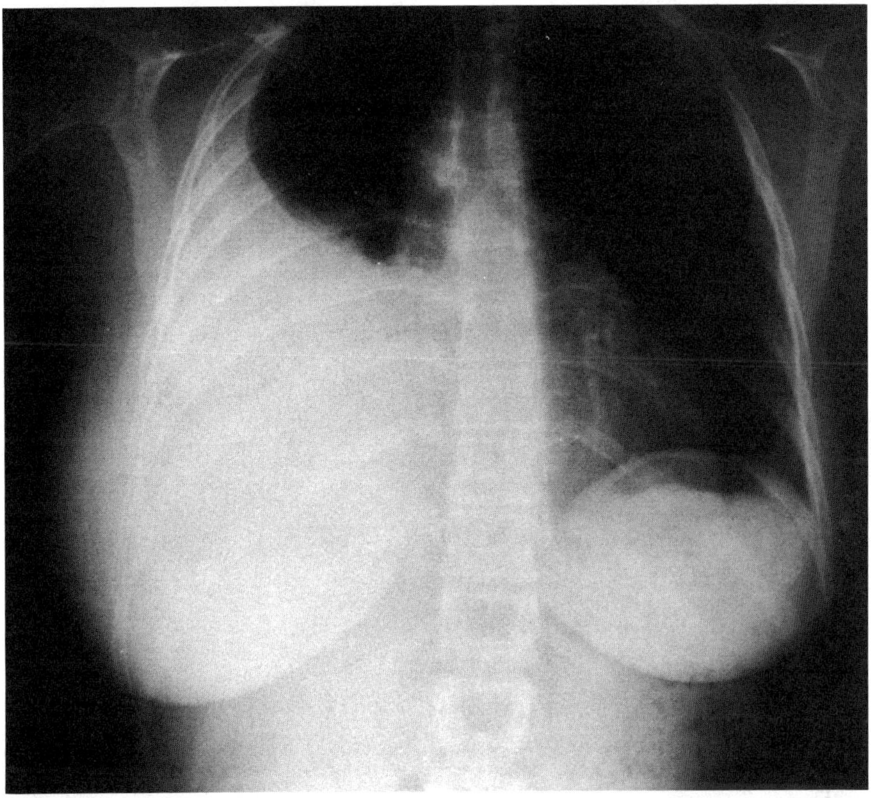

Figure 4 Chest radiograph shows right massive pleural effusion.

of a relapse or chronic form of systemic brucellosis. Fever (99-101°F) and cough are not always present. Patients with chronic localized pulmonary brucellosis are usually asymptomatic and are discovered during a routine chest x-ray and medical check-up (Tables 1, 2).

Physical examination of the chest may show clinical findings according to the pathological abnormality in the lungs. Patients with solitary granuloma, localized encysted interlobar effusion, hilar lymphadenopathy, millet-seed calcification, and pleural and septal thickening have normal findings on physical examination. Fine and coarse crepitations and rhonchi, when present, are mostly basal. Pleural rub is usually present in pleurisy. Diminished air entry with dullness on percussion is elicited in patients with pleural effusion or empyema.

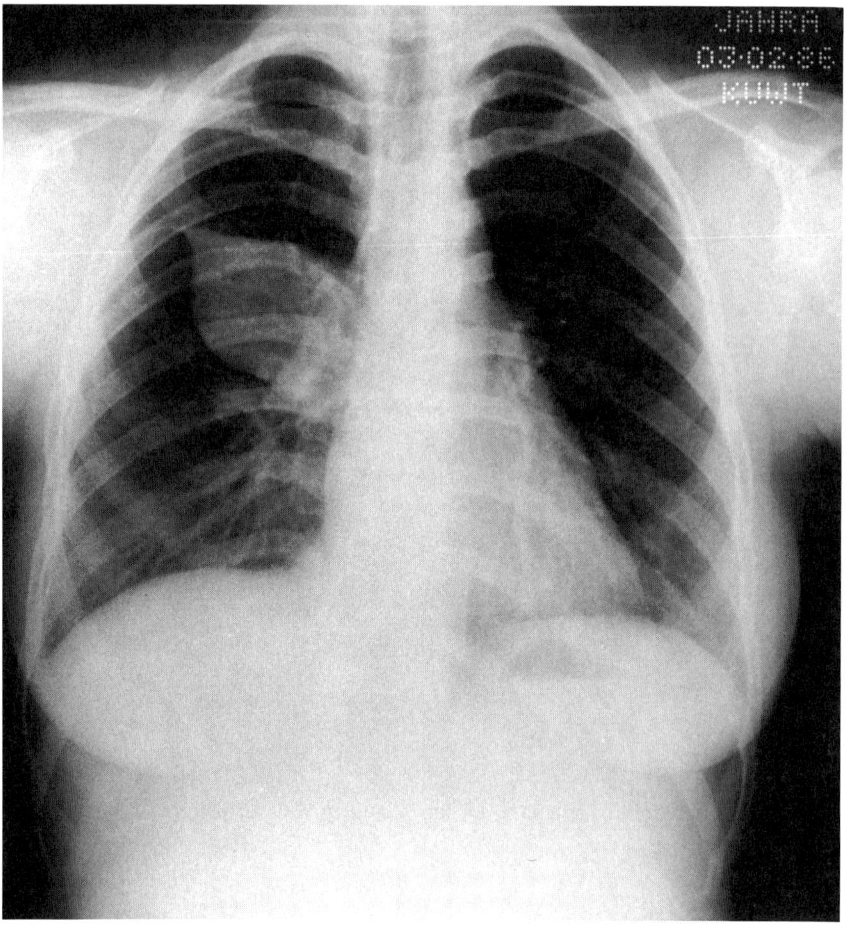

Figure 5 Chest radiograph shows encysted interlobar effusion.

VI. Diagnostic Techniques

The diagnosis of pulmonary brucellosis is based on a combination of clinical features, epidemiological evidence, culture, and serologic tests. The hematologic and non-*Brucella* biochemical findings are not diagnostic. The clinical features are diverse and nonspecific, as mentioned earlier in the chapter, and they overlap with those of a variety of infectious and noninfectious diseases

Table 3 Clinical and Radiographic Lesions Encountered in Patients with Acute and Chronic Pulmonary Brucellosis

Acute Lesions[a]	Chronic Lesions[a]
Generalized	Generalized
Bronchitis	Bronchitis
Bronchopneumonia	Bronchopneumonia
Interstitial pneumonitis	Perihilar and peribronchial infiltrations
Soft miliary mottlings	Millet-seed calcifications
Diffuse parencymal nodulation	Parenchymal nodulations
Hilar and paratracheal lymphadenopathy	Hilar and paratracheal lymphadenopathy
	Interstitial lung fibrosis
Localized	Localized
Pneumonia (consolidation)	Single granuloma "coin lesion"
Pneumonitis	Atelectasis (segmental or lobar)
Pleural effusion	Abscess
Encysted interlobar effusion	Empyema
Empyema	Lung zone fibrosis
Abscess	Pleural or septal thickening
Pneumothorax	
Pyopneumothorax	
Granuloma	

[a]Lesions could be single or combined.

(Buchanan et al., 1974a,b; Pfischner et al., 1957; Samra et al., 1983; Young, 1983). These features together with epidemiological evidence of exposure to *Brucella* would alert the physician to the possibility of brucellosis. However, the definitive diagnosis is established by recovering *Brucella* in culture (e.g., from blood, bone marrow, body fluids, or tissues), seroconversion from negative to positive, demonstrating fourfold increase in titer or the presence of high titers. These *Brucella* culture and serological tests are not without problems. For example, culture is time-consuming and of low yield (15-50%) when disease is in the acute stage and of very low yield (around 5%)

in the chronic stage of brucellosis. Bone marrow cultures may give a higher yield than blood cultures. In patients with localized brucellosis, cultures of purulent material or tissue usually result in more positive cultures than blood. In addition, in patients with pulmonary brucellosis, *Brucella* could be recovered from pleural and empyema fluid but rarely from sputum (Harris et al., 1962; Greer, 1956; Lulu et al., 1988; Vanni, 1925; Weed et al., 1952).

Due to the severe limitations of culture results, serological investigations have been heavily relied on in the diagnosis of brucellosis. Several serological tests have been used, including agglutination tests with or without 2-mercaptoethanol treatment (Alton et al., 1975; Araj et al., 1988a,b; Kerr et al., 1966), and tests to detect nonagglutinating antibodies such as Coombs' (McDevitt, 1973), indirect fluorescent antibodies (Edwards et al., 1970), radioimmunoassay (Parratt et al., 1977), counterimmunoelectrophoresis (Diaz et al., 1976), and, most recently, the enzyme-linked immunosorbent assay (ELISA; Araj et al., 1986a; Sippel et al., 1982; Magee, 1980). The majority ($\geqslant$ 97%) of patients with acute brucellosis show positive results in any of these tests. Agglutination tests on slides or in tubes, although most commonly used in *Brucella* serodiagnosis, suffer from high (up to 40%) false-negative results, especially in patients with chronic or localized infection (Araj et al., 1988b). ELISA is the most reliable and is considered the test of choice, especially for patients with chronic or complicated stages of the disease. In addition, ELISA provides antibody profiles. Patients with acute brucellosis show on ELISA either an elevation in IgM alone, which is uncommon, or together with IgG and IgA, which is common and occurs in 97% of patients. Patients with chronic brucellosis have consistently elevated IgG and IgA levels, but IgM antibodies are present in fewer than 33% of the patients.

In our experience, the fourfold increase in titers between two specimens tested 10-14 days apart is uncommon. Because of the vague and nonspecific nature of the disease, many patients fail to seek medical help early in the course, during which their antibody levels might already have been elevated. The significant serological titers should be determined for the population in a given geographic location because background titers could be present in asymptomatic individuals in *Brucella* endemic areas (Araj et al., 1986a; Williams, 1982). It is also important to keep in mind that significantly elevated antibody levels may persist for a long time in treated and cured patients. Thus, results of serological tests need to be interpreted in light of the clinical signs and symptoms. Although the diagnostic significance of *Brucella*-specific immunoglobulins is well established, follow-up studies are needed to determine their prognostic significance. Monitoring the antibody titers is helpful in differentiating potential cure from relapse (Araj et al., 1988a,b; Araj et al., 1986a,b; Pellicer et al., 1988).

VII. Differential Diagnosis

The clinical and radiographic presentation of patients with pulmonary brucellosis resembles that of many infectious and noninfectious diseases (Paratzky, 1936; Williams, 1982). These include infection with mycobacteria, fungi, *Chlamydia, Rickettsia,* sarcoidosis, carcinoma, extrinsic allergic alveolitis, fibrosing alveolitis, radiation pneumonitis, pneumonitis, pneumoconiosis, and connective tissues disorders. The radiographic picture is often helpful in limiting the spectrum of the differential diagnosis (Patel et al., 1988; Shaw et al., 1981; Davis et al., 1965; Haden and Kyger, 1946; Hunninghake and Fauci, 1979; Jacobson and Gilson, 1972; Nicholson, 1972). Blood, sputum, and pleural fluid should be submitted for culture to exclude aerobic and anaerobic bacteria, mycobacteria, and *Legionella.* Serological tests, antigen detection tests, or nucleic acid probes are helpful in the diagnosis of bacteria (e.g., *Chlamydia, Legionella, Rickettsia,* and *Mycoplasma*), viruses (e.g., Epstein-Barr), and fungi (e.g., *Cryptococcus neoformans, Histoplasma capsulatum,* and *Coccidioides immitus*) as well as connective tissue disorders. The skin tests are helpful in excluding the diagnosis of tuberculosis and sarcoidosis. Tissue biopsy from lymph nodes, pleura, lung, bone marrow, or liver should be obtained for histopathological studies and culture of the causative organisms (Weed et al., 1952). Other investigations such as a complete hemogram, measurement of erythrocyte sedimentation rate, and renal and liver function tests are of use in the differential diagnosis of some of these diseases. Bronchoscopy may be necessary to obtain bronchial aspirates and biopsies, and for relieving bronchial obstruction if present.

Pleural fluid analysis for cytological, cellular, and biochemical content may help to identify pleural effusion and empyema.

VIII. Treatment

Treatment of brucellosis is prolonged. If started early, it prevents complications, relapses, and chronicity since *Brucella* is an intracellular pathogen and relatively inaccessible to antibiotics (Farrell and Robertson, 1980; Feiz et al., 1973; Havas, 1980; Lubani et al., 1989a,b; Smith, 1976).

Different drug regimens have been used in the treatment of brucellosis depending on duration of illness, severity, presence of pregnancy, and tolerance to drugs. In patients with acute pulmonary disease, monotherapy with oxtetracycline (0.5 g four times daily), doxycycline (200 mg once daily), or rifampicin (600-900 mg once daily) for 6 weeks is effective. Trimethoprim-sulfamethoxazole (TMP/SMX, 160/800 mg twice daily) alone has a high relapse rate (around 50%) in adults and children. In pregnant patients, TMP/SMZ could be used in midtrimester up to near term and rifampicin from the first trimester. Use of the aminoglycosides should be avoided if possible. Nevertheless, the decision regarding treatment must be assessed on an individual basis during pregnancy, taking into consideration the risks and benefits of giving or withholding antibrucella antibiotics. Ceftriaxone and cefotaxime could be useful since they demonstrate high activity against *Brucella* spp. (Lubani et al., 1989a; Lulu et al., 1988; Williams, 1982; Young, 1983).

In patients with extrapulmonary complications, severe and toxic illness, with no response to the monotherapy within 10 days of treatment, or chronic pulmonary brucellosis, a combination of two drugs should be instituted. The joint FAO/WHO committee (1986) recommends a combination of doxycyclin plus rifampicin. It is convenient and patients tend to comply better. Other effective combinations include, tetracycline plus intramuscular streptomycin (1 g, once daily) or gentamicin (80 mg, three times daily), TMP/SMX plus streptomycin or gentamicin, and rifampicin plus streptomycin or gentamicin. The oral drugs are used for 6 weeks while the streptomycin or gentamicin is used for 10 days, except in patients with chronic brucellosis in whom the combination of oral antibiotic must be extended for a 12 week course once or repeatedly. A triple-drug (rifampicin, tetracycline, and streptomycin) regimen has been used in complicated cases and chronic brucellosis. In patients with chronic generalized pulmonary fibrosis and millet-seed calcification, treatment is not indicated. These lesions are inactive and healed. In cases with a solitary pulmonary nodule, so-called "coin lesion," surgical removal by exploratory thoracotomy is resorted to as a diagnostic and therapeutic measure (Lulu et al., 1988; Mousa et al., 1987).

In cases of acute empyema, antibiotic treatment should be accompanied by repeated aspiration. In case of failure or in chronic empyema, intercostal tube drainage is indicated.

In children ($\leqslant$ 8 yrs) a combination of TMP/SMX (8/40 mg/kg/day orally in two divided doses) for 3 weeks along with gentamicin (5 mg/kg/day intramuscularly in two divided doses) over the first 5 days is the recommended treatment. Other regimens could include rifampicin (20 mg/kg/day) alone for 3 weeks or together with gentamicin. In children older than 8 years, doxycycline (4 mg/kg/day orally in two divided doses) or oxytetracycline (30 mg/kg/day orally in two divided doses) over 3 weeks along with gentamicin during the first 5 days is recommended.

In acute pulmonary brucellosis, clinical response to treatment is usually noted within 7-10 days of starting therapy, while the radiographic resolution is delayed to 4-8 weeks (Lulu et al., 1988; Mousa et al., 1987). In chronic active pulmonary brucellosis, the clinical response is observed within 2-3 weeks while radiographic resolution takes months. Residual fibrosis may occur.

In all patients, a chest radiograph should be obtained on admission and at the end of treatment. Chest x-ray films should be taken again every 4 months for about 2 years, to detect a possible relapse.

IX. Prognosis

Patients with acute brucellosis and those with acute pulmonary complications usually have an excellent prognosis. Early diagnosis and proper treatment result in rapid cure, and minimize complications and relapses of the disease. Complications such as respiratory insufficiency and secondary infection with pyogenic bacteria that may occur in patients with generalized chronic pulmonary brucellosis are avoidable with early diagnosis and management.

Mortality is rare in brucellosis (FAO/WHO Report 1986; Williams, 1982; Young, 1983). Before antibiotics were available, mortality occurred in less than 3% of all cases with brucellosis and with the introduction of antibiotics it became even more rare (≤ 1%). The course is fatal (85%) in patients with endocarditis, often associated with severe congestive heart failure, and those with severe neurologic complications (Salata, 1988).

X. Prevention

The key to preventing brucellosis is eradicating the disease from animals through proper implementation of control policy. The policy should include testing of imported and local domestic animals (e.g., sheep, goats, cows, camels), slaughtering positive reactors and compensating farmers for this, as well as vaccinating young seronegative animals. In countries where the incidence of brucellosis is still high, public education regarding the avoidance of unpasteurized or unboiled milk or its products is important. Protective measures against contact or aerosol infection should be taken by persons at high occupational risk (e.g., veterinarians, abattoir employees, and workers at clinical or research laboratories).

XI. Summary

Pulmonary complications of brucellosis are rare and could be easily missed due to the lack of awareness of this disease among physicians, especially in developed countries. The incidence of respiratory symptoms in brucellosis ranges from 4.5% in children up to 31% in adults. Pulmonary complications are less frequently encountered (0-16%). Lung involvement is believed to be through the bloodstream regardless of the microorganism's portal of entry.

Based on the duration of respiratory symptoms and signs, pulmonary brucellosis could be conveniently categorized into two clinical types: acute ($\leqslant 3$ months duration) or chronic (> 3 months). The chronic form is thought to be due to delayed diagnosis and/or inappropriate treatment. Many antimicrobial drugs are available for the treatment of pulmonary brucellosis. The cure rate is high in the acute form, while the chronic form requires repeated courses to achieve satisfactory results. The prognosis of treated patients is excellent, especially in the acute form. Mortality is very low ($\leqslant 1\%$). In patients with unexplained pulmonary manifestations, brucellosis should be considered in the differential diagnosis especially, in areas where the disease is still endemic.

References

Alausa, O. K. (1980). Brucellosis: socio-economic problems and control in various countries. *Trop. Geogr. Med.* **32**:5-11.

Al-Kandari, S., Al-Enizi, A. A., and Christie, A. B. (1987). Brucellosis a continuing problem—epidemiology. *Postgrad. Doc. Middle East* **11**: 499-504.

Alton, G. G., Jones, L. M., and Pietz, D. E. (1975). *Laboratory Techniques in Brucellosis*, 2nd ed. Geneva, World Health Organization Monograph series No. 55.

Araj, G. F., Lulu, A. R., Mustafa, M. Y., and Khateeb, M. I. (1986a). Evaluation of ELISA in the diagnosis of acute and chronic brucellosis in human beings. *J. Hyg.* **97**:457-469.

Araj, G. F., Lulu, A. R., Saadah, M. A., Mousa, A. M., Strannegard, I. L., and Shakir, R. A. (1986b). Rapid diagnosis of central nervous system brucellosis by ELISA. *J. Neuroimmunol.* **12**:173-182.

Araj, G. F., Brown, G. M., Haj, M. M., and Madhvan, N. V. (1988a). Assessment of Brucellosis Card Test in screening patients for brucellosis. *Epidemiol. Infect.* **100**:389-398.

Araj, G. F., Lulu, A. R., Khateeb, M. I., Saadah, M. A., and Shakir, R. A. (1988b). ELISA versus routine tests in the diagnosis of patients with systemic and neurobrucellosis. *Acta Pathol. Microbiol. Immunol. Scand.* **96**:171-176.

Beatty, O. A. (1937). Manifestations of undulant fever in the respiratory tract. *Am. Rev. Tuberc.* **36**:283-289.

Bogart, F. B. (1936). Pulmonary changes in undulant fever. *South. Med. J.* **29**:1-9.

Buchanan, T. M., Faber, L. C., and Feldman, R. A. (1974a). Brucellosis in the United States 1960-1972; an abattoir-associated disease, Part I. Clinical features and therapy. *Medicine* **53**:403-413.

Buchanan, T. M., Hendricks, S. l., Patton, C. M., and Feldman, R. A. (1974b). Brucellosis in the United States 1960-1972; an abattoir-associated disease, Part III. Epidemiology and evidence for acquired immunity. *Medicine* **53**:427-439.

Chavez, C. A., and Veach, G. E. (1976). Localized pulmonary nodule due to Brucella suis. *J. Kansas Med. Soc.* **77**:434-437.

Davis, E. W., Peabody, J. W., and Katz, S. (1965). The solitary pulmonary nodule: A 10 year survey based on 215 cases. *J. Thorac. Surg.* **32**:728.

De Mello, M. T., Aronson, M., and Elberg, S. S. (1967). In vivo infection of monkey alveolar histiocytes with airborne *Brucella melitensis. Ann. Microbiol.* **12**:55 (1964); abstracted in *Bull. Hyg.* (*London*) **42**:338.

Diaz, R., Marvi-Poma, E., and Rivero, A. (1976). Comparison of counterimmunoelectrophoresis with other serological tests in the diagnosis of human brucellosis. *Bull. W.H.O.* **53**:417-424.

Di Pace, I. (1928). Etiology of bronchitis and pleuritis observed in undulant fever. *Riforma Med.* **44**:1057-1060.

Economidow, J., Kalafatas, P., Vatopoulou, T., Petropoulou, D., and Kattamis, C. (1976). Brucellosis in two thalassaemic patients infected by blood transfusion from the same donor. *Acta. Haematol.* **55**:244-249.

Edwards, J. M. B., Tannahill, A. J., and Bradstreet, C. M. P. (1970). Comparison of the indirect fluorescent antibody test with agglutination, complement fixation and Coombs tests for Brucella antibody. *J. Clin. Pathol.* **23**:161-165.

Elberg, S. S., and Henderson, D. W. (1948). Respiratory pathogenicity of brucella. *J. Infect. Dis.* **45**:271-282.

Elson, K. A., and Ingelfinger, F. J. (1942). Eosinophilia and pneumonitis in chronic brucellosis; report of two cases. *Ann. Intern. Med.* **16**:995-1002.

FAO/WHO Expert Committee on Brucellosis. (1986). 6th Report Technical report series No. 740., Geneva, World Health Organization.

Farrell, I. D., and Robertson, L. R. (1980). The treatment of brucellosis. *J. Antimicrob. Chemother.* **6**:695-697.

Feiz, J. M., Sabbaghian, H., and Sohrabi, F. (1973). A comparative study of the therapeutic agents used for treatment of acute brucellosis. *Br. J. Clin. Pract.* **27**:410-413.

Gotuzzo, E., Alarcon, G. S., Bocanegra, T. S., Carrillo, C., Guerra, J. C., Rolando, I., and Espinoza, L. R. (1982). Articular involvement in human brucellosis: a retrospective analysis of 304 cases. *Semin. Arthritis Rheum.* **12**:245-255.

Greer, A. E. (1956). Pulmonary brucellosis. *Dis. Chest* **29**:508-519.

Haden, R. L., and Kyger, E. R. (1946). Pulmonary manifestations of brucellosis. *Cleve. Clin. Q.* **13**:220-227.

Hagebusch, O. E., and Frei, C. F. (1940). Undulant fever in children. *Am. J. Clin. Pathol.* **11**:497-515.

Harris, M. M., Hendricks, S. L., Gorman, G. W., and Held, J. R. (1962). Isolation of *Brucella suis* from air of slaughter house. *Public Health Rep.* **77**:602-604.

Harvey, W. A. (1948). Pulmonary brucellosis. *Ann. Intern. Med.* **28**:768-781.

Havas, L. (1980). Problems and new developments in the treatment of acute and chronic brucellosis in man. *Acta Trop.* **37**:281-286.

Hendricks, S. L., Borts, I. H., Heeren, R. H., Hausler, W. J., and Held, J. R. (1962). Brucellosis outbreak in an Iowa packing house. *Am. J. Public Health* **52**:1166-1178.

Hughes, M. L. (1897). *Mediterranean, Malta or Undulant Fever.* New York, McMillan and Company.

Hunninghake, G. W., and Fauci, A. S. (1979). Pulmonary involvement in the collagen vascular diseases. *Am. Rev. Respir. Dis.* **119**:471-503.

Jacobson, G., and Gilson, J. C. (1972). Present status of UICC-Cincinnati. Classification of radiographic appearances of pneumoconiosis. *Ann. N.Y. Acad. Sci.* **200**:552-570.

Johnson, R. M. (1935). Pneumonia in undulant fever. *Am. J. Med. Sci.* **189**: 483-486.

Kaufmann, A. F., Fox, M. D., Royce, J. M., Anderson, D. C., Potter, M. E., Martone, W. J., and Patton, C. M. (1980). Airborne spread of brucellosis. *Ann. N.Y. Acad. Sci.* **353**:105-114.

Kerr, W. R., Coghlan, J. D., Payne, D. J. H., and Robertson, L. (1966). The laboratory diagnosis of chronic brucellosis. *Lancet* **2**:1181-1183.

Lafferty, R. H., and Phillips, C. C. (1937). Pulmonary changes in patients suffering from Malta fever. *South Med. J.* **30**:595-600.

Lubani, M. M., Dudin, K. I., Sharda, D. C., Mandhar, D. S., Araj, G. F., Hafiz, H. A., et al. (1989a). A multicenter therapeutic study of 1100 children with brucellosis. *Pediatr. Infect. Dis. J.* **8**:75-78.

Lubani, M. M., Lulu, A. R., Araj, G. F., Khateeb, M. I., Qurtom, M. A. F., and Doudin, K. I. (1989b). Pulmonary brucellosis. *Q. J. Med.* **71**:319-324.

Lulu, A. R., Araj, G. F., Khateeb, M. I., Mustafa, M. Y., Yusuf, A. R., and Fenech, F. F. (1988). Human brucellosis in Kuwait: a prospective study of 400 cases. *Q. J. Med.* **66**:39-54.

Macdonald, R. H. (1939). Acute empyema with *Brucella abortus* as the primary causative agent. *J. Thorac. Surg.* **9**:92-94.

Magee, J. T. (1980). An enzyme-labelled immunosorbent assay for *Brucella abortus* antibodies. *J. Med. Microbiol.* **13**:167-172.

Mathur, T. N. (1960). Brucellosis simulating respiratory illness. A report of eleven cases. *Indian J. Med. Sci.* **14**:610-618.

Matyas, Z., and Fujikura, T. (1984). Brucellosis as a world problem. *Dev. Biol. Stand.* **56**:3-20.

McDevitt, D. G. (1973). The relevance of antihuman globulin (Coombs) test and the complement fixation test in the diagnosis of brucellosis. *J. Hyg.* **68**:173-187.

Miller, C. D., Songer, J. R., and Sullivan, J. F. (1987). A twenty five year review of laboratory acquired human infections at the National Animal Disease Center. *Ann. Ind. Hyg. Assoc. J.* **48**:271-275.

Mousa, A. m., Elhag, K. M., Khogali, M., and Sugathan, T. N. (1987). Brucellosis in Kuwait: a clinico-epidemiological study. *Trans. R. Soc. Trop. Med. Hyg.* **81**:1020-1021.

Mousa, A. M., Elhag, K. M., Khogali, M., and Marafie, A. A. (1988). The nature of human brucellosis in Kuwait: study of 379 cases. *Rev. Infect. Dis.* **10**:211-217.

Nicholson, D. P. (1972). Extrinsic allergic pneumonias. *J. Med.* **53**:131-136.

Paratzky, M. (1936). Undulant fever: pulmonary findings simulating tuberculosis. *Med. Res.* **144**:11-14.

Parratt, D., Nielson, K. H., White, R. G., and Payne, D. J. H. (1977). Radioimmunoassay of IgM, IgG and IgA brucella antibodies. *Lancet* **1**: 1075-1078.

Patel, P. J., Al-Suhaibani, H., Al-Aska, A. K., Kolawole, T. M., and Al-Kassimi, F. A. (1988). The chest radiograph in brucellosis. *Clin. Radiol.* **39**:39-41.

Pellicer, T., Ariza, J., Fox, A., Pallares, R., and Gudiol, F. (1988). Specific antibodies detected during relapse of human brucellosis. *J. Infect. Dis.* **157**:918-924.

Pfischner, W. C. E., Ishuk, K. G., Neptune, E. M., Fox, S. M., Farid, Z., and Nor el Din, G. (1957). Brucellosis in Egypt: a review of experience with 228 patients. *Am. J. Med.* **22**:915-929.

Ramah, S. J., Chomet, D., McLean, J., and Lemke, C. (1959). Pulmonary granuloma due to brucellosis. *J.A.M.A.* **170**:1665-1667.

Robinson, F. H. (1938). Discussion of pulmonary changes in patients suffering from Malta fever. *South. Med. J.* **75**:247-250.

Salata, R. A. (1988). Brucellosis. In *Cecil Textbook of Medicine*, 18th ed. Philadelphia, W.B. Saunders, pp. 1676-1679.

Samra, Y., Shaked, Y., Hertz, M., and Altmon, G. (1983). Brucellosis: difficulties in diagnosis and a report on 38 cases. *Infection* **11**:310-312.

Schirger, A., Nichols, D. R., Martin, W. J., Wellmon, W. E., and Weed, L. A. (1960). Brucellosis: experience with 224 patients. *Ann. Intern. Med.* **52**:827-837.

Sharda, D. C., and Lubani, M. (1986). A study of brucellosis in childhood. *Clin. Pediatr.* **25**:492-495.

Shaw, R. A., Fass, R. J., and Perkins, R. L. (1981). Roentgenogram of the month; fever, weight loss and hilar adenopathy in a microbiologist. *Chest* **79**:587-588.

Shipley, F. M. (1945). Pulmonary manifestations of brucellosis. *Bull. School Med. Univ. Maryland.* **30**:80-83.

Sippel, J. E., Masry, N. A., and Farid, Z. (1982). Diagnosis of human brucellosis with ELISA. *Lancet* **2**:19-21.

Smith, C. C. (1976). Treatment of human brucellosis. *Scott. Med. J.* **21**: 132-135.

Spink, W. W. (1956). *The Nature of Brucellosis.* Minneapolis, University of Minnesota Press, pp. 145-190.

Stanec-Paulinic, M., Cec, V., and Mehle, J. (1983). Brucellosis in spouses and the possibility of interhuman infection. *Infection* **6**:313-314.

Vanni, V. (1925). Malta fever simulating tuberculosis. *J.A.M.A.* **85**:934-936.

Webb, W. A., and Thorougham, J. C. (1966). Solitary pulmonary nodule due to *Brucella suis. Dis. Chest* **49**:222-224.

Weed, L. A., Dahlin, D. C., Pugh, D. G., and Ivins, V. C. (1952). Brucella in tissue removed at surgery. *Am. J. Clin. Pathol.* **22**:10-12.

Weed, L. A., Sloss, P. J., and Clagett, O. T. (1956). Chronic localized pulmonary brucellosis. *J.A.M.A.* **161**:1044-1047.

Williams, E. (1982). *Brucellosis. Practioner* **226**:1507-1517.

Wise, R. I. (1980). Brucellosis in the United States, past, present and future. *J.A.M.A.* **244**:2318-2322.

Young, E. J. (1983). Human brucellosis. *Rev. Infect. Dis.* **5**:821-842.

6

Pulmonary Problems During Makkah Pilgrimage (Hajj)

FEISAL A. EL-KASSIMI

King Saud University
College of Medicine
Riyadh, Saudi Arabia

I. Introduction

The yearly pilgrimage (Hajj) to Makkah and adjoining sites is a unique event during which between 1 and 2 million pilgrims flock to the holy sites near the western coast of the Arabian Peninsula, lying at a latitude of 20 degrees north. Hajj rituals take place in a desert valley surrounded by sunbaked hills, where temperatures in the shade exceed 45°C (113°F) in the summer with a relative humidity of 25-50%. Many of those rituals have to be performed during the day, in the open, and entail protracted physical exertion by pilgrims who are mostly unacclimated to hot weather. This situation is liable to produce a host of medical emergencies, the most serious of which is heat stroke. To appreciate the magnitude of the task facing the Health Services, one has to know that in addition to the 3000 hospital beds already existing in the Makkah region, more than 1400 temporary emergency beds had to be created and increased to 2500 in 1986 (Seraj et al., 1987). These are equipped with facilities to deal with serious emergencies, and they offer doctors and researchers working there the opportunity to make valuable medical observations.

Although Hajj gives rise to the usual pulmonary complications associated with any large human gathering, such as respiratory tract infections, some unique observations were recorded on the effect of heat stroke on the lung, which will be discussed under the following headings: Abnormalities of Respiratory Drive and Acid-Base Balance, Adult Respiratory Distress Syndrome, and Hemodynamic and Oxygenation Abnormalities.

Heat stroke is characterized by a rectal temperature in excess of 40.0°C (104°F) after exposure to hot conditions, deterioration of level of consciousness, and usually dry, flushed skin (Shibolet et al., 1976). Implicit in the definition is the exclusion of other highly febrile conditions, such as malaria. Heat stroke produces multiple organ derangement with coma, disseminated intravascular coagulation (DIC), circulatory collapse, and respiratory failure as the main features. The heat stroke in Hajj is mainly of the exertional type, which is more likely to give rise to DIC, rhabdomyolysis, and uremia than is the nonexertional type.

II. Abnormalities of Respiratory Drive and Acid-Base Balance

Mustafa and co-workers (1983a) studied the arterial blood gas levels of 233 pilgrims to Makkah and found that 9% had primary hyperventilation with low $PaCO_2$ as the only abnormality, with 2 cases of overt tetany as a result of respiratory alkalosis (Table 1). Several earlier reports have described hyperventilation in patients with heat stroke (Leithead, 1964; O'Donnell, 1975; Costrini et al., 1979; Sprung et al., 1980). Extreme heat has been shown to cause hyperventilation in resting subjects (Gaudio and Abramson, 1968). Mustafa et al. attributed the finding to tachypnea. This is supported by studies on hyperthermic exercising fowl (Gleeson and Brackenbury, 1984), which documented increased respiratory frequency.

In Mustafa et al.'s same study, 24% of pilgrims with heat stroke had hyperventilation secondary to metabolic acidosis. This is in line with earlier studies that documented lactic acidosis in humans with heat stroke (Sprung et al., 1980) and in exercising fowl in which isothermic exercise produced less lactoacidosis than hyperthermic exercise (Gleeson and Brackenbury, 1984), a condition simulating the physically demanding rituals of Hajj. The rise of lactic acid in goats paralleled the rise of temperature (Feistkorn et al., 1984). Pilgrims with base deficit greater than 5 mmol/L had double the mortality rate of those with no base deficit, which supports the findings of Hart et al. (1982) that heat stroke with lactic acidosis has an unfavorable prognosis.

Another 28 cases (12%) showed hypercapnia and hypoxemia, associated in some with lobar or segmental collapse that the authors attributed

Table 1 Arterial Blood Gas Abnormalities of 233 Heat Stroke Victims: 1982 Pilgrimage

Pathophysiological findings	Number	%
Hyperventilation (primary) $PaCO_2 < 35$ mmHg	20	9
Hyperventilation (secondary to acidosis) $PaCO_2 < 35$ mmHg Base deficit > 5 mmol/L	58	24
Hypoventilation $PaCO_2 > 44$ mmHg $PaO_2 < 90$ mmHg	28	12
Hypoxemia without CO_2 retention $PaO_2 < 90$ mmHg (on 28% O_2) $PaCO_2 < 44$ mmHg	94	40[a]
Normal	33	15

[a] $PaO_2 < 60$ mmHg in 17%.
Source: Mustafa et al., 1983a.

to retention of secretions and inhalation of vomitus. However, in six cases among this group the chest x-ray was normal but the patients had very shallow breathing, and administration of oxygen resulted in correction of hypoxemia. The hypercapnia and shallow breathing in these six cases were taken as evidence of depression of the respiratory center necessitating the use of mechanical ventilation.

Lastly, 40% were hypoxemic while breathing 28% oxygen with normal or low $PaCO_2$, a finding that will be discussed under the next heading. Only 33 cases (15%) had normal arterial blood gases and acid-base balance.

Temperature must be corrected whenever arterial blood gases are measured in hyperthermic patients. In general, a rise of 1°C will increase the PaO_2 by 6%, and will decrease the pH by 0.0147 (Bradley et al., 1956).

III. Adult Respiratory Distress Syndrome

A. Incidence and Clinical Picture

In the last century, Osler (1892) wrote about the pulmonary complications of heat stroke: "The blood is usually fluid; the lungs are intensely congested." Austin and Berry (1956) found that out of 17 heat stroke patients who died, 8 had "left ventricular failure" and two had "anoxic nephrosis." These were possibly cases of a yet unrecognized entity: adult respiratory distress syndrome (ARDS). Soliman et al. (1983) were the first to describe ARDS as a complication of heat stroke on the basis of observations made during the Hajj seasons of 1981 and 1982; 10 of 40 patients with heat stroke developed the syndrome. They attributed ARDS to pulmonary aspiration of gastric contents. They committed the ethically questionable act of managing comatose patients in the supine position to prove that the incidence of ARDS in that group (65%) is higher than in the group nursed in the left lateral head-down position (35%). Their paper did not mention whether their methods were approved by any ethics committee. Moreover, pulmonary artery wedge pressure measurements were not done in any patients in their series to exclude pulmonary edema of cardiac origin, particularly in view of the fact that 4 of their 40 cases had developed acute myocardial infarction. Yaqub et al. (1986) described one case of ARDS in pilgrims on the basis of hypoxemia and a chest radiograph showing "bilateral opacities consistent with adult respiratory distress syndrome," without documenting wedge pressure or response of hypoxemia to oxygen inhalation.

We were the first (El-Kassimi et al., 1986) to use the Swan-Ganz catheter to document the presence of ARDS in 12 of 52 pilgrims with heat stroke selected randomly. All patients with ARDS cases had PaO_2 <50 mmHg that did not correct with oxygen inhalation. All chest x-rays (Fig. 1) showed bilateral diffuse micronodular, reticular, or alveolar infiltrate.

B. Pathogenesis

All of the 12 patients with ARDS in the above series (El-Kassimi et al., 1986) had DIC, compared to only 1 among the 40 patients without ARDS. The conclusion was that the coagulopathy may be an essential mediator of lung damage in heat stroke. The authors suggested that screening heat stroke victims for DIC may identify patients at increased risk of developing overt ARDS and allow early institution of measures that may possibly improve survival. Further support for an association between the DIC of heat stroke and lung damage can be found in an earlier study on heat stroke (Wright, Reppert, and Cuttino, 1946). Of six patients with postmortem lung findings typical of what is now ARDS ("severe multiple pulmonary hemorrhages, severe bilateral pulmonary edema"), five had low platelet levels with coagulation abnormalities, and one who died shortly after admission had massive gastrointestinal bleeding. That paper, however, did not recognize any link between the lung condition and the coagulation disorder. Bone and colleagues (1976) observed that among a group of patients with ARDS secondary to trauma or sepsis, more than half had either DIC or a drop of platelet levels below 50%, and they concluded that DIC was a complication of ARDS. Reviewing all

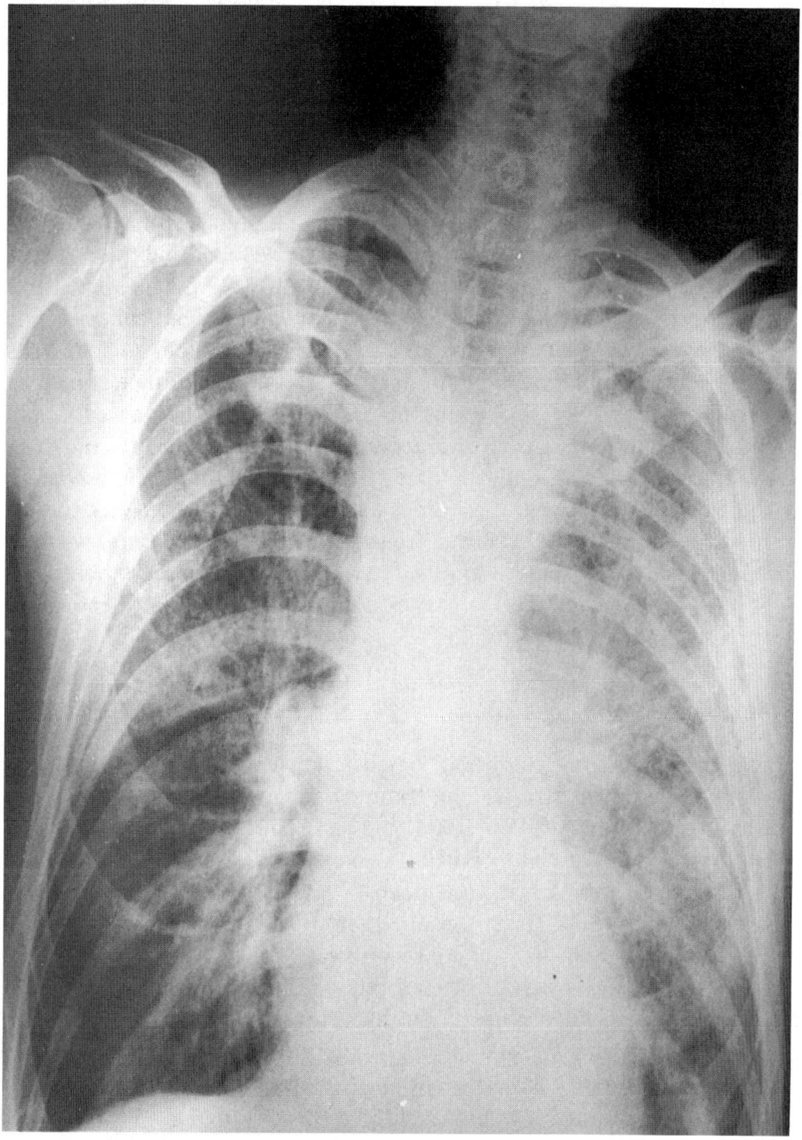

Figure 1 A posteroanterior chest roentgenogram shows diffuse bilateral ground glass haziness and nodular infiltrate. (Author's personal collection-Pilgrimage season 1985)

the available evidence that DIC can trigger lung damage and ARDS is beyond the scope of this chapter, but it is worth citing the work of Luterman et al. (1977), who showed that ARDS could be produced in rabbits by infusion of fragment D of human fibrin split products, while the infusion of human fibrinogen or human albumin had no such effect.

Hyperthermia could exert a direct cellular effect resulting in capillary leak and pulmonary edema. Heat is documented to cause increased cell permeability in mouse fibroblasts (Hayat and Friedberg, 1986). Mustafa et al. (1986) have demonstrated that isolated lungs developed pulmonary edema when infused with blood-free solution at 43°C (109.4°F), while perfusion at lower temperatures produced no change. There was no significant rise in pulmonary capillary pressure at 43°C (109.4°F) or 45°C (113°F). Also the clearance of [^{125}I]albumin across pulmonary arterial endothelial cells increased threefold at 45°C (113°F). During the Hajj of 1982 (Al-Khawashki et al., 1983), the rectal temperature of 172 pilgrims admitted to Mina and Arafat Heat Stroke Centres was higher than 42°C (107°F) in 75% and higher than 43°C (109.4°F) in 16% of cases. Since all the patients are actively cooled in air-conditioned ambulances during transport to the medical centers, the core temperatures must have been significantly higher at the onset of heat stroke, and therefore a direct effect of hyperthermia on the lung, independent of DIC, cannot be ruled out.

C. Pathological Findings

To our knowledge, lung biopsy or postmortem studies were not performed on pilgrims with heat stroke. The Islamic doctrine considers autopsy to be desecration of dead bodies unless doctors can prove convincingly that the information sought is likely to contribute to the welfare of future patients and cannot be obtained by less drastic means. Pulmonary edema, with (Knochel et al., 1961) or without (Harris et al., 1985) myocardial infarction, was described in human subjects who died with heat stroke, and experimentally in hyperthemic dogs (Amsterdam et al., 1986). The histopathological findings in a woman who died with malignant hyperthermia following general anesthesia with halothane showed alveolar exudates and infiltration by macrophages (Kimura et al., 1985). The latter finding might explain a report (Tonami et al., 1985) of diffuse lung uptake of ^{99m}Tc tin colloid in a patient with heat stroke. A repeat 7 days after the initial scan showed no lung uptake. In another study on 10 marathon runners with fatal exertional heat stroke who developed severe DIC, the lungs showed diffuse hemorrhage with blood in the trachea and bronchi. On microscopic examination there were widespread microthrombi in pulmonary capillaries and arterioles (Chao et al., 1981).

IV. Hemodynamic and Oxygenation Abnormalities

A. Cardiac Output

Al-Harthi et al. (1989) studied the hemodynamics of 13 pilgrims with heat stroke and found the cardiac index to be raised with decreased total peripheral vascular resistance in all cases, with no significant rise in pulmonary vascular resistance. These findings are similar to previous Western studies on fit marine recruits with exertional heat stroke (O'Donnell and Clowes, 1972). However, the cardiac output tends to be low in the elderly (Sprung, 1979). We can safely conclude that the hypotension that occurs in 17% of Makkah heat stroke victims (Al-Khawashki et al., 1983), who are usually previously healthy, is caused by peripheral vasodilatation in the majority of cases rather than low cardiac output or hypovolemia. The systemic vascular resistance index correlated inversely with rectal temperature in pilgrims with heat stroke (Al-Harthi et al., 1989).

B. Fluid Balance

Al-Harthi et al. (1989) described five pilgrims who developed pulmonary edema associated with increased cardiac index (5.29 +/− [SD] 5.6 L/min/m^2) and normal or raised pulmonary capillary wedge pressure (PCWP). They concluded that the pulmonary edema was aggravated by fluid overloading. The fluid administration in those patients with pulmonary edema was 1200-1800 ml of 0.9% NaCl in the first 4 h, compared with 400-1200 ml for those without. None of the patients had low PCWP before administration of fluid. The standard treatment at the Makkah Heat Stroke Centres included the administration of 3-4 L of crystalloids quickly (Khogali et al., 1983), which was suspected to be excessive by Seraj et al. (personal communication), who found that only 500-2500 ml (average 1060 ml) were needed to normalize the central venous pressure and stabilize blood pressure in all 34 pilgrims. Eight American marine recruits with exertional heat stroke had mostly high central venous pressures when measured half an hour after collapse (O'Donnell and Clowes, 1972). We believe that the hypovolemia of heat stroke at Hajj is mild in the majority of cases and that only 1 L of crystalloids should be adequate to correct it in the majority of cases.

C. Oxygenation Studies

Although 40% of pilgrims with heat stroke (Mustafa et al., 1983a) develop hypoxemia resistant to oxygen inhalation, implying a degree of physiological pulmonary shunting, only a fraction of those progress to ARDS. Studies of heat-stressed animals (Barnas and Rautenberg, 1984) and humans subjected to therapeutic hyperthermia for cancer (Cronau et al., 1984; Eisler et al., 1985) document increased oxygen delivery and oxygen consumption, probably as a result of increased metabolic rates.

The increased oxygen delivery occurs despite hypoxemia, increased shunt fraction (Qs/Qt), and widened arterial-alveolar oxygen gradient (Eisler et al., 1985), and is achieved by augmenting the cardiac output (Eisler et al., 1985).

V. Prognosis

Although 85% of pilgrims with heat stroke are deeply comatose on admission (Al-Khawashki et al., 1983), 70% show early recovery after cooling. Mortality figures from various Heat Stroke Centres in Makkah varied from 5 to 18% (Yaqub et al., 1986; Khogali et al., 1983; Al-Aska et al., 1987a; Khogali, 1983; Khogali and Weiner, 1980). The following signs were associated with poor prognosis: prolonged cooling time, prolonged coma, generalized bleeding (Al-Khawashki et al., 1983) or DIC (El-Kassimi et al., 1986), anuria, or hypotension refractory to fluid therapy (Al-Khawashki et al., 1983).

Pulmonary disturbances in particular have an ominous significance. In one series (Mustafa et al., 1983a), the mortality was 0% in patients with normal arterial blood gases, rising to 23% if hypoxemia only was present, to 36% if hypoxemia was associated with CO_2 retention. The mortality was 50% in the group with $PaO_2 < 90$ mmHg (on 28% oxygen), and a base deficit > 5 mmol/L. In another series (El-Kassimi et al., 1986) the mortality in pilgrims with ARDS (proven by Swan Ganz catheters) was 75%.

VI. Management

A. Cooling

The single most important measure is to bring the patient's temperature to near normal in as short a time as possible. The various Heat Stroke Centres in Makkah continue cooling until the rectal temperature drops to between 38°C (100.4°F) and 39°C (102.2°F), since hypothermia was noted to develop if cooling is continued to 37°C (98.6°F). There is ample evidence that rapid cooling improves prognosis. Prolonged cooling time was found to be associated with increased mortality in pilgrams (Al-Khawashki et al., 1983; Mustafa et al., 1983b), as well as a higher incidence of DIC, which, in turn, was associated with greater hypoxemia and mortality (Mustafa et al., 1983b). Experimental studies on animals showed that dogs maintained a higher PaO_2, a lower $PaCO_2$, and a more physiological pH when cooled 1.7 times faster than controls (Barker et al., 1986), although there was no noticeable difference in the severity of microscopic changes of pulmonary edema between the two groups. In another study (White et al., 1987), dogs experienced a quicker and more complete return to baseline cardiac indices and a lower incidence of mortality and neurological deficits when the rate of cooling was doubled. There is also general agreement that adverse outcome in classic heat stroke in humans correlates with increased duration of hyperthermia (Graham et al., 1986; Vicario et al., 1986) and delayed cooling while the initial rectal temperatures on admission did not correlate with outcome (Al-Khawashki et al., 1983; Hart et al., 1982) or the likelihood of developing ARDS (El-Kassimi et al., 1986). Only few studies (Austin and Berry, 1956; Tucker et al., 1985) found a correlation between initial temperature on admission and mortality.

In practice, only three methods of cooling have acquired universal acceptance and are discussed here.

Ice-Water Immersion

This should be done while the skin is massaged vigorously to prevent the intense cutaneous vasoconstriction that inevitably accompanies such treatment. Although many authors continue to recommend its use (Clowes and O'Donnell, 1974), ice-water immersion has been totally abandoned at Hajj. Immersion in cold water is uncomfortable to the semiconscious patient and to the attendants rubbing his skin. Profuse diarrhea frequently occurs in hyperthermic patients, who also might have generalized fits with loss of sphincter control. If any of these happens while the patient is in the tub, the procedure becomes highly unpleasant. Ice-water immersion also interferes with the use of life-saving procedures such as continuous rectal temperature monitoring, intravenous hydration, cardiac monitoring, defibrillation, or external cardiac massage.

Body Cooling Unit

The body cooling unit (BCU) was designed by Khogali and Weiner (1980) specifically for use at the Makkah Hajj and first tested during the 1978 season. Finely atomized water under pressure, at 15°C (59°F), is sprayed over the whole nude body surface from above and below. The spray is combined with the delivery of air warmed at 46°C (114.8°F) and blown over the body surface to maintain cutaneous vasodilatation, and ensure a high rate of heat loss from core to skin. The physiological principle of keeping the skin surface relatively warm to encourage dissipation of body heat was established long before (Wyndham et al., 1959). Although the BCU allows reasonable freedom to monitor patients and administer fluids while cooling is in progress, it is expensive, occupies a large space, and in trials done during the

Hajj season of 1985 was found to be no more effective than simple fanning (Al-Harthi et al., 1986; Al-Aska et al., 1987a).

Simple Fanning and "King Saud University Bed"

The patient is transferred to an air-conditioned room (25°C, 77°F) where his nude body is covered by large pieces of thin gauze soaked in tap water. Three ordinary household fans are used to blow air as fast as is tolerated by the patient and attendants (Al-Harthi et al., 1986). Later the fans were mounted on a special bed fitted with a nonabsorbable surface, which allows excess water and loose bowel movements to be washed away into a special drainage pipe. This trolley, called the "King Saud University Bed" (Al-Aska et al., 1987b) is slowly replacing the BCU.

Other methods such as gastric lavage, high-frequency jet ventilation cooling, ice packs, or the "Duo Therm" cooling blanket (American Medical Systems, Indianapolis, IN) are not routinely in use during Hajj. Gastric lavage was found in a canine model to be less efficacious than fanning (White et al., 1987) and other methods are either impractical or not yet fully evaluated.

B. Other Considerations in Management

Since DIC may be a mediator of lung damage, the Makkah Heat Stroke Centres have adopted the policy of administering fresh frozen plasma to patients with DIC. Although DIC of heat stroke was reported to improve with heparin (Weber and Blakely, 1969), no controlled trials have prove its usefulness. Moreover, 20% of heat stroke cases in Makkah pilgrims display increased fibrinolytic activity (Mustafa et al., 1983b) with little or no evidence of DIC; such patients are likely to be harmed by receiving heparin. For these reasons, the use of heparin is not popular at the Hajj Centres, although small doses (up to 10,000 units/day) were tried.

Mechanical ventilation was used for the treatment of ARDS and was followed by recovery in 25% of cases (El-Kassimi et al., 1986). The indications for its use are similar to those for ARDS in general. Adequate oxygenation is vital in view of increased work of the heart, the tendency to develop myocardial infarction, and the fact that hyperthermia of 41°C (105.8°F) is documented to reduce the affinity of adult and fetal blood to bound oxygen in humans (Gilbert et al., 1985). Intubation and ventilation might rarely be needed for central alveolar hypoventilation (Mustafa et al., 1983a), or for a patient in a deep coma.

One to 1½ L of 0.9% NaCl could safely be administered over 4 h. A central venous line or, preferably, Swan-Ganz catheter should be used only in those who remain hypotensive thereafter. This allows one to classify hypotensive cases into either the hyperdynamic-increased peripheral resistance category or the hypodynamic category, in a manner that could rationalize management. Dopamine, digoxin, or dobutamine (Editorial, 1982) is recommended, but there are no documented studies on their efficacy in treating the shock of heat stroke. Great care should be exercised when digoxin is given because of the high incidence of hypokalemia and uremia. Isoproterenol (1 μg/min) reversed shock and improved the cardiac index in a patient with exertional heat stroke who had hypotensive status with raised central venous pressure (O'donnell and Clowes, 1972). The cardiac index increased from 1.7 to 7.1 L/min/m^2 after it had failed to respond to intravenous fluids and cooling (O'Donnell and Clowes, 1972).

The infusion of 10% glycerol lengthened the survival time and reduced the peak intracranial pressure in rabbits with heat stroke (Shih et al., 1984), implying that cerebral edema determines the time of death. The role of glycerol has not yet been assessed in humans. However, this information strengthens the need to avoid fluid overloading in heat stroke victims.

Chlorpromazine is useful in patients with shivering, spasticity, or convulsions, which increase the metabolic rate and delay cooling.

Table 2 shows that the incidence and mortality of heat stroke during Hajj have declined. The improvement coincided with a campaign of health education, free distribution of iced water to all pilgrims, and the sharp increase in the number of temporary emergency beds in the Hajj area from 1400 to 2500 (Seraj et al., 1987).

Table 2 Analysis of Heat Stroke in Foreign Pilgrims

Year	Period of Hajj	No. of Foreign Pilgrims	No. of Heat Stroke Cases	Heat Stroke per 10,000 Pilgrims	Male/ Female Ratio	Mortality (%)
1980	19th October	812,812	176	2.2	N/A	N/A
1981	8th October	879,368	478	5.4	N/A	N/A
1982	27th September	853,555	1,119	13.1	70:30	N/A
1983	16th September	1,005,060	1,365	13.5	60:40	11.9
1984	5th September	919,671	1,058	11.5	52:48	12.6
1985	25th August	851,761	2,087	24	50:50	10.0
1986	14th August	856,718	594	6.9	57:43	8

Source: Seraj et al., 1987.

References

Al-Aska, A., Yaqub, B. A., Al-Harthi, S. S., and Al-Dalaan, A. (1987a). Rapid cooling in management of heat stroke: clinical methods and practical implications. *Ann. Saudi Med.* **7**:135-138.

Al-Aska, A. K., Abu-Aisha, H., Yaqub, B., Al-Harthi, S. S., and Sallam, A. (1987b). Simplified cooling bed for heat stroke (letter). *Lancet* **1** (8529):381.

Al-Harthi, S. S., Yaqub, B. A., Al-Nozha, M., and Al-Aska, A. (1986). Management of heat stroke patients by rapid cooling at Mecca pilgrimage (Hajj 1404)—comparing a conventional method with a body cooling unit. *Saudi Med. J.* **7**:369-376.

Al-Harthi, S. S., El-Deane, M. S., Akhtar, J., and Al-Nozha, M. M. (1989). Hemodynamic changes and intravascular hydration state in heat stroke. *Ann. Saudi Med.* **9**:378-383.

Al-Khawashki, M. I., Mustafa, M. K. Y., Khogali, M., and El-Sayed, H. (1983). Clinical presentation of 172 heat stroke cases seen at Mina and Arafat—September 1982. In *Heat Stroke and Temperature Regulation.* Edited by M. K. Khogali and J. R. S. Hales. Sydney, Australia, Academic press, pp. 99-108.

Amsterdam, J. T., Syverud, S. C., Barker, W. J., Bills, G. R., Goltra, D. D., Armao, J. C., and Hedges, J. R. (1986). Dantrolene sodium for treatment of heat stroke victims: lack of efficacy in a canine model. *Am. J. Emerg. Med.* **4**:399-405.

Austin, M. G., and Berry, J. W. (1956). Observation on one hundred cases of heat stroke. *J.A.M.A.* **161**:1525-1529.

Barker, W. J., Church, F., Amsterdam, J. T., Syverud, S. A., Hedges, J. R., and Huff, J. S. (1986). High-frequency jet ventilation cooling in a canine hyperthermia model. *Ann. Emerg. Med.* **15**:680-684.

Barnas, G. M., and Rautenberg, W. (1984). Cardiovascular and blood gas changes during panting responses induced by ambient or spinal cord heating in the pigeon. *Respir. Physiol.* **57**:89-101.

Bone, R. C., Francis, P. B., and Pierce, A. (1976). Intravascular coagulation associated with the adult respiratory distress syndrome. *Am. J. Med.* **61**:585-589.

Bradley, A. F., Stupfel, M., and Severinghaus, J. W. (1956). Effect of temperature on PCO_2 and PO_2 of blood in vitro. *J. Appl. Physiol.* **9**:201-204.

Chao, T. C., Sinniah, R., and Pakiam, J. E. (1981). Acute heat stroke deaths. *Pathology* **13**:145-156.

Clowes, G. H. A., and O'Donnell, T. F. (1974). Current concepts: heat stroke. *N. Engl. J. Med.* **291**:564-567.

Costrini, A. M., Pitt, H. A., Gustafson, A. B., and Uddin, D. E. (1979). Cardiovascular and metabolic manifestations of heat stroke and severe heat exhaustion. *Am. J. Med.* **66**:296-302.

Cronau, L. H., Bourke, D. L., and Bull, M. (1984). General anesthesia for whole-body hyperthermia. *Cancer Res.* (*suppl.*) **44**:4873s-4877s.

Editorial (1982). Management of heat stroke. *Lancet* **2**:910-911.

Eisler, K., Landauer, B., Hipp, R., Kolb, E., Lange, J., Siewert, J. R., Zänker, K., and Blümel, G. (1985). Enfahrunger mit der Ganzkörperhyperthermie. *Anaesthesist* **34**:299-303.

El-Kassimi, F. A., Mashhadani, S., Abdullah, A. K., and Akhtar, J. (1986). Adult respiratory distress syndrome and disseminated intravascular coagulation complicating heat stroke. *Chest* **90**:571-574.

Feistkorn, G., Nagel, A., and Jessen, C. (1984). Circulation and acid base balance in exercising goats at different body temperatures. *J. Appl. Physiol.* **57**:1655-1661.

Gaudio, R., and Abramson, N. (1968). Heat-induced hyperventilation. *J. Appl. Physiol.* **25**:742-746.

Gilbert, R. D., Lis, L., and Longo, L. D. (1985). Temperature effects on oxygen affinity of human fetal blood. *J. Dev. Physiol.* **7**:299-304.

Gleeson, M., and Brackenbury, J. H. (1984). Effects of body temperature on ventilation, blood gases and acid base balance in exercising fowl. *Q.J. Exp. Physiol.* **69**:61-72.

Graham, B. S., Lichtenstein, M. J., Hinson, J. M., and Theil, G. B. (1986). Nonexertional heat stroke—physiologic management and cooling in 14 patients. *Arch. Intern. Med.* **146**:87-90.

Harris, J. R., Blake, P. A., Cruz, J. G. R., and Jones, T. S. (1985). Fatal heat-related illness in naval cadets in Ecuador. *Int. J. Epidemiol.* **14**: 438-440.

Hart, G. R., Anderson, R. J., Crumpler, C. P., Shulkin, A., Reed, G., and Knochel, J. P. (1982). Epidemic classical heat stroke: clinical characteristics and course of 28 patients. *Medicine* **61**:189-197.

Hayat, H., and Friedberg, I. (1986). Heat-induced alterations in cell membrane permeability and cell inactivation of transformed mouse fibroblasts. *Int. J. Hyperthermia* **2**:369-378.

Khogali, M. (1983). Epidemiology of heat illnesses during the Makkah Pilgrimages in Saudi Arabia. *Int. J. Epidemiol.* **12**:267-273.

Khogali, M., and Weiner, J. S. (1980). Heat stroke: report of 18 cases. *Lancet* **2**:276-278.

Khogali, M., El-Sayed, H., Amar, M., El-Sayad, S., Al-Habashi, S., and Mutwali, A. (1983). Management and therapy regimen during cooling and in the recovery room at different heat stroke treatment centers. In *Heat Stroke and Temperature Regulation.* Edited by M. K. Khogali and J. R. S. Hales. Sidney, Australia, Academic Press, pp. 149-156.

Kimura, H., Yoshida, K., Ohsawa, M., Arai, T., and Tsujimura, T. (1985). An autopsy case of malignant hyperthermia. *Forensic Sci. Int.* **27**:25-30.

Knochel, J. P., Beisel, W. R., Herndon, E. G., Gerard, E. S., and Barry, K. G. (1961). The renal, cardiovascular, hematologic and serum electrolyte abnormalities of heat stroke. *Am. J. Med.* **30**:299-309.

Leithead, C. S. (1964). Heat illness-II. Heat illness and some related problems. *WHO Chron.* **18**:288-304.

Luterman, A., Manwaring, D., and Curreri, P. W. (1977). The role of fibrinogen degradation products in the pathogenesis of the adult respiratory distress syndrome. *Surgery* **82**:703-709.

Mustafa, M. K. Y., Khogali, M., and Gumaa, K. (1983a). Respiratory pathophysiology in heat stroke. In *Heat Stroke and Temperature Regulation.* Edited by M. K. Khogali and J. R. S. Hales. Sydney, Australia, Academic Press, pp. 119-127.

Mustafa, M. K. Y., Khogali, M., Gumaa, K., and Abu Al-Nasr, N. M. (1983b). Disseminated intravascular coagulation among heat stroke cases. In *Heat Stroke and Temperature Regulation.* Edited by M. K. Khogali and J. R. S. Hales. Sydney, Australia, Academic Press, pp. 109-117.

Mustafa, K. Y., Selig, W. M., Burhop, K. E., Minnear, F. L., and Malik, A. B. (1986). Hyperthermia - induced pulmonary edema. *J. Appl. Physiol.* **60**:1980-1985.

O'Donnell, T. F. (1975). Acute heat stroke—epidemiologic, biochemical, renal, and coagulation studies. *J.A.M.A.* **234**:824-828.

O'Donnell, T. F., and Clowes, G. H. A. (1972). The circulatory abnormalities of heat stroke. *N. Engl. J. Med.* **287**:734-737.

Osler, W. (1892). *Principles and Practice of Medicine.* New York, Appleton and Company, pp. 1017.

Seraj, M. A., Channa, A. B., Sharif, A. Y., Kadiwal, G. H., and Jamjoom, A. (1987). Heat related illnesses during the Hajj (pilgrimage)—emerging role of the anesthesiologist. *Middle East J. Anesthesiol.* **9**:255-276.

Shibolet, S., Lancaster, M. C., and Danon, Y. (1976). Heat stroke: a review. *Aviat. Space Environ. Med.* **47**:280-301.

Shih, C. J., Lin, M. T., and Tsai, S. H. (1984). Experimental study on the pathogenesis of heat stroke. *J. Neurosurg.* **60**:1246-1252.

Sprung, C. L. (1979). Hemodynamic alternation of heat stroke in the elderly. *Chest* **75**:362-366.

Sprung, C. L., Portocarrero, C. J., Fernaine, A. V., and Weinberg, P. F. (1980). The metabolic and respiratory alterations of heat stroke. *Arch. Intern. Med.* **140**:665-669.

Soliman, S. M., Abu-Taleb, Z., Khogali, M., and El-Sayed, H. (1983). Pulmonary aspiration and adult respiratory distress syndrome in 40 cases of heat stroke. In *Heat Stroke and Temperature Regulation*. Edited by M. K. Khogali and J. R. S. Hales. Sydney, Australia, Academic Press, pp. 129-138.

Tonami, N., Taki, J., Hisada, K., and Katsuki, K. (1985). Diffuse lung uptake of technetium-99m tin colloid in heat stroke: case report. *Clin. Nucl. Med.* **10**:769-771.

Tucker, L. E., Stanford, J., Graves, B., Swetnam, J., Hamburger, S., and Anwar, A. (1985). Classical heat stroke: clinical and laboratory assessment. *South Med. J.* **78**:20-25.

Vicario, S. J., Okabajue, R., and Haltom, T. (1986). Rapid cooling in classic heat stroke: effect on mortality rates. *Am. J. Emerg. Med.* **4**:394-398.

Weber, M. B., and Blakely, J. A. (1969). The haemorrhagic diathesis of heat stroke—a consumption coagulopathy successfully treated with heparin. *Lancet* **1**:1190-1192.

White, J. D., Riccobene, E., Nucci, R., Johnson, C., Butterfied, A. B., and Kamath, R. (1987). Evaporation versus iced gastric lavage treatment of heat stroke: comparative efficacy in a canine model. *Crit. Care Med.* **15**:748-750.

Wright, D. O., Reppert, L. B., and Cuttino, J. T. (1946). Purpuric manifestations of heat stroke—studies of prothrombin and platelets in twelve cases. *Arch. Intern. Med.* **77**:27-36.

Wyndham, C. H., Strydom, N. B., Cooke, H. M., Maritz, J. S., Norrison, J. F., Fleming, P. W., and Ward, J. S. (1959). Methods of cooling subjects with hyperpyrexia. *J. Appl. Physiol.* **14**:771-776.

Yaqub, B. A., Al-Harthi, S. S., Al-Orainey, I. O., Laajam, M. A., and Obeid, M. T. (1986). Heat stroke at the Mekkah pilgrimage: clinical characteristics and course of 30 patients. *Q. J. Med.* **59**:523-530.

7

Pulmonary Eosinophilic Syndromes in the Tropics
A Clinical Approach

CHARANJIT LAL, GURDIP S. FLORA, and OM P. SHARMA

Los Angeles County-University of Southern California Medical Center
Los Angeles, California

I. Introduction

The eosinophil was first described by Paul Ehrlich in 1879 and was so named because of the intense staining of its granules with the dye eosin (Hirsch and Hirsch, 1980). However, only in the last 10 years have we learned about the intricacies of the structure and function of this mysterious cell and its role in human disease (Spry, 1985).

The eosinophil is derived from an, as yet, unidentified precursor cell in the bone marrow. T lymphocytes or eosinophilopoietic factors secreted by T lymphocytes and unknown genetic factors are involved in regulating the production of eosinophils (Spry, 1985; Vadas, 1982). The eosinophil passes through several stages before entering the bloodstream, where it undergoes a late differentiation stage termed "activation." It acquires an increased capacity to kill and to metabolize oxygen and glucose (Parwaresch et al., 1976; Bass et al., 1980). The half-life of a blood eosinophil in humans is 3-8 h. After a brief stay in the blood, the eosinophils move into various tissues, including the skin, bronchial mucosa, gastrointestinal tract, lactating mammary glands, vagina, uterus, and connective tissues (Ringoen, 1938; Rytomma,

1960). There they reside for a few days before being destroyed by macrophages (Rytomma, 1960; Ross and Klebanoff, 1966; Speirs and Osada, 1962).

The normal level of eosinophils is approximately 4% in the blood and 5% in the bone marrow. The upper limit of normal absolute eosinophil count is about 350/mm^3 (Rud, 1947). The number of eosinophils is highest late at night and lowest in the early morning hours (Best et la., 1953). In women, the count rises during menstruation and decreases thereafter until the onset of the next menstrual cycle (Oathak and Kahali, 1957).

The eosinophil is slightly larger than the neutrophil and ranges from 12 to 17 μm in diameter. Its nucleus is usually bilobed and lacks a nucleolus. The cytoplasm is rich in organelles and possesses well-developed mitochondria and Golgi bodies. Eosinophilic granules are characteristically orange to deep red. Under the electron microscope, the mature eosinophil reveals two types of granules: smaller, round, homogeneous granules that produce arylsulfatase and acid phosphatase; and larger granules that contain an electron-dense core (the internum) and produce major basic protein (Gleich et al., 1974). The granules contain an array of hydrolytic enzymes including sulfatase, acid phosphatase, peroxidases, phospholipase, betaglucuronidase, acid beta-glycosophosphatase, ribonuclease, and cathepsin. They do not contain lysozyme and phagocytin (Archer and Hirsch, 1981).

The eosinophil serves at least two functions: first, it can inactivate mediators released from mast cells and modulate IgE-mediated type I reactions; second, it can damage the larval stages of some helminthic parasites (Butterworth and David, 1981). The eosinophils also make large amounts of slow-releasing substance-A (SRS-A), and leukotrienes, particularly leukotriene-C4 (Henderson et al., 1984). The efficiency of the helminthicidal activity of eosinophils is enhanced by leukotriene B4 and eosinophil chemotactic factors of anaphylaxis (ECF-A). The finding of elevated concentrations of specific eosinophil constituents in sputum and lung tissues of patients with asthma and other inflammatory lung diseases of suspected allergic origin emphasizes the importance of eosinophils in normal lung function and lung diseases. Whether eosinophils produce sufficient leukotrienes to affect the lungs of patients with asthma is not known. Activated eosinophils in such patients could produce toxic substances that could damage the pulmonary epithelium (Gleich et al., 1985; Sun et al., 1985). The platelet-activating factor (PAF) released from eosinophils is also thought to be involved in the pathogenesis of asthma (Gleich and Loegering, 1982).

The association between pulmonary infiltrates and blood eosinophilia is recognized as "pulmonary eosinophilia" or "pulmonary infiltration with eosinophilia" (PIE). The term *PIE syndromes* was coined in 1952 (Reeder and Goodrich, 1952). In the same year, Crofton and associates classified the pulmonary eosinophilias into five clinical groups: Loeffler's syndrome, prolonged pulmonary eosinophilia, pulmonary eosinophilia with asthma, tropical eosinophilia, and periarteritis nodosa (Crofton et al., 1952). The classification was arbitrary and based primarily on the clinical manifestations. The recent advances in allergy and immunology have made Crofton's classification obsolete. The number of PIE syndromes have increased since Loffler's first description in 1932 (Loffler, 1932). More recently added entities include Churg-Strauss syndrome, allergic bronchopulmonary aspergillosis (ABPA), and hypereosinophilic syndrome. It is logical to develop a causative classification of pulmonary eosinophilias (Fig. 1). However, recommended classifications have their limitations, whether based on clinical features, cause, or anatomical and pathological features. The differential diagnosis of pulmonary eosinophilias is outlined in Table 1.

PIE appears to result from the introduction of foreign material into the human body by different routes including ingestion, infections, inhalation, skin contact, and vaginal absorption. Most cases of tropical pulmonary eosinophilia are allergic reactions to filarial infestations, whereas various helminths have been implicated in more temperate latitudes. Control of human parasites and vectors has resulted in a decrease in the more benign form of the disease (Loeffler's syndrome or simple pulmonary eosinophilia), but eosinophilic pneumonias continue to pose a major problem in parts of the world

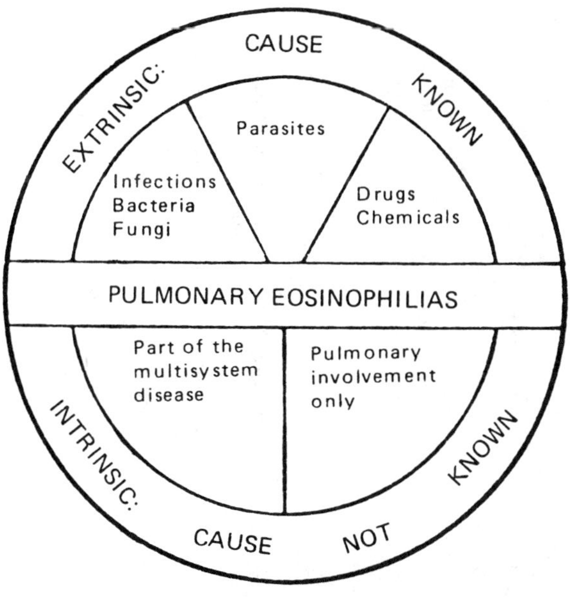

Figure 1 Classification of pulmonary eosinophilias.

Table 1 Differential Diagnosis of Pulmonary Eosinophilias

Disease	History	Clinical Features	Laboratory Tests	Chest Radiograph Studies	Lung Histological Findings
Tuberculosis	History of contact with tuberculosis	Fever, cough, weight loss	Tuberculin skin test may be positive. Sputum, urine, and bone cultures may show acid-fast bacilli	Cavity, soft infiltrate, hilar adenopathy, and miliary infiltrate	Caseating granulomata
Coccidioidomycosis	Recent travel or residence in an endemic area	Usually asymptomatic, but fever, chills, cough, and erythema nodosum may occur	Coccidioidin skin test positive. Coccidioidin complement-fixation and precipitin tests positive	Hilar adenopathy, infiltration	Granulomatous lesion with necrosis
Histoplasmosis	Recent travel or residence in an endemic area	Usually asymptomatic, but fever, chills, cough, and erythema nodosum may occur	Histoplasmin skin test positive. Complement-fixation test may be helpful	Any of the above, and calcification	Granulomatous lesion with necrosis
Brucellosis	Farm worker, drinking raw milk, or working in a slaughterhouse	Fever, weight loss, and night sweats	Brucella skin test positive. Complement-fixation antibodies. Positive blood culture	Nonspecific changes	Granulomatous lesion
Allergic bronchopulmonary aspergillosis	Atopic host with asthma	Fever, episodic wheezing, sputum plugs	Elevated serum IgE, precipitating antibody to *Aspergillus*. Types I and III responses on skin tests	Transient infiltrates, bronchiectasis	Not applicable
Tropical eosinophilia	Native of India or Southeast Asia	Fever, night sweats, nocturnal wheezing, and cough	Filarial skin test positive. Filarial complement-fixation test positive	Miliary infiltrate	Eosinophilic infiltrate with giant cells and granulomata

Parasites	Residence in endemic area	Fever, anemia	Stool examination may show ova	Nonspecific changes	Nonspecific celular response
Drug-induced	Relevant drug intake	Fever, tightness in chest, dyspnea	Eosinophilia	Nonspecific changes	Cellular infiltrates
Loeffler's syndrome	—	Fever, dry cough lasting less than 1 month	Mild eosinophilia	Transient infiltrate	Eosinophilic infiltrates
Chronic eosinophilic pneumonia	Occurs mostly in adult women	Fever, cough, night sweats, weight loss, persistent weakness	Eosinophilia	Peripherally located infiltrates	Eosinophilic, monocytic, and histiocytic infiltrates in alveoli and interstitial tissues
Wegener's granulomatosis and polyarteritis nodosa	Multisystem involvement	Fever, malaise, weight loss	Raised sedimentation rate and hyperglobulinemia	Infiltrates, cavity formation, single or multiple nodules	Necrotic lesions surrounded by giant cells, lymphocytes, plasma cells, and eosinophils
Sarcoidosis	Occurs frequently in young people	Dyspnea, fever, iritis, skin lesions	Hypercalcemia, hypergammaglobulinemia, positive Kveim test	Bilateral hilar adenopathy, with or without infiltration	Noncaseating granuloma
Eosinophilic granuloma	Occurs mostly in children and young adults	Fever, malaise, bone pains, diabetes insipidus	Occasional anemia	Nodular, diffuse lesions, honeycombing, pneumothorax	Aggregates of mature eosinophils and mononuclear cells
Hypereosinophilic syndrome	Occurs in adults	Weakness, cough, dyspnea, neurologic, cardiac, and skin manifestations	Eosinophilia for 6 months, anemia, and thrombocytopenia	Infiltrates, effusion	Eosinophilic infiltrates

where the human population is still heavily parasitized. Drugs and elements in the environment have also become important causes of pulmonary eosinophilia. The causes of pulmonary eosinophilia in the tropics are essentially similar to those in temperate climates, except that parasitic infestations and tuberculosis are more common in the tropics.

II. Extrinsic Pulmonary Eosinophilias

Those diseases in which the cause is known are listed in Table 2 and discussed in the following sections.

Table 2 Extrinsic Pulmonary Eosinophilias

Cause	Disease
Infections	
Mycobacteria	Tuberculosis
Aspergillus	Allergic bronchopulmonary aspergillosis
	Bronchocentric granulomatosis
Coccidioides	Coccidioidomycosis
Histoplasma	Histoplasmosis
Parasites	
Filaria sp.	Tropical eosinophilia
Strongyloides	
Schistosoma	
Ascaris	Pneumonitis
Trichinella	
Ancylostoma	
Paragonimus	
Drugs	
Sulfonamides	
Penicillin	
Nitrofurantoin	
Radiotherapy	
Irradiation	Radiation pneumonitis
Chemicals	
Nickel	Nickel toxicity
Insect bite	
Scorpion	

A. Tuberculosis

Schwarz noted a characteristic undulating response of eosinophils that correlated with the activity level of tuberculosis. Most patients with acute fulminating disease or miliary spread showed eosinopenia, especially in the presence of fever, with a rising eosinophil count as they recover (Schwarz, 1914). Patients with pulmonary and pleural tuberculosis who improved without therapy showed eosinophilia up to 14% of the leukocyte count. In 1943, Muller reported a study of 7,000 eosinophil determinations in 1,000 patients with tuberculosis (Muller, 1943). The eosinophil count correlated with the activity of the disease. Eosinophilia was present in about 14% of the patients who were doing well. Eosinophilia was twice as frequent in men as in women, with the incidence in women being about 6%. Muller also reported the development of eosinophilia after tuberculin injection in infected patients and suggested it to be a hypersensitivity reaction that might serve as a protective function. Pulmonary eosinophilia has also been reported with atypical mycobacteriae such as *Mycobacterium simiae* (Wright et al., 1983).

B. Fungal Infections

With the exception of coccidioidomycosis, fungal infections generally do not cause eosinophilia. Peripheral eosinophilia with primary coccidioidomycosis infection occurs in up to 88% of patients (Drutz and Catanzaro, 1978). Pulmonary eosinophilia represents a hypersensitivity reaction to coccidioidomycosis and not a host defense mechanism (Lombard et al., 1987). In the early stages of this infection, eosinophilia is present in 5-18% of patients. After 4 weeks, the levels gradually decline (Dickson and Gilford, 1938; Wilett and Weiss, 1943). Eosinophilia is more likely to occur if the patient has other allergic or hypersensitivity manifestations such as erythema nodosum, erythema multiforme, urticaria, or arthritis. Eosinophil counts as high as 20-25% are not unusual (Wilett and Oppenheim, 1946). Fiese indicated that very high eosinophil counts are often associated with pulmonary infiltrations and may herald dissemination (Fiese, 1958). Lonky and associates observed eosinophilia in 11 of 28 patients (39%) who had acute coccidioidomycosis (Lonky et al., 1976). Pulmonary eosinophilia due to coccidioidomycosis should be suspected in patients either living in or with a history of travel to an endemic area with positive skin and serological tests. Lung biopsy specimens may or may not show the organisms (Lombard et al., 1987).

Histoplasma capsulatum infection is endemic in many parts of the world and is also known to produce transient pneumonitis with peripheral eosinophilia.

C. Allergic Bronchopulmonary Aspergillosis

ABPA was first described in England in 1952 (Hinson et al., 1952). It is most commonly caused by *Aspergillus fumigatus*, but other *Aspergillus* species have also been implicated (Akiyama et al., 1987). Hypersensitivity to fungi other than of the *Aspergillus* species has been reported to produce a clinical syndrome identical to ABPA (Benatar et al., 1980; McAleer et al., 1981; Hendrick et al., 1982). ABPA is found almost exclusively in atopic asthmatic individuals. It causes an acute migratory infiltration of the lungs with a variety of irreversible changes that cause chronic lung dysfunction. The disease can occur at any age. In general, patients with ABPA associated with long-standing asthma and frequent episodes of pulmonary infiltrates are at higher risk of developing chronic lung disease. Cor pulmonale occurs in about 1% of these patients.

ABPA usually manifests with a low-grade fever, wheezing, cough productive of golden-brown sputum plugs, and progressive dyspnea. Examination reveals a prolonged expiratory phase and diffuse rhonchi. Patients may complain of chest pain, malaise, weight loss, and blood-streaked sputum. Chest radiographs may show transient pulmonary infiltrates, usually involving the upper lobes. Mucus plugs may cause segmental, lobar, or total collapse of the lung. "Tram-line" shadows, "gloved-finger" shadows, or "ring" shadows due to inflammation and thickening of bronchial wall are frequently seen. In early stages of ABPA, loss of volume of upper lobes, honeycombing, and extensive bronchiectasis may be present. Bronchography may reveal a characteristic saccular dilatation of the proximal bronchi (McCarthy et al., 1970; Fig. 2).

The pathogenesis of ABPA is believed to involve the inhalation, trapping, and subsequent germination of fungal spores of *Aspergillus fumigatus*. Following germination, the organisms vegetate in the bronchial lumen and produce high concentrations of antigens. The immunological reaction is thought to involve a combination of immediate type I or IgE-mediated hypersensitivity, as evidenced by the presence of immediate skin reactions and high levels of IgE and also possibly an Arthus reaction, manifested by skin test reactions, precipitating antibodies, fever, and a late decline in forced expiratory volume in 1 s (FEV1) to inhaled *Aspergillus*. It is also possible that the intense eosinophilic infiltrates represent late phage IgE-dependent response. Based on this hypothesis, mast-cell-derived chemotactic factors such as eosinophilic chemotactic factor of anaphylaxis (ECF-A) and leukotriene B4 liberated during intense type I IgE-mediated reactions would result in later accumulation of eosinophils in the pulmonary parenchyma and bronchial lining tissues. Eosinophils, in turn, could further stimulate the mast cells to release mediators and directly damage pulmonary tissues via liberation of major basic protein and other eosinophil cationic proteins. Furthermore,

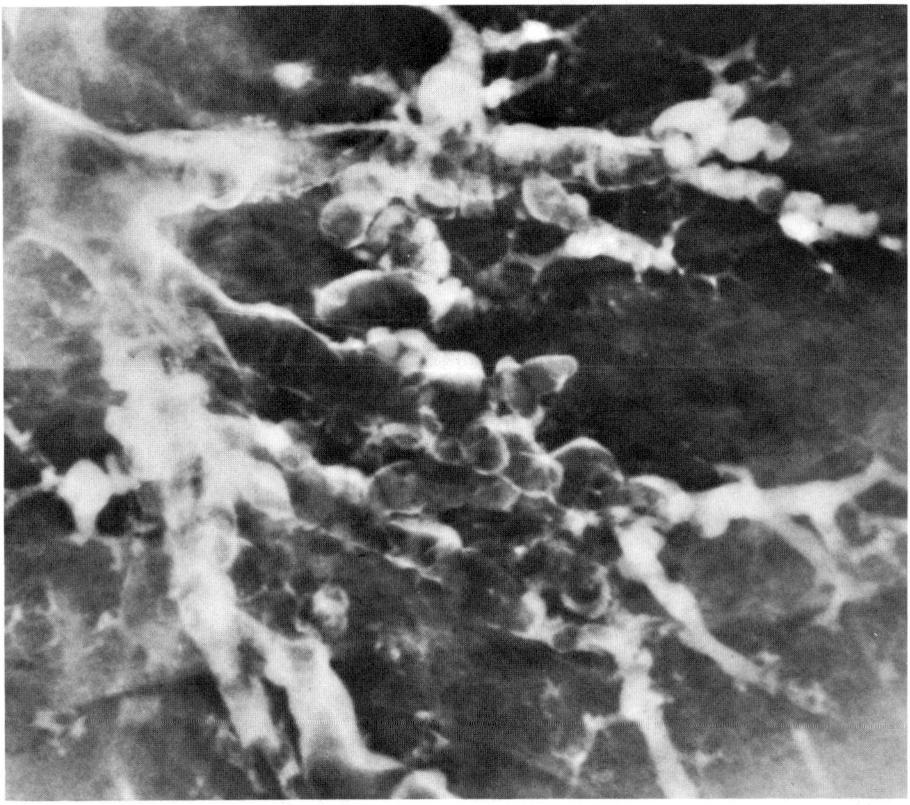

Figure 2 Extensive saccular bronchiectasis in a young man with asthma and allergic bronchopulmonary aspergillosis. Because of the availability of high-resolution computed tomography, conventional bronchography is rarely used.

leukotriene C4 released from eosinophils could cause bronchoconstriction and increased mucus production. The immune complex injury produces bronchietasis. The presence of IgE is essential in enhancing the tissue-damaging effect of immune complexes.

Histological study of lung tissue shows irregular bronchi filled with mucus, inflammatory cells, and *Aspergillus* hyphae. The bronchial walls and peribronchial parenchyma are infiltrated with mononuclear cells and eosinophils. Lung parenchyma from areas of consolidation shows large number of eosinophils, multinucleated giant cells, and granuloma formation (Slavin, 1985).

Several clinical conditions including tuberculosis, hypersensitivity pneumonitis, atopic asthma with recurrent pneumonia, and other PIE syndromes can be confused with ABPA. No single clinical, radiographic, or laboratory finding is pathognomonic for ABPA. The important diagnostic criteria include a history of asthma with peripheral blood eosinophilia in excess of 500/mm^3, immediate skin reactivity and precipitating antibodies to *Aspergillus* species, serum IgE level greater than 2000 ng/ml, a history of transient or fixed pulmonary infiltrates, and central bronchiectasis (Safirstein et al., 1973; Rosenberg et al., 1977). Lesser criteria include the presence of *Aspergillus* hyphae in the sputum, a history of expectoration of brown plugs or flecks, and late-phase skin reactivity to *Aspergillus* antigen. The presence of six of the seven primary criteria makes the diagnosis very likely. If all seven are met, the diagnosis is certain (Fig. 3).

The natural history of patients with ABPA is not completely understood. The disease can be organized into five clinical stages. The acute stage is characterized by bronchospasm, eosinophilia, migratory infiltrates on the chest radiograph, positive *Aspergillus* skin test, and increased serum IgE levels. The remission stage, following therapy with corticosteroids, is characterized

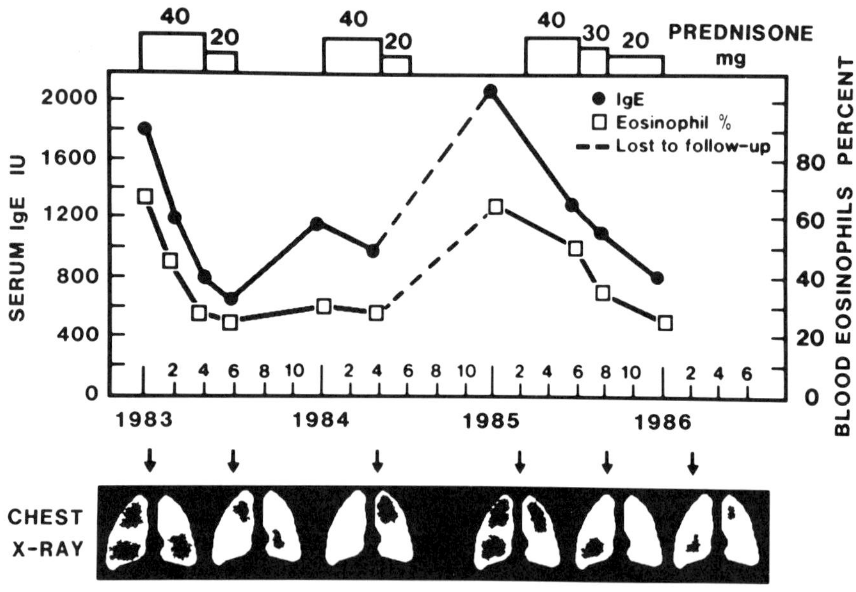

Figure 3 Serum IgE determination is not only useful in diagnosing allergic bronchopulmonary aspergillosis but the test also reflects the course of the disease and the response to corticosteroids, as shown here.

by resolution of symptoms, clearing of pulmonary infiltrates, and a decrease in the serum IgE levels. Corticosteroids can be slowly tapered off at this time. The exacerbation stage includes recurrence of some or all of the clinical and laboratory abnormalities of the acute stage. Treatment with corticosteroids usually again causes an improvement. The corticosteroid-dependent asthmatic stage consists of patients who require long-term maintenance corticosteroid therapy to control their asthma or to prevent exacerbation of ABPA or both. The fibrotic lung disease stage of ABPA occurs in inadequately treated or long-standing cases of ABPA. In some of these patients, the disease progresses to cor pulmonale, respiratory failure, and death (Patterson et al., 1982).

The mainstay of treatment of ABPA is corticosteroids. In untreated cases, irreversible fibrosis and bronchiectasis may occur. In acute disease, 40-60 mg of oral prednisone daily is the usual dosage. As the clinical symptoms and chest radiographs improve, the dosage is tapered off over the next 3 months and then discontinued if the disease is clinically resolved. Serum IgE levels are important in monitoring the activity of the disease (Halwig et al., 1984). Close follow-up is needed because radiographic infiltrates and increased levels of serum IgE may occur in asymptomatic patients. Asymptomatic or symptomatic exacerbations should be treated in the same manner as the acute stage. Inhaled costicosteroids, disodium cromoglycate, and immunotherapy have not proved to be effective. Recently, ketoconazole has been tried with some success (Shale et al., 1987).

D. Bronchocentric Granulomatosis

Bronchocentric granulomatosis (BCG) is characterized by the presence of bronchocentric granulomatous lesions in the bronchial mucosa, particularly in the mucosa of the conducting airways (Liebow, 1973). BCG appears to affect primarily persons with bronchial asthma. The atopic patients are generally younger, have peripheral eosinophilia, and their mucus plugs contain fungal hyphae. The nonatopic patients are a much more heterogenous group. They lack tissue eosinophilia. Approximately one-half of the patients in one series had asthma along with eosinophilia and serological evidence of exposure to *Aspergillus* and other fungal species (Katzenstein et al., 1975). *Aspergillus* was recovered from the sputum of several patients, and eosinophils and degraded fungal hyphae were present within necrotizing granulomas in their lungs. Although immunological mechanisms in BCG are not clearly understood, the basic abnormality seems to be a hypersensitivity reaction to fungi. Serum precipitin antibodies are found in about 40% of atopic patients.

The chest radiograph may show infiltrates, nodular lesions, or atelectasis. Rarely, it may produce an ARDS-like syndrome (Brooker and Sharma,

1982). Although BCG is clearly defined pathologically, it is difficult to diagnose clinically. The disease often causes few respiratory symptoms.

On microscopic examination the necrotizing granulomas have a bronchocentric distribution and destroy bronchioles. The lesion consists of heavy eosinophilic and plasma cell infiltrates surrounded by palisading epitheloid cells. In some isntances foreign body giant cells are present. Special stains often reveal fungal hyphae within the necrotic centers. Unlike the findings in Wegener's granulomatosis, vasculitis is not a prominent feature of bronchocentric granulomatosis and veins are not involved. Chondritis is present when the larger bronchi are involved (Katzenstein et al., 1975).

Corticosteroids are helpful in patients with BCG who also have asthma. The prognosis is not so favorable in nonatopic patients.

E. Chronic Brucellosis

Chronic brucellosis has been reported to be associated with pulmonary infiltrates and eosinophilia (Elsom and Ingelfinger, 1942). Patients usually have fever, peripheral eosinophilia up to 40%, and bilateral pulmonary infiltrates. The chest roentgenographic abnormality may be out of proportion to the clinical presentation. Although parahilar infiltrates and diffuse pneumonic patches are frequent, the occurrence of pleural effusion, pleural thickening, and cavitary disease has been described. Lesions on the chest radiograph may simulate tuberculosis. In diagnosing this infection, knowledge of the patient's history is important, particularly with regard to exposure to animals or animal products and to residence in a rural area. The diagnosis may be confirmed by blood or bone marrow cultures. Brucella agglutination tests showing a fourfold or greater increase in antibody titers indicate recent infection. The treatment of choice is a combination of streptomycin and tetracycline. Corticosteroids may be helpful.

F. Parasitic Infestations

Almost all metazoan infestations are accompanied by eosinophilia. Because of the high prevalence of worm infestations in the tropics, pulmonary eosinophilia as a manifestation of parasitic disease is not uncommon. Ascariasis, schistosomiasis, ancylostomiasis, trichinosis, paragonimiasis, and strongyloidiasis can all cause chronic pulmonary eosinophilia. The pulmonary infiltrates appear during larval migration through the lungs and are usually transitory. Symptoms are mild and self-limiting and include wheezing, cough, hemoptysis, and dyspnea. The pulmonary eosinophilia is thought to be a hypersensitivity response to the parasites in sensitized individuals, as evidenced by high serum IgE levels. There is no permanent lung damage with these infestations. Stool specimens should be examined for ova and parasites.

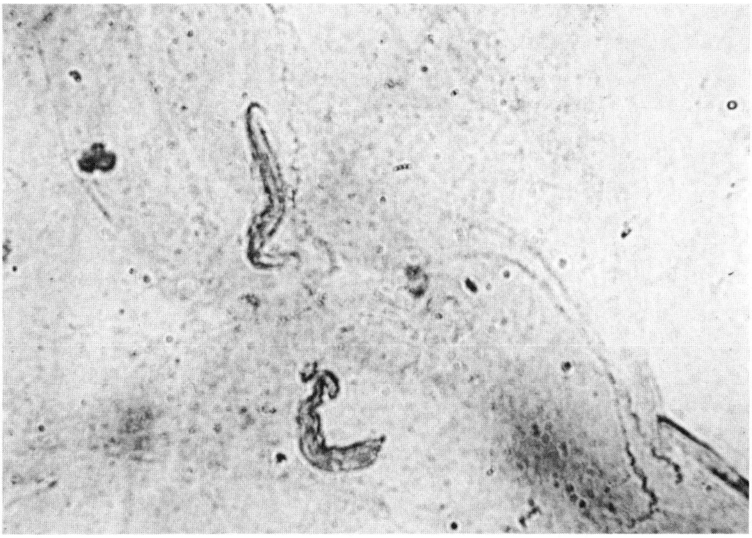

a

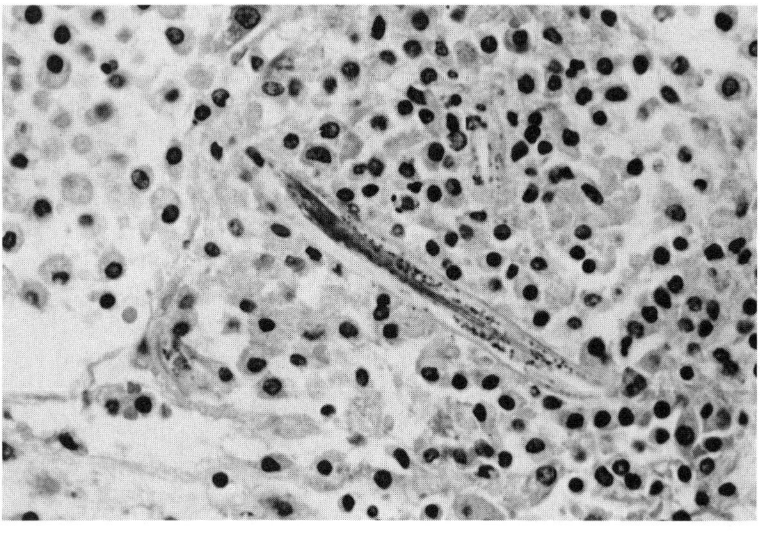

b

Figure 4 *Strongyloides stercoralis* larvae. a. In sputum (hematoxylin and eosin, × 75). b. In a lung biopsy specimen (hematoxylin and eosin, × 100).

Also blood, sputum, and gastric lavage should be examined for microfilariae. Lung biopsies are rarely necessary (Fig. 4). Treatment consists of the appropriate antihelminthic drugs.

G. Tropical Pulmonary Eosinophilia

Tropical eosinophilia (TE) is a clinical syndrome characterized by respiratory symptoms and peripheral eosinophilia. The disease is believed to be a cryptic filarial infection. Although the illness has a geographic distribution similar to bancroftian and Malayian filariasis, it is more often recognized in Asia, particularly on the Indian subcontinent (Frimodt-Moller and Barton, 1940).

TE is thought to be a hypersensitivity reaction to degenerating microfilariae trapped in the lungs (Neva and Ottesen, 1978). Histopathological examination of the lung initially shows histocytic infiltrates in the interstitium and alveoli that may later progress to eosinophilic pneumonias and chronic nodular interstitial disease with mixed cell infiltrates, granulomatous reaction, and fibrosis. The disease may remit spontaneously (Joshi et al., 1969).

The onset of illness is gradual, sometimes with fatigue, low-grade fever, night sweats, and weight loss. Cough, often at night, wheezing, dyspnea, and tightness of the chest are the main symptoms. Occasionally chest pain may occur. Physical examination may reveal diffuse rhonchi and scattered rales. In children, peripheral lymphadenopathy and hepatosplenomegaly are prominent. Pericarditis with or without effusion and central nervous system involvement have been reported (Singh et al., 1974; Ravindran, 1979).

Laboratory studies show leukocytosis and marked eosinophilia with absolute eosinophil counts often more than 20,000/mm^3. Serum IgE levels are elevated to usually greater than 1000 units/ml (normal, less than 300 units/ml). Antifilarial antibodies are present in blood but microfilariae are almost never found. The chest roentgenogram may be normal or show a variety of abnormalities including generalized ground glass haziness often misdiagnosed as miliary tuberculosis; reticulonodular pattern involving mainly the middle and lower lung zones; mild hilar adenopathy with perihilar haze resembling sarcoidosis; and interstitial nodular pattern (Fig. 5). Patchy consolidations, cavity formation, and pleural effusion have been reported (Jain and Beniwal, 1984; Nath and Jain, 1984; Boornazian and Fagan, 1985). The lung function tests commonly show a restrictive pattern but in 25-30% of patients airway obstruction is present (Udwadia, 1975; Nasarajah, 1972).

It is prudent to always think of pulmonary eosinophilia in a patient who has a history of prolonged stay in an endemic area and presents with cough, wheezing, and eosinophilia (Lal and Sharma, 1989). Markedly elevated levels of IgE and antifilarial antibodies establish the diagnosis. Bron-

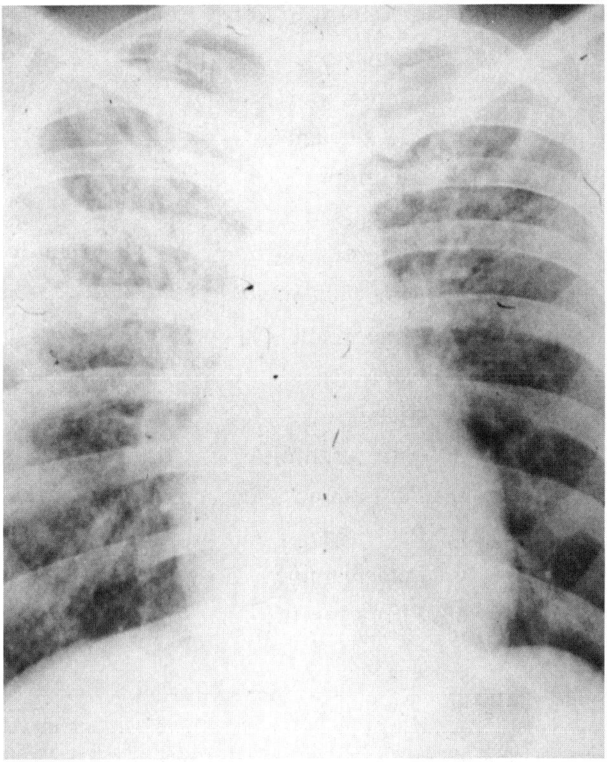

Figure 5 Bilateral nodular pulmonary infiltrates in a patient with tropical eosinophilia. Because of the distribution of the infiltrate in the middle and upper lung fields, the appearance can be misdiagnosed as pulmonary tuberculosis.

choscopy, bronchoalveolar lavage, and lung biopsy are neither indicated nor helpful.

Diethylcarbamazine citrate is the treatment of choice. A daily dosage of 8-12 mg/kg body weight in divided doses for 8-16 days usually results in total relief (Spry and Kumaraswami, 1982). Relapses can occur, but usually respond to a second course of treatment. Hypotension, urticaria, and other allergic reactions may occur. Patients should be hospitalized for close observation. Corticosteroids and antihistaminics have also been used.

H. Drug-Induced Pulmonary Eosinophilia

A large number of drugs have been associated with pulmonary eosinophilia (Table 3). Low-grade fever, dry cough with or without wheezing, and severe

Table 3 Drugs and Chemicals Known to Cause Pulmonary Eosinophilia

Amiodarone	Isoniazid	Phenytoin
Aspirin	Imipramine	Pituitary snuff
Azathioprine	Mecamylamine	Procarbazine
Azulfidine	Mesantoin	Streptomycin
Beclomethasone	Melphalan	Sulfonamides
Beryllium	Methotrexate	Sulfonylureas
Bleomycin	Methylphenidate	Tetracycline
Carbamazepine	Minocycline	Thiazides
Chlorpromide	Naproxen	Tolseran
Clofibrate	Nickel	
Dantrolene	Nitrofurantoin	
Disodium cromoglycate	Para-aminosalicyclic acid (PAS)	
Tetracycline	Penicillin	
Gold salts	Penicillamine	
Hydralazine	Phenylephrine	

dyspnea and peripheral eosinophilia may be present. Chest examination may show wheezing and crackles. Pulmonary infiltrates are usually diffuse and patchy. On pulmonary function testing, most patients show a decrease in DLCO but no obstruction or restriction. In chronic cases, however, the lung function tests may reveal a restrictive pattern because of fibrosis. In most cases the lung infiltrates and symptoms improve after discontinuation of the offending drug (Rosenow, 1972). Corticosteroids do not appear to affect the outcome of drug-induced acute pulmonary eosinophilia.

Nitrofurantoin is the drug most commonly associated with pulmonary eosinophilia, probably because of its frequent use in the prophylaxis and treatment of urinary tract infections. Nitrofurantoin is unique in that it can cause acute, subacute, and chronic reactions (Sovijarvi et al., 1977). The acute phase usually begins 2 h to 10 days after the start of nitrofurantoin treatment. Clinical symptoms include dry cough, fever, and dyspnea. Radiographically documented lung involvement is usually diffuse but sometimes can be patchy. In addition to the peripheral eosinophilia, a characteristic finding is the development of eosinophilic pleural effusion that is not seen with other drugs causing pulmonary eosinophilia. Symptoms and signs usually resolve after discontinuation of nitrofurantoin. However, remission is sometimes slow and may require corticosteroid therapy. The subacute and chronic phases develop insidiously and run a course resembling chronic interstitial pneumonitis.

On histological examination, obliterative pulmonary vasculitis and granulomatous interstitial inflammation with fibrosis occurs that can result in permanent lung damage. In addition to stopping the offending agent, steroid therapy may be helpful in these cases to stop the progression of the disease (Sovijarvi et al., 1977).

Loeffler's syndrome following ingestion of a nickel coin and after inhalation of nickel carbonyl fumes has also been reported (Sunderman and

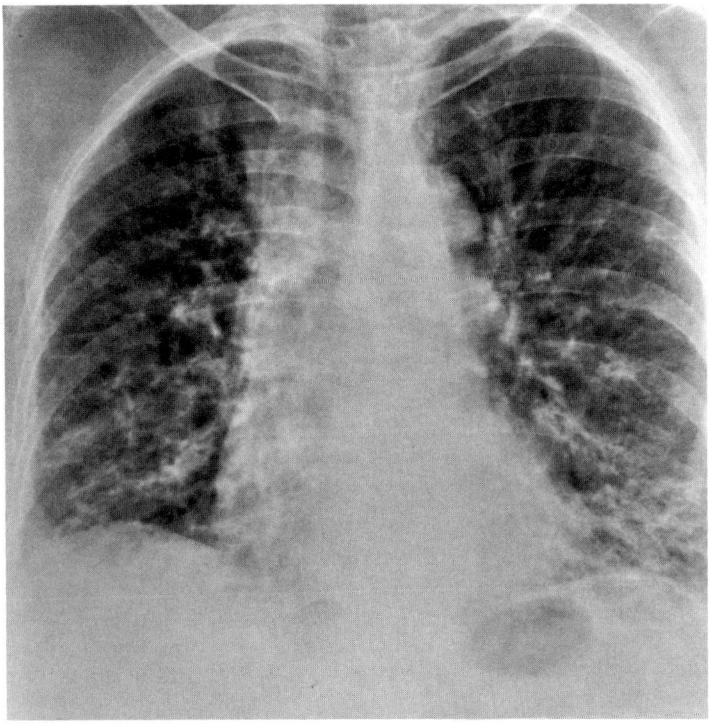

Figure 6a A patient with rheumatoid arthritis developed cough, fever, chest tightness, eosinophilia and pulmonary infiltrates, while receiving gold injections. She was diagnosed as having gold pneumonitis.

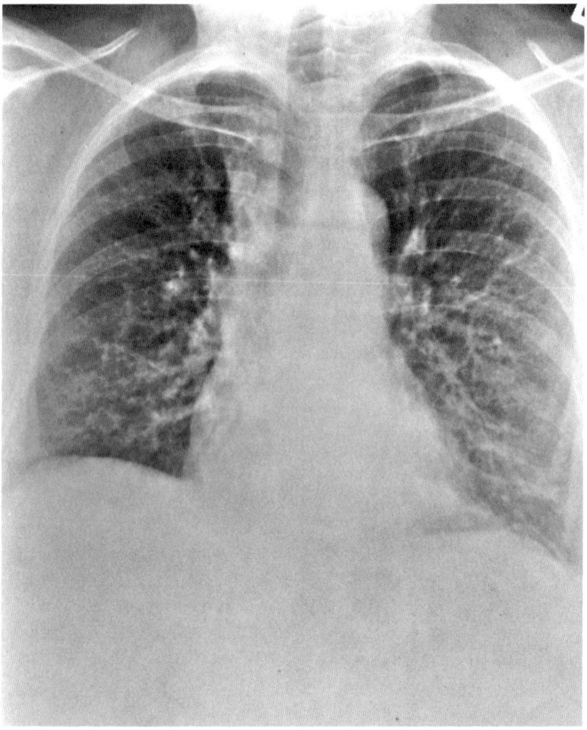

Figure 6b The patient responded to corticosteroids. Gold therapy was discontinued.

Sunderman, 1961; Gray, 1982). Treatment with gold for rheumatoid arthritis may result in gold pneumonitis characterized by cough, fever, chest tightness, pulmonary infiltrates, and eosinophilia (Fig. 6).

III. Intrinsic Pulmonary Eosinophilias

These include diseases in which the cause is unknown and are discussed in the following sections.

The term intrinsic (also known as idiopathic or cryptogenic) pulmonary eosinophilia is reserved for pulmonary eosinophilia in which there is no evidence of bacterial infection, fungal hypersensitivity, parasitic infestation, or drug reaction. As many as 20% of cases of pulmonary eosinophilia are unexplained and fall into this category (McCarthy and Pepys, 1973).

A. Loeffler's Syndrome

In 1932, Loffler described a syndrome consisting of transient fleeting pulmonary infiltrates, minimal or no respiratory symptoms, and peripheral blood eosinophilia (Loffler, 1932). Respiratory symptoms, when present, usually consist of dry cough or scanty mucoid expectoration, and wheezing with or without mild dyspnea. Low-grade fever and myalgia may also be present. Chest radiographic examination reveals fleeting homogeneous, peripheral nonsegmental densities that appear and disappear over a period of 1-2 days. Serial chest x-rays usually suggest the diagnosis. The disease is benign and self-limiting and usually subsides within 3-4 weeks. The cause of the syndrome was not known at the time of the report by Loeffler, but circumstantial evidence suggested it to be due to the *Ascaris* larvae. In some cases of Loeffer's syndrome, careful examination may reveal an extrinsic cause, in which case the term *Loeffler's syndrome* should not be used.

B. Chronic Eosinophilic Pneumonia

The clinical and pathological features of chronic eosinophilic pneumonia were first described in 1969 (Carrington et al., 1969). Although no age group is exempt, the age distribution for this disease peaks in the fifth decade. It is twice as common in women as in men. The clinical picture is that of an infection characterized by high-grade fever, weight loss, night sweats, and severe progressive dyspnea. Most of the patients are white women. About 50% of the patients may have asthma that may accompany or precede the clinical picture.

Peripheral eosinophilia is seen in about two-thirds of the patients. Erythrocyte sedimentation rate, serum IgE levels, and platelet levels may be elevated (Frigas et al., 1981; Enokihara et al., 1985; Grantham et al., 1986; Gonzales et al., 1986). Chest radiography shows peripheral infiltrates termed "photographic negative of pulmonary edema" in about two-thirds of the patients (Gaensler and Carrington, 1977). Unusual chest x-ray findings include pleural effusions, migratory pulmonary infiltrates, cavitary lesions, and an ARDS-like picture. Normal chest x-rays have also been reported (Fig. 7).

On histological examination the interstitial tissue and alveoli are infiltrated with eosinophils, lymphocytes, plasma cells, and macrophages. Multinucleated histiocytic giant cells with eosinophilic granules and Charcot-Leyden crystals are also present in the airspaces.

In more severe illness, the lung volumes, diffusing capacity, and arterial oxygenation are decreased. These values may improve with steroid therapy. The role of bronchoalveolar lavage, transbronchial lung biopsy, and open lung biopsy in the diagnosis of chronic eosinophilic pneumonia is controversial.

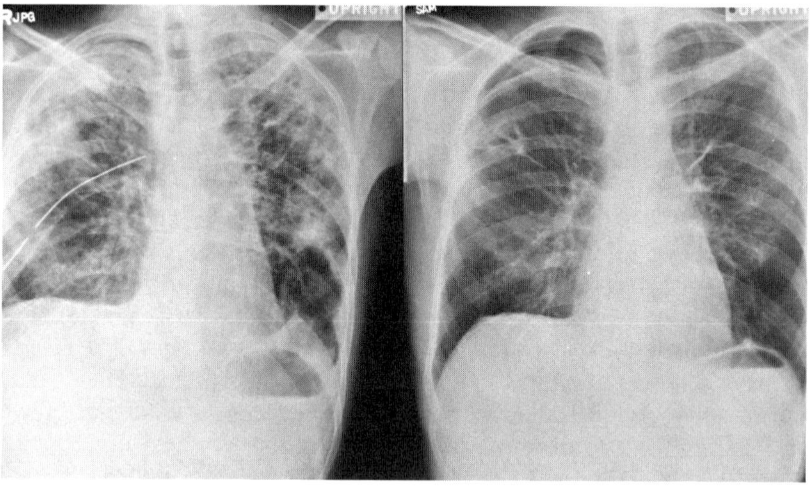

(a) (b)

Figure 7 a. Typical bilateral peripheral infiltrates in a patient with chronic eosinophilic pneumonia. b. Clearing of the chest x-ray film occurred after a short course of prednisone.

In patients with the classic clinical presentation of constitutional symptoms, peripheral infiltrates, and eosinophilia, a diagnostic trial of corticosteroids is all that is needed (Dines, 1978). Infectious diseases such as tuberculosis, histoplasmosis, coccidioidomycosis, and brucellosis, which can produce similar clinical pictures, should be excluded before therapy with corticosteroids is begun.

Corticosteroid therapy results in dramatic clinical, radiographic, and physiological improvement, usually within a few days. The chest radiograph clears within 1-2 weeks. The usual corticosteroid dosage is 20-40 mg of prednisone daily (Pearson and Rosenow, 1978). Relapses may occur, and in those cases pulmonary lesions are usually identical in size, shape, and location to those of the initial episode. The duration of steroid therapy should be individualized because some patients may need corticosteroids for a long period of time.

C. Acute Eosinophilic Pneumonia

Badesch and associates recently described a syndrome in a young man characterized by an acute febrile illness, severe respiratory insufficiency, and diffuse bilateral infiltrates on chest radiograph. There was no evidence of an infectious cause. Eosinophilic pneumonia was diagnosed by bronchoalveolar lavage and confirmed by transbronchial biopsy. The patient showed rapid improvement with corticosteroid therapy (Badesch et al., 1989). Although the cause of this acute eosinophilic pneumonia is unknown, a hypersensitivity reaction has been suggested as a possible mechanism.

Allen and associates studied four patients with acute eosinophilic pneumonia and described the clinical characteristics of the syndrome. The disease is distinct from other types of idiopathic eosinophilic lung disease in its acute presentation in previously healthy patients and in its failure to recur after cessation of corticosteroid therapy. Patients present with an acute febrile illness, severe hypoxemia, diffuse pulmonary infiltrates, increased number of eosinophils in bronchoalveolar lavage (BAL), and an absence of infection and previous atopic illness. The illness resolves rapidly after treatment with corticosteroids. There are no residual abnormalities on chest radiograph or pulmonary function tests several months after treatment, and BAL shows less than 1% eosinophils (Allen et al., 1989).

D. Allergic Granulomatosis and Angiitis (Churg-Strauss Syndrome)

Allergic granulomatosis and angiitis is a multisystem disease characterized by the presence of asthma, fever, eosinophilia, and vascular lesions similar to that seen in polyarteritis nodosa (Churg and Strauss, 1951). In 1957, Rose and Spencer reviewed a large number of cases of polyarteritis nodosa and separated out cases of allergic granulomatosis and angiitis previously classified in the same group (Rose and Spencer, 1957). The syndrome is characterized clinically by multisystem symptoms, asthma, and blood eosinophilia, and pathologically by a combination of necrotizing vasculitis and extravascular granulomas (Lanham et al., 1984). The cause of Churg-Strauss syndrome is unclear. Because it occurs only in allergic individuals it is thought to be due to an antigen-antibody reaction. IgG and IgE levels are increased in the serum in some cases. Immune complexes containing IgE were recently demonstrated in the sera but not in the blood vessel walls.

Although the disease occurs in patients between the ages of 20 and 40, it also affects children and the elderly. The male to female ratio is 1:1. Allergic granulomatosis is invariably preceded by asthma and allergic rhinitis or, rarely, by sensitization to a drug. A shorter duration between the onset of asthma and the onset of vasculitis is a bad prognostic sign (Chumbley et al., 1977). Fever is a common presenting symptom. Weight loss, malaise, and anemia may occur. Splenomegaly, hepatomegaly, and lymphadenopathy are not uncommon.

Pulmonary infiltrates appear in about two-thirds of the patients (Lanham et al., 1984). Chest radiographic findings are nonspecific and may show migratory pulmonary infiltrates resembling Loeffler's syndrome, bilateral nodular infiltrates that may rarely cavitate, or diffuse interstitial disease. Hilar lymphadenopathy is infrequent. Pleural effusions with pleural fluid eosinophilia occur in about one-third of the cases. Pleuritis without pleural effusion is occasionally seen.

The other organs involved include the cardiovascular system manifested by pericarditis, myocardial infarction, or congestive heart failure. Cardiac involvement is the most common cause of death (Lanham et al., 1984). Nervous system involvement is manifested by peripheral neuropathy, usually mononeuritis multiplex. The cranial nerves, such as the optic nerve, may also be involved. Development of coma, convulsions, and cerebrovascular accidents may occur.

Involvement of the skin is manifested by palpable purpura, urticaria, nodules, and ulcerations. Involvement of the gastrointestinal tract may cause gastric ulcers, bowel perforation, and gastric obstruction. Renal involvement is mild compared to that seen in polyarteritis nodosa and Wegener's granulomatosis; it is manifested by hematuria and proteinuria. Nephrotic syndrome, renal failure, and hypertension are uncommon. Patients can also develop hypertension. Arthralgias and myalgias, when present, are migratory. True arthritis is rare.

Laboratory examination shows leukocytosis with marked eosinophilia (20-80%). Anemia and high erythrocyte sedimentation rate are frequent, particularly during the vasculitic phase. IgG and IgE levels are likewise elevated during the vasculitic phase. Rheumatoid factor levels are moderately elevated in a number of patients. Hypocomplementemia and immune complexes in the serum are found occasionally.

On histological examination the hallmarks of the disease are necrotizing extravascular granulomas and vasculitis of the small arteries and veins. There is initially a tissue invasion by eosinophils, followed by necrosis of this exudate and the tissues, and finally the development of granulomas that may heal completely or leave a scar. The vasculitis is predominantly eosinophilic.

Prior to the introduction of corticosteroids, Churg-Strauss syndrome was invariably fatal. High-dosage steroid therapy (60-100 mg prednisone/day) in the acute phase may lead to clinical improvement. Pulse therapy with methylprednisone has been used in patients who are not responsive to prednisone (MacFadyen et al., 1987). A 5 year survival has been reported in 62% of patients treated with corticosteroids in one series (Chumbley et al., 1971). In a small percentage of patients in whom steroid therapy is ineffective, immunosuppression with cyclophosphamide or azathioprine has been used, usually with good results.

E. Polyarteritis Nodosa

Polyarteritis nodosa (PAN) is a systemic vasculitis that can also involve the lungs. It was originally considered to be associated with systemic angiitis, eosinophilic pneumonia, and granulomatous disease. In 1951, Churg and Strauss differentiated from PAN 14 patients with asthma, fever, disseminated vasculitis, and eosinophilia. This illness had a fulminating and often fatal course. Rose and Spencer reviewed 111 cases with PAN and separated out those with allergic granulomatosis and angiitis previously described in this group (Rose and Spencer, 1957).

PAN mainly affects young men. Clinical features include fever, malaise, weight loss, and skin lesions such as purpura, urticaria, nodules, or ulcerations. Patients may develop asthma, hypertension, hematuria, mononeuritis, or polyneuritis. Leukocytosis is present in about two-thirds of the cases but eosinophilia is rare. Erythrocyte sedimentation rate is high. Hepatitis B antigenemia has been reported in 30% of the patients. The primary lesion of polyarteritis nodosa is a neutrophilic cellular infiltrate that involves small and medium-sized arteries.

PAN is differentiated from Churg-Strauss syndrome by neutrophil, rather than eosinophil, predominance, lack of extravascular granulomas, involvement of medium-sized arteries in addition to smaller arteries, and lack of elevated levels of IgE. Also, asthma is less common in patients with PAN than in those with Churg-Strauss syndrome.

Untreated PAN is usually fatal. Use of corticosteroids and cyclophosphamide has been reported to prolong survival.

F. Eosinophilic Granuloma of the Lung

Eosinophilic granuloma is one of the three closely related disorders grouped under the term *Histiocytosis X*, the other disorders being Letterer-Siwe disease and Hand-Schüller-Christian disease (Lichtenstein, 1953). The latter two diseases are characterized by similar histiocytic infiltrations of multiple organs. They affect different age groups and often have poor prognosis. The new nomenclature for this group of disorders is "Langerhans' cell granulomatosis."

Letterer-Siwe disease almost invariably becomes evident before 2 years of age, and clinically presents with fever and weight loss, causing death within a few years.

Hand-Schüller-Christian disease, a slowly progressive illness, affects older infants and young adults. It is characterized by disseminated eosinophilic granulomatous nodules in the skin, bones, lymph nodes, and abdominal viscera.

Primary pulmonary histiocytosis X, or eosinophilic granuloma of the lung, is a disease of the third or fourth decade, but has been reported in patients at the extremes of age. It usually involves the lung or bones or both organs together without further dissemination. The incidence in males and females is about equal. It is uncommon in blacks and rare in Asians.

About 25% of patients are clinically asymptomatic, and the disease is discovered on routine chest radiograph. Common symptoms are nonproductive cough, dyspnea, and chest pain. Fever, wheezing, weight loss, and hemoptysis occur rarely. Ten to 20% of patients develop a pneumothorax either initially or during the course of the disease. Half of them develop recurrent or bilateral pneumothoraces. Diabetes insipidus occurs in 15% and eosinophilic granuloma of the bone in 20% of the patients. Almost all the patients are cigarette smokers.

Results of physical examination are usually unremarkable. Clubbing of digits is rare. Chest roentgenogram is abnormal in almost all patients with the disease. It shows interstitial lung disease involving the middle and upper zones with sparing of the costophrenic angles. The radiographic pattern may vary from micronodular or reticulonodular to cystic, with honeycombing. Occasionally, nodules greater than 1 cm, solid or cavitating, may be seen on the chest radiograph. Large cysts and bullae may cause hyperinflation.

Pulmonary function testing shows decreased compliance and DLCO in the early stages of the disease. In later stages, with cystic changes and bullae formation, evidence of airway obstruction appears.

On gross examination, the lungs show diffuse, irregular, grayish white or yellow nodules with occasional cavitations, less than 20 mm in diameter. Other findings include granulomatous polypoid lesions of the airways and pleural plaques. On microscopic examination the changes vary with the extent of the disease. The pathological findings of histiocytosis X can be classified into three phases:

Early Exudative Phase

The pulmonary pathological findings in this stage include filling of alveoli with histiocytes and other inflammatory cells.

Intermediate Phase

This is characterized by stellate granulomatous infiltrates consisting of histiocytes, eosinophils, and other inflammatory cells along the alveolar septae. Vascular and bronchial involvement by granuloma with resultant arteriolar and bronchiolar obliteration, respectively, may also occur. The diagnostic cell is the large histiocyte with an indented nucleus and eosinophilic cytoplasm. On electron microscopic examination, the histiocyte shows "x bodies" or "Birbeck granules" 40-45 nm wide. These "x bodies" are nonspecific and can be seen in many other tissues including Langerhans' cells of the skin, bronchoalveolar cell carcinomas, and hypersensitivity pneumonitis. These histiocytic cells are rare in the BAL of patients with other interstitial lung diseases but are found in large numbers in the BAL of patients with eosinophilic granuloma.

Advanced Fibrotic Stage

This stage presents no histological features to permit the diagnosis of histiocytosis.

The diagnosis of histocytosis X may be suggested by the presence of recurrent pneumothoraces and a typical x-ray picture. Transbronchial lung biopsy can be diagnostic. Diagnostic yield is probably less than 50%. BAL may show histiocytes with typical "x bodies"; they constitute 2-20% of the cells. The percentage of neutrophils and or lymphocytes is also increased. If no diagnosis can be made based on the above techniques, open lung biopsy is required.

Asymptomatic cases require no treatment. Most asymptomatic cases apparently occur and resolve without coming to the attention of the physician. Corticosteroids are the treatment of choice if symptoms such as dyspnea are present or there is evidence of progression of the disease. Although most patients respond to corticosteroid therapy, the disease can progress to cor pulmonale and respiratory failure in a small number of patients. A trial of vincristine, vinblastine, or cyclophosphamide should be considered in patients whose disease is unresponsive to corticosteroids. Bony lesions may respond to radiation therapy. Surgical pleurodesis may be helpful in patients with recurrent pneumothoraces. The overall prognosis in adults is very good, with the mortality rate being less than 5%.

G. Hypereosinophilic Syndrome

Hypereosinophilic syndrome is a multisystem disease characterized by persistent eosinophilia of more than 1500/mm^3 for at least 6 months and lack of evidence of infection, allergy, parasitic infestation, or hypersensitivity. Patients have bone marrow and blood eosinophilia and infiltration of multiple organs by mature eosinophils. The most commonly involved organs include the heart, central nervous system, muscles, and lungs. The disease can range from a benign condition consisting of hypereosinophilia, lung involvement, and angioedema to a fatal disease resembling eosinophilic leukemia.

The hypereosinophilic syndrome usually affects men in their third to sixth decades. The clinical features depend on the organ involved. Pulmonary involvement occurs in 40-50% of patients (Chused et al., 1975; Hardy and Anderson, 1968). Patients may show local or diffuse infiltrates as well as pleural effusion on chest radiography. The most common pulmonary symptom is paroxysmal nocturnal cough associated with sweating and scanty viscous sputum. A diagnosis of asthma is usually suspected, but no airflow obstruction is seen on pulmonary function testing. This could be due to the margination of large numbers of eosinophils into the pulmonary vasculature.

The cardiovascular system is the most commonly involved organ and restrictive cardiomyopathy and endocardial fibrosis are the most common causes of death. Central nervous system involvement is associated with chronic disability and poor prognosis.

Laboratory tests show an elevated leukocyte count, usually between 10,000 and 50,000/mm^3, with 30-70% eosinophils. About one-third of patients may have myeloblasts in the peripheral blood. Histological studies show infiltration of multiple organs with mature eosinophils.

The causes and pathogenesis of this syndrome are unknown. The diagnosis is made by the presence of persistent eosinophilia of more than 1500/mm^3 for at least 6 months; signs and symptoms of several involvement of organ systems; and lack of evidence of allergies, parasites, neoplastic, infections, autoimmune, or other causes of hypereosinophilia (Chused et al., 1975). Biopsies of the bone marrow and involved organ may be helpful in excluding neoplasm and confirming the diagnosis.

Corticosteroids are the mainstay of treatment. Patients whose disease is unresponsive to corticosteroids may benefit from treatment with hydroxyurea or vincristine (Parillo et al., 1978). Leukopheresis has been tried with successful results (Fauci, 1982).

H. Sarcoidosis

Sarcoidosis is a multisystem disease of unknown cause that most commonly affects young adults. The hallmark of this disease is noncaseating, epithelioid granulomatous involvement of more than one organ. The lungs are involved in about 80% of the patients. At the time of diagnosis, about 50% of the patients are asymptomatic and about 25% have pulmonary symptoms. The mean incidence of eosinophilia in sarcoidosis is about 24%, the range being from about 10% to as high as 7% (Sharma, 1984).

References

Akiyama, K., Takizawa, H., Suzuki, M., Miyachi, S., et al. (1987). Allergic bronchopulmonary aspergillosis due to *Aspergillus oryzae*. *Chest* **91**: 285-286.

Allen, J. A., Pacht, E. R., Gadek, J. E., and Bruce Davis, W. (1989). Acute eosinophilic pneumonia as a reversible cause of noninfectious respiratory failure. *N. Engl. J. Med.* **321**:569-574.

Archer, G. T., and Hirsch, J. G. (1981). Isolation of granules from eosinophil leucocytes and study of their enzyme content. *J. Exp. Med.* **304**: 154-156.

Badesch, D. B., King, T. E., Jr., and Schwarz, M. I. (1989). Acute eosinophilic pneumonia: a hypersensitivity phenomenon? *Am. Rev. Respir. Dis.* **139**:249-252.

Bass, D. A., Grover, W. H., Lewis, J. C., et al. (1980). Comparison of human eosinophils from normals and patients with eosinophilia. *J. Clin. Invest.* **66**:1255-1273.

Benatar, S. R., Allan, B., Hewitson, R. P., and Don, P. A. (1980). Allergic bronchopulmonary stemphyliosis. *Thorax* **35**:515-518.

Best, W. R., Kark, R. M., Muehreke, R. C., and Samter, M. (1953). Clinical value of eosinophil counts and eosinophil response tests. *J.A.M.A.* **151**: 702-706.

Boornazian, J. S., and Fagan, J. M. (1985). Tropical pulmonary eosinophilia associated with pleural effusions. *Am. J. Trop. Med. Hyg.* **34**(3):473-475.

Brooker, A., and Sharma, O. P. (1982). Bronchocentric granulomatosis and adult respiratory distress syndrome. *Br. J. Dis. Chest* **76**:189-193.

Butterworth, A. E., and David, J. R. (1981). Eosinophil function. *N. Engl. J. Med.* **304**:154-156.

Carrington, C. D., Addington, W. W., Goff, M. A., et al. (1969). Chronic eosinophilic pneumonia. *N. Engl. J. Med.* **280**:787-798.

Chumbley, L. C., Harrison, E. G., Jr., and DeRemee, R. A. (1971). Allergic granulomatosis and angiitis (Churg-Strauss syndrome). *Mayo Clin. Proc.* **52**:477-484.

Chumbley, L. C., Harrison, E. G., Jr., and De Remee, R. A. (1977). Allergic granulomatosis and angiitis. Report and analysis of 30 cases. *Mayo Clin. Proc.* **52**:477-484.

Churg, J., and Strauss, L. (1951). Allergic granulomatosis, allergic angiitis and periarteritis nodosa. *Am. J. Pathol.* **27**:277-301.

Chusid, M. J., Dale, D. C., West, B. C., and Wolff, S. M. (1975). The hypereosinophilic syndrome: analysis of fourteen cases with review of the literature. *Medicine* (*Baltimore*) **54**:1-27.

Crofton, J. W., Livingston, J. L., Oswald, N. C., and Roberts, A. T. U. (1952). Pulmonary eosinophilia. *Thorax* **7**:1-35.

Dickson, E. C., and Gilford, M. A. (1938). Coccidioidomycosis: the primary type of infection. *Arch. Intern. Med.* **62**:853-871.

Dines, D. E. (1978). Chronic eosinophilic pneumonia: a roentgenographic diagnosis (editorial). *Mayo Clin. Proc.* **53**:129-130.

Drutz, D. J., and Catanzaro, A. (1978). Coccidioidomycosis: part 2. *Am. Rev. Respir. Dis.* **118**:727-771.

Elsom, K. A., and Ingelfinger, F. J. (1942). Eosinophilia and pneumonitis in chronic brucellosis: a report of two cases. *Ann. Intern. Med.* **16**:995-1002.

Enokihara, H., Hamaguchi, H., Sakamaki, H., Hazama, S., et al. (1985). Specific production of eosinophil colony stimulating factor from sensitized T cells from a patient with allergic eosinophilia. *Br. J. Haematol.* **59**:85-91.

Fauci, A. (1982). The idiopathic hypereosinophilic syndrome. *Ann. Intern. Med.* **97**:78-92.

Fiese, M. (1958). *Coccidioidomycosis.* Charles C. Thomas, Springfield, IL.

Frigas, E., Loegering, D. A., Solly, G. O., Farrow, G. M., and Gleich, G. J. (1981). Elevated levels of the eosinophil granule major basic protein in the sputum of patients with bronchial asthma. *Mayo Clin. Proc.* **56**:345-353.

Frimodt-Moller, C., and Barton, R. M. (1940). A pseudo-tuberculosis condition associated with eosinophilia. *Indian Med. Gaz.* **75**:607-613.

Gaensler, E. A., and Carrington, C. D. (1977). Peripheral opacities in chronic eosinophilic pneumonia: the photographic negative of pulmonary edema. *Am. J. Roentgenol.* **128**:1-13.

Gleich, G. J., and Loegering, D. A. (1982). Immunobiology of esosinophils. *Annu. Rev. Immunol.* **2**:429-259.

Gleich, G. J., Loegering, D. A., Kueppers, F., et al. (1974). Physiochemical and biological properties of the major basic protein from guinea pig eosinophil granules. *J. Exp. Med.* **140**:113-332.

Gleich, G. J., Loegering, D. A., and Adolphson, C. R. (1985). Eosinophils and bronchial inflammation. *Chest* **87** (Jan suppl.):105-135.

Gonzales, E. B., Swedo, J. L., Rajaraman, S., Daniels, J. C., and Grant, J. A. (1986). Ultrastructural and immunohistochemical evidence for release of eosinophil granules in vivo: cytotoxic potential in chronic eosinophilic pneumonia. *J. Allergy Clin. Immunol.* **79**:755-762.

Grantham, J. G., Meadows, J. A., and Gleich, G. J. (1986). Chronic eosinophilic pneumonia; evidence for eosinophilic degranulation and release of major basic protein. *Am. J. Med.* **80**:89-94.

Gray, J. (1982). Loffler's syndrome following ingestion of a coin. *Can. Med. Assoc. J.* **127**:999-1000.

Halwig, J. M., Greenberger, P. A., and Patterson, R. (1984). Allergic bronchopulmonary aspergillosis. *Immunol. Allergy Pract.* **8**:292-301.

Hardy, W. R., and Anderson, R. E. (1968). The hypereosinophilic syndromes. *Ann. Intern. Med.* **68**:1220-1229.

Henderson, W. R., Harley, J. B., and Fauci, A. S. (1984). Arachidonic acid metabolism in normal and hypereosinophilia syndrome human eosinophils: generation of leukotrienes B4, C4 and 15-lipooxygenase pathway products. *Immunology* **51**:679-686.

Hendrick, D. J., Ellithorpe, D. B., Lyon, F., et al. (1982). Allergic bronchopulmonary helminthosporosis. *Am. Rev. Respir. Dis.* **126**:935-938.

Hinson, K. F. W., Moon, A. J., and Plummer, N. S. (1952). Bronchopulmonary aspergillosis: a review and report of eight cases. *Thorax* **7**:317-333.

Hirsch, J. G., and Hirsch, B. I. (1980). Paul Ehrlich and the discovery of the eosinophil. In *The Eosinophil in Health and Disease.* Edited by A. A. F. Mahmoud and K. F. Austen. Grune and Stratton, New York, p. 3.

Jain, V. K., and Beniwal, O. P. (1984). Unusual presentation of tropical pulmonary eosinophilia. *Thorax* **39**:634-635.

Joshi, V. V., Udwadia, F. E., and Gadgil, R. K. (1969). Etiology of tropical eosinophilia: a study of lung biopsies and review of published reports. *Am. J. Trop. Med. Hyg.* **18**:231-240.

Katzenstein, A., Liebow, A. A., and Friedman, P. J. (1975). Bronchocentric granulomatosis, mucoid impaction, and hypersensitivity reactions to fungi. *Am. Rev. Respir. Dis.* **111**:497-537.

Lal, C., and Sharma, O. P. (1989). Everything that wheezes is not asthma. A tale of an Indian businessman. *Chest* **96**:1418-1419.

Lanham, J. G., Elkon, K. B., Pusey, C. D., and Hughes, G. R. (1984). Systemic vasculitis with asthma and eosinophilia: a clinical approach to the Churg-Strauss syndrome. *Medicine* **63**:65-81.

Lichtenstein, L. (1953). Histiocytosis X: integration of eosinophilic granuloma of the bone, "Letterer-Siwe disease," and Schuller-Christian disease" as related manifestations of a single nosologic entity. *Arch. Pathol.* **56**:84.

Liebow, A. A. (1973). Pulmonary angiitis and granulomatosis. *Am. Rev. Respir. Dis.* **108**:1-18.

Loffler, W. (1932). Zur differential-diagnose der lungeninfiltrierungen: II. Uber fluchtige succedan-infiltrate (mit eosinophile). *Beitr. Klin. Tuberk.* **79**:368-382.

Lombard, C. M., Tazelaar, H. D., and Krasne, D. L. (1987). Pulmonary eosinophilia in coccidioidal infections. *Chest* **91**:734-736.

Lonky, S. A., Catanzaro, A., Moser, K. M., and Einstein, A. (1976). Acute coccidioidal pleural effusion. *Am. Rev. Respir. Dis.* **114**:681-688.

MacFadyen, R., Tron, V., Kashmiri, M., and Road, J. D. (1987). Allergic angiitis of Churg and Strauss syndrome: response to pulse methylprednisolone. *Chest* **91**:629-631.

McAleer, R., Kroenert, D. B., Elder, J. L., and Froudist, J. H. (1981). Allergic bronchopulmonary disease caused by *Curvularia lunata* and *Drechslera hawaiiensis. Thorax* **36**:338-344.

McCarthy, D. S., and Pepys, J. (1973). Cryptogenic pulmonary eosinophilia. *Clin. Allergy* **3**:339-351.

McCarthy, D. S., Simon, G., and Hargreave, D. F. D. (1970). The radiological appearances in allergic bronchopulmonary aspergillosis. *Clin. Radiol.* **21**:366-375.

Muller, G. L. (1943). *Clinical Significance of the Blood in Tuberculosis.* Commonwealth Fund, New York, pp. 95-121.

Nasarajah, M. S. (1972). Pulmonary function in tropical eosinophilia. *Thorax* **27**:185-187.

Nath, J., and Jain, V. K. (1978). Atypical presentation of pulmonary eosinophilia. *Indian J. Chest Dis. Allied Sci.* **20**:141-144.

Neva, F. A., and Ottesen, E. A. (1978). Tropical (filarial) eosinophilia. *N. Engl. J. Med.* **298**:1129-1131.

Oathak, C. L., and Kahali, R. S. (1957). Cyclic variations in the eosinophil count during the phases of the menstrual cycle. *J. Clin. Endocrinol. Metab.* **17**:862-869.

Parillo, J. E., Fauci, A. S., and Wolff, S. M. (1978). Therapy of the hypereosinophilic syndrome. *Ann. Intern. Med.* **89**:162-172.

Parwaresch, M. R., Walle, A. J., and Arndt, D. (1976). The peripheral kinetics of human radiolabelled eosinophils. *Virchows Arch.* (*Cell. Pathol.*) **21**:57-66.

Patterson, R., Greenberger, P. A., Radin, R. C., and Roberts, M. (1982). Allergic bronchopulmonary aspergillosis: staging as an aid to management. *Ann. Intern. Med.* **96**:286-291.

Pearson, D. J., and Rosenow, E. C. III (1978). Chronic eosinophilic pneumonia (Carrington's): a follow-up study. *Mayo Clin. Proc.* **53**:73-78.

Ravindran, M. (1979). Tropical eosinophilia presenting with neurological features. *Br. Med. J.* **2**:1262.

Reeder, W. H., and Goodrich, B. E. (1952). Pulmonary infiltrate with eosinophilia (PIE syndrome). *Ann. Intern. Med.* **36**:1217-1240.

Ringoen, A. R. (1938). Eosinophil leukocytes and eosinophilia. In *Handbook of Hematology*, vol. 1. Edited by H. Downey. London, Hamish Hamilton Medical Books, p. 181.

Rose, G. A., and Spencer, H. (1957). Polyarteritis nodosa. *Q. J. Med.* **26**: 43-81.

Rosenberg, M., Patterson, R., Mintzer, R., Cooper, B. J., et al. (1977). Clinical and immunologic criteria for the diagnosis of allergic bronchopulmonary aspergillosis. *Ann. Intern. Med.* **86**:405-414.

Rosenow, E. C. III (1972). The spectrum of drug-induced pulmonary disease. *Ann. Intern. Med.* **77**:977-991.

Ross, R., and Klebanoff, S. J. (1966). The eosinophil leukocyte. Fine structure studies of changes in the uterus during the estrous cycle. *J. Exp. Med.* **124**:653-659.

Rud, F. (1947). The eosinophil count in health and in mental disease: a biometrical study. *Acta Psychiatr. Neurol.* **22** (Suppl. 40):1-433.

Rytomma, T. (1960). Organ distribution and histochemical properties of eosinophil granulocytes in the rat. *Acta Pathol. Microbiol. Scand.* **50**: (Suppl 140):1-118.

Safirstein, B. H., D'Souza, M. F., Simon, G., Tai, E. H. C., and Pepys, J. (1973). Five-year follow-up of allergic bronchopulmonary aspergillosis. *Am. Rev. Respir. Dis.* **108**:450-459.

Schwarz, E. (1914). Die Lehre von der allgemeinen und ortlichen eosinophilie. *Ergeb. Allg. Pathol. Anat.* **7**:137-787.

Shale, D. J., Faux, J. A., and Lane, D. J. (1987). Trial of ketoconazole in non-invasive pulmonary aspergillosis. *Thorax* **42**:26-31.

Sharma, O. P. (1984). *Sarcoidosis: Clinical Management.* Butterworth, London and Boston, 1984.

Singh, M. M., Sharma, S. K., and Patney, R. I. M. (1974). Tropical eosinophilic pericarditis. *Indian Heart J.* **26**:261-263.

Slavin, R. G. (1985). Allergic bronchopulmonary aspergillosis. *Clin. Rev. Allergy* **3**:167-182.

Sovijarvi, A. R. A., Lemola, M., Stenius, B., and Idanpaan-Hekkila, J. (1977). Nitrofurantoin-induced acute, subacute, and chronic pulmonary reactions. *Scand. J. Respir. Dis.* **58**:41-50.

Speirs, R. S., and Osada, Y. (1962). Chemotactic activity and phagocytosis of eosinophils. *Proc. Soc. Exp. Biol. Med.* **109**:929-932.

Spry, C. J. F. (1985). New properties and roles for eosinophils in disease. *J. R. Soc. Med.* **78**:844-847.

Spry, C. J. F., and Kumaraswamy, V. (1982). Tropical eosinophilia. *Semin. Haematol.* **19**:107-115.

Sun, X. H., Davis, W. B., Fukuda, Y., et al. (1985). Experimental polymyxin-B induced interstitial lung disease characterized by an accumulation of cytotoxic eosinophils in the alveolar structures. *Am. Rev. Respir. Dis.* **131**:103-108.

Sunderman, F. W., and Sunderman, F. W., Jr. (1961). Loffler's syndrome associated with nickel sensitivity. *Arch. Intern. Med.* **107**:405-408.

Udwadia, F. E. (1975). *Pulmonary Eosinophilia: Progress in Respiratory Research*, Vol. 7. S. Karger, Basel, pp. 35-155.

Vadas, M. A. (1982). Genetic control of eosinophilia in mice: genes expressed in bone marrow-derived cells control high responsiveness. *J. Immunol.* **128**:691-695.

Wilett, F. M., and Oppenheim, E. (1946). Pulmonary infiltrations with associated eosinophilia. *Am. J. Med. Sci.* **212**:608-612.

Wilett, F. M., and Weiss, A. (1945). Coccidioidomycosis in southern California: report of a new endemic area with a review of 100 cases. *Ann. Intern. Med.* **23**:349-375.

Wright, J. L., Pare, P. D., Hammond, M., and Donevan, R. E. (1983). Eosinophilic pneumonia and atypical mycobacterial infection. *Am. Rev. Respir. Dis.* **127**:497-499.

8

Pleuropulmonary Amebiasis

KAMLESH PANDYA and OM P. SHARMA

Los Angeles County-University of Southern California Medical Center
Los Angeles, California

Amebiasis is an infection caused by the protozoan *Entamoeba histolytica.* The disease has a variable picture and may cause acute or chronic symptoms. At one extreme it may remain an asymptomatic infestation, whereas at the other it can blossom into a multisystem disorder involving liver, thorax, brain, and almost any other tissue systems. Frequently the major presenting symptoms are pulmonary in nature; diarrhea is absent or mild. Delay in diagnosis remains a major factor in the severity of the illness, so familiarity with the pleuropulmonary complications of amebiasis is very important.

I. History

Entamoeba was first described in 1875 by Losch of St. Petersburg, Leningrad, Russia (Fig. 1). He named the organism *Amoeba coli* (Losch, 1875; translated from original, 1975). During the following years, Kartulis (in Egypt, 1886), Koch and Gaffky (in Egypt, 1887), and Halva (in Prague, 1887) linked ameba to dysentery and liver abscess. In the United States, Osler was the first to report in 1890 the association of amebic dysentery and liver abscess. Simon (1890) described a patient in whom the liver abscess had ruptured

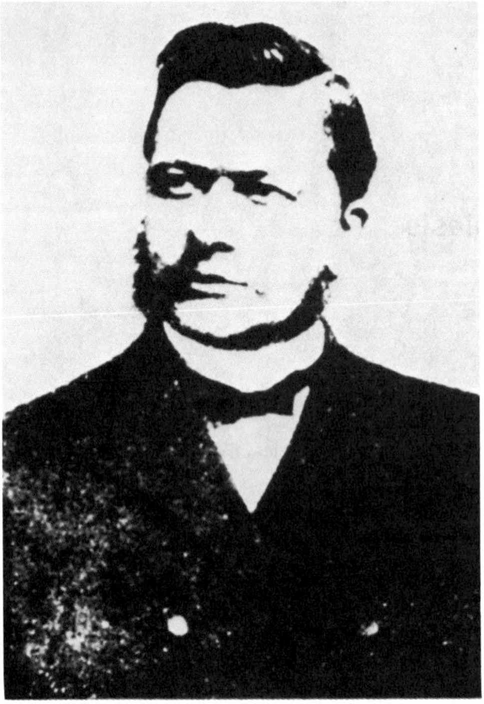

Figure 1 Fedor Aleksandrovich Lesh (Losch): 1840-1903.

into the lung; *Amoeba coli* were observed in the sputum. Schaudinn in 1903 first named the species *Entamoeba histolytica* (tissue-destroying) and differentiated it from *Entamoeba coli*. The cyst stage was discovered by Quincke and Ross in 1893. Further studies revealed that the cyst was the infective stage, and that not all persons infected with *E. histolytica* became ill.

Losch treated his patients who had amebiasis with quinine enemas. In the early 19th century, Indian physicians used ipecacuanha for the treatment of dysentery. Later, the active ingredient of ipecacuanha was found to be emetine. In 1912, Rogers, in Calcutta, first treated amebic dysentery and liver abscess with emetine injections. Subsequently, chloroquine (Conan, 1948), dihydroemetine (Brossi et al., 1959), and metronidazole (Powell et al., 1966) were introduced.

II. Parasitological Characteristics

Entamoeba histolytica, a protozoan, is a parasite that moves by producing pseudopods. The organism has a life cycle with three distinct stages: trophozite, precyst, and cyst. The cyst is the infective stage, which remains viable in water up to 4 weeks. If ingested, usually from fecally contaminated food, water, and fingers, it passes through the stomach. Excystation occurs in the lower small bowel. Four trophozoites are formed from a cyst. Trophozoites multiply and move along the intestinal canal until conditions favorable for colonization are found; commonly in the large bowel, particularly the cecal area. Once in the colon, *E. histolytica* can remain either a commensal or become a pathogen. In the presence of diarrhea, the parasite does not become encysted. However, if bowel evacuation is not rapid, the trophozites that travel toward the rectum discharge food vacuoles and other cytoplasmic inclusions and become precysts. The precyst then acquires a wall and develops into a mature quandrinucleate cyst. Both precyst and cyst are infective. *E. histolytica* is the only species of genus *Entameba* that produces disease in humans. Thus, it is important to differentiate *E. histolytica* from other ameba in this genus, which include *E. coli*, *E. hartmani, E. polecki,* and *E. gingivalis.*

Host-parasite interactions that determine invasiveness are not completely known, but include the protozoal strain and its virulence, bacterial flora of the intestine, and host immunity, both humoral and cell-mediated. In some countries including France, Guatemala, Iraq, Great Britain, South Africa, and India, *E. histolytica* tends to be aggressive and preferentially involves the chest (Herrera-Llerandi, 1966). Alcoholism and malnutrition, although without any definite evidence, have frequently been blamed as host factors that promote invasive amebiasis. Use of immunosuppressive drugs in experimental animals promotes the development of amebic liver abscess (Biagi et al., 1963). Clinical observations in humans suggest that these drugs may also stimulate invasiveness. In nonendemic regions, where amebic dysentery is often diagnosed as ulcerative colitis, the immunosuppression associated with administration of corticosteroids has resulted in disseminated disease. Fulminant amebiasis during pregnancy or the immediate postpartum period has been described (Lewis and Antia, 1969).

III. Immunological Aspects

The human immune mechanisms that develop with amebic infection are not completely understood. Both humoral and cell-mediated immune responses are induced by *E. histolytica* (Salata and Ravdin, 1988).

A. Humoral Immunity

Antibody

The complex humoral response to amebic infection results primary in IgG antibody production; however IgM antibody may also appear. Several studies have demonstrated the development of IgA antibody in intestinal amebiasis; however, it persists only a short time. Antigenic determinants capable of eliciting an antibody response occur in subcellular fractions of trophozoites containing ribsosomal, lysosomal, and soluble cytoplasmic matter, as well in material derived from the trophozoite surface. Antibody titers usually begin to rise 1 week after inoculation and reach the maximum in about 2 weeks. In general, the growth of the amebic abscess parallels antibody production; animals with larger abscesses have the highest antibody titers (Ghadirian and Meerovitch, 1978a,b; Norman et al., 1979; Gold et al., 1978). Antibody titer does not correlate with the clinical outcome (Trissl, 1982; Krupp and Powell, 1971). Since antibody titers rise with the severity of the disease, the humoral response does not seem to be protective. In vitro studies have show that amebic tropozoites repeatedly aggregate, ingest, or shed, attached human antibodies to the ameba (Aust-Kettis and Sundqvist, 1978; Calderon et al., 1980). One or mroe of these mechanisms may be used by the parasite to escape human humoral host defenses and cause invasive disease. At present, the presence of serum antibodies serves more as a marker for invasive disease (Sargeaunt et al., 1978; Shetty et al., 1988).

Immune Complexes

The role of circulating immune complexes in invasive disease is not known. Despite the demonstration of serum immune complexes, manifestations of immune complex-related disease have generally been absent. In amebiasis, local immune complex formation may relate to the pathogenesis of invasive disease (Ravi et al., 1975; Mahajan and Ganguly, 1980).

Complement

Many studies have shown that the complement system plays an important role in the defense against invasive amebiasis. Ameba in the presence of serum can activate complement by the alternative pathway, resulting in lysis of the ameba by terminal complement components C5-C0 (Huldt et al., 1979; Ortiz et al., 1978). Capin demonstrated that hamsters depleted of complement with cobra venom developed extensive hepatic lesions (Capin et al., 1980). Calderon and Schreiber (1985) investigated the contribution of classic and alternative pathway in complement activation by ameba. They showed that both pathways were activated by *E. histolytica*; the contribution from the classic pathway was greater. However, it is not known how ameba survive in tissues in the presence of complement-induced lysis. Perhaps the continuous turnover of parasite cell membrane components, accompanied by changes in distribution of complement receptors, influence their survival in the host. Reed et al. (1983) observed that pathogenic strains of *E. histolytica* were resistant to human complement, while nonpathogenic strains were susceptible.

B. Cell-Mediated Immunity

Animal studies reveal that cell-mediated immunity plays an important role in protecting the body against ameba. In hamsters, T-cell depletion by thymectomy or pretreatment with antithymocyte serum results in the production of larger amebic liver abscess and widespread lesions (Ghadirian and Meerovitch, 1981a,b). Depleting the experimental animals of macrophages either by injecting silica particles (Ghadirian and Meerovitch, 1982; Stern et al., 1984) or antimacrophage serum (Ghadirian et al., 1983) produces similar results. Chemically induced immunosupression or pretreatment with antilymphocyte serum results in the formation of hepatic lesion in mice (Wijesundera, 1980). Immunosuppressed guinea pigs, when inoculated with ameba cecally, develop deep penetrating cecal ulcers and metastasis abscess in the liver (Vinayak et al., 1982). In rats, administration of corticosteroids or irradiation induces deep amebic ulcers in the cecum (Vinayak et al., 1979). Protection against invasive amebiasis has been demonstrated with bacillus calmette-Gúerin (BCG) vaccination, or prior infection with *Trichinella spiralis* (Ghadirian et al., 1980; Krupp and Powell, 1971).

In human patients, cell-mediated immune responses develop during invasive amebiasis (Ortiz-Ortiz et al., 1975; Savant et al., 1973). In patients treated for amebic liver abscess, Salata et al. (1986) have characterized T-lymphocyte phenotypes and their response to mitogens and amebic antigens. They also studied gamma interferon generation in supernatants of immune lymphocytes stimulated with amebic antigen, and the ability of amebic antigen-elicited lymphokine to activate macrophage in vitro and kill virulent amebic trophozoites (Salata and Ravdin, 1986). Cell-mediated immune mechanisms against *Entamoeba histolytica* have been well reviewed recently (Salata and Ravdin, 1988).

IV. Incidence

E. histolytica has a worldwide distribution. About one-tenth of the worlds population is infected with *E. histolytica*. Every year 35-50 million cases of symptomatic amebiasis are reported. Amebiasis is responsible for 40,000-100,000 deaths annually (Walsh, 1984). The disease is endemic in Mexico, the western portion of South America, South Africa, Egypt, parts of the Middle East, India, and Southeast Asia. It is prevalent in tropical areas, where invasive disease is more frequent and severe. As much as 50% of the prevalence has been reported from developing countries (Walsh, 1986). Poor sanitation and lack of hygiene are responsible for this prevalence. Transmission is mainly by the fecal-oral route.

In the United States, the prevalence of amebiasis is less than 5%. Antiamebic antibodies were found in 2% of 6,195 random specimens, 4% of healthy U.S. military recruits, and 1% of 3,033 general hospital patients (Cuyadrado and Kagan, 1967; Melvin and Mata, 1971; Chacon Zamora et al., 1978). It is estimated that more than 100,000 cases of clinical amebiasis occur annually in the United States (Walsh, 1986). The incidence is higher in institutionalized individuals, people living in slum areas, immigrants from endemic areas, and homosexuals. In latter group, the prevalence rates have ranged from 20 to 36% (Healy, 1986). An interesting finding is that in homosexuals the infection is caused by organisms of low virulence and invasive disease is uncommon (Sargeaunt et al., 1983; Ortega et al., 1984). A minor epidemic was reported from Colorado, where the spread of disease was related to use of an enema in a chiropractic clinic (Istre et al., 1982).

V. Pleuropulmonary Complications

The incidence of pleuropulmonary complications of amebiasis varies considerably (Table 1). In 1935, Oschner and DeBakey reported an incidence of 13.5% in their 59 cases of amebic liver abscess. An incidence of 15.7% was found in another series of 95 patients with amebic liver abscess (Oschner and DeBakey, 1936). Radke (1951) found only one patient with pulmonary disease in 101 cases of amebiasis. Webster observed an incidence of 6.3% among 95 patients with intestinal amebiasis reported in 1956 and 4.02% among 249 patients reported in 1959. In the latter series, 9 of 48 patients with amebic liver abscess had pleuropulmonary complication. Shaw (1949) estimated that 15% of his patients with amebic liver abscess had thoracic involvement. Twenty percent of DeBakey and Oschner's (1951) patients with amebic liver abscess had intrathoracic extension. In an analysis of 2074 cases of amebic abscess, Adams was able to separate out 146 cases with rupture into the chest (Adams and MacLeod, 1977). In one study of fatal amebiasis, 41 of 90 cases with amebic liver abscess had rupture; in 22 disease extended into the lung (Kean et al., 1956).

It appears that pleuropulmonary complications occur more frequently in developing countries. Nwafo and Egbue (1981) reported that 38 (86%) of 44 patients with amebic liver abscess had thoracic involvement; however, they included 14 patients with isolated smooth elevation of right hemidiaphragm and 10 patients with serous pleural effusion. Adeyemo and Aderounmu (1984) reported 22 (67%) out of 33 patients with amebic liver abscess who

Table 1 Incidence of Pleuropulmonary Complications

Author	Number of Patients with			Incidence of Pleuropulmonary Complications
	Amebiasis	ALA	PPA	
Oschner, 1935	388	59	7	11.9% of ALA 1.8% of amebiasis
Oschner and DeBakey, 1936		95	15	15.7% of ALA
DeBakey and Oschner, 1951		176	35	19.9% of ALA
Radke, 1951	101		1	0.99% of amebiasis
Kean et al., 1956		90	22	24.4% of ALA
Webster, 1956	95	24	6 (5 of these pt. had ALA)	20.8% of ALA 6.3% of amebiasis
Webster, 1960	249	48	10 (9 of these pt. had ALA)	18.8% of ALA 4.02% of amebiasis
Adams and MacLeod, 1977		2074	146	7.03% of ALA
Verghese et al., 1979	1534	686	23	3.35% of ALA
Nwafo and Egbue, 1981		44	38	86% of ALA
Adeyemo and Aderounmu, 1984		33	22	66.7% of ALA

ALA, amebic liver abscess; PPA, pleuropulmonary amebiasis.

had pleuropulmonary involvement. They also included in their series seven patients with elevated diaphragms only and five patients with serous pleural effusion. Verghese and colleagues (1979), after having excluded patients with serous pleural effusion, found that pleuropulmonary complications occurred in only 23 (3.35%) of 686 patients with amebic liver abscess.

Pleuropulmonary amebiasis, like amebic liver abscess, occurs predominantly in men. The reported male/female ratio varies from 9:1 to 15:1 (Bookless, 1950; Oschner and DeBakey, 1936). No age is exempt, but the disease commonly affects people between the ages of 20 and 50 years (Daniels and Childress, 1956; Kubitschek et al., 1985).

VI. Pathogenesis

Pulmonary involvement is almost always secondary to intestinal infection, although a few isolated case reports suggest that the organism might have been inhaled before producing bronchial and pulmonary changes (Mathew and Avantachari, 1964; Minetto and Prinotti, 1965).

From the intestines, amebae reach the lung in one of the following ways:

Trophozoites invade the portal circulation and travel to the liver via the portal vein. Hepatic abscesses may form by lytic activity of the parasites. Progression of the abscess may incorporate the diaphragm and pleuropulmonary complications may then occur by direct extension. As the hepatic abscess enlarges upwards, adhesions are formed between the surface of liver and the diaphragm and, later, the diaphragm and the base of the lung. Thus, the involvement of the pleura or the lung depends upon the extent to which the subdiaphragmatic and pleural spaces have been obliterated by adhesions. A perforation in the pleural space leads to an amebic empyema, in which a rupture into the lung may produce an abscess, a consolidation, or a hepatobronchial fistula. Most pleuropulmonary complications are due to direct extension of amebic liver abscess. Hepatic abscesses may also induce inflammatory changes in the adjacent areas without causing definite parasitic invasion or perforation (Rhode et al., 1979).

Hematogeneous dissemination occasionally occurs that takes place either through the portal system and hepatic veins or through the inferior hemorrhoidal veins and inferior vena cava.

In rare cases, the route is via the lymphatic stream locally (thence to the inferior vena cava) or through the thoracic duct and then to the superior vena cava, producing lung lesions.

Ochsner and DeBakey first classified pleuropulmonary amebiasis into hematogenous pulmonary abscess without liver involvement (14.3%), hematogenous pulmonary abscess and an independent liver abscess (10.4%), pulmonary abscess extending directly from a liver abscess (37.2%), bronchohepatic fistula with little pulmonary involvement (19.6%), and empyema extending from a liver abscess (17.6%). There are four main types of pleuropulmonary involvement: serous effusion with or without atelectasis, consolidation or lung abscess, empyema, and hepatobronchial fistula.

VII. Clinical Features

Because pleuropulmonary amebiasis is secondary to amebic liver abscess, it behooves us to know clinical features of amebic liver abscess. The liver abscess may appear acutely or, more commonly, follow an insidious course.

Patients complain of malaise, fever, night sweats, abdominal discomfort, anorexia, and/or pain in the right hypochondrium. Infrequently, an abrupt onset may produce a clinical picture of acute abdomen. Sometimes patients experience ill health and weight loss for many months; in a small number of patients, fever may be the first and only manifestation (DeCock and Reynolds, 1987).

Chest symptoms are present in approximately one-quarter of the patients with amebic liver abscess. Pulmonary symptoms occasionally dominate the clinical presentation. Chest symptoms depend upon the type and extent of pleuropulmonary involvement. Inflammation of pleura may cause pleura chest pain, right shoulder pain, hiccups, or nonproductive cough. Sudden rupture of a liver abscess into the chest may produce tearing sensation in the chest, which sometimes may be followed by dyspnea, cough, or even collapse. Patients with a hepatobronchial fistula usually cough up "anchovy paste," chocolate-colored, or creamy contents of amebic liver abscess.

The liver is tender and enlarged in 9 of every 10 patients. The point of maximum tenderness can often be detected, either in the intercostal space or over the enlarged liver. The dullness to percussion with diminished air entry at the right base is usually due to a raised diaphragm or accumulation of pleural fluid. Percussion may demonstrate a fixed raised diaphragm. A large abscess may produce visible bulging in the right intercostal space or hypochondrium. Diarrhea occurs in less than 20% of the patients.

VIII. Laboratory Abnormalities

A. Routine Blood Tests

Normochromic anemia is common. Leukocytosis occur in about three-quarters of patients; bands may be seen. Eosinophilia is rare. Although the alkaline phosphatase, serum glutamic oxaloacetic and serum glutamic pyruvic transaminase levels are often elevated, the normal value of these tests by no means excludes diagnosis of liver or pulmonary amebiasis. Bilirubin levels are usually normal. Hypoalbuminimia is present in more than half of the patients.

B. Serological Testing

More than 90% of patients with pleuropulmonary amebiasis or amebic liver abscess have positive antiamebic antibody titers. Occasionally the antibody test is negative in the very early course of the disease, but it almost always become positive if repeated after 1-2 weeks. A positive serological result, however, does not differentiate between active tissue invasion and previous infection. Serological tests may be positive for 2 years or more after effective treatment.

Available serological tests include complement fixation, immunodiffusion, indirect fluorescent antibody (IFA), indirect hemagglutination (IHA), counterimmunoelectrophoresis (CIE), and enzyme-linked immunosorbent assay (ELISA). The IHA test is highly sensitive and easily available. A serological titer of 1:512 is suggestive, but not diagnostic, of invasive disease. A latex agglutination slide test, which is also commercially available, is useful for quick and easy screening.

IX. Roentgenographic Examination

The roentgenographic features of pleuropulmonary amebiasis are not specific for the disease. However, the combination of roentgenographic features, history, and physical examination may suggest the diagnosis of pleuropulmonary amebiasis. The abnormalities are usually limited to the right side of the chest.

A. Chest Roentgenogram

Elevation of the right hemidiaphragm is among the common findings. This abnormality occurs in about 50% of patients with amebic liver abscess, but the reported incidence varies between 30 and 86% (Nanda and Hoon, 1976; Nwafo and Egbue, 1981). The lateral chest radiograph may show a diaphragmatic hump situated anteriorly, posteriorly, or in the middle of the diaphragm. The anterior locations are common.

A triangular area of consolidation with its base against the diaphragm and the apex pointing upwards toward the hilum may be present. Cavitation may occur in the consolidated area.

A hazy crescentic shadow, less dense than the liver, may be seen above the right dome of the diaphragm.

Pleural effusion can be small, moderate, or massive. Small effusions might be seen only on lateral or lateral decubitus films. Occasionally, they produce only a minor blunting of the right costophrenic angle (Fig. 2). If a hepatobronchial fistula is formed, an air-containing cavity may be present under the diaphragm.

Occasionally, a pulmonary abscess may be seen distant from the liver. This may occur in any lobe and usually indicates a hematogenous dissemination. Fluoroscopy of the diaphragm may reveal decreased or absent diaphragmatic motility. Diagnostic pneumoperitoneum, which differentiates the elevated diaphragm due to liver abscess from the pleural effusion caused by primary pulmonary disease, is rarely used nowadays.

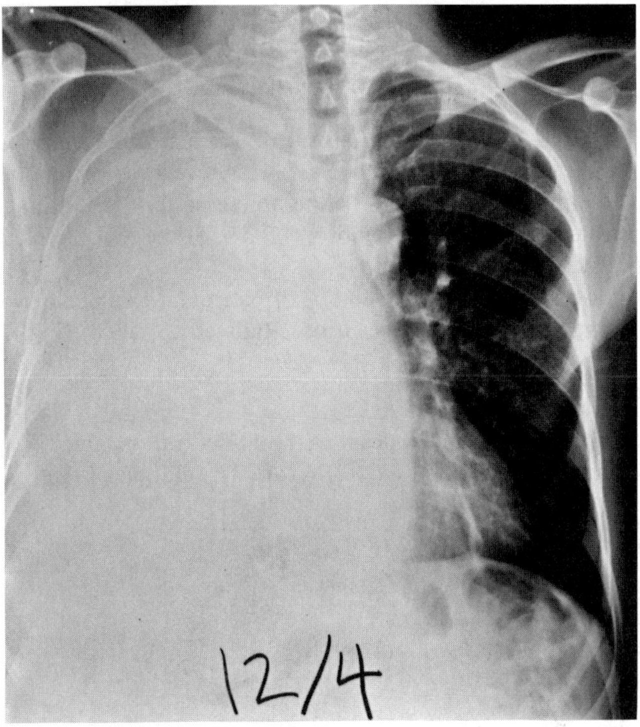

Figure 2 Chest x-ray film shows massive pleural effusion due to amebic empyema.

B. Ultrasound

Technological advances, noninvasiveness, diagnostic accuracy, and cost-effectiveness have made ultrasound a test of choice. About one-third of patients with amebic liver abscesses have the ultrasound pattern that is highly suggestive, although not pathognomonic, of hepatic amebic abscess (Ralls et al., 1982). The following are the characteristic features of a amebic liver abscess.

1. It is round or oval.
2. It has no significant wall echoes (abrupt transition from normal hepatic parenchyma to the amebic lesion).
3. It is less echogenic than normal hepatic parenchyma. Fine, homogeneous, low-level echoes are seen throughout the lesion at high gain.

4. It is located peripherally.
5. Distal sonic enhancement of echoes is observed behind the lesions (increased through-transmission).

Ralls et al. tell us that when all of the above features are present, sonographers should consider amebic liver abscess, even when the diagnosis is not suspected clinically. Although the complete pattern is seen in only one-third of patients with amebic liver abscess, 90% of the lesions fulfill at least three of the five criteria given above.

Pleural disease was present in 18.9% of patients with amebic liver abscess who underwent ultrasound examination (Ralls et al., 1988) (Fig. 3).

C. Computer Tomography

Amebic liver abscess typically appears as a well-defined, rounded, low-density lesion on a computed tomographic (CT) scan. The margin of the abscess may

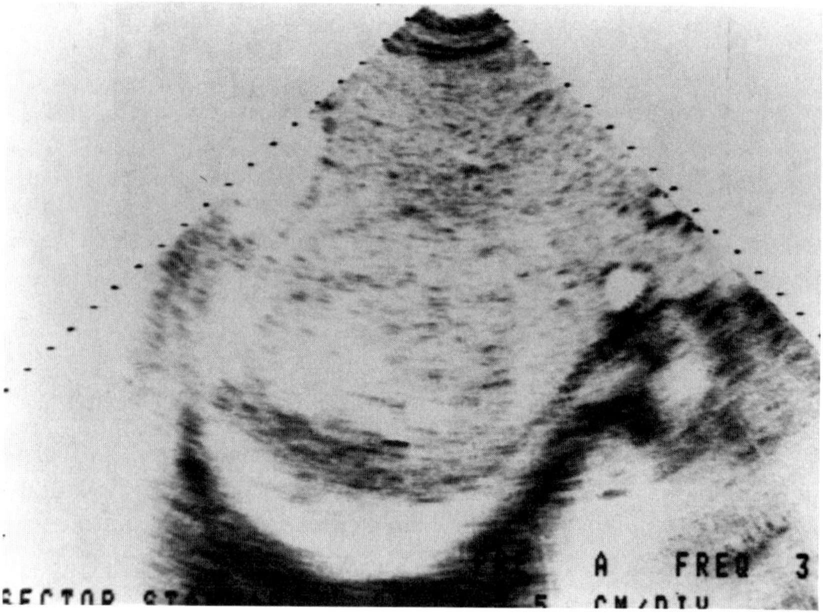

(a)

Figure 3 Ultrasound scan of liver shows a large amebic liver abscess (A) eroding through the diaphragm and pleural effusion due to rupture of amebic liver abscess in to pleural space. a. Transverse view. b. Longitudinal view.

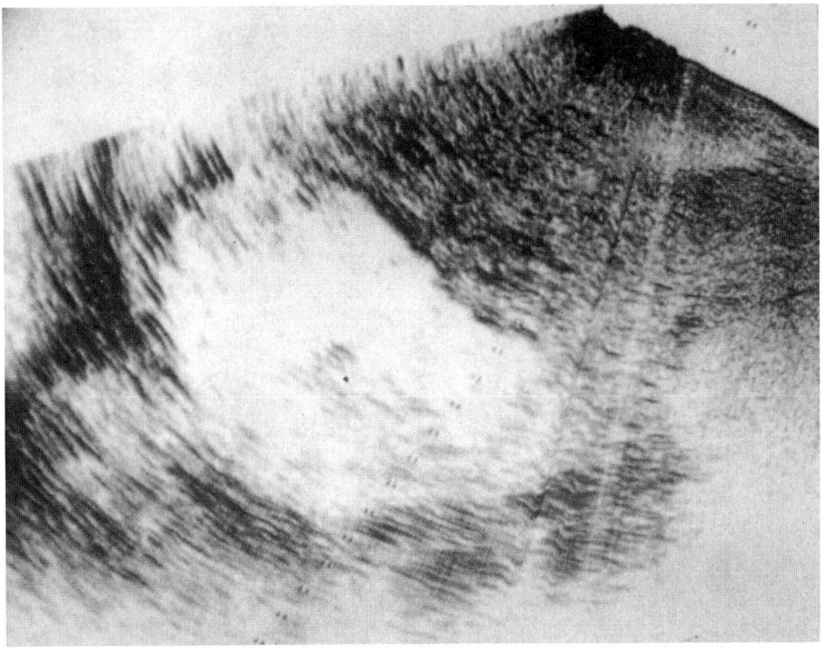

(b)

be smooth or nodular and one or more internal septa may be present. Occasionally, a dense rim around the periphery of the amebic liver abscess may be seen after enhancement (Baert et al., 1980). A feature of amebic liver abscess that helps to differentiate it from other focal hepatic lesions is its tendency to extend beyond the surface of the liver. Radin and co-workers (1988) found that only 5 of their 23 patients (21%) did not have any extrahepatic extension; pleural effusion was present in 9 (39%) patients. Although CT is superior to ultrasound in determining the extent of disease, it is less specific and more expensive (Fig. 4).

D. Magnetic Resonance Imaging

Magnetic resonance imaging (MRI) is used for imaging amebic liver abscess, but sufficient data on characterisitc patterns are not available. Ralls and colleagues (1987b) studied 12 patients with amebic liver abscess. They were not able to identify any specific patterns to differentiate an amebic liver abscess from other hepatic lesions. One patient with amebic empyema showed increased pleural intensity on both T1- and T2-weighted images, compared

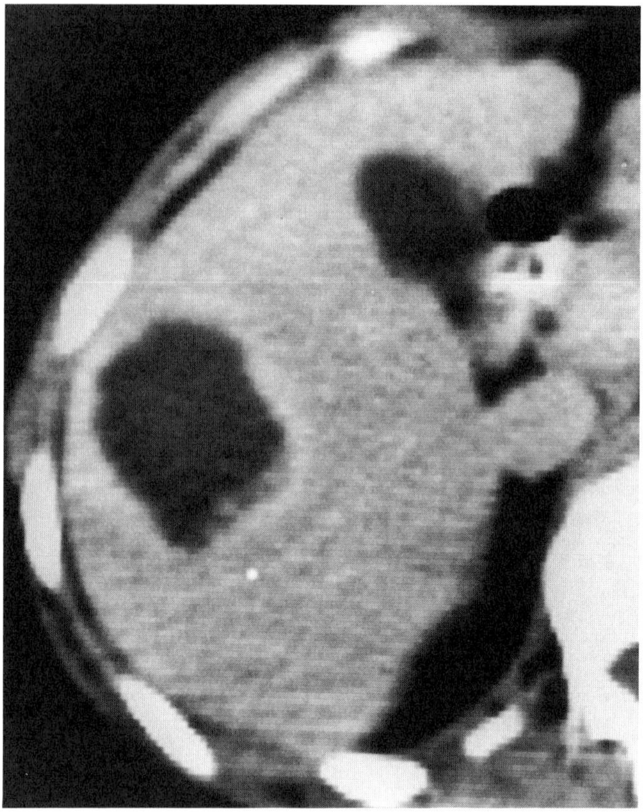

Figure 4 Enhanced CT scan shows an amebic liver abscess. Wall is hyperdense compared with hepatic parenchyma.

to low signal intensity with T1-weighted sequence and a high signal intensity with T2-weighted sequence in patients with sympathetic effusions (Fig. 5).

E. Nuclear Medicine Scans

The following nuclear medicine procedures are generally used for the diagnosis of amebic liver abscess (Ralls et al., 1988; Czerniak et al., 1963; Marberg and Czerniak, 1964).

Technetium 99m-labeled sulfur colloid scan is sensitive for the detection of a amebic liver abscess; however, its specificity is poor. Amebic liver defects are difficult to differentiate from pyogenic or echinococcal abscesses and neoplasms. In a proper clinical setting, the information might be helpful. The test is easy to perform and requires less than 1 h to complete.

Gallium 67 citrate scan is used to complement the sulfur colloid scan. It is useful for imaging neoplastic and inflammatory lesions. Gallium 67 citrate

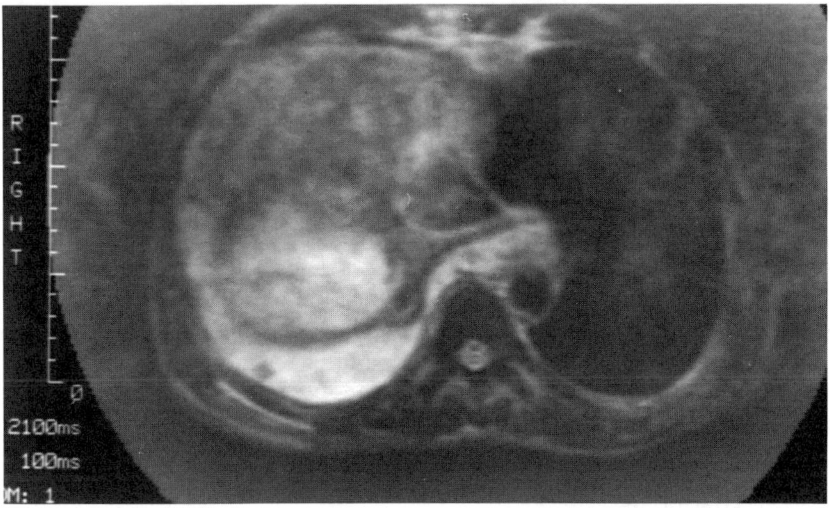

(a)

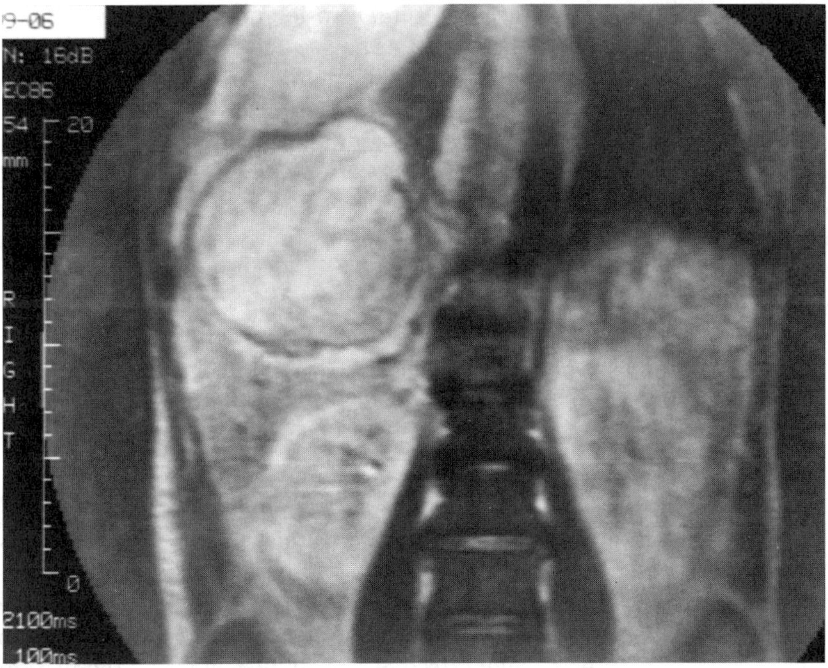

(b)

Figure 5 MRI scan shows a liver abscess and pleural effusion. a. Axial section. b. Coronal section.

concentrates poorly in an amebic abscess. Unlike a pyogenic abscess and a primary hepatocellular carcinoma, an amebic liver abscess generally concentrates gallium at the periphery of the abscess. Gallium scans usually take up to 48 h to complete.

The technetium 99m dimethyl-imidodiacetic acid (dis-IDA) scan, which is widely used in patients with right upper quadrant pain, can be helpful in the diagnosis of a amebic liver abscess. The agent is taken up by hepatocytes and secreted in the biliary tree. Thus, the liver, bile ducts, and the gallbladder can be studied simultaneously. An abscess is detected as a focal liver defect. Because of the large size and peripheral location of an amebic liver abscess, detection with the Dis-IDA scan is quite reliable and comparable to results with sulfur colloid scanning. Remedios and colleagues (1986) showed rim enhancement in 9 of 17 patients undergoing dis-IDA scan. None of the 25 patients with nonamebic liver lesion showed this ring enhancement.

X. Diagnosis

Pleuropulmonary amebiasis should be included in the differential diagnosis of patients with unexplained right pleural effusion or consolidation, particularly in individuals who either live in or have come from an endemic area.

Demonstration of *E. histolytica* from sputum, bronchoalveolar lavage fluid, or pleural fluid establishes the diagnosis of pleuropulmonary amebiasis. Unfortunately, *E. histolytica* is present in less than 10% of patients. *E. gingivalis*, an oral commensal, should be differentiated from *E. histolytica*. An ultrasound (US) scan, a liver scan or a CT scan is helpful in confirming the presence of a liver abscess. The US and CT studies may also demonstrate small pleural effusions. Serological tests should be always performed in patients with suspected pleuropulmonary amebiasis. Once the diagnosis is established, the patient is treated with antiamebic drugs. If the patient responds to the treatment, the diagnosis of amebiasis is established. A pyogenic infection might also occasionally respond to metronidazole therapy.

XI. Treatment

In the past, emetine was the mainstay of treatment for pleuropulmonary amebiasis. Although effective, the drug is very toxic. Chloroquine and metronidazole have revolutionized the therapy of invasive amebiasis. Both drugs are highly effective and have only a few serious side effects. Although both drugs were found to be equally effective in a study comparing the two for the treatment of amebic liver abscess (Cohen and Reynold, 1975), they have not been compared in the treatment of pleuropulmonary amebiasis. Intravenous metronidazole is superior to intramuscular dehydroemetine (Satpathy et al., 1988; Ralls et al., 1987a; Maharaj et al., 1987).

A. Metronidazole

This is currently the drug of choice (Finegold, 1980). Cameron (1978) gave 400-800 mg three times a day for 10-14 days. Only 6 of his 145 patients required a repeat course of therapy; 4 of these 6 patients had secondary infections. We use the drug at a dosage of 750 mg three times a day or 35-50 mg/kg/day in pediatric patients for 10-14 days. Side effects include nausea, anorexia, metallic taste, dizziness, and a disulfiram-like reaction with alcohol. Long-term use might cause vertigo, ataxia, and peripheral neuropathy. A transient leukopenia is occasionally observed. Carcinogenicity and teratogenicity have been observed under experimental conditions. However, this has not been a significant problem in practical terms. Metronidazole acts as a radiation sensitizer, so it should be used with caution in patients receiving radiation treatment. Although metronidazole is both a tissue and a luminal amebicide, its luminal amebicidal activity is not dependable.

B. Chloroquine

This is a tissue amebicidal agent. The usual dosage is 1 g/day for 2 days followed by 500 mg/day for 20 days. Side effects are nausea, abdominal discomfort, and pruritus. Retinopathy, an uncommon complication, usually occurs with its long-term use.

C. Emetine

Emetine is the oldest as well as the most effective amebicidal drug. Emetine has no luminal amebicidal action. The usual dosage is 1 mg/kg/day, to a maximum of 60 mg/day for 10 days by intramuscular or subcutaneous injection. The therapy can be repeated after 1 month. Side effects include pain and necrosis at the injection site, nausea, vomiting, diarrhea, renal impairment, cardiotoxicity, peripheral neuropathy, autonomic blockage, hypotension, and cardiac arrhythmias.

D. Dihydroemetine

Dihydroemetine is a synthetic preparation with action similar to that of emetine but with less cardiotoxicity. The daily dosage is 1.25 mg/kg/day, up to a maximum of 90 mg/day, given by either intramuscular or subcutaneous route.

It is commonly believed that serous pleural effusion should be medically treated. Therapeutic thoracentesis is required for a large pleural effusion. Occasionally an amebic liver abscess may rupture and discharge all its contents into an airway, producing a dramatic improvement. The patient should be treated with antiamebic drugs, postural drainage, and physiotherapy. Bronchoscopy is rarely needed. Persistent bronchohepatic fistula may require a second course of antiamebic drugs (Ibarra-Perez, 1981). Bacterial superinfection, which is common in patients with bronchopleural fistula, responds to appropriate antibiotic therapy (Eggleston et al., 1978).

XII. Empyema

The treatment of amebic empyema is controversial. Surgical management has played a major role in patients with advanced disease (Table 2). Ibarra-Perez and Selman-hema (1977) cautioned that even though both emetine and metronidazole were effective, patients remained toxic and dyspneic as long as the chest remained undrained. He recommended drainage with a large-bore chest tube connected to strong suction.

Verghese et al. (1979) commented that thickening occurred that was out of proportion to the duration of the disease and required closed thoracotomy with insertion of a large tube. Continuous suction was required. He found repeated chest taps inadequate. Ragaheb and colleagues (1976) described five patients with empyema who, despite repeated chest tube thoracentesis and drainage, required decortication. Rasaretnam et al. (1974) reported that even though the response to closed thoracotomy was dramatic, complete lung expansion was achieved in only 37% of patients. They reported that if complete expansion did not occur by the 9th day, it would probably not occur and decortication would be necessary.

On the other hand, Stephen and Uragoda (1970) mentioned that amebic infection differs from pyogenic infection in that tissue reaction is minimal, unless secondary bacterial infection is present. They recommended repeated needle aspirations. Chest tube insertion was indicated if pus was very thick or failed to diminish. In this series of 22 patients with empyema, only 1 required decortication. The patient also had a secondary infection. Imari (1965) treated five patients with empyema using repeated aspiration and two courses of emetine therapy at 10-day intervals. Adams and MacLeod (1977) treated all their patients with pleural effusion using aspiration and amebicidial drugs. Surgical intervention was rarely required. Greaney and co-workers (1985) stated that rupture of amebic abscess (into thorax and peritoneum) can be managed without recourse to percutaneous or surgical drainage. However, that paper reported on only two patients with empyema; one patient underwent chest tube insertion, thoracotomy, and decortication. No information was given about the second patient.

Table 2 Published Series in Which Surgical Management Played a Major Role

Author	Thoracic Complications	Comments
Adeyemo and Aderounmu, Nigeria (1984)	Serous PE:5 Empyema:7 HB fistula:3	All empyema:CT; serous effusion: TH; all HB fistula: postural drainage and bronchoscopy
Verghese et al. India (1979)	Pleura effusion:13 Lung abscess:4 Both:6	20 CT, 3 OT, 1 D, 1 TP, 1 open drainage of liver abscess and repeated TH, 3 rib resection
Cameron, Natal (1978)	Serous PE:12 Amebic empyema:35	Diagnostic TH 4 TH, 31 CT
	Mixed bacterial and amebic empyema:20	12 OT, 8 D
	Lung abscess and infiltrate:72	7 OT (2 for diagnostic purpose)
Ibara-Perez et al. Mexico (1977)	Empyema:88 3 undiagnosed	75 CT, 7 OT, 31 D
Ragaheb et al. Egypt (1976)	Empyema:5 Lung abscess:3	Conservative treatment failed in all patients. All empyema patients had TH, 3 had CT; all patients still required D. Lobectomy for all abscesses
Le Roux Natal (1969)	Empyema:37	37 CT, 2 OT, 3 D. Patients who required OT and D were secondarily infected
Tokaro and Bond, U.S.A. and India (1958)	Empyema:2 Lung abscess:4 HB fistula:1	1 CT, 4 OT, 1 lobectomy, 1 conservative treatment
Vickers et al. India (1982)	Empyema:24 Serous effusion:5	17 TH, 20 CT, 3 OT, 2 D
Rasaretnam et al. Ceylon (1974)	Empyema:31	1 TH, 3 TH and D, 13 CT, 14 CT and D

CT, chest tube; OT, open thoracotomy; D, decortication; TH, thoracentesis; TP, thoracoplasty; PE, pleural effusion; HB, hepatobronchial fistula.

XIII. Summary

Although amebiasis may occur in all parts of the world, the disease occurs predominantly in tropical and subtropical countries where environmental sanitation is poor. In endemic areas, the overall prevalence rate may approach 40%. The disease is, however, not restricted to the tropics; outbreaks have been reported in Indian settlements in Canada and in Oslo in the winter. High prevalence rates of *E. histolytica* have been reported from northern Europe.

Pleuropulmonary amebiasis is usually an extension or complication of hepatic involvement. The tissue amebicides are effective in eradicating ameba from the involved organs. Surgical involvement is rarely required.

There is no evidence that prophylactic treatment is effective in preventing intestinal amebiasis in travelers.

References

Adams, E. B., and MacLeod, N. (1977). Invasive amebiasis 11. *Medicine* **56**:325-334.

Adeyemo, A. O., and Aderounmu, A. (1984). Intrathoracic complications of amoebic liver abscess. *J. R. Soc. Med.* **77**:16-21.

Aust-Kettis, A., and Sundqvist, K. G. (1978). Dynamics of the interaction between *Entamoeba histolytica* and components of the immune response. Capping and endocytosis; influence of inhibiting and accelerating factors; variation of the expression of surface antigens. *Scand. J. Immunol.* **71**:35-44.

Baert, A. L., Wackenheim, A., and Jeanmart, L. (1980). *Atlas of Pathological Computer Tomography*, Vol 2. *Abdominal Computer Tomography.* New York, Springer-Verlag, p. 116.

Biagi, F. F., Robledo, E., Servin, H., and Marvan, G. (1963). Influence of some steroids in the experimental production of amebic hepatic abscess. *Am. J. Trop. Med. Hyg.* **12**:318-320.

Bookless, A. S. (1950). Thoracic amoebiasis. *J. Royal Army Med. Corps.* **94**:52-60.

Brossi, A., Baumann, N., and Choparddit, J. (1959). Syntheseversuche in der Emetine-Reihe: 4. mitteilung Racemisches 2-Dehydroemetine. *Helv. Chim. Acta* **42**:772.

Calderon, J., and Schreiber, R. D. (1985). Activation of the alternative and classical complement pathways by *Entamoeba histolytica. Infect. Immun.* **50**(2):560-565.

Calderon, J., de Lourdes Munoz, M., and Acosta, H. M. (1980). Surface redistribution and release of antibody-induced caps in Entamoebae. *J. Exp. Med.* **151**:184-193.

Cameron, E. W. J. (1978). The treatment of pleuropulmonary amebiasis with metronidazole. *Chest* **73**:647-650.

Capin, R., Capin, N. R., Carmona, M., and Ortiz-Ortiz, L. (1980). Effect of complement depletion on the induction of amebic liver abscess in the hamster. *Arch. Invest. Med(Mex).* **11**(Suppl. 1):173-180.

Chacon-Zamora, A. V., Ocampa Mora, R., Soto, C., and Beauregard, R. (1978). Current status of intestinal parasitism in the Puriscal area (Costa Rica). *Acta Med. Costarric.* **21**:271-273.

Cohen, H. G., and Reynold, T. B. (1975). Comparison of metronidazole and chloroquine for the treatment of amoebic liver abscess. *Gastroenterology* **69**:35-41.

Conan, N. J., Jr. (1948). Chloroquine in amebiasis. *Am. J. Trop. Med.* **28**: 107-110.

Cuyadrado, R., and Kagan, I. G. (1967). The prevalence of antibodies to parasitic diseases in sera of young Army recruits from the United States and Brazil. *Am. J. Epidemiol.* **86**:330-340.

Czerniak, P., Lubin, E., Djaldetti, M., and de Vries, A. (1963). Scintilligraphic follow-up of amoebic abscesses and hydatid cysts of the liver. *J. Nucl. Med.* **4**:35-44.

Daniels, A. C., and Childress, M. E. (1956). Pleuropulmonary amebiasis. *Calif. Med.* **85**:369-375.

DeBakey, M. E., and Ochsner, A. (1951). Hepatic amebiasis: a 20 year experience and analysis of 263 cases. *Int. Abstr. Surg.* **92**:209-231.

DeCock, K. M., and Reynolds, T. B. (1987). Amebic and pyogenic liver abscess. In *Diseases of the Liver*. Edited by L. Schiff and E. Schiff. Philadelphia, J. B. Lippincott, pp. 1235-1253.

Eggleston, F. C., Verghese, M., Handa, A. K., and Gill, S. S. (1978). The result of surgery in amebic liver abscess: experiences in eighty-three patients. *Surgery* **83**:536-539.

Finegold, S. (1980). Metronidazole. *Ann. Intern. Med.* **93**:585-587.

Ghadirian, E., and Meerovitch, E. (1978a). Vaccination against hepatic amebiasis in hamster. *J. Parasitol.* **64**(4):742-743.

Ghadirian, E., and Meerovitch, E. (1978b). Behavior of axenic IP-106 strain of *Entamoeba histolytica* in golden hamster. *Am. J. Trop. Med. Hyg.* **27**(2, pt. 1):241-247.

Ghadirian, E., and Meerovitch, E. (1981a). Effect of immunosuppression on the size and metastasis of amoebic liver abscesses in hamsters. *Parasite Immunol.* **3**:329-338.

Ghadirian, E., and Meerovitch, E. (1981b). Effect of splenectomy on the size of amoebic liver abscesses and metastatic foci in hamster. *Infect. Immun.* **31**:571-573.

Ghadirian, E., and Meerovitch, E. (1982). Macrophage requirement for host defense against experimental hepatic amoebiasis in hamster. *Parasite Immunol.* **4**:219-225.

Ghadirian, E., Meerovitch, E., and Hartmann, D. P. (1980). Protection against amebic liver abscess in hamsters by means of immunization with amebic antigen and some of its fractions. *Am. J. Trop. Med. Hyg.* **29**:779-784.

Ghadirian, E., Meerovitch, K., and Kongshavn, P. A. L. (1983). Role of macrophages in host defense against hepatic amoebiasis in hamster. *Infect. Immun.* **42**:1017-1019.

Gold, D., Norman, L. G., Maddison, S. E., and Kagan, I. G. (1978). Immunological studies on hamsters against *Entamoeba histolytica*. *J. Parasitol.* **64**:866-873.

Greaney, G. C., Reynolds, T. B., and Donnovan, A. J. (1985). Ruptured amebic liver abscess. *Arch. Surg.* **120**:555-561.

Healy, G. R. (1986). Immunologic tools in the diagnosis of amebiasis: Epidemiology in the United States. *Rev. Infect. Dis.* **8**:239-246.

Herrera-Llerandi, R. (1966). Thoracic repercussions of amebiasis. *J. Thorac. Cardiovasc. Surg.* **52**:361-375.

Huldt, G., Davies, P., Allison, A. C., and Shorlemmer, H. U. (1979). Interaction between *Entamoeba histolytica* and complement. *Nature* **277**: 214-216.

Ibarra-Perez, C. (1981). Thoracid complication of amebic abscess of the liver. *Chest* **79**:672-677.

Ibarra-Perez, C., and Selman-Lema, M. (1977). Diagnosis and treatment of amebic "empyema." *Am. J. Surg.* **134**:283-287.

Imari, A. J. (1965). Pleuropulmonary amebiasis in Iraq. *Dis. Chest* **47**:17-19.

Imperato, P. J. (1981). A historical overview of amebiasis. *Bull. N.Y. Acad. Mec.* **57**:175-187.

Istre, G. R., Kreiss, K., Hopkins, R. S., Healy, G. R., Benziger, M., Canfield, T. H., Dickinson, P., Englert, T. R., Compton, R. C., Mathews, H. M., and Simmons, R. A. (1982). An outbreak of amebiasis spread by colonic irrigation at a chiropractic clinic. *N. Engl. J. Med.* **307**:339-342.

Kean, B. H., Gilmore, H. R., and Van Stone, W. W. (1956). Fatal amebiasis: report of 148 fatal cases from Armed Forces Institutes of Pathology. *Ann. Intern. Med.* **44**:831-843.

Krupp, I. M., and Powell, S. J. (1971). Comparative study of the antibody response in amebiasis. *Am. J. Trop. Med. Hyg.* **20**:421-424.

Kubitschek, K. R., Peters, J., Nickeson, D., and Musher, D. M. (1985). Amebiasis presenting as pleuropulmonary disease. *West. J. Med.* **142**: 203-207.

Le Roux, B. T. (1969). *Pleuro-pulmonary amoebiasis. Thorax* **24**:91-101.

Losch, F. A. (1875). Massenhafte Entwickelung Von Amoeben in Dickdarm. *Arch. Pathol. Anat.* **65**:196-211.

Losch, F. A. (1975). Massive development of amebas in the large intestine (translated from the original). *Am. J. Trop. Med. Hyg.* **24**:383-392.

Lewis, E. A., and Antia, A. U. (1969). Amebic colitis: review of 295 cases. *Trans. R. Soc. Trop. Med. Hyg.* **63**:633-638.

Mahajan, R. C., and Ganguly, N. K. (1980). Amoebic antigen in immunodiagnosis and prognosis of amoebic liver abscess. *Trans. R. Soc. Trop. Med. Hyg.* **74**:300-302.

Maharaj, B., Mzikayise, L., Peregrine, L., and Pudfin, L. C. (1987). The conservative management of amoebic liver abscess complicated by thoracic extension. *Trop. Geogr. Med.* **39**:299-302.

Marberg, K., and Czerniak, P. (1964). Observations of isotope hepatoscanning in diagnosis and treatment of amoebic liver infection. *Ann. Intern. Med.* **60**:66-78.

Mathew, N. T., and Ananthachari, M. C. (1964). Pleuropulmonary amoebiasis. *J. Assoc. Physicians. India* **12**:839-44.

Melvin, D. M., and Mata, L. J. (1971). Intestinal parasites in a Mayan-Indian village of Guatemala. *Rev. Latinoam. Microbiol.* **13**:15-19.

Minetto, E., and Prinotti, C. (1965). Etat de mal asthmatique dans un cas d'amebiase bronchique. *Ann. Otolaryngol. (Paris).* **82**:223-225.

Nanda, R. B., and Hoon, R. S. (1976). Amoebic liver abscess. *Med. J. Armed Forces India* **32**:404-412.

Norman, L., Gold, D., and Kagan, I. G. (1979). The serological response of hamster to experimental liver inoculations with *Entamoeba histolytica* as measured by indirect hemagglutination test and enzyme linked immunosorbent assay. *Am. J. Trop. Med. Hyg.* **28**(2):198-205.

Nwafo, D. C., and Egbue, M. O. (1981). Intrathoracic manifestations of amoebiasis. *Ann. R. Coll. Surgeons Engl.* **63**:126-128.

Ochsner, A., and Debakey, M. (1935). Diagnosis and treatment of amebic abscess of liver: study based on 4484 collected and personal cases. *Am. J. Digest. Dis. Nutr.* **2**:47-51.

Ochsner, A., and DeBakey, M. (1936). Pleuropulmonary complications of amebiasis. *J. Thoracic Surg.* **5**:225-258.

Ortega, H. B., Borchardt, K. A., Hamilton, R., Ortega, P., and Mahood, J. (1984). Enteric pathogenic protozoa in homosexual men from San Francisco. *Sex. Transm. Dis.* **11**:59-63.

Ortiz-Ortiz, L., Zamacona, G., Sepulveda, B., and Capin, N. R. (1975). Cell mediated immunity in patients with amebic abscess of the liver. *Clin. Immunopathol.* **4**:127-134.

Ortiz-Ortiz, L., Capin, R., Capin, N. R., Sepulveda, B., and Zamacona, G. (1978). Activation of the alternative pathway of complement by *Entamoeba histolytica. Clin. Exp. Immunol.* **34**:10-18.

Powell, S. J., Wilmont, A. J., MacLeod, I., and Elsdon-Dew, R. (1966). Metroniadazole in amoebic dysentery and amoebic liver abscess. *Lancet* **2**:1329-1331.

Radin, D. R., Rall, P. W., Colleti, P. M., and Halls, J. (1988). CT of amebic liver abscess. *AJR* **150**:1297-1301.

Radke, R. A. (1951). Amebiasis with hepatic abscess and pleuropulmonary involvement. *U.S. Armed Forces Med. J.* **2**:437-444.

Ragaheb, M. I., Ramadan, A. A., and Khalil, M. A. H. (1976). Intrathoracic presentation of amebic liver abscess. *Ann. Thorac. Surg.* **22**:483-489.

Ralls, P. W., Colleti, P. M., Quinn, M. F., and Halls, J. (1982). Sonographic findings in hepatic amebic abscess. *Radiology* **145**:123-126.

Ralls, P. W., Barnes, P. F., Johnson, M. B., DeCock, K. M., Radin, D. R., and Halls, J. (1987a). Medical treatment of hepatic amebic abscess: rare need for percutaneous drainage. *Radiology* **165**:805-807.

Ralls, P. W., Henley, D. S., Colletti, P. M., Benson, R., Raval, J. K., Radin D. R., Boswell, W. D., and Halls, J. M. (1987b). Amebic liver abscess: *MR imaging*. **165**:801-804.

Ralls, P. W., Colleti, P. M., and Halls, J. M. (1988). Imaging in hepatic amebic abscess. In *Amebiasis. Human Infection by Entamoeba histolytica.* Edited by J. I. Ravdin. New York, Churchill Livingstone.

Rasaretnam, R., Paul, A. T. S., and Yoganathan, M. (1974). Pleural empyema due to ruptured amoebic liver abscess. *Br. J. Surg.* **61**:713-715.

Ravi, V. V., Mithal, S., Malaviya, A. N., and Tandon, B. N. (1975). Immunologic studies in amoebic liver abscess. *Indian J. Med. Res.* **63**:1732-1736.

Reed, S. L., Sargeaunt, P. G., and Braude, A. I. (1983). Resistance to lysis by human serum of pathogenic *Entamoeba histolytica. Trans. R. Soc. Trop. Med. Hyg.* **77**:248-253.

Remedios, P. A., Colleti, P. M., and Ralls, P. W. (1986). Cholescintigraphic rim enhancement in hepatic amebic abscess. *Radiology* **160**:395-398.

Rhode, F. C., Prieto, O., and Riveros, O. (1979). Thoracic complications of amoebic liver abscess. *Br. J. Dis. Chest.* **73**:302-304.

Rogers, L. (1912). The rapid cure of amoebic dysentery and hepatitis by hypodermic injections of soluble salts of emetine. *Br. Med. J.* **1**:14-24.

Salata, R. A., and Ravdin, J. I. (1986). Review of human immune mechanisms directed against *Entamoeba histolytica. Rev. Infect. Dis.* **8**:261-272.

Salata, R. A., and Ravdin, J. I. (1988). Human cell mediated immune mechanisms directed against *Entamoeba histolytica.* In *Amebiasis. Human Infection by Entamoeba histolytica.* Edited by J. I. Ravdin. New York, Churchill Livingstone, pp. 471-479.

Salata, R. A., Martinez-Palomo, A., Murray, H. W., Conales, L., Trevino, N., Segovia, E., Murphy, C. F., and Ravdin, J. I. (1986). Patients treated for amebic liver abscess develop cell-mediated immune mechanisms effective in vitro against *Entamoeba histolytica. J. Immunol.* **136**:2633-2639.

Sargeaunt, P. G., Oates, J. K., MacLennan, I., Oriel, J. D., and Goldmeier, D. (1983). *Entamoeba histolytica* in male homosexuals. *Br. J. Vener. Dis.* **59**:193-195.

Sargeaunt, P. G., Williams, J. E., and Grene, J. D. (1978). The differentiation of invasive and noninvasive *Entamoeba histolytica* by isenzyme electrophoresis. *Trans. R. Soc. Trop. Med. Hyg.* **72**:519-521.

Satpathy, B. K., Acharya, S. K., and Satpathy, S. (1988). Comparative study of intravenous metronidazole and intramuscular dehydroemetine in amoebic liver abscess. *J. Indian Med. Assoc.* **86**(2):38-40.

Savant, T., Viriyanond, P., and Nimitmong Kol, N. (1973). Blast transformation of lymphocytes in amebiasis. *Am. J. Trop. Med. Hyg.* **22**:705-710.

Shaw, R. R. (1949). Thoracic complications of amebiasis. *Surg. Gynecol. Obstet.* **88**:753-762.

Shetty, N., Das, P., Pal, S. C., and Prabhu, T. (1988). Observations on the interpretation of amoebic serology in endemic areas. *J. Trop. Med. Hyg.* **91**:222-227.

Simon, C. E. (1890). Abscess of the liver: perforation into the lung; *Amoeba coli* in sputum. *Bull. Johns Hopkins Hosp.* **1**:97.

Stephen, S. J., and Uragoda, C. G. (1970). Pleuro-pulmonary amoebiasis. *Br. J. Dis. Chest* **64**:96-106.

Stern, J. J., Grasbill, J. R., and Drutz, J. J. (1984). Murine amebiasis: the role of the macrophage in host defense. *Am. J. Trop. Med. Hyg.* **18**(1): 67-77.

Tokaro, T., and Bond, W. (1958). Pleuropulmonary, pericardial, and cerebral complications of amebiasis. A twenty year survey. *Int. Abst. Surg.* **107**(3):209-229.

Trissl, D. (1982). Immunology of *Entamoeba-histolytica* in human and animal hosts. *Rev. Infect. Dis.* **4**:1154-1184.

Verghese, M., Eggleston, F. C., Handa, A. K., and Singh, C. H. (1979). Management of thoracic amebiasis. *J. Thorac. Cardiovasc. Surg.* **78**: 757-760.

Vickers, P. J., Bohra, R. C., and Sharma, G. C. (1982). Hepatopulmonary amebiasis—a review of 40 cases. *Int. Surg.* **67**:427-429.

Vinayak, V. K., Chitkara, N. L., and Chhuttani, P. M. (1979). Effect of corticosteroid and irradiation on caecal amoebic infection in rats. *Trans. R. Soc. Trop. Med. Hyg.* **73**(3):266-268.

Vinayak, V. K., Sawhney, S., Jain, P., Chung, S., and Chakravarti, R. M. (1982). Immunosuppression and experimental amoebiasis in guinea pigs. *Ann. Trop. Med. Parasitol.* **76**(3):309-316.

Walsh, J. A. (1984). Estimating the burden of illness in the tropics. In *Tropical and Geographical Medicine.* Edited by K. S. Warren and A. A. F. Mahmoud. New York, McGraw-Hill.

Walsh, J. A. .(1986). Problem in recognition and diagnosis of amebiasis: estimation of the global magnitude of morbidity and mortality. *Rev. Infect. Dis.* **8**:228-238.

Webster, B. H. (1956). Pulmonary complications of amebiasis. *Dis. Chest* **30**:315-325.

Webster, B. H. (1960). Pleuropulmonary amebiasis. A review with an analysis of ten cases. *Am. Rev. Respir. Dis.* **81**:683-688.

Wijesundra, M., and De, S. (1980). Hepatic amoebiasis in immunodepressed mice. *Trans. R. Soc. Trop. Med. Hyg.* **74**:216-218.

9

Pulmonary Manifestations in Chagas' Disease

NEWTON M. BETHLEM, ALFRED LEMLE, and EDSON A. SAAD

Hospital-Universitario de Universidade
Federal de Rio de Janeiro
Rio de Janeiro, Brazil

I. Background

American trypanosomiasis, described for the first time by Brazilian scientist Carlos Chagas (1909), is an endemic disease of rural populations, caused by a protozoan, *Trypanosoma cruzi*, which is transmitted to humans by a blood-sucking bug of the subfamily Triatominae. It is a widespread human infection, being reported from the southern United States to Argentina, and a major public health problem in Latin America where, in endemic areas from Mexico to Argentina, an estimated 10-12 million people are infected (Brenner, 1982). In Brazil alone more than 6 million people are affected. More than 50 million people are exposed to infection in the New World.

II. Distribution of the Chagas' Disease Vector

American trypanosomiasis was originally an infection of wild mammals of the American continent, with apparently multiple foci, and became a zoonosis when the reduviid insect vectors adapted to human dwellings. It is noticeable that the Amazon region (Fig. 1: white area on the map) is a barrier between

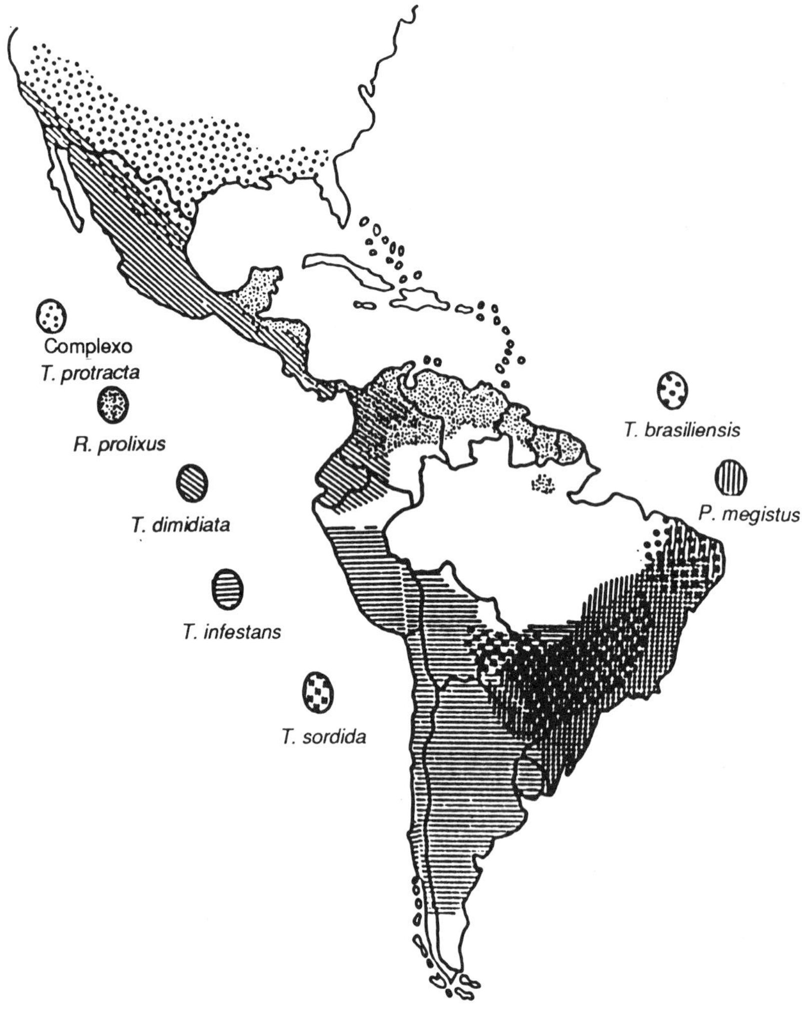

Figure 1 Vector distribution in Chagas' disease in the American continent.

two kinds of main vectors: the *Panstrongilus megistus* and *Triatoma infestans* to the south and *Rhodnius prolixus* to the north. With the rapid and progressive human occupation of the Amazon, epidemiological conditions have been created for the expansion of more infecting *P. Megistus-Triatoma* to the north in the near future, which may be of importance for the United States. Despite the presence of some reduviid vectors, as well as several types of *Trypanosoma cruzi*-infected wild animals (Kagan et al., 1966), only three autochthonous cases of Chagas' disease in the United States have been reported (Woody and Woody 1955; Schiffler et al., 1984). The general quality of housing and the absence of bugs that readily become domiciliary certainly explain the rarity of *Trypanosoma cruzi* transmission to humans in the United States—a situation that might be changed if other vectors came into the scene.

III. Wild Cycle and Domiciliary Cycles in Transmission of the Disease

The disease was initially one of wild animals including armadillos, opossums, rats and other rodents, and racoons. In the absence of animals, the disease cycle may occur between the insect and humans (Fig. 2). Transmission between one insect and another has been suggested and transmission from human to human occurs both transplacentally and as a result of blood transfusions. Other domestic animals might participate in the cycle and some of them may become infected by eating small rodents (Zeledon, 1974).

Infection is usually acquired by humans in the mud and wood houses of rural areas, where blood-sucking bugs live. During or after sucking human

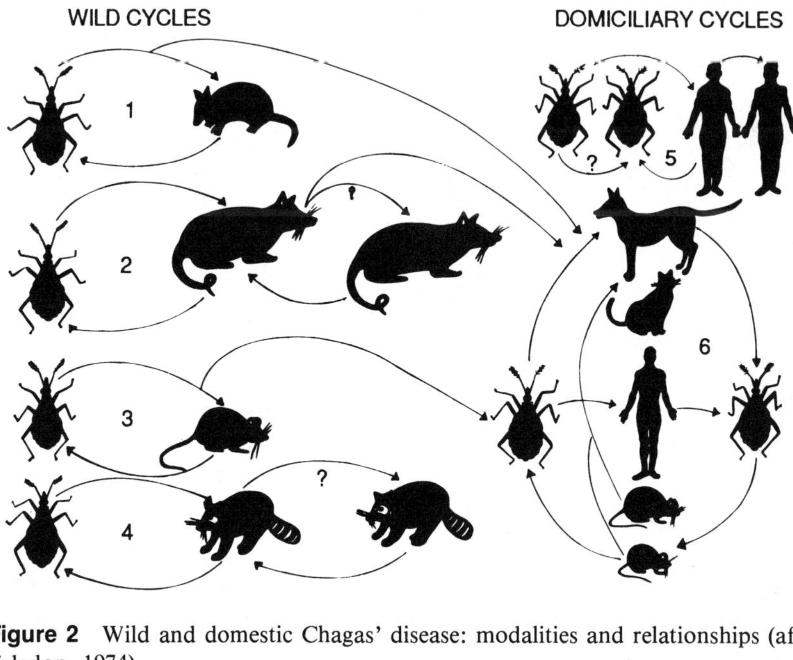

Figure 2 Wild and domestic Chagas' disease: modalities and relationships (after Zeledon, 1974).

blood at night, the bugs eliminate excreta with parasites that penetrate the skin of the arms or mucous membranes due to the host scratching or rubbing after receiving a bite.

IV. Life Cycle of the Parasite

Metacyclic forms of the parasite (Fig. 3A) eliminated with insect feces penetrate human skin and reach the blood (B), from where they penetrate the tissue. In tissue cells (C) they multiply by binary division and transform into the leishmania forms (Fig. 4). The infected cell ruptures (D), releasing the *trypanosomas* into the blood. Once again, the parasite invades other cells and waits to be ingested by other bugs. In the bug these blood forms transform themselves into crytidial forms, which multiply by binary division in the duodenum and differentiate themselves into metacyclic trypanosoma (H).

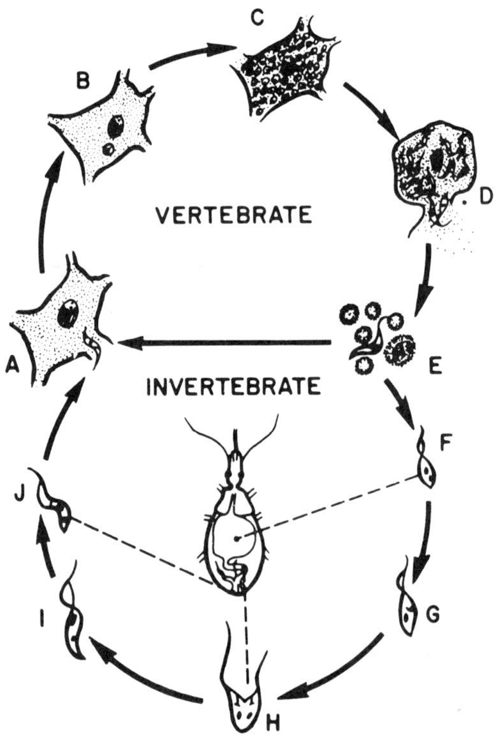

Figure 3 Life cycle of *Trypanosoma cruzi* in the vertebrate and invertebrate.

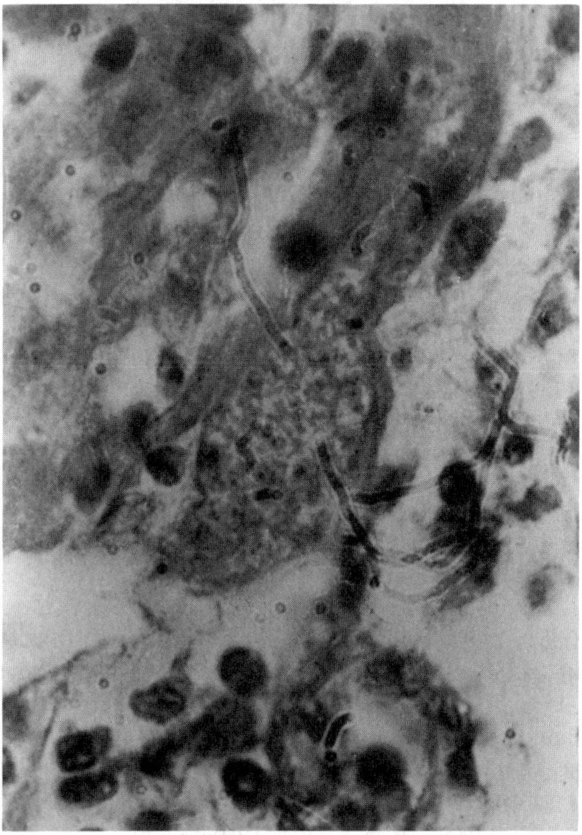

Figure 4 Leishmania forms of *T. cruzi* in myocardial fibers, where they develop and form a pseudocyst that may later rupture.

V. North American Problem

In recent years, the number of persons estimated to have migrated to the United States from Central America is probably 500,000-2 million (Passel & Woodrow, 1984; Department of State, 1984). In Washington, D.C., alone there are about 150,000 legal and undocumented Central Americans. This is an important problem for three reasons:

1. Occurrence of Chagas' disease in these people, who will need medical care (Kirchhoff and Neva, 1985)

2. Possibility of congenital transmission
3. Risk of disease transmission by blood transfusion

Of a selected group of 205 emigrants from Nicaragua and El Salvador living in Washington, D. C., 4.9% were found to be infected by *Trypanosoma cruzi*. Antibody specifics for the 72 and 90 kilodalton (Kda) surface glycoproteins of the parasite tested by immunoprecipitation and electrophoresis showed that these persons were truly infected with *T. cruzi*. Since enzyme-linked immunosorbent assay (ELISA) may cross-react with leishmaniasis, xenodiagnosis was performed in 60% of the infected migrants and showed *Trypanosoma cruzi* in the blood of 33%. Thus, physicians in the united States should be aware of Chagas' disease when caring for Latin-American migrants. It has been estimated that in South America 2-5% of infants born to women with chronic Chagas' disease are infected with the parasite (Schmunis and Szarfman, 1977). In the United States, two cases have been reported (Kirchhoff et al., 1987). No epidemiological data on congenital transmission of *T. cruzi* in Central America are available.

The other important issue relating to the presence of persons with chronic *T. cruzi* infection in the United States is the possibility of transmission of the organism by blood transfusion. Transfusion-related transmission of Chagas' disease is an important public health problem in Brazil and Bolivia (Amato Neto et al., 1968; Maekelt, 1973; Schmunis, 1984). In South America, there is a 12-18% probability that the recipient will become infected when *T. cruzi*-contaminated blood is transfused (Coura et al., 1966; Rassi and Rezende, 1975; Bergoglio, 1972). No data are available from Central America. The problem persists in certain regions because donated blood comes from migrants who are unaware of their seropositivity and it is not tested for antibody to the parasite.

The current situation with *T. cruzi*-infected Salvadoran and Nicaraguan immigrants in the United States is analogous, since most of them are unaware of their disease (Kirchhoff et al., 1987). As they become more integrated in the society they may volunteer to donate blood, when problem of transmission might become relevant.

In the last few years, the incidence of Chagas' disease has been decreased by governmental action to interrupt transmission through better housing and application of insecticides, as in Brazil, or incidental depletion of reduviid population due to spraying of insecticides for malaria vector control, as in southeastern Mexico (Goldsmith et al., 1985).

Figure 5 shows *Triatoma infestans* distribution in Brazil in the period 1975-1983 and 1986, showing how effective the action against vectors of Chagas' disease can be.

Figure 6 shows the diminishing incidence of Chagas' disease as measured by seropositivity in school children in São Paulo State, Brazil, coincident with partial interruption of transmission of Chagas' disease.

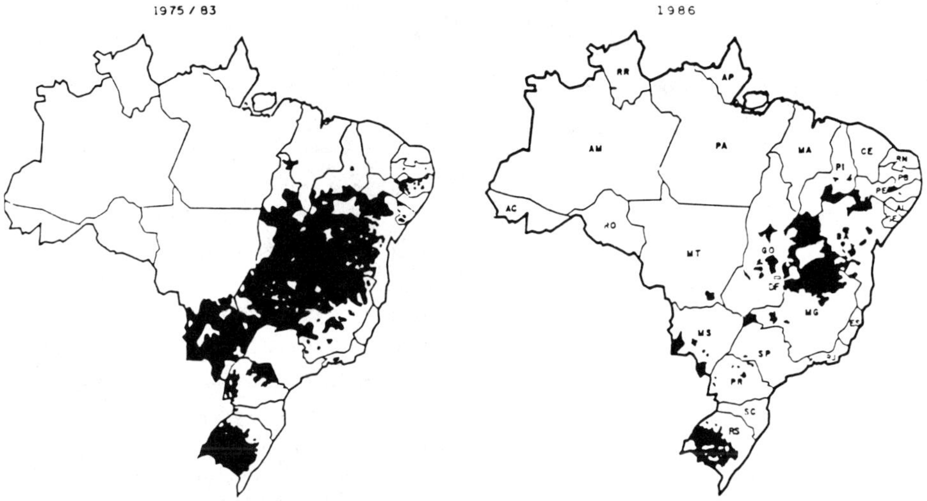

Figure 5 Distribution of *Triatoma infestans* in Brazil in 1975-1983 and 1986 shows a remarkable decrease in prevalence due to prophylactic measures.

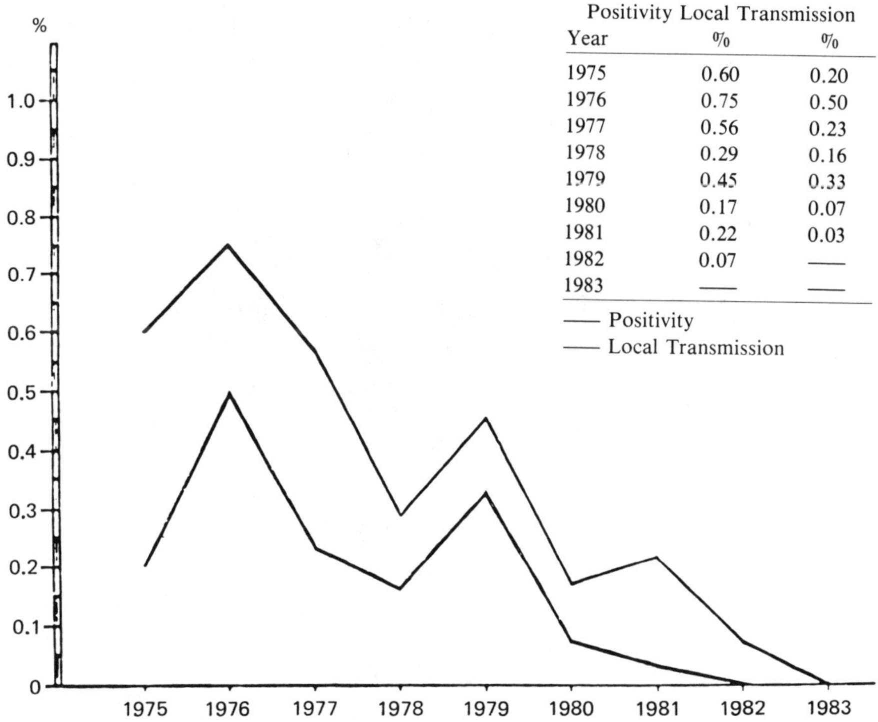

Year	Positivity %	Local Transmission %
1975	0.60	0.20
1976	0.75	0.50
1977	0.56	0.23
1978	0.29	0.16
1979	0.45	0.33
1980	0.17	0.07
1981	0.22	0.03
1982	0.07	—
1983	—	—

Figure 6 Incidence of positive Machado-Guerreiro reaction in school children in São Paulo, Brazil, shows decrease in coincident with reduction in vector distrubution (after Souza et al., 1985). (Courtesy of Dias, J. C. 1989).

VI. Clinical Presentation

A. Acute Phase

This affects predominantly children in rural areas, and is characterized by a febrile illness in which the portal of entry of the parasite can be recognized by inflammation of the body parts that remain uncovered during sleep. Romana (1935) described the typical unilateral edema of the palpebra, with conjunctivitis and auricular lymph node enlargement found in persons with *T. cruzi* inoculation. The disease may cause only a febrile illness, an acute myocarditis, with or without heart failure, and meningoencephalitis. The symptoms usually subside between 2 and 4 weeks. Cardiac failure may occur at any time within the first 6 months. Death occurs in 10% of the cases, either from heart failure or meningoencephalitis (Laranja et al., 1956). The acute phase may pass unnoticed, since many adults with chronic Chagas' disease or positive serological tests deny a typical history of this phase.

B. Chronic Disease

Why certain patients never develop clinical disease, while others do, in more or less time, is unknown. Table 1 shows the evolution of acute to chronic Chagas' disease.

The heart is the organ most commonly affected in chronic Chagas' disease. Chronic Chagas' heart disease results from continued myocardial cell

Table 1 Principal Clinical Forms of Chagas' Disease in Patients Followed Since the Acute Phase in Bambui, Brazil, According to Evolution Time[a]

		Principal detected clinical forms (%)				
				Digestive		
Evolution time since acute phase (years)	Number of patients	Indeterminate	Cardiac[b]	Esophagus	Colon	Pulmonary bronchi
10-20	68	60.3	33.8	10.3	7.4	unknown
21-30	73	39.7	39.3	17.8	21.9	unknown
31-40	31	32.3	58.1	19.4	25.8	unknown

([a]) World Health Organization criteria, Caracas, 1971.
([b]) 90% in initial evolutive degree.
Source: Dias, 1982.

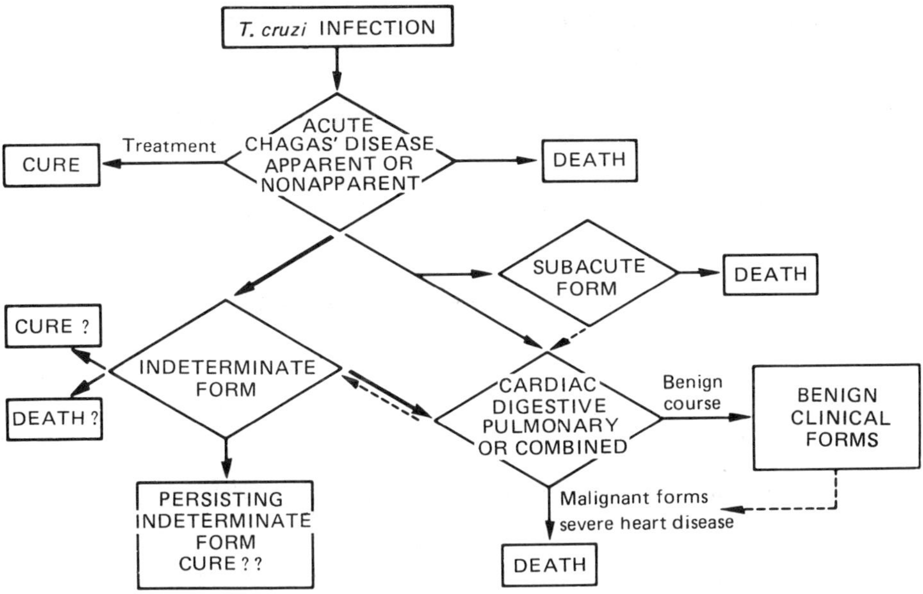

Figure 7 Natural history of Chagas' disease (from Dias, 1982).

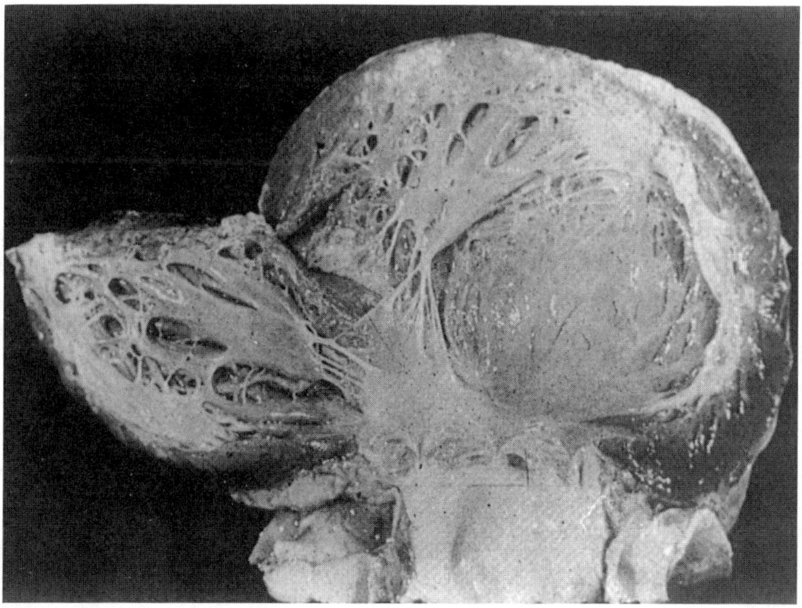

Figure 8 Heart in Chagas' cardiomyopathy. Note the aneurysm of the cardiac apex.

destruction by the leishmania forms of the parasite. It occurs usually in people aged 20-40 years. Figure 7 shows the natural history of Chagas' disease and its heart and lung manifestations. Pathological examination shows fibrosis, inflammatory mononuclear cell infiltration, and a high incidence of intracardiac thrombi Andrade & Andrade (197a). Most characteristic is the vortical lesion, an aneurysm of the apex that is usually small, but may be large (Fig. 8). Other affected organs are salivary glands, esophagus, stomach, colon, and bronchi.

VII. Pulmonary Manifestations of Chagas' Disease

Except for bronchiectasis, which is due to direct infection by *T. cruzi*, lung manifestations are rather uncommon and secondary to infection of other organs, as described in the following sections.

A. Pulmonary Manifestations Secondary to Megaesophagus

Esophageal lesions result from muscle fiber parasitism and destruction of eosphageal neurons, causing circular muscle layer hypertrophy, fibrosis of myoenteric plexus, and esophageal dilatation.

In approximately 17% of the cases there is associated cardiopathy. The prevalence of megaesophagus is around 7% in endemic areas. The association of megaesophagus, heart enlargement, and poorly vascularized lungs may be recognized by radiographic examination and is unique to Chagas' heart disease (Fig. 9, 10).

Patients complain of dysphagia, odynophagia, regurgitation, heartburn, singultus, constipation, and coughing. Fifty percent of the patients regurgitate. Esophageal content is distributed according to density, liquids and fats being in the upper part. In a recumbent position, there will be a reflux to mouth and nose with coughing and suffocation. Aspiration to the lungs of the liquid content and fat is common and provokes pneumonia or bronchopneumonia. This may be a most prominent manifestation of megaesophagus. A correct diagnosis may be suspected based on a previous history of coughing spells and suffocation in recumbency, by the association with hiccups, and by finding pneumonia plus megaesophagus, clear lung fields, and cardiomegaly (Fig. 9).

B. Pulmonary Manifestations Secondary to Cardiopathy

Pulmonary Congestion

In patients with congestive cardiomyopathy, Chagas' disease patients with heart failure may have pulmonary congestion, with enlarged upper lobe veins,

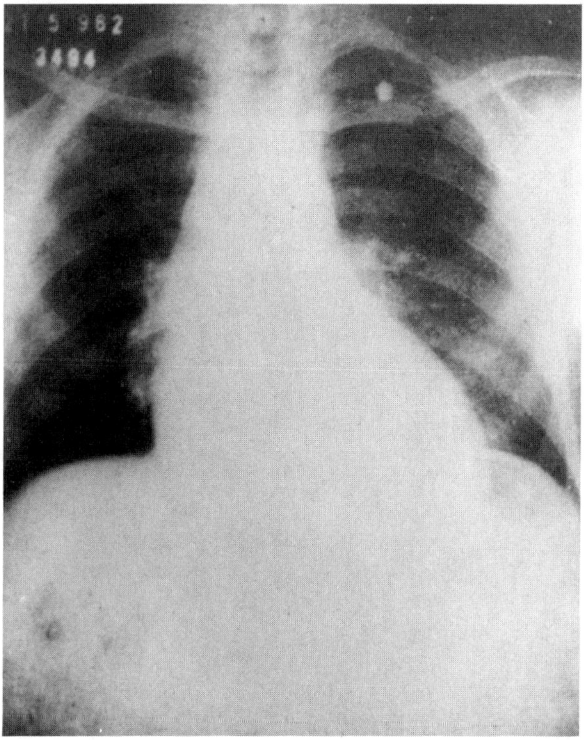

Figure 9 Chest radiograph in Chagas' disease. Note the increase in heart volume and clear lung fields. Abnormal, rightward curved, and deviated right border plus absent air in the gastric fundus are diagnostic of associated megaesophagus. This combination is diagnostic of Chagas' disease with heart and digestive system involvement.

enlarged hilus, Kerley's B lines, and alveolar congestion. The most common feature is, however, clear lung fields even in patients with profound heart failure, probably due to the predominance of right ventricular failure (Fig. 11). Unilateral or bilateral pleural effusion may occur.

Pulmonary Thromboembolism

Pulmonary thromboembolism occurs in about 75% of patients with Chagas' cardiomyopathy, which is about the same incidence as congestive idiopathic cardiomyopathy in the same endemic area, and distinctly higher than the incidence in patients with endomyocardial fibrosis. Pulmonary embolism is more common in patients with cardiac failure (Fig. 12), but it may occur in

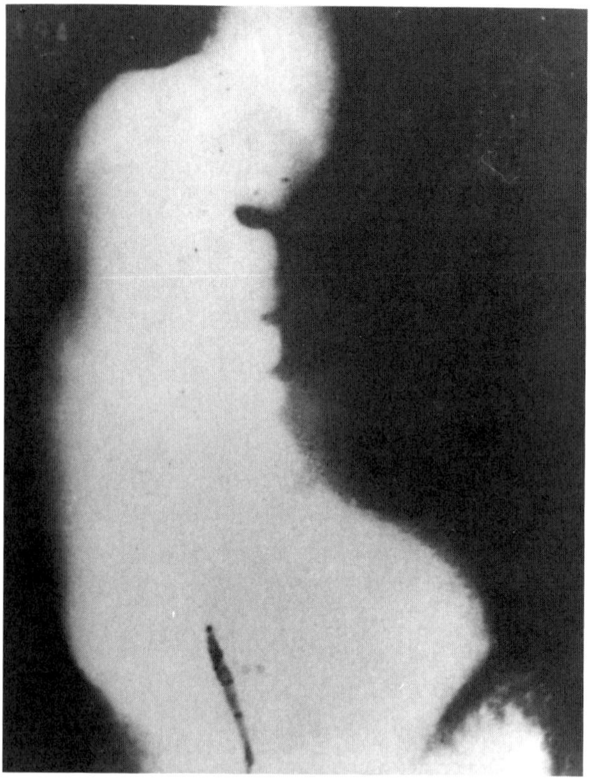

Figure 10 Same patient as Figure 9 with megaesophagus.

patients with cardiomegaly, without signs of decompensation (Fig. 13). Emboli of the legs or abdominal veins may occur, but most frequently they originate from the heart itself.

In a series of 208 autopsies, mural thrombi were found in 56% of cases in the right atrium, 47% in the apex of the left ventricle, 13% in the left atrium and apex of right ventricle, 10% in the left ventricle endocardium, and 1.5% in the right ventricle endocardium. In only 24% of cases were cardiac thrombi not found (Koeberle, 1962). Echocardiography may detect thrombi in the left ventricle, but only very rarely in the atria or right ventricle. Comparison with patients showing idiopathic congestive cardiomyopathy in the same areas shows identical proportions of intrathoracic thrombi. Incidence of thromboembolism is also increased by the frequent occurrence in those patients of atrial fibrillation and localized endocarditis. The clinical spectrum

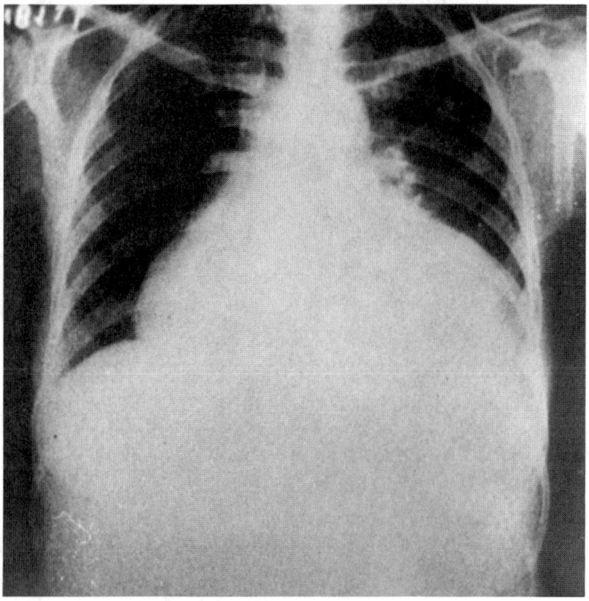

Figure 11 Chest x-ray in Chagas' cardiomyopathy. Note the enlarged heart but clear lung fields.

of thromboembolism is similar to that in other diseases. Chest pain and hemorrhagic sputum are very suggestive. Cardiac failure is aggravated by thromboembolism, and acute cor pulmonale may occur. Sudden death may occur due to massive pulmonary embolism.

Treatment is the same as for embolism in other diseases. Prophylaxis by anticoagulants, antiplatelets, or vena cava umbrella may be tried, but the value of these agents is not proved beyond a reasonable doubt.

C. Pneumonitis and Pulmonary Fibrosis Due to Amiodarone Treatment of Arrhythmias

High-grade arrhythmias are very common in Chagas' heart disease and their best treatment is amiodarone.

Pulmonary toxicity has been described with chronic use of this drug (Rotmensch et al., 1980; Dantas et al., 1983; Moura et al., 1984). Lung complications affect up to 6% of the patients who use the drug on a chronic basis (Martin and Rosenow, 1988). In Chagas' heart disease, in which it is widely used, lung complications are very rare (Lorga and Rassi, (1989) personal

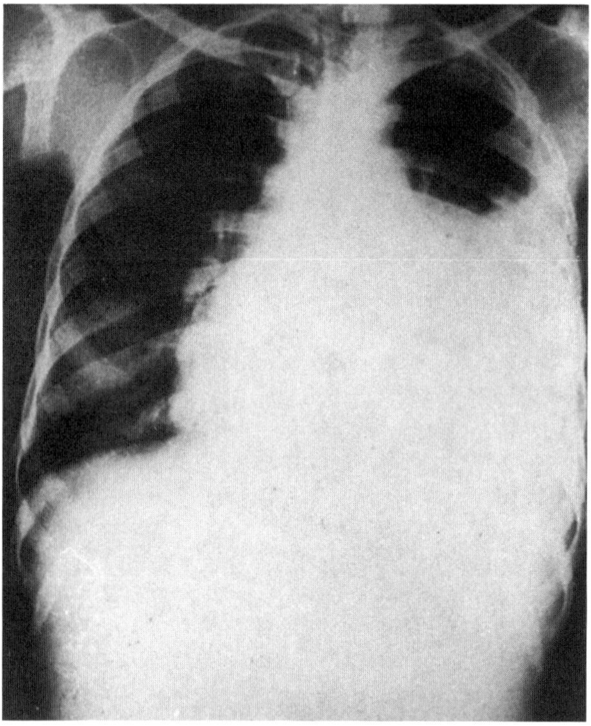

Figure 12 Pulmonary thromboembolism in patients with Chagas' heart disease with cardiomegaly and cardiac failure. Pleural effusion was secondary to massive left-sided thromboembolism. Despite severe failure, note clear right lung fields.

communication) but a few fatal cases have been described (Mady, C. (1989), personal communication).

The clinical course may be subacute, with shortness of breath, nonproductive cough, and weight loss. X-ray shows interstitial infiltrates in both lung lower fields (Fig. 14).

Respiratory functional tests show a restrictive ventilatory insufficiency, with hypoxemia and low carbon monoxide diffusional capacity (Martin and Rosenow, 1988).

In patients with cardiac failure as in Chagas' disease, clinical and x-ray findings due to passive pulmonary congestion may be very similar to those due to amiodarone pneumonitis. In these cases the pulmonary clearance of diethylene triamine pentacetate-Technetium 99m (DTPA-Tc99m) is a very sensitive technique for diagnosis and monitoring of treatment (Terra Filho et al., 1987, 1990; Terra Filho, 1989).

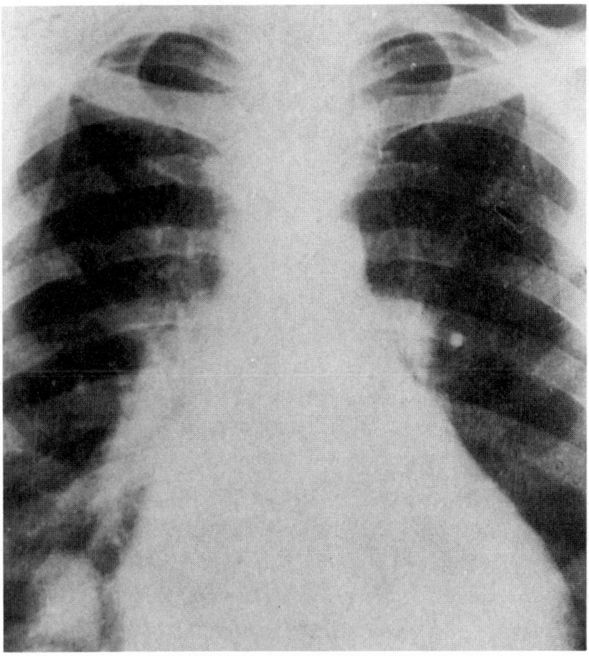

Figure 13 Chagas' heart disease thromboembolism. Despite enlarged heart, the patient was not in cardiac failure.

D. Aspiration Pneumonia

Aspiration pneumonia is a common occurrence in patients with long-standing megaesophagus due to Chagas' disease.

Since most patients with the digestive form of Chagas' disease usually have less severe cardiac manifestations and survive longer, huge esophageal dilatation is quite common, with dysmotility and delayed emptying, achalasia, and aperistalsis, thus favoring the reflux of esophageal contents and pneumonia (Figs. 15, 16).

As with megaesophagus due to other causes, food and liquid content of the esophagus may be aspirated at any time or even during sleep; death may ensue in rare cases.

These pneumonias are more frequently due to anaerobic organisms and may be associated with aerobic mixed flora or gram-negative bacilli. Offending microorganisms are identified as in any other pulmonary anaerobic infections.

Lung abscess, necrotizing pneumonia, and empyema are rarely found as complications of Chagas' disease megaesophagus.

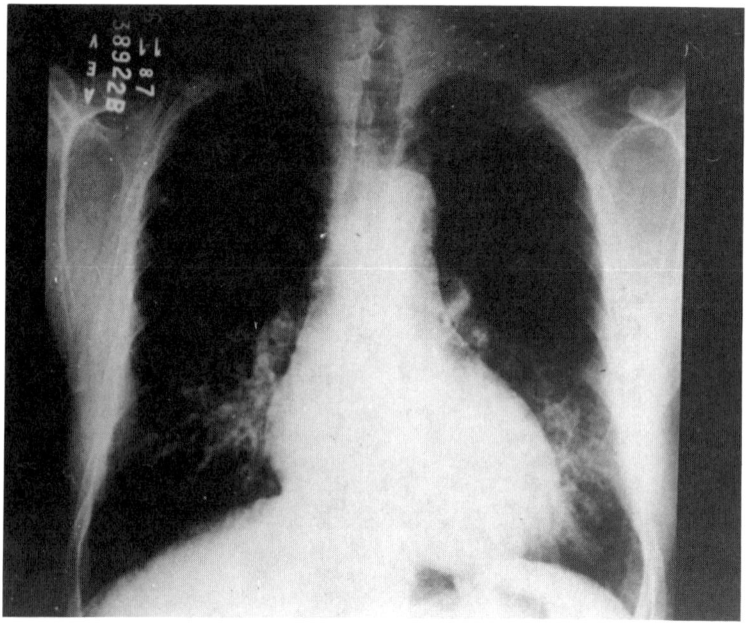

Figure 14 Amiodarone pneumonitis as complication of treatment of high-grade arrhythmia in Chagas' heart disease. Respiratory failure was successfully treated with steroids. (Courtesy of Dr. Charles Mady. Institute do Coraças. University of São Paulo)

E. Chagas' Disease Bronchopathy

The tracheobronchial tree may show morphological and physiological changes in Chagas' disease. Their incidence is not known, not is it known how many patients with acute cases will develop respiratory manifestations (Table 1), or their natural history. It is also possible that different strains of the parasite involve different risks of developing respiratory Chagas' disease, since they have been described almost exclusively in Brazil and Argentina (Estevez et al., 1967).

However, despite their minor clinical significance, the respiratory lesions of Chagas' disease represent a model of disease in which lesions of the autonomic nervous system result in bronchiectasis of a peculiar configuration, more rarely megabronchi and megatrachea, and in functional bronchomotor disturbance, characterized by abnormal sensitivity of the bronchial muscles to vagotonic drugs.

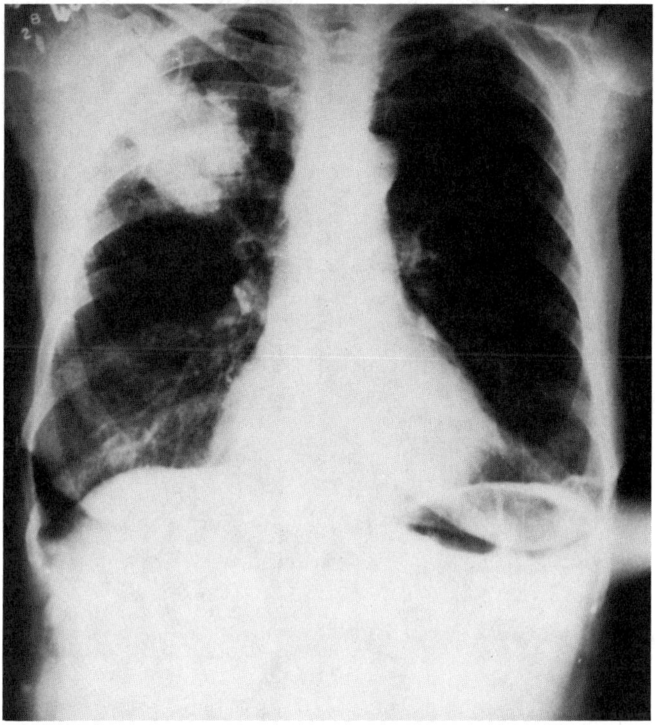

Figure 15 Findings in a 67-year-old woman with achalasic megaesophagus and positive Machado-Guerreiro reaction. Chest x-ray shows opacity in the right upper lobe posterior segment. Gram-negative flora were found in sputum. Penicillin treatment was effective in 7 days.

Bronchiectasis

Similarly to the digestive system, the tracheobronchial tree may be affected uncommonly by lesions that result in dilatation (Koeberle, 1962; Terra Filho, 1982) (Fig. 17).

In 250 autopsied cases of patients with chronic Chagas' disease, Koeberle (1959) found 13 cases of bronchiectasis, compared to 69 cases of megacolon and 61 of megaesophagus.

There were also seven cases of megalogastrium, two of megaduodenum, two of megajejunum, two of megagallbladder and, one of megaureter, as testimony to the more diffuse nature of the disease.

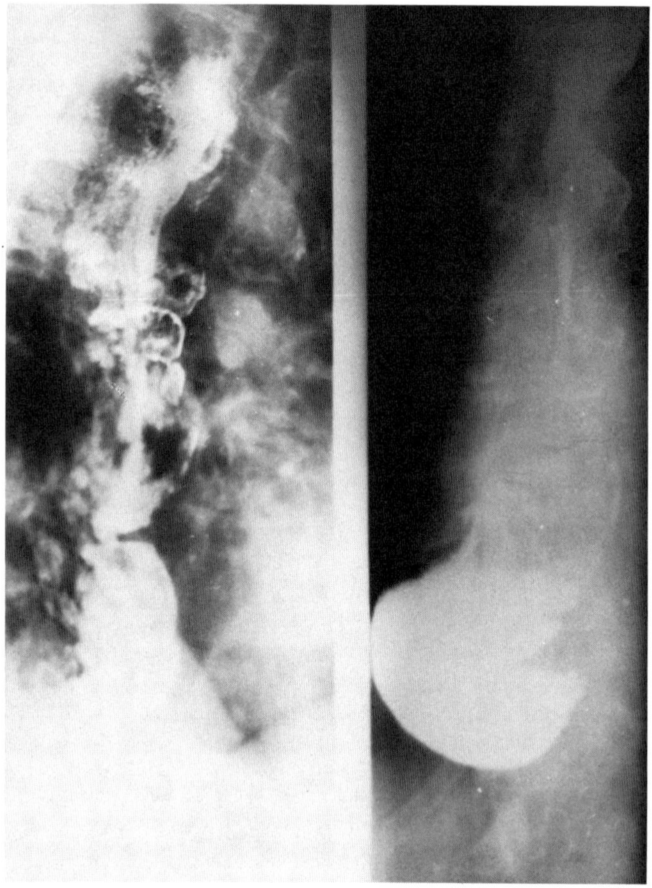

Figure 16 Marked dilatation of esophagus with severe tortuosity (Chagasic dolicomegaesophagus) in the same patient as in Figure 15.

Lima Pereira (1969) autopsied 40 patients, of whom 1 had diffuse dilatation of the tracheobronchial system and 2 had diffuse bronchiectasis without dilatation of the trachea or the main bronchi. In another study, Lima Pereira and Almeida (1979) found a significant enlargement of the tracheal circumference in patients with Chagas' disease, as compared to patients without Chagas' disease.

The pathogenesis is the same as in the digestive system. The fundamental lesion is a denervation of the nervous plexi of the parietal muscle layers (Fig. 18). Koeberle (1959) found 5-65 (average, 30) ganglionic cells in bronchial

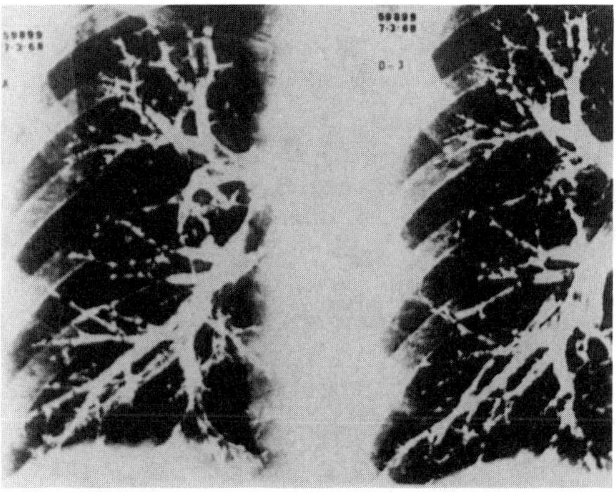

Figure 17 Bronchiectasis in Chagas' disease. A. Bronchogram shows diffuse bronchial dilation, made more evident. D.3: Results 3 min after methacholine injection (courtesy of Dr. Clivis Simao and Prof. Dalmo S. Amorim, Medical Faculty of Ribeirao Preto, Sao Paulo University).

wall muscle of patients with Chagas' disease, compared to an average of 251 cells in controls. In the Chagas' disease patients, the cells also show degenerative changes. The ganglionic cells give rise to bronchoconstricting parasympathetic nervous fibers, and their destruction produces predominance of a relaxed tonus, leading to bronchial dilatation. The localization of those dilations is dependent on intraluminal pressures. Diffuse or localized dilations of the trachea and bronchi have been described (Fig. 17).

Lima Pereira (1969) described several types of lesions. Patients without bronchial dilatation had a variable and inconstant (58 8% of these cases) decrease in ganglionic neurons. When the decrease was slight, there was a proliferation of Schwann's cells, fibrosis, and, rarely, a chronic ganglionitis with lymphocytic infiltration and neuronal atrophy. When denervation was severe, with or without bronchial dilatation, there was chronic ganglionitis and periganglionitis (Fig. 19). Neurons showed nuclear pyknosis, cariolisis, and chromatolisis, but normal-looking neurons were also present. Nervous fibers showed a round cell infiltration and occasional hypotrophy. These findings confirm Koeberle's earlier studies, although the correlation between bronchial dilatation and ganglionic denervation was less marked in Lima Pereira's material. This investigator observed a general correlation between bronchial denervation and other "megas."

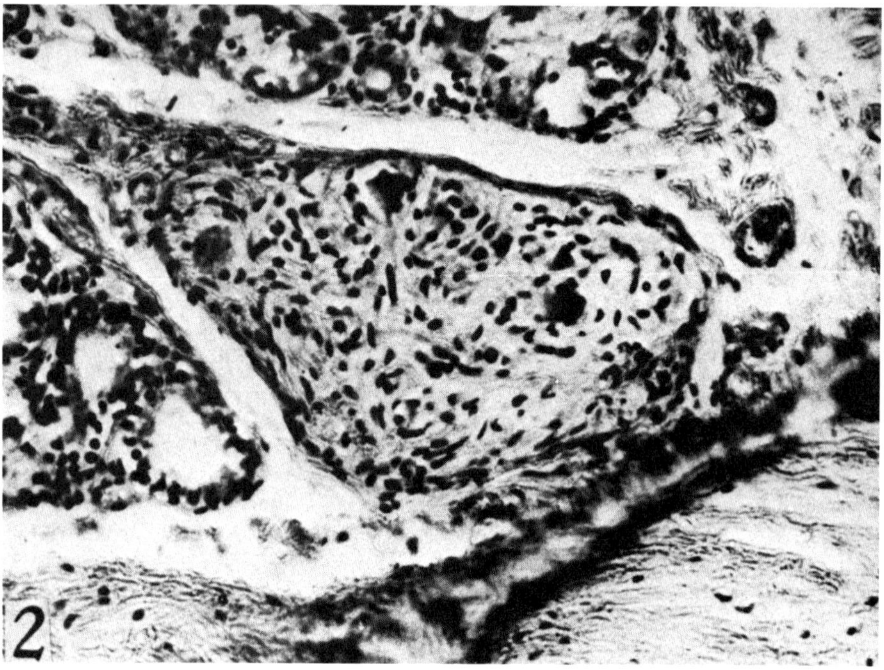

Figure 18 Bronchial wall ganglia with diminished number of neurons and residual nodules (from Lima Pereira, 1969, by courtesy of the author).

It is assumed that denervation is caused by the development and rupture of pseudocysts and destruction of leishmanial forms that have been found in muscular layers of bronchi, as well as in pulmonary arteries and veins (Koeberle, 1959).

The real significance of bronchiectasis in Chagas' disease remains unclear. Clinical manifestations are not prominent among these patients. Other pathological studies do not show an increased incidence of these lesions (Vianna and Vianna, 1978). On the other hand, bronchographic studies confirm Koeberle's findings. Souza Filho (1966) found several changes among 50 patients with a positive Machado-Guerreiro reaction, sometimes involving the whole tracheobronchial tree. The trachea appeared elongated and tortuous in some cases. In others, there was constriction of the bronchi, followed by dilatation. At times, the bronchial walls appeared irregular and fringed.

In another study, Simao (1970) found a 28.6% incidence of bronchial dilatations in 35 patients with Chagus' disease. These dilatations were cylindrical or saccular, and were regionally distributed, with irregular contours.

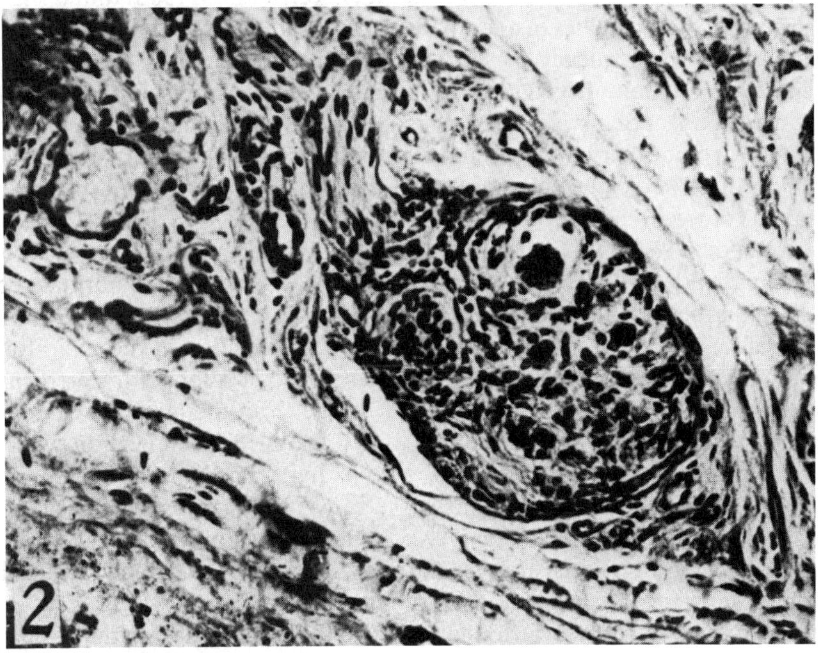

Figure 19 Bronchial wall ganglia with extensive denervation, ganglionitis, and periganglionitis (From Lima Pereira, 1969, by courtesy of the author).

The lack of correlation between bronchographic and some pathological findings might be explained by the observation that mean diameters in the Chagas' disease patients do not appear to differ from those with no bronchiectatic disease (Simao, 1970; Manco and Terra Filho, 1974).

Bronchomotor Functional Disturbances

According to Cannon's principle, the bronchial musculature vagal denervation could generate a bronchomotor hyperreactivity to the appropriate stimuli. This would not necessarily alter basal airway function. However, data on this subject are conflicting.

Manco and colleagues (1976) found a decrease in forced expiratory volume in 1 s (FEV_1) in 19 patients with Chagas' disease compared to 48 controls. Tavares et al. (1981) reported a reduction in maximum expiratory flows at 25 and 50% (V_{max25}, V_{max50}) and of the forced vital capacity (FVC) but not of FEV_1 in 40 patients. Vargas (1979) found no spirometric changes in his

19 patients, and our findings agree with this. Terra Filho (1982) found slight spirometric abnormalities in a few patients, comparable to a group of normals, well within the frequency of spirometric abnormalities to be found in the general population. This author also used more sensitive methods, such as the measurement of airways resistance, dead space ventilation, closing volume, and flow volume curves before and after patients breathed a mixture of 80% helium in 20% oxygen. No consistent abnormalities were found in the 22 patients studied.

Godoy (1964) used a pneumograph to study the amplitude and frequency of 82 patients with a positive Machado-Guerreiro test and 22 normals before and after administration of methacholine. In 40.2% of the patients abnormalities appeared that were consistent with elongation of the expiratory phase and increase in thoracic circumference. Correlation with electrocardiographic abnormalities was not good. Aside from the method, Godoy's study has the shortcoming of having used a methacholine injection, which could have caused digestive effects, such as hypermotility and hypersecretion. These could have had an influence on ventilatory performance.

Manco et al. (1967) studied 11 patients with chronic Chagas' disease and cardiac or digestive symptoms but without cardiac failure and 7 controls using a spirometer and a methacholine spray. A statistically significant decrease in the mean FEV_1 was found (−23.1%) that was absent in the normals (−7.3%). One of the patients had dyspnea during the test, which improved rapidly with a bronchodilator. Later, in a larger study, Manco and colleagues (1976) confirmed these findings.

Using more sensitive, albeit less specific, methods besides spirometry, Terra Filho (1982) studied 22 patients with Chagas' disease, of whom 14 had manifestations of cardiac or digestive involvement, and 17 normals. The studies were done before and after the administration of three increasingly concentrated sprays of methacholine (1.25, −2.50, and 5.00 mg dissolved in 2 ml). No significant differences were found between the two groups. No explanation for the difference between these findings and those of Manco et al. (1967) was found. In a later paper, Terra Filho et al. (1986) attributed these differences to technical factors, such as lack of standardization of pharmacological and spirographic tests. Another possible factor is the difference between sample formation in these studies, since the proportion of patients with cardiac and digestive manifestations was not the same.

Other drugs besides methacholine are being tested. Terra Filho et al. (1986) studied the effects on specific airways conductance (SGaw) of atropine in correlation with cardiac autonomic control, as evaluated by changes in respiratory sinus arrhythmia and heart rate. After the injection of 0.04 mg/kg of atropine sulfate intravenously, cardiac autonomic control seemed to be well preserved in 6 of the 16 patients studied (group I), and in 10 there appeared to be variable degrees of loss of vagal regulation (Group II). There was no difference in airways response in the two groups: SGaw increased by

32.3% in group I and by 31.0% in group II. Changes in expiratory flows were also similar, suggesting that a residual vagal tonus persists in the airways of Chagas' disease patients, even in the presence of cardiac autonomic control impairment. There were no controls in this study.

Calcium blocking agents have not been studied in this context. We had the opportunity to record the effects of nifedipine, a well-known calcium antagonist with completely studied pharmacological effect in asthmatic subjects (Molho et al., 1987), on the spirometric findings of two patients with Chagas' disease (Table 2). Both were male, aged 41 and 45, and, despite caridac involvement, had no signs of heart failure and no past history of bronchopulmonary disease. One also had a megacolon. Both were light smokers. Spirometry was normal before nifedipine: FEV_1 was 97% and 112% of predicted; $FEF_{25\text{-}75}$ was 85% and 76%, V_{max25} was 93% and 131%, and V_{max50} was 80% and 67%, respectively. After nifedipine was administered, (20 mg sublingually), there was no significant change in FEV_1 or V_{max}, but the maximum expiratory flows at low lung volumes fell slightly after 30 and 45 min

Table 2 Results of Spirometry in Two Patients with Chagas' Disease Before and After 20 mg of Sublingual Nifedipine [a]

Patient	J.V.B.			A.O.		
	Pre	45′	60′	Pre	45′	60′
FVC (1)	3.90	4.17	4.17	4.68	4.62	4.77
FEV_1 (1)	3.32	3.39	3.39	4.08	3.82	3.91
FEV_1/FVC	85	81	81	87	82	82
$FEF_{25\text{-}75}$ (1/s)	3.74	3.14	2.92	3.49	3.24	3.01
$FEF_{75\text{-}85}$ (1/s)	1.03	0.64	0.61	1.03	0.92	0.81
V_{max} (1/s)	8.26	10.3	8.5	11.4	9.2	10.0
$V_{max}50$ (1/s)	4.47	3.95	3.34	3.96	3.96	3.98

[a] All results are in absolute values. For percent of predicteds, see text.

Abbreviations: FVC = forced vital capacity;
FEV_1 = forced expiratory volume in 1 s;
$FEF_{25\text{-}75}$ = forced expiratory flow, between 25 and 75% of FVC;
$FEF_{75\text{-}85}$ = forced expiratory flow, between 75 and 85% of FVC;
V_{max} = peak flow;
V_{max50} = maximum expiratory flow, 50% of FVC.

in both cases, and were still reduced after 60 min. The decrease in maximum expiratory flows rates after nifedipine administration has been noted in some asthmatic subjects and the reasons for this are unclear (Henderson et al., 1983).

References

Andrade, Z. A., and Andrade, S. G. (1979). Patologia da Doenca de Chagas. In *Trypanosoma cruzi* e *Doenca de Chagas*. Edited by Z. Brenner and Z. A. Andrade. Editora Guanabara Koogan, Rio de Janeiro.

Amato Neto, V., Doles, J., Rassi, A., Borges, A. P., Rezende, J. M., and Gomes, M. C. O. (1968). Relato de novos casos de transmissao da doenca de Chagas por transfusao de sangue. *Rev. Inst. Med. Trop. S. Paulo* **101**:46.

Bergoglio, R. M. (1972). Perfil clinico de la enfermedad de Chagas postransfusional. *Rev. Med. Cordoba* **60**:123.

Brenner, Z. (1982). Recent developments in the field of Chagas' disease. *Bull. W.H.O.* **60**:463.

Chagas, C. (1909). Nova trypanosomiase humana. *Gaz. Med. Bahia* **40**:433.

Coura, J. R., Nogueira, E. S., and da Silva, J. R. (1966). Indices de transmissao da doenca de Chagas por transfusao de sangue de doadores na fase cronica da doenca. *O Hospital* **69**:991.

Dantas, J. C., Pinheiro Neto, J., and Sampaio, W. P. (1983). Pneumonia intersticial associada ao uso de amiodarona. Relato de um caso. *Arq. Bras. Cardiol.* **40**:406.

Dias, J. C. P. (1982). Docena de Chagas em Bambui, Minas Gerais, Brasil. Estudo clinico-epidemiologico a partir da fase aguda, entre 1940 e 1982. Tese, Fac. Med. da Universidade Federal de Minas Gerais, Belo Horizon te, Brasil.

Estevez, J. A., Isoardi, O., Kuschnir, E., Montenegro, C. I., and Podio, R. B. (1967). Studio de la fauncion pulmonar en la cardiopatia chagasica cronica. I. En reposo y despues de la administracion de drogas simpatico y para simpaticomimeticas. *Arq. Bras. Cardiol.* **20**:79.

Godoy, R. A. (1964). Hipersensibilidade da musculatura bronquica a metacolina na forma cronica da molestia de Chagas. *Rev. Goiana Med.* **10**: 91.

Goldsmith, R. S., Narate, R. J., Zarate, L. G., Kagan, I., and Jacobson, L. B. (1985). Clinical and epidemiologic studies of Chagas' disease in rural communities in Oxaca State and a seven-year follow up. I. Cerro del Aire. *Bull. Pan Am. Health Organ.* **19**:120.

Henderson, A. F., Heaton, R. W., Dunlop, L. S., and Costello, J. F. (1983). Effects of nifedipine on antigen-induced bronchoconstriction. *Am. Rev. Respir. Dis.* **127**:549-553.

Kagan, I., Norman, L., and Allain, D. (1966). Studies on *Trypanosoma cruzi* isolated in the United States: a review. *Rev. Biol. Trop.* **14**:55.

Kirchoff, L. V., and Neva, F. A. (1985). Chagas' disease in Latin American immigrants. *J.A.M.A.* **254**:3058.

Kirchoff, L. V., Gam, A., and Gillam, F. C. (1987). American trypanosomiasis (Chagas' disease) in Central American immigrants. *Am. J. Med.* **82**:915.

Koeberle, F. (1959). Chagas-bronchiektasie. *Tropenmed. Parasitol.* **10**:304.

Koeberle, F. (1962). Patologia da Molestia de Chagas. *Med. Cardiol.* **1**:73.

Laranja, F. S., Dias, E., Nobrega, G., and Miranda, A. (1956). Chagas' disease: a clinical epidemiologic and pathological study. *Circulation* **14**:1035.

Lima Pereira, F. E. (1969). Contribution a l'étude des lesions du systéme nerveux autonome des bronches principales dans les formes chroniques de la maladie de Chagas (Trypanosomiase Americaine). **25**:887-905.

Lima Pereira, F. E., and Almeida, H. O. (1979). Variacoes da circumferencia da traqueia em chagasicos cronicos. *Rev. Assoc. Med. Bras.* **25**:197-198.

Maekelt, G. A. (1973). Aspectos seroepidemiologicos de la enfermedad de Chagas en Venezuela. *Arch. Venez. Med. Trop. Paras. Med.* **5**:95.

Manco, J. C., and Terra Filho, J. (1984). Comprometimento das vias aereas na forma cronica da doenca de Chagas. *J. Pneumol.* **10**:243-247.

Manco, J. C., Godoy, R. A., Gallo, L., Jr., and Amorim, D. S. (1967). Resposta ventilatoria a metacolina na forma cronica da doenca de Chagas. Resultados preliminares de estudo espirografico. *Arq. Bras. Cardiol.* **20**:175.

Manco, J. C., Gallo, L., Jr., and Amorim, D. S. (1976). Alteracoes funcionais pulmonares na Molestida de Chagas. Estudo espirografico. *Arq. Bras. Cardiol.* **29** (Supl. 1):132.

Martin, W. J. II, and Rosenow, E. C. III (1988). Amiodarone pulmonary toxicity. Recognition and pathogenesis—parts I and II. *Chest* **93**:1067, **92**:1242.

Molho, J., Guzman, C. K., Katz, I., Lidgi, M., and Chaniac, A. (1987). Nifedipine in asthma. Dose-related effect on resting bronchial tone. **91**:667-670.

Moura, A., Choma, L., and Bendlach, L. I. (1984). Amiodarona e infiltrado pulmonar alveolo-intersticial difuso. Relato de um caso. *Arq. Bras. Cardiol.* **42**:213.

Rassi, A., and Rezende, J. M. (1975). Prevention of transmission of T. cruzi by blood transfusion. In *New Approaches to Trypanosomiasis Research* (Scientific Publication no 318) Washington, Pan American Health Organization, pp. 273-278.
Romana, C. (1935). Acerca de un sintoma inicial de valor para el diagnostico de forma aguda de la Enfermedad de Chagas. La conjunctivitis esquizotripanosica unilateral (Hipotesis sobre puerta de entrada conjuntival de la enfermedad). *Public Mepra* **22**(16):28.
Rotmensch, H. H., Liron, M., Tupilski, M., and Raniado, S. (1980). Possible association of pneumonitis with amiodarone therapy. *Am. Heart J.* **100**:412.
Schiffler, R. J., Mansur, G. P., Navin, T. R., and Khanchit, L. (1984). Indigenous Chagas' disease (American Trypanosomiasis) in California. *J.A.M.A.* **251**:2983.
Schmunis, G. A. (1984). Chagas' disease and blood transfusion. In *Infection Immunity and Blood Transfusion.* Edited by R. Y. Dodd and L. F. Barker. New York, Alan R. Liss, pp. 127-145.
Schmunis, G. A., and Szarfman, A. (1977). La enfermedad de Chagas congenita. *Medicina* (B. Aires) **37**:47.
Simao, C. (1970). Estudo da broncropatia chagasica atraves da bronchografia associada a prova da metacolina. Tese, Faculdade de Medicina de Ribeirao Preto, Universidade de Sao Paulo.
Souza Filho, C. A. (1966). Estudo radiologico da bronclopatia chagasica (nota previa). *Rev. Paul. Med.* **68**:133.
Tavares, P., Vianna, L. G., and Oliveira, S. M. (1981). Maximal expiratory flow-volume curve in chronic chagasic patients with megaesophagus with or without megacolon. *J. Pneumol.* **7**:67.
Terra Filho, J. (1982). Estudo funcional das vias aereas em individuos portadores da forma cronica da Molestia de Chagas. Tese Faculdade de Medicina de Ribeirao Preto, Universidade de Sao Paulo.
Terra Filho, M. (1989). Estudo com radioaerossol de DTPA-Tecnecio 99m em pacientes portadores de pneumopatia por amiodarona. Ph. Thesis, University of Sao Paulo.
Terra Filho, J., Gallo, L., Jr., Macliel, B. C. Marin Neto, J. A., Manco, J. C. (1986). Estudo functional das vias aereas na forma cronica da Doenca de chagas. **12**:91-100.
Terra Filho, M., Meneguetti, J. C., Cuckier, A., Camargo, E. E., Fliss, E., Soares, J. Jr., Romeiro-Neto, M., and Vargas, F. S. (1987). Estudo com radioaerossol de DTPA- Tecnelio 99m em pacientes portadores de pneumopatia por amiodarona. Resultados preliminares. *Rev. Hosp. Clin. Fac. Med. S. Paulo* **42**:78.

Terra Filho, M., Vargas, F. S., Cuckier, A., Teixeira, L. R., Carvalho Pinto, R. M., and Pileggi, F. (1990). Amiodarone induced pneumonitis. *Arq. Bras. Cardiol.*, in press.

Vargas, F. S. (1979). Mecanica respiratoria em pacientes chagasicos sem insuficiencia cardiaca. *Dissertation*, Faculdade de Medicina, Universidade de Sao Paulo.

Vianna, L. G., and Vianna, A. L. (1978). Broncoectasia e pneumonia chagasica. *Rev. Inst. Med. Trop. S. Paulo* **20**:64-68.

Woody, N. C., and Woody, H. B. (1955). American trypanosomiasis (Chagas' disease). First indigenous case in the United States. *J.A.M.A.* **159**:676.

Zeledon, R. (1974). Epidemiology, modes of transmission and reservoir hosts of Chagas' disease. In *Trypanosomiasis and Leishmaniasis with Special Reference to Chagas' disease.* Ciba Found. Symp. 20 (new series). Excerpta Medica, pp. 51-77.

10

Hydatid Disease of the Lung
Diagnosis and Management

SURRENDER N. DHAR

Chest Disease Hospital
Kashmir, India

CHAND WATTAL

Sheri Kashmir Institute of
Medical Sciences
Kashmir, India

I. Incidence and Natural History

Hydatid disease in humans is caused by the larval stage of *Echinococcus granulosus* (dog tapeworm) or *E. multilocularis*, which belongs to the family Taenidae in the order Cyclophyllidia of cestodes. *Echinococcus* infection is a cyclozoonosis, that is, a parasitic disease that humans share with other vertebrates but that requires at least one other vertebrate host to complete its cycle (Redford, 1984).

Although hydatid disease is world wide in its distribution, it is most commonly found in countries where sheep and cattle raising constitute important industries. It is prevalent in temperate as well as tropical climates. The disease occurs in Europe except Scandinavia, northern and eastern Africa, the Middle East, much of Canada and Australasia, and southern and western South America (Redford, 1984; Matossian et al., 1977; Imari, 1962; Tusckka, 1969; Rausch, 1960; Schills, 1960). *E. multilocularis* is common in North America, the Soviet Union, Japan, parts of central Europe, and Turkey (Matossian et al., 1977; Tusckka, 1969; Rausch, 1960). Schills (1960) has summarized the worldwide distribution of *E. granulosus.*

The life cycle of the worm is spent in two hosts. The definitive hosts are dog, wolf, fox, and jackal. The adult worm lives in the small intestine of these animals, who discharge a large number of eggs in their feces. These are taken up in turn by the intermediate hosts: sheep, pigs, horses, goats, and humans. Humans are an accidental host. The larvae develop in these animals and give rise to the echinococcal cyst. Humans are usually infected by the intimate handling of an infected dog, especially by children.

The liver (60-70%) and the lungs (20-30%) are the most frequently involved organs (Chatterjee, 1980; Redford, 1984; Tusckka, 1969; Crofton and Douglas, 1961).

After having settled down in tissue, the embryo generates an active cellular reaction consisting of monocytes, macrophages, giant cells, and eosinophils. This defensive reaction destroys a large number of parasites. The embryos that escape destruction develop into hydatid cysts. The cellular reaction gradually disappears followed by the appearance of fibroblasts that give rise to fibrous tissue. This fibrous layer around the cyst, known as the pericyst, may become sclerosed or calcified and the parasite within, owing to lack of nutrition, may die or degenerate. Rate of growth is slow, taking about 3 months to reach 4-5 mm in diameter and 5-6 months to become 20 mm. In *E. multilocularis* the cyst is an alveolar or honeycombed structure. A benign sylvatic form of the disease, in which the usual invasive character is lacking, has been reported from indigenous Alaskans (Wilson et al., 1968).

II. Diagnosis

Diagnosis is relatively easy if the typical radiological features are present. However, a high degree of suspicion is necessary when a patient is seen with atypical clinical and radiographic presentations. Hydatid disease should be included in the differential diagnosis of any localized obscure pulmonary lesion occurring in a person in an endemic area. Apart from the clinical picture, radiological and immunological features form the basis of the diagnosis.

A. Clinical Diagnosis

No clinical features are characteristic of lung hydatid cyst, except in an unusual situation in which a patient has expectorated the contents of a cyst and is able to describe these to the doctor. The slimy membranous fluid with a salty taste is diagnostic of hydatid fluid. Hemoptysis is uncommon.

Humans are remarkably tolerent to the organism and wall off the cyst, which calcifies in nearly 3.5% of cases (Chatterjee, 1980; Redford, 1984). Many lesions are noted only at autopsy. There is a latent period of 1-2 years before the cysts can be detected, but this can extend up to 50 years. There is no apparent sex preponderance.

Symptoms and signs due to echinococcosis arise due either to compression of the surrounding tissues where the worm is lodged or the complications such as rupture and infection in the cyst itself. Large cysts (Fig. 1) occupying the whole hemithorax maybe found in the lung mainly because the surrounding tissue yields to pressure. The cyst may erode bronchi, blood vessels, mediastinal structures, or even the chest wall (Chatterjee, 1980; Redford, 1984; Crofton and Douglas, 1961; Le Roux, 1972). Rupture into the pleural cavity may lead to pleural effusion and hydropneumothorax (Kaul et al., 1981; Dhar and Kaul, 1988) or even tension pneumothorax (Baker and Al Omeri, 1969; Comellan et al., 1979). Pulmonary cyst may be found accidentally when a chest roentgenogram is taken for evaluation of an unrelated illness (Crofton and Douglas, 1961). More than 90% of our patients were asymptomatic. The symptoms usually are related to the presence of the

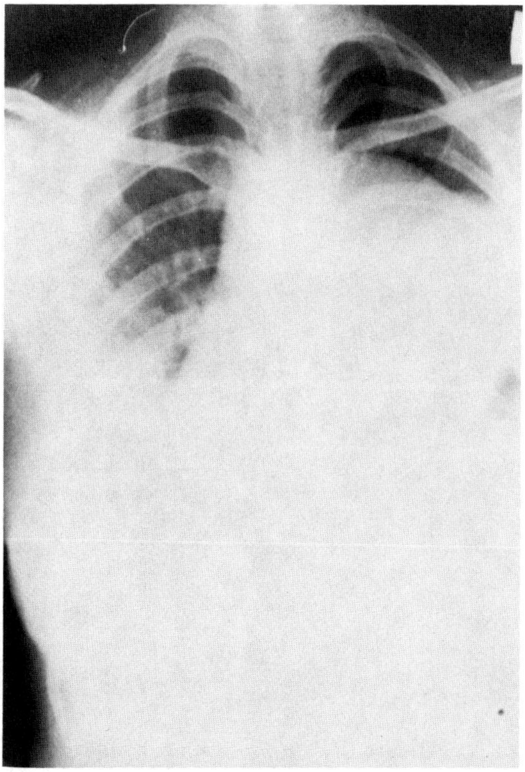

Figure 1 Bilateral hydatid cysts in a young woman. Patient was successfully operated on both sides.

cyst (Kaul et al., 1981; Dhar and Kaul, 1988). The benign salvatic form usually is asymptomatic and is discovered in association with other diseases such as tuberculosis (Wilson et al., 1968).

Cough with or without hemoptysis occurs in 60% of patients. The other symptoms are related to the presence of a complication such as consolidation, lung abscess, pyopneumothorax, or tension pyopneumothorax. Pyopneumothorax occurs in up to 15% of complicated cases (Crofton and Douglas, 1961). In our series of 80 patients seen over a period of 4 years (1979-1983), 8 presented with lung abscess, 3 with undiagnosed lung infiltrate, and 6 with consolidations. Eight patients had pleural involvement. Mediastinal

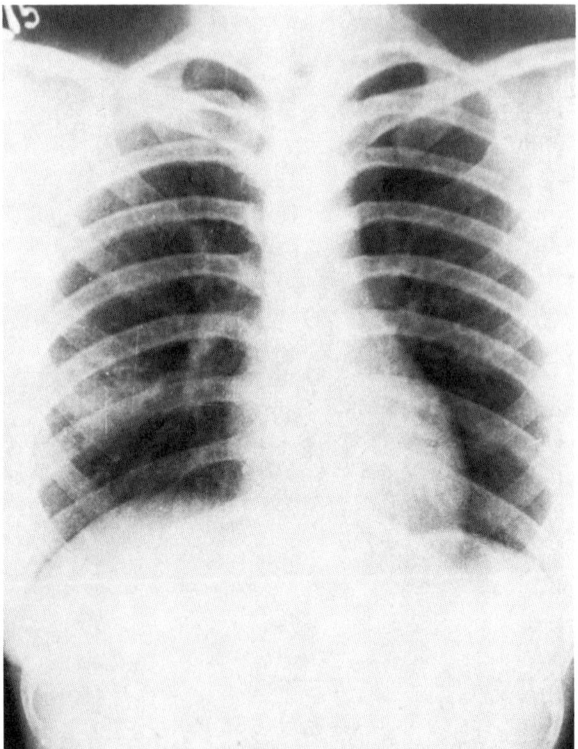

a

Figure 2 Patch of pneumonitis in right lower zone. a. The patch of pneumonitis turned into a round area with a small breakdown. b. The half-empty lung abscess from the patch of consolidation seen in a. After complete healing, the evolutionary cycle was repeated again.

hydatid cyst is rare, and the diagnosis is established only on thoracotomy (Kaul et al., 1981). Twenty-five percent of the lung lesions are bilateral. There is an increased incidence of right lung involvement, with a preponderance in the right lower lobe (Baker and Al Omeri, 1969). Upper lobe involvement occurred in about 30% of cases.

The presentation of the disease in endemic areas may vary (Chatterjee, 1980; Redford, 1984; Imari, 1962). Localized pulmonary opacities of different sizes and shapes may defy diagnosis. A persistent pneumonitis or lung abscess should raise suspicions (Fig. 2). Pain due to destruction of the first rib or even Horner's syndrome may occur due to upper lobe involvement (Omeri and Wasif, 1984; Singh et al., 1983).

Spontaneous cure with coughing out of the hydatid membrane is reported occasionally (Crofton and Douglas, 1961). We encountered such a phenomenon in at least three cases (Fig. 3). In yet another case of multiple hydatid cysts, one of the hydatids was removed surgically and one on the other side was coughed out 4 months later.

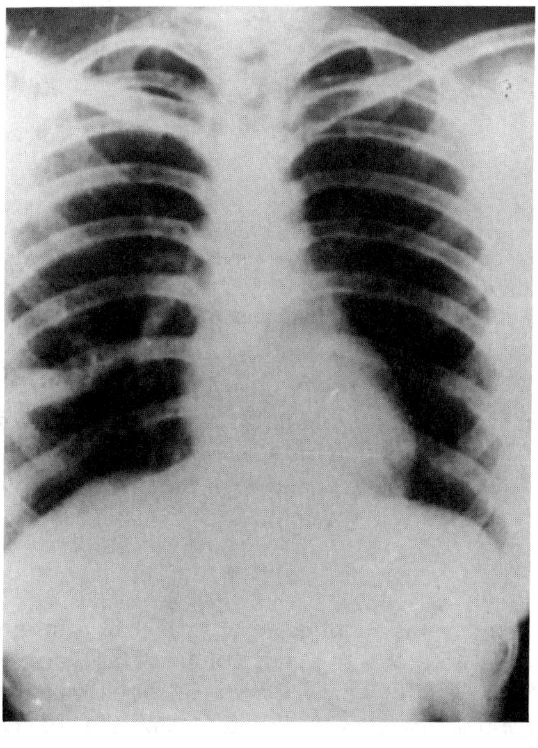

b

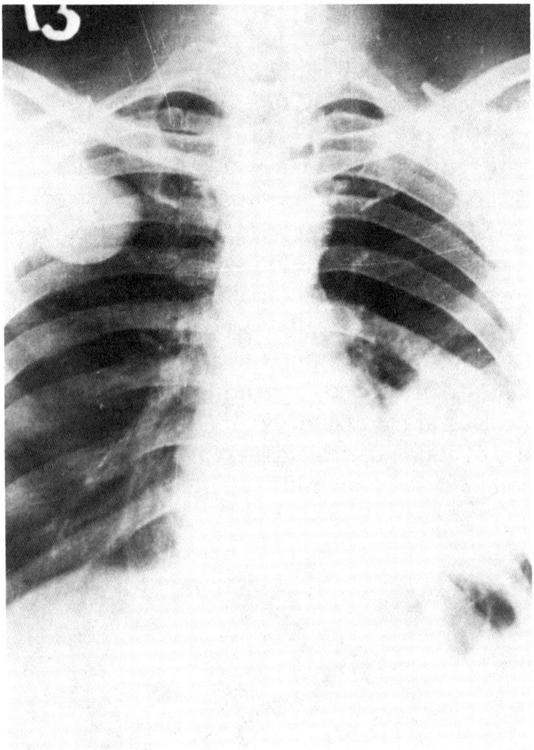

a

Figure 3 Bilateral cysts (reproduced by courtesy of *Seminars in Respiratory Medicine*, New York, Thieme Medical Publishers, 1988). a. One of the cysts is surgically removed, leaving a scar and surrounding area of pneumonitis.

The residual space after the hydatid has been coughed out may leave a patch of bronchiectasis that may subsequently lead to infection and bleeding. Postoperative complications and sequelae are more often encountered when the cysts are large and multiple.

Case 1

A 55-year-old woman was admitted with occasional pain in the right side of her chest along with productive cough of 6 months' duration, fever for 3 months, and hemoptysis for 2 days. On examination the patient had normal vital signs. The respiratory rate was 22/min. Examination of chest showed the right base to be dull with feeble breath sounds. There was no pleural friction

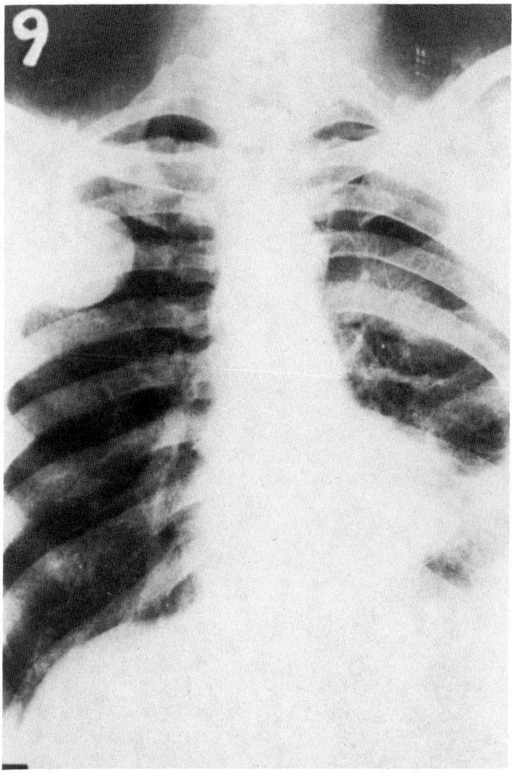

b

rub. Cardiovascular and other systems were normal. A chest roentgenogram showed pleural effusion on the right side (Fig. 4). Attempts at needle aspiration failed three times. A course of broad-spectrum antibiotics was given for 2 weeks. A repeat chest roentgenogram did not reveal any change. Aspiration with a wide-bore needle yielded a few drops of thick pus. Smear examination did not show AFB or any other organism. She underwent rib resection with a presumptive diagnosis of thick empyema. After manipulation, daughter cysts came out and a liver cyst communicating with pleural space through the diaphragm was observed. A more complete surgical resection and closing of the diaphragmatic opening was performed.

Case 2

A 40-year-old woman presented with a history of right lower chest pain, fever, cough, and occasional hemoptysis of 3 months' duration.

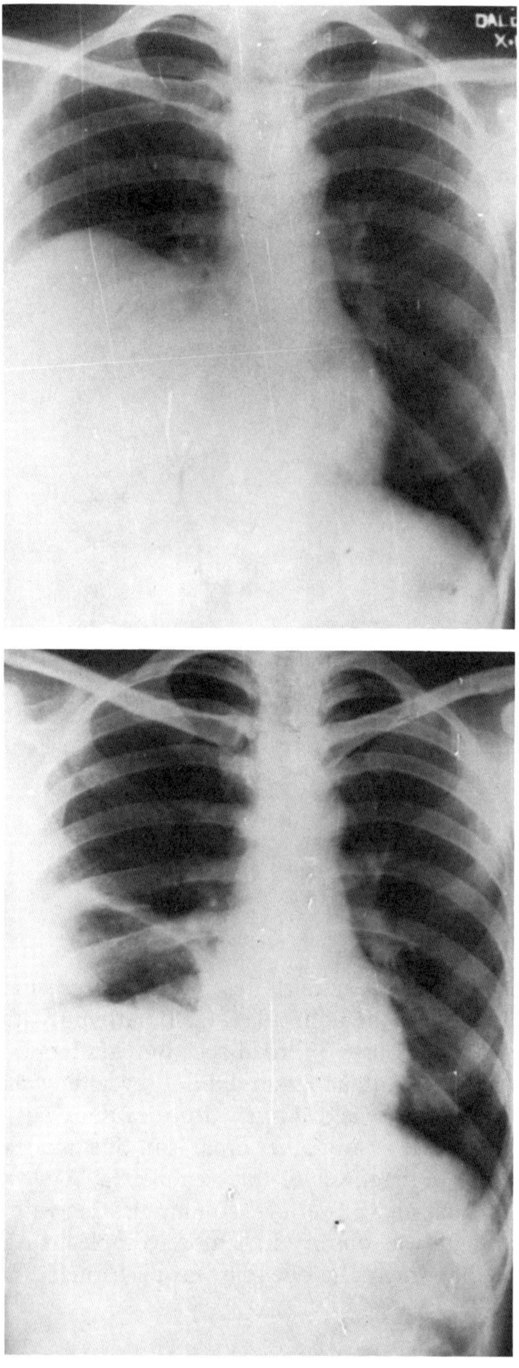

a

b

Figure 4 Intra-abdominal hydatid cyst rupturing into the lungs and simulating a pleural effusion.

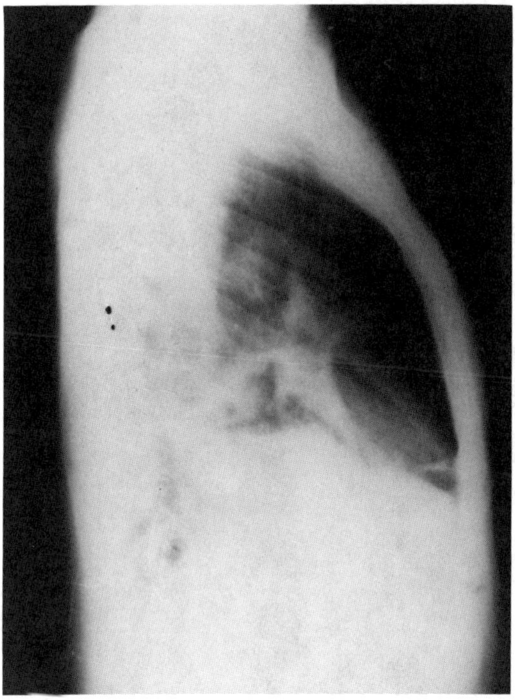

c

There was an exaggeration of pain on deep respiration. The patient was slightly pale and febrile with a 3 cm hepatomegaly. Chest examination showed percussion dullness from the fourth space downwards, which merged with the hepatic dullness. A chest x-ray showed a cyst in the right lower lobe (Fig. 5). Ultrasound examination of the liver showed normal findings. She had mild anemia and a raised erythrocyte sedimentation rate. Casoni's intradermal test was negative. A course of antibiotics for 1 week improved her general condition. She left the hospital against medical advice. Three months later, however, she developed hemoptysis and shock. At this time she also coughed up small cysts with blood. The appearance of the membrane was characteristic. She was managed conservatively. Chest x-ray at this time revealed a half-empty chest (Fig. 5). She was given preoperative Albendazole for 3 weeks, followed by surgical removal of the cyst.

B. Radiological Diagnosis

The pulmonary diagnosis can usually be made by x-rays that show well-defined solitary or multiple lesions (LeRoux, 1972; Kaul et al., 1981). The

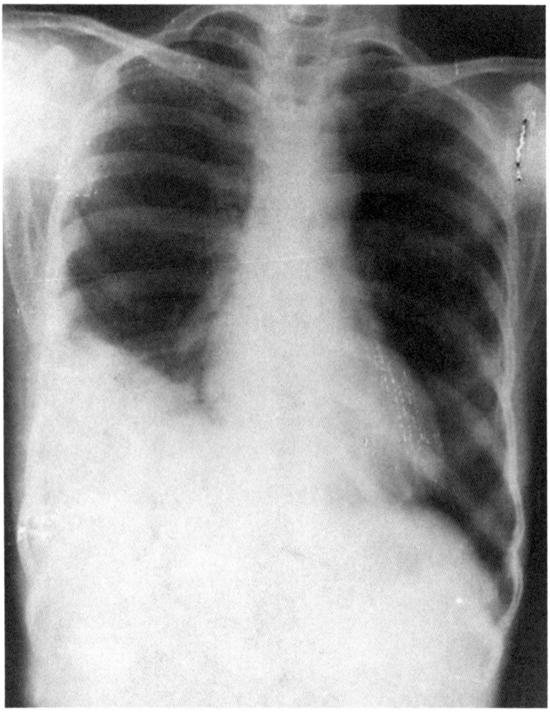

Figure 5 Huge cyst in right lower zone. Posteroanterior view of the same cyst when half empty through spontaneous expectoration of cyst contents.

lesions are usually round but are occasionally associated with an area of pneumonitis or atelectasis (Fig. 6). When the parasite dies, the lesion may calcify. Polycystic lesions of *E. multilocularis* infections may show budding of cyst walls.

A few radiographic signs are specific and diagnostic; however, these occur infrequently. An air leak between the adventitious and the laminated membranes may give rise to a "crescent," "double arch" (Fig. 7), or "water lily" (Fig. 8) appearance (Chatterjee, 1980; Redford, 1984; Crofton and Douglas, 1961). Thin- and thick-walled cavities need to be differented from other pulmonary abscesses, although a clear "hair line" edge indicates that the underlying lesion is hydatid disease. In nearly one-quarter of cases pleural reaction may occur and it may occasionally be difficult to differentiate from a pleural effusion (Redford, 1984; Crofton and Douglas, 1961).

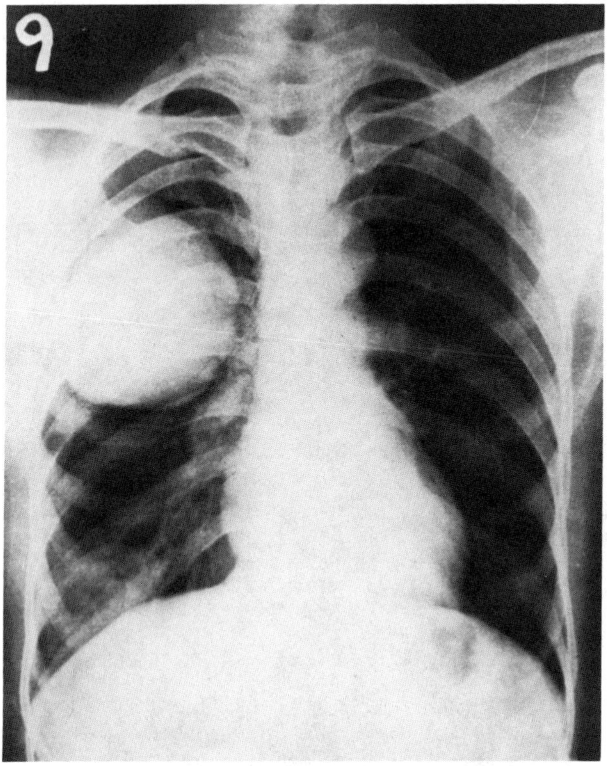

Figure 6 Solitary hydatid cyst in the right lower zone with an area of pneumonitis.

Next to radiography, computed tomography and ultrasound are helpful in establishing the diagnosis of hydatids (Redford, 1984; Crofton and Douglas, 1961). These methods are especially useful in cases of liver and other organ involvement. We have used ultrasound examination to exclude liver hydatid even when the liver was not enlarged.

Sonography accurately demonstrates cysts that may be single or multiple, uni- or multilocular, and thin or thick walled (Earnest et al., 1983). Daughter cysts, either single or multiple, initially present as localized thickening of the cyst wall or small, solid echogenic areas on sonography. Separation of the laminated membrane from the pericyst may produce a floating membrane appearance. Infected pulmonary cysts are usually poorly defined and may contain internal echoes and air and air-fluid levels (Dusaj et al., 1988). Echocardiography is useful for diagnosing cardiac hydatid. It may even show the pathognomonic daughter cyst in the brood capsule (Earnest et al., 1983).

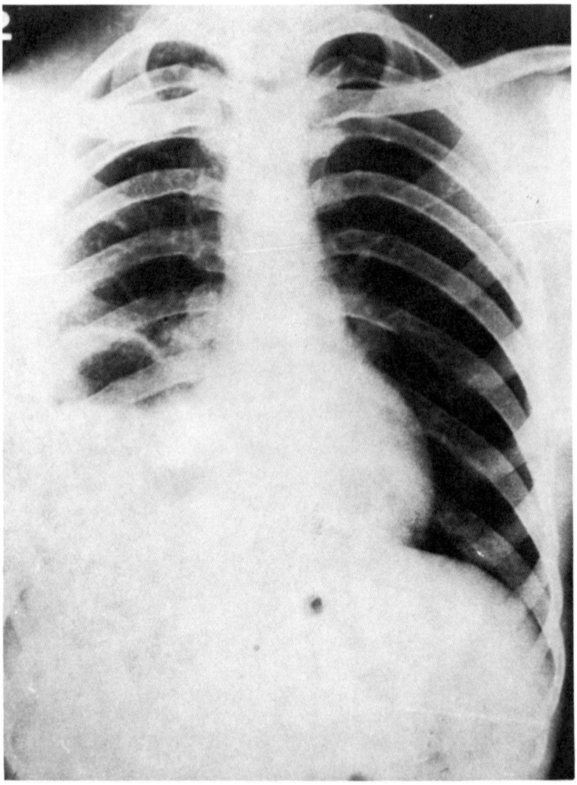

Figure 7 Double arch sign (reproduced by courtesy of *Seminars in Respiratory Medicine*, New York, Thieme Medical Publishers, 1988).

C. Immunodiagnosis

Considerable progress has been made in the field of immunodiagnosis of hydatid disease, particularly lung echinococcosis. It is known that pulmonary cyst patients are poor reactors (Chematai et al., 1981; Mahajan et al., 1976; Kagan, 1968; Todorov et al., 1979a; Pini et al., 1983; Theofilopoulos and Dixon, 1980). Some believe that the permeation of immunocompetent cells in pulmonary cysts is limited because of the formation of a tougher cyst germinal membranes. This allows only minimal antigenic leak from the cyst to the general circulation, resulting in impaired antibody production (Richard-Lenoble et al., 1978). Others (Pini et al., 1983; Theofilopoulos and Dixon, 1980; Chematai et al., 1981) believe that the incidence of formation of circulating immune complexes is much higher in lung hydatid disease but it somehow interferes with the specific immunoglobulin estimation.

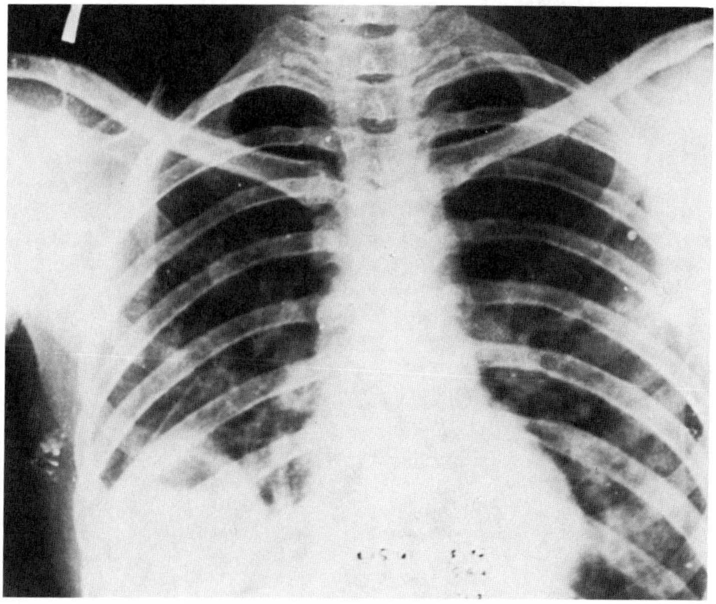

Figure 8 The water-lily sign (adapted from *Seminars in Respiratory Medicine*, New York, Thieme Medical Publishers, 1988).

The immunodiagnosis of hydatid disease is currently based on the detection of anti-*Echinococcus* antibodies. Various workers have used different types of antigens and detecting systems (Craig et al., 1988). Casoni's intradermal test is still being performed but the test is rapidly becoming obsolete (Todorov et al., 1979a,b).

In our experience, only 50% of pulmonary cases gave a positive response to Casoni's test. The overall sensitivity of Casoni's test is about 65%. It does detect about 71% of liver hydatid cases, but the percentage of false-positive results in our hands was about 16% (Table 1; Wattal et al., 1986a). The World Health Organization (1979) suggests that the test be replaced by a serological test that detects hydatid-specific IgE antibodies. It has been reported that hydatid-specific IgE-enzyme-linked immunosorbent assay (ELISA) does not correlate with Casoni's intradermal test. Although specific IgE estimation was 87% sensitive, the false-positive rate was as high as 57.14% because of its cross reaction with cases of ascariasis and taeniasis (Table 2; Wattal et al., 1988). Other workers have also found that detection of parasite-specific IgE by ELISA is less sensitive than either intradermal tests or in vitro basophil histamine release (Hamilton et al., 1981; Lunde and Ottesen, 1980). In Turkana, 100 hydatid-proved cases were investigated by Chematai and

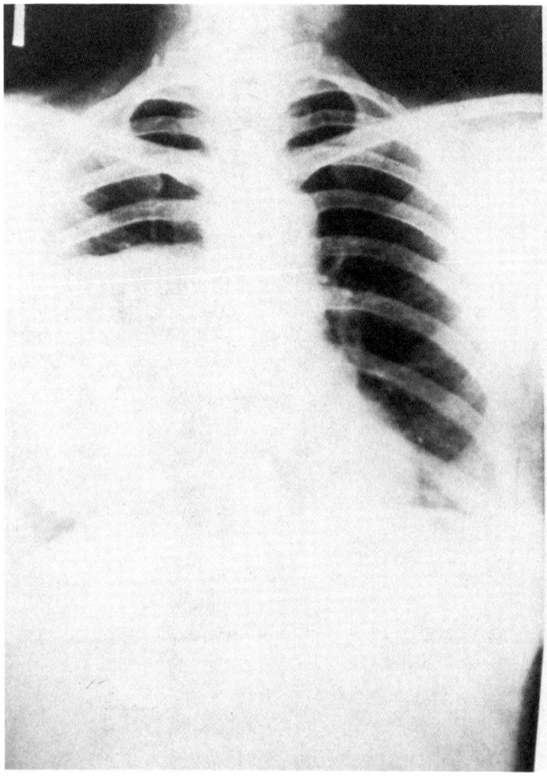

a

Figure 9 Large hydatid cyst (reproduced by courtesy of *Seminars in Respiratory Medicine*, New York, Thieme Medical Publishers, 1988). a. Cyst seen as double cyst in lateral view (reproduced by courtesy of *Seminars in Respiratory Medicine*, New York, Thieme Medical Publishers, 1988).

co-workers (1981; Okelo and Chematai, 1981; Okelo and Kyobe, 1981) using immunoelectrophoresis (IEP) and double diffusion gel (DD) precipitin tests to detect antibodies to arc 5 antigen, which was the most specific test available at that time. They also used indirect hemagglutination (IHA) test, Latex agglutination (LA), and complement fixation test (CFT). Although highly specific, decreased sensitivity is a recognized problem for the arc 5-IEP and DD-5 tests and up to 35% of pulmonary hydatid-proved cases may be arc-5 negative. CFT and LA tests are more likely to give nonspecific and false-positive reactions (Dighero and Bradstreet, 1979; Rickard, 1984). The IHA test is still useful but has poor reproducibility (Mahajan et al., 1976). Using

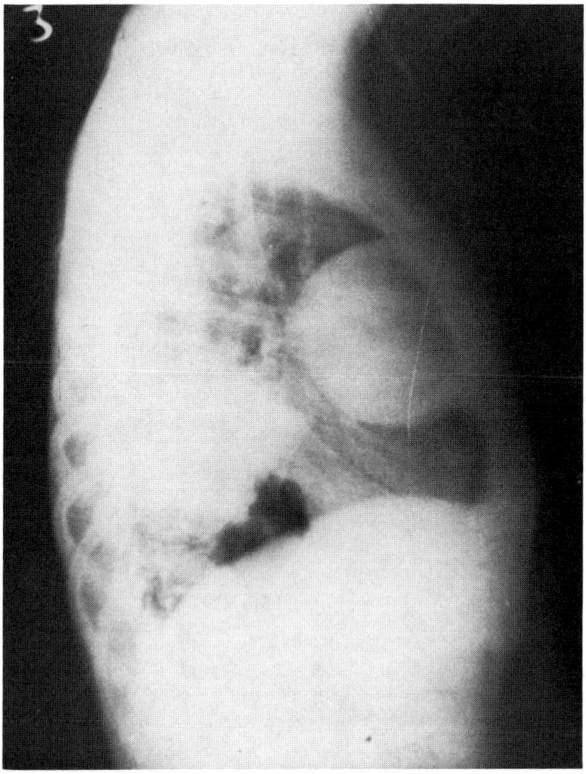

b

Table 1 Immunological Profile of 46 Surgically Proven Cases of Hydatid Disease

Cyst Localization	No. of Cases Tested	No. (%) of Cases Positive in Casoni's Test	No. (%) of Cases Positive in IHA[a]	No. (%) of Cases Positive in IFA[b]	No. (%) of Cases Positive in IgG ELISA[c]
Lung	22	11 (50)	13 (59)	18 (81)	22 (100)
Liver	21	15 (71.4)	16 (76.2)	129	21 (100)
Multiple cysts	3	3 (100)	3 (100)	3 (100)	3 (100)

[a]Titers ⩾ 80.
[b]Titers ⩾ 32.
[c]Titers ⩾ 160.
Source: Adapted from Wattal et al., 1986a.

Table 2 Sensitivity and Specificity of Casoni's Intradermal Test Compared to Specific IgE and IgG-ELISA Using Human Hydatid Cyst Fluid Antigen

Serum samples	Number	Casoni's intradermal Test (≥2 cm²)	IgE ELISA (Titer ≥ 1:10)	IgG ELISA (Titer ≥ 1:160)
Surgically proven hydatid cases				
Lung	7	3 (42.8)	6 (85.71)	7 (100)
Liver	16	13 (81.25)	14 (87.5)	15 (93.75)
Total	23	16 (69.56)	20 (86.95)	22 (95.65)
Nonhydatid cases				
Taeniasis and ascariasis	8	0	5 (62)	0
Bronchogenic and esophageal carcinoma	2	2 (100)	2 (100)	1 (50)
Lung and liver abscesses	4	0	1 (25)	0
Total	14	2 (14.28)	8 (57.14)	1 (7.14)
Normal healthy subjects	10	1 (10)	0	0

Figures in parentheses indicate percentage positive.
Source: Adapted from Wattal et al., 1988.

hydatid cyst fluid antigen as well as soluble scolex antigen, we detected overall 70% of cases but, again, the test's sensitivity in detecting pulmonary echinococcosis remained 59%, with a false-positive rate of 5.7% (Wattal et al., 1986a).

Like other workers (Craif et al., 1986) we also found the IFA test useful in detecting cases of hydatid disease. It could detect 81% of pulmonary and 90% of liver involvement using tagged polyimmunogloblin-FITC. The false-positive rate obtained was 3% (Wattal et al., 1986a). The poly-IFA test remained positive up to 5 years after operation, but the specific IgM-IFA test shows negative results within 6 weeks after operation. A seroconversion or demonstration of rising titer for specific IgM antibodies to echinococcal antigen might be a reliable indicator of recurrence or reinfection in patients who have undergone surgery (Wattal et al., 1986a).

Other parasitic infections that cross-react and produce false-positive results include *Taenia solium* cysticercosis, filariasis, fascioliasis, and schistosomiasis (Farag et al., 1975; Matossian et al., 1979; Ben-Ismail et al., 1980). We have not seen such infections in our population; however, infestation with *T. saginata* occasionally occurs (Craig et al., 1986). In Kashmir, the other endemic helminthic infection is ascariasis, and in our cross-absorption studies with larva stage 2 of *A. lumbricoides*, the IFA test was found not to affect the echinococcal immunofluorescence results (Fig. 10; Wattal et al., 1986b).

Since the development of heterologous immunoenzymatic techniques, several authors have reported the benefits of these tests in the immunodiagnosis of parasitic diseases (Engvall and Perlmann, 1977). Various authors have studied the application of ELISA for the immunodiagnosis of human hydatidosis using total antigens (Farag et al., 1975; Matossian et al., 1979; Speiser, 1980; Gottstein et al., 1984) or antigens purified at different grades (Farag et al., 1975; Iacona et al., 1980; Tassi et al., 1982). We, like others (Coltorti, 1986; Iacona et al., 1980; Wattal et al., 1986a), have found specific IgG/IgM ELISA to be the most sensitive and specific using hydatid fluid antigen. The sensitivity and specificity were improved if soluble scolex antigen was used (Wattal et al., 1986a; Table 1). Detection of specific IgG by ELISA was found to be more sensitive and specific than the determination of specific IgE antibodies (Wattal et al., 1988; Table 2). IgM-ELISA is also useful in detecting recurrence of reinfection. The sensitivity and specificity of specific IgG-ELISA remain the same regardless of the site of cyst localization (Table 1). The ELISA test has a less than 2% rate of false-positive reactions in cases of Hodgkin's disease and hepatocellular carcinoma, ELISA is helpful in the serodiagnosis of pulmonary hydatid disease.

The presence of cryoglobulins (Bombardieri et al., 1973), the occurrence of immune complexes in sera of hydatid cases (Bekhti et al., 1977; Richard-Lenoble et al., 1978; D'Amello et al., 1983), and the association of glomerulonephritis because of hydatidosis (Ibarrola et al., 1981; Bekhti et al., 1977; Kunju, 1982) all point to the possibility that the hydatid cyst-derived circulating antigen may occur in humans. The first reports of identification of specific circulating antigen in human echinococcosis were from a Greek patient with a ruptured hydatid cyst (Tselentis et al., 1981) and a Russian patient (Leikina et al., 1982). The use of ELISA for the detection of specific circulating antigens with affinity-purified rabbit or human antisera could result in useful information on antibody-borderline or -negative hydatid cases (Craig and Nelson, 1984; Craig et al., 1986). Its detection in combination with ELISA will increase the overall sensitivity in detecting hydatid cases, and more so in pulmonary ones.

However, with the immunochemical and physiochemical procedures currently available it has not been possible to obtain adequately purified

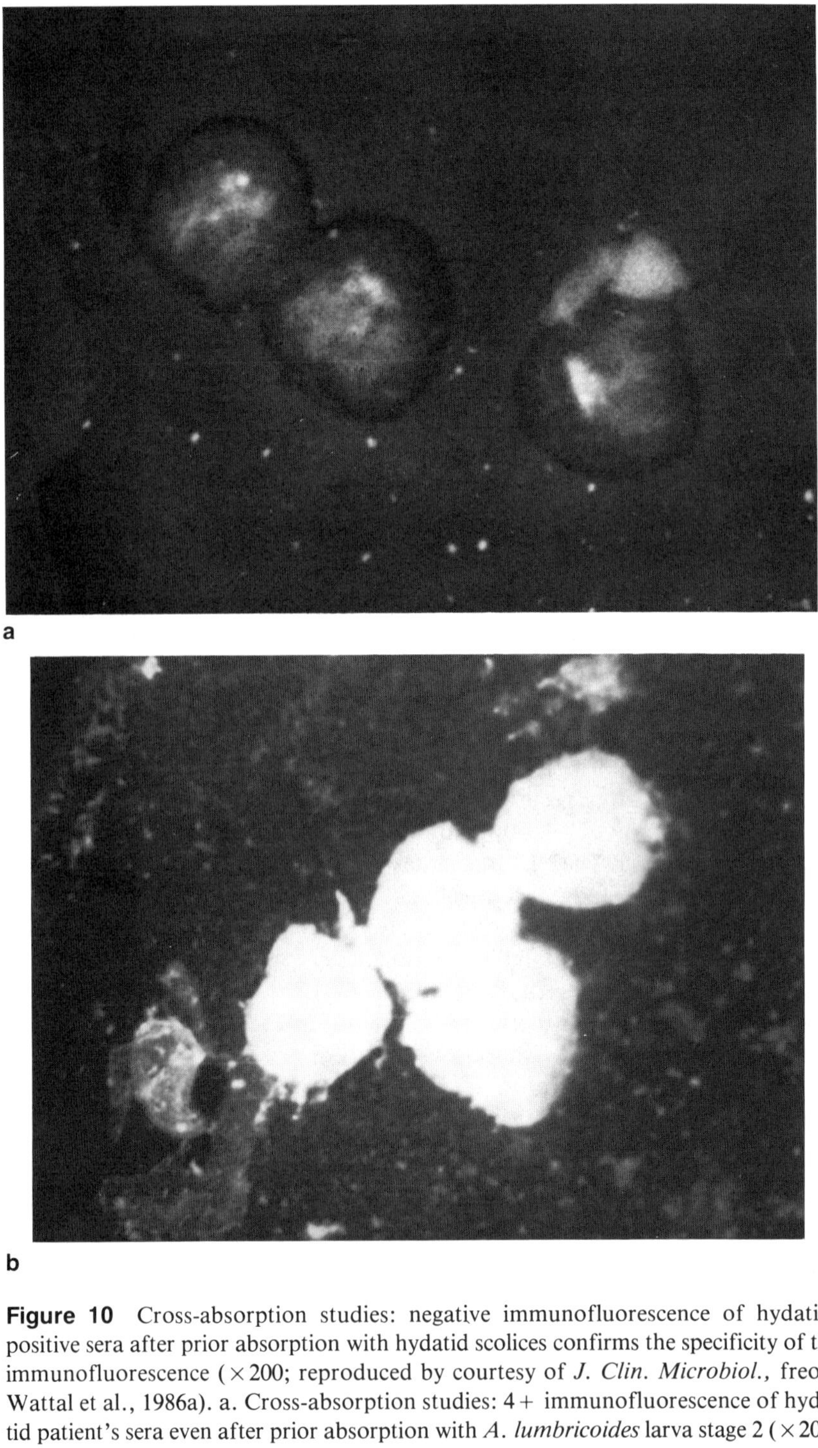

a

b

Figure 10 Cross-absorption studies: negative immunofluorescence of hydatid-positive sera after prior absorption with hydatid scolices confirms the specificity of the immunofluorescence (×200; reproduced by courtesy of *J. Clin. Microbiol.,* freom Wattal et al., 1986a). a. Cross-absorption studies: 4+ immunofluorescence of hydatid patient's sera even after prior absorption with *A. lumbricoides* larva stage 2 (×200; reproduced by *J. Clin. Microbiol.,* from Wattal et al., 1986a).

antigens in the amounts required for diagnostic purposes. The finding of hybridomas producing monoclonal antibodies against species-specific parasitic epitopes capable of inducing antibodies during the disease in a high proportion of patients would be a significant contribution to solving the problem. The possibility of developing competition enzyme immunoassays (EIA) using monoclonal antibodies and patient's antibodies against the same specific epitope would eliminate the need for a diagnostic titer and allow the best use of ELISA's diagnostic sensitivity.

To sum up, it is advisable to use a battery of tests to increase the chances of detecting pulmonary hydatid cases. We prefer the following tests for screening purposes; enzyme immunoassay (ELISA), IFA, and IHA.

III. Management

A. Surgical

Surgery is still the mainstay of management, although the medical treatment of hydatid disease is a fast developing area. Before benzimidazole was available, the majority of symptomatic hydatid cysts, if surgery was not performed, were fatal (Amir Jehad et al., 1975). In the natural history of the evolution of hydatid disease, there is a latent period of several years but once the cyst becomes symptomatic there is a rapid deterioration (Earnest et al., 1983). The type of surgery depends upon the extent of lung disease and the presence or absence of complications. Conservative surgery with preservation of healthy lung tissue is preferred (Barett and Thomas, 1952; Barett, 1947; Walcott et al., 1958; Sarsam, 1971). Enucleation is the procedure of choice for a simple cyst.

From 1979 to 1983, 71 surgical procedures were performed at the Chest Disease Hospital. The majority required only enucleation (Kaul et al., 1981). It has been our practice to inflate the compressed lung, after all the fistulae have been sutured in the bed of the cavity (left after removal of the cyst), so that if proper inflation occurs, no lung resection is needed. Sometimes one may encounter an infected bronchial stump. In such a situation, particularly if a portion of lung is diseased, a segmental resection or lobectomy is indicated. Five of our 71 patients required only lobectomy; 3 other patients had lobectomy with decortication. Even though we encountered many large cysts, some occupying the whole hemithorax, only two patients required pneumonectomy. In both cases, the lung parenchyma of all the lobes of the affected lung had been destroyed by chronic hydatid cysts. After conservative surgery, patients developed left to right shunt that was corrected by a pneumonectomy.

The cyst wall is a fragile white membrane that may rupture on enucleation, with the spilling of hydatid fluid over the lung tissue. Apart from the possibility of causing anaphylactic shock, it may also cause spread of disease to the adjoining area. For this reason several techniques have been used to sterilize the contents of the cyst before enucleation is attempted and to strengthen the friable cyst membrane to allow a controlled evacuation. CO_2 gas through a steel cone is used to freeze the tissue over the site of incision (Redford, 1984; Matossian et al., 1977). Sterilization is achieved by aspiration of 10 ml fluid followed by injection of 10 ml of a scolicide. Formaline, alcohol, and 20% hypertonic saline have all been used as scolicides, but 10% aqueous iodine or 5% silver nitrate is the least toxic (Saidi and Nazian, 1971). We use 20% saline, leaving it for 10 min inside the cyst followed by aspiration of the whole cyst and extrusion of laminated membrane. This ensures sterilization and prevents dissemination to the surrounding tissue.

B. Medical Treatment

There is a 1-3% reported incidence of surgical mortality for hydatid disease of the lung (Barett, 1947; Barrett and Thomas, 1952; Sarsam, 1971). The incidence of complications after surgery is such that the search for a drug cure is always worthwhile (Fitzpatrick, 1951). The discovery of an effective oral or parenteral medication able to destroy the parasite and sterilize the cyst, for use alone or in combination with surgery, is a cherished hope. The introduction of mebendazole was a step towards this. This synthetic benzimidazole derivative is related to the veterinary anthelminthics thiabendazole and cambendazole. It is effective against several nematodes and cestodes (Theinpont, Vanpanijs and Hermans 1974). The drug is active against the larval stages of *E. granulosus* and *E. multilocularis.* It kills the parasite by limiting its glucose uptake and depleting its glycogen (Editorial, 1979). In experiments, mebendazole has a better effect on the germinal membrane of the larvae in white mice infected with *E. granulosus.* It not only sterilizes the cyst but also retards the growth of intraperitoneal cysts. In vitro mebendazole diffuses passively through the cyst membrane of *E. granulosus* and produces the ultrastructural changes of germinal cells. Ever since Bekhti and his colleagues (1977) reported good results with mebendazole, a widespread scepticism has prevailed. Mebendezole pentrates large hydatid cysts in humans, but the amount that diffuses remains scanty (Morris and Gould, 1982). Our experience also has been discouraging, especially with large inoperable cysts. A dosage of 200 mg/kg or more needs to be used for several months must before any noticeable improvement in cyst size occurs. Although serious side effects are uncommon with mebendazole, hemotopoietic depression and increased transaminase activity have been reported. Fever is common in the first few days of treatment (Murray-Lyon and Reynolds, 1979). Despite the initial promising results with mebendazole, the drug is of limited clinical use (Morris et al., 1987).

Albendazole, another benzimidazole carbonate is found to be very effective in clinical and animal studies. Albendazole achieves much higher concentrations of one of its principal metabolites, albendazole sulfoxide, which is believed to be the active agent (Saimot et al., 1983). The drug is well absorbed and high tissue, cyst, and intracyst levels are attained. Although it is premature to conclude that albendazole offers a cure of hydatid disease, the drug is well tolerated in 30 day courses separated by 2 week intervals and given at a dosage of 10-14 mg/kg/day (Saimot et al., 1983). Surgical management of hydatid disease is associated with recurrence in 10% of patients. Albendazole given preoperatively sterilizes cysts and kills most of the protoscolices within the cysts. This reduces and prevents recurrences (Morris, 1987). The optimum dosage and duration of preoperative and postoperative therapy are being evaluated (Davidson et al., 1988). The reason for conflicting reports about therapies is the lack of understanding of the natural history of the disease. The search for an effective drug must nonetheless continue. Until then, preventive programs in affected countries, if implemented properly, are the best answer for this global problem.

References

Amir Jehad, A. K., Frdin, R., Farzad, A., and Bakshandeh, K. (1975). Clinical echinococcosis. *Ann. Surg.* **182**:402-408.

Baker, F., and Al Omeri, M. M. (1969). Echinococcal tension pneumothorax. *Thorax* **24**:547-549.

Barett, N. R. (1947). The treatment of pulmonary hydatid disease. *Thorax* **3**:21-24.

Barett, N. R., and Thomas, D. (1952). Pulmonary hydatid disease. *Br. J. surg.* **40**:222-224.

Beggs, I. (1985). The radiology of hydatid disease. *AJR* **54**:335-338.

Bekhti, A., Schaaps, J. P., Capron, M., Dessaint, J. P., Santofo, F., and Capron, A. (1977). Treatment of hepatic hydatid disease with mebendazole—preliminary results in four cases. *Br. Med. J.* **2**:1047-1051.

Ben-Ismail, R., Carme, B., Niel, G., and Gentilini, M. (1980). Nonspecific serological reactions with echinococcosis granulosus antigens: role of P_1 antibodies. *Am. J. Trop. Med. Hyg.* **29**:239-245.

Bomdardieri, S., Theichner, A., and Bicari, G. (1973). Cryoglobulinemia in echinococcosis. *Proc. Soc. Exp. Biol. Med.* **142**:941-945.

Chatterjee, K. D. (1980). *Parasitology*. Calcutta, India, Chatterjee Medical Publishers, pp. 121-128.

Chematai, A. K., Bowry, T. R., and Ahmad, Z. (1981). Evaluation of five immunodiagnostic techniques in echinococcus patients. *Bull. W.H.O.* **59**:767-772.

Coltorti, E. A. (1986). Standardization and evaluation of an enzyme linked immunosorbent assay as a screening test for the seroepidemiology of human hydatidosis. *Am. J. Trop. Med. Hyg.* **35**(5):1000-1005.

Comellan, S. J., Jowelth, A. W., and Wilson, R. S. E. (1979). Hydatid disease presenting as tension pneumothorax. *Br. J. Dis. Chest* **73**:405-408.

Craig, P. S., and Nelson, G. S. (1984). Detection of specific circulating antigen. *Ann. Trop. Med. Parasitol.* **78**:219-227.

Craig, P. S., Zeyhle, E., and Romig, T. (1988). Hydatid disease: research and control in Turkana II. The role of immunological techniques for the diagnosis of hydatid disease. **80**:183-192.

Crofton, J., and Douglas, A. (1961). *Respiratory Diseases.* London, Blackwell Scientific Publications, pp. 439.

D'Amello, R., Pontesilli, O., Palmisano, I., Pezzello, M., Vullo, V., Delia, S., De Rose, F., Sorice, F., and Aiuti, F. (1983). Detection and partial characterization of circulating immune complexes in hydatid disease. *J. Clin. Microbiol.* **18**:1021-1026.

Davidson, R. N., Boyceson, A. D. M., Cowie, A. G. A., and MacManus, D. P. (1988). Pre-operative mebendozole therapy and hydatid cyst (letter). *Br. J. Surg.* **75**(4):391-

Dhar, S. N., and Kaul, B. L. (1988). Hydatid disease of the lung. *Semin. Respir. Med.* **9**:409-413.

Dighero, H. W., and Bradstreet, C. M. P. (1979). The serological diagnosis of hydatid disease I. The routine use of latex agglutination and complement fixation in diagnosis. *J. Helminthol.* **53**:283-286.

Dusaj, J. A., Pant, K., and Bhagat, R. (1988). Ultrasonographic appearance in a case of hydatid disease. *Indian J. Chest Dis. Allied Sci.* **30**(3): 205-209.

Earnest, A., Cikes, I., and Radsvanovic, N. (1983). Two dimensional echocardiographic study of a cardiac hydatid cyst. *Am. J. Cardiol.* **52**(10): 1361-1363.

Editorial (1979). Medical treatment of hydatid disease. *Br. Med. J.* **10**:563.

Engvall, E., and Perlmann, P. (1971). Enzyme linked immunosorbent assay (ELISA): quantitative assay of immunoglobulin G. *Immunochemistry* **8**:871-874.

Farag, H., Bout, D., and Capron, A. (1975). Specific immunodiagnosis of hydatidosis by enzyme linked immunosorbent assay (ELISA). *Biomedicine* **23**:276-278.

Felgner, P. (1978). Antibody activity in stic ELISA as compared to other quantitative immunological tests in sera of echinococcosis cases. *Tropenmed. Parasitol.* **29**:417-422.

Fitzpatrick, S. C. (1951). Sequelae of treatment of hydatid cyst of lung. *Aust. N.Z. J. Surg.* **20**:278-280.

Gottstein, B., Eckert, J., and Woodtli, W. C. (1984). Determination of parasitic specific immunoglobulins using ELISA in patients with echinococcosis treated with mebendazole. *Z. Parasitenkd.* **70**:385-389.

Hamilton, R. G., Hussain, R., and Oltesen, E. A. (1981). The quantitation of parasite specific human IgG and IgE in sera: evaluation of solid phase RIA & ELISA methodology. *J. Immunol.̀ Methods* **44**:104-114.

Iacona, A., Pini, C., and Vicari, G. (1980). ELISA in the serodiagnosis of hydatid disease. *Am. J. Trop. Med. Hyg.* **29**:95-102.

Ibarrola, A. S., Sobrini, B., Guisantes, J., Pardo, J., Diez, J., Monfa, J. M., and Purroy, A. (1981). Membranous glomerulonephritis secondary to hydatid disease. *Am. J. Med.* **70**:311-315.

Imari, A. J. (1962). Pulmonary hydatid disease in Iraq. *Am. J. Trop. Med.* **II**:481-490.

Kagan, I. G. (1976). Serodiagnosis of hydatid disease. In *Immunology of Parasitic Infections.* Edited by S. Cohen and E. H. Sadus. Oxford/London, Blackwell Scientific Publishers, pp. 130-142.

Kaul, B. L., Dhar, S. N., Chowdhary, K. L., Daljit, S., Ashaq, H., Malik, N. A., and Sapru, R. (1981). Pulmonary hydatid disease—abstracts. The 4th Congress of Association of Thorocic & Cardiovascular Surgeons of Asia, p. 30.

Kunju, A. (1982). Glomerulonephritis following chemotherapy of hydatid disease with mebendazole. *East Afr. Med. J.* **59**:404-409.

Le Roux, B. T. (1972). Pulmonary hydatid disease. *Thorax* **27**:;365-367.

Leikina, E. S., Kovrova, E. A., and Krasovskaya, N. N. (1982). Detection of circulating antigens in the blood stream of patients with hydatid disease, alveococcosis and trichinosis. *Med. Parazitol.* (Mosk.) **51**:7-15.

Lunde, M. N., and Ottesen, E. A. (1980). ELISA for detection of IgM and IgE antibodies in human schistosomiasis. *Am. J. Trop. Med. Hyg.* **29**: 82-87.

Mahajan, R. C., Ganguly, N. K., and Chitkara, N. L. (1976). Evaluation of immunodiagnostic techniques in hydatid disease. *Indian J. Med. Res.* **64**:405-409.

Matossian, R. M., Richard, M. D., and Smith, J. D. (1977). Hydatidosis—a global problem of increasing importance. *Bull. W.H.O.* 455-499.

Matossian, R. M., Maclaren, M. L., Drapu, C. C., Bradstreet, C. M., Dighero, M. W., Kane, G. J., Madeinly, L. M., and Rikard, M. D. (1979). The serodiagnosis of human hydatid disease 2. Additional studies on selected sera using indirect haemogglutination (IMA); enzyme linked immunosorbent assay (ELISA) and defined antigen substrate spheres (DASS). *J. Helminthol.* **53**:28-291.

Morris, D. L. (1987). Pre-operative albendazole therapy for hydatid cyst. *Br. J. Surg.* **74**:805-806.

Morris, D. L., and Gould, S. E. (1982). Serum and cyst concentration of mebendazole and flubendazole in hydatid disease. *Br. Med. J.* **285**(ii): 175.

Morris, D. L., Dykes, P. W., Dickson, B., Marriner, S. E., Bojen, J. A., and Burrows, F. G. O. (1983). Albendazole in hydatid disease. *Br. Med. J.* **286**:103-104.

Morris, D. L., Chinnery, J. B., Georgious, G., Stamatateries, G., and Golematis, B. (1987). Penetration of albendazole sulphoxide into hydatid cysts. *Gut* **28**:75-80.

Murray-Lyon, I. M., and Reynolds, K. W. (1979). Complication of mebendazole treatment for hydatid disease. *Br. Med. J.* **2**:1111-1112.

Okelo, G. B. A., and Chematai, A. K. (1981). Treatment of hepatic hydatid disease with mebendazole, report of 16 cases. *East Afr. Med. J.* **58**: 608-610.

Okelo, G. B. A., and Kyobe, J. (1981). A three year review of human hydatid disease seen at the Kenyatta National Hospital. *East Afr. Med. J.* **58**:695-710.

Omeri, A. L. M., and Wasif, S. A. (1984). Surgical management of hydatid disease of lung. *J. R. Coll. Surg. Edinb.* **29**(4):218-220.

Papadimitrion, J., and Mandrekas, A. (1970). The surgical treatment of hydatid disease of the liver. *Br. J. Surg.* **57**:431-433.

Pini, C., Pastore, R., and Valesini, G. (1983). Circulating immune complexes in sea of patients infectred with *Echinococcus granulosus. Clin. Exp. Immunol.* **51**:572-578.

Rausch, R. L. (1960). Recent studies on hydatid disease in Alaska. *Parasitology* **2**:391-396.

Redford, A. J. (1984). Hydatid disease. In *Oxford Text Book of Medicine.* Edited by Worthwall, Ladingham, and Warrell. New York, Oxford University Press, p. 442.

Richard-Lenoble, D., Smith, M. D., Loisy, M., and Verroust, P. J. (1978). Human hydatidosis: evaluation of three serodiagnostic methods the principal subclass of specific immunoglobulin and the detection of circulating immune complexes. *Ann. Trop. Med. Parasitol.* **72**:553-560.

Rickard, M. D. (1984). Serological diagnosis and post operative surveillance of human hydatid disease. I. Latex agglutination and immunoelectrophoresis using crude fluid antigen. *Pathology* **10**:207-210.

Saidi, F., and Nazarian, I. (1971). Surgical treatment of hydatid cysts by freezing of the cyst wall and installation of 0.5 percent silver nitrate solution. *N. Engl. J. Med.* **284**:1346-1350.

Saimot, A. G., Gernieux, A. C., Hary, J. H., Meulmans, A., Giovanangeli, M. D., Delaitre, B., and Couland, J. P. (1983). *Lancet* **2**:652-656.

Sarsam, A. (1971). Surgery of pulmonary hydatid cyst. *J. Thorax Cardiovasc. Surg.* **62**(4):663-667.

Schills, E. (1960). Echinococcus in North America. *Am. J. Intern. Med.* **52**:464-414.

Singh, R. P., Saxena, S., Narang, R. K., and Katiyar, S. K. (1983). Horner's syndrome due to hydatid cyst. *Indian J. Chest Dis. Allied Sci.* **26**(2): 119-122.

Speiser, F. (1980). Application of ELISA for the diagnosis of filariasis and echinococcosis. *Tropenmed. Parasitol.* **31**:459-466.

Tassi, C., Baldelli, F., Dottorini, S., and Pauluzzi, S. (1982). Specificita degli anticropi della classe IgM rilevabili nell' infezione idatidea umana. *Boll Ist Siroter. Milan.* **61**:499-504.

Theofilopoulos, A. N., and Dixon, F. J. (1980). Immune complexes in human diseases. *Am. J. Pathol.* **100**:530-538.

Todorov, T., Dakov, J., Kosturkova, M., Tenev, S., and Dimitrov, A. (1979a). Immunoreactivity in pulmonary echinococcosis I. A comparative study of immunodiagnostic test. *Bull. W.H.O.* **57**:735-740.

Todorov, T., Raicev, I., Tenev, S., Kosturkova, M., Dakov, I., and Dimitrov, A. (1979b). Immunoreactivity in pulmonary echinococcosis II. Evaluation of antibody response. *Bull. W.H.O.* **57**:741-750.

Tselentis, J., Plataris, J., Giannopolos, A., Golematis, B., and Melissinos, K. (1981). Ruptured echinococcal cysts and their immunological diagnosis. *Acta Microbiol. Hellen.* **26**:339-342.

Tusckka, O. (1969). Hydatid cyst—occurrence in central California. *Am. J. Surg.* **118**:569-572.

Walcott, M. W., Harris, S. H., Briggs, J. N., Dobell, A. R. C., and Brown, R. K. (1958). Hydatid disease of lung. *J. Thorac. Cardiovasc. Surg.* **62**:465-469.

Wattal, C., Malla, N., Khan, I. A., and Agarwal, S. C. (1986a). Comparative evaluation of enzyme linked immunosorbent assay for the diagnosis of pulmonary echinococcosis. *J. Clin. Microb.* **24**(1):41-46.

Wattal, C., Malla, N., Khan, I. A., and Agarwal, S. C. (1986b). In vitro development and hatching of *A. lumbricoides* var. *hominis* eggs. *Indian J. Med. Res.* **83**:257-264.

Wattal, C., Chandermohan, and Agarwal, S. C. (1988). Evaluation of specific immunoglobulin E by enzyme linked immunosorbent assay in hydatid disease. *Int. Arch. Allergy Appl. Immunol.* **87**:98-100.

Wilson, J. F., Diddams, A. S., and Rausch, R. L. (1968). Cystic hydatid disease in Alaska. *Am. Rev. Respir. Dis.* **98**:1-8.

World Health Organization (1979). Parasitic zoonosis. WHO Tech. Report Series, No. 637. Geneva, WHO.

11

The Lung and AIDS in Developing Countries

JAMES TUCHSCHMIDT and BISHER AKIL

Los Angeles County-University of Southern California Medical Center
Los Angeles, California

I. Introduction

The heat and congestion of Nairobi were now far behind. It was September and the drizzle that had begun to fall marked the beginning of the rainy season. The showers to come would bring a welcome coolness to Uganda and restore life to this parched land. Barely visible in the dim light, a young cachectic woman lay on a cot in the corner. Her eyes stared from sunken orbits and small beads of perspiration formed on her forehead. Thin frail legs, which surely could not support her weight, protruded from beneath a blanket. A meager and ineffective cough would periodically disturb her rest. She had been this way for months, unable to eat because of the pain that swallowing produced and always the crampy diarrhea.

Prostitution had provided food, shelter, and clothing for her children. Her customers were truck drivers, salesman, soldiers—men separated from their families by economic hardship, looking for work, a better life. Having never finished her primary education, she was simply earning a living, unknowingly passing the acquired immunodeficiency syndrome (AIDS) virus to her lovers. Now she was sick and modern medicine had nothing to offer. She had come home to die.

Although AIDS is not a tropical disease, it certainly is no stranger to the tropics. The first reported cases of AIDS came from the United States in 1981 (Centers for Disease Control, 1981), but current data would suggest that the human immunodeficiency virus (HIV) existed in Africa as early as 1959. This is not to presume that HIV originated in sub-Saharan Africa, for clearly no such facts support this contention. Sudden increases in cases of cryptococcal meningitis, Kaposi's sarcoma (KS), and chronic diarrhea occurred in central Africa during the late 1970s and early 1980s. In the Caribbean, and Haiti in particular, there have been a growing number of AIDS patients. From Brazil to the Philippines, AIDS has become an international health problem. However, many underdeveloped Third World countries are ill-equipped and financially restrained, making the battle against AIDS all but impossible.

II. Epidemiology

It has been estimated that 5 million people are infected with HIV worldwide, with 2 million of these residing in the United States. Because many developing countries lack financial resources and sophisticated laboratory technology, their data on the incidence of AIDS are perhaps distorted and difficult to interpret. Furthermore, in many of these countries the stigmata of AIDS have significant political implications. However, the World Health Organization (WHO) has reported 151,790 cases from 175 countries in May, 1989; Africa 23,262 (Burundi 1,408, Congo 1,250, Kenya 2,732, Malawi 2,586, Rwanda 987, Uganda 5,998, Tanzania 4,158, Zambia 1,296), the Americas 105,612 (Brazil 5,712, Canada 2,449, Haiti 1,849, Mexico 2,158, United States 89,501), Europe 21,136 (France 6,409, West Germany 3,086, Italy 3,494, Netherlands 791, Spain 2,165, Switzerland 806, United Kingdom 2,192), Oceania 1,411 (Australia 1,270, New Zealand 119), Japan 97, and Israel 79 (WHO, 1989).

A. Africa

The nations making up sub-Saharan Africa have reported the majority of that continents' cases. AIDS was recognized in Africa as an epidemic of KS in Zaire, Zambia, and Uganda (Taylor et al., 1971; Biggar et al., 1984; Clumeck et al., 1984), as a wasting condition in Zaire, Uganda, Tanzania (Serwadda et al., 1985), as an outbreak of esophageal candidiasis in Rwanda in 1983 (Van de Perre et al., 1984), and as a sudden increase in cryptococcal meningitis in Kinshasa, Zaire beginning in 1978 (Piot et al., 1984).

The incidence of AIDS in adults in Kinshasa (age-corrected) is approximately 2000 cases per million. Those affected with AIDS are primarily over

Table 1 Reported AIDS Cases by Country

Africa	
Burundi	1,408
Congo	1,250
Kenya	2,732
Malawi	2,586
Rwanda	987
Uganda	5,998
Tanzania	4,158
Zambia	1,296
Americas	
Brazil	5,712
Canada	2,449
Haiti	1,849
Mexico	2,158
US	89,501
Europe	
France	6,409
West Germany	3,086
Italy	3,494
The Netherlands	791
Spain	2,165
Switzerland	806
UK	2,192
Oceania	
Australia	1,270
New Zealand	119
Japan	97
Isreal	79

Source: World Health Organization, 1989.

20 years old with a mean age of 33.6 years. Unlike the epidemic encountered in the United States, the majority of these patients are heterosexuals, with no history of intravenous drug abuse or blood transfusion (Piot et al., 1987). But most have had multiple sexual contacts (32 vs. 3 in controls) and/or exposure to prostitutes (81% vs. 34% of controls). Men and women are equally affected (1:1.3), however female patients are more likely to be unmarried

(61% vs. 36%). Eighty percent describe undergoing medical injections, ritual scarification, or tattooing, with instruments that may not have been adequately sterilized; only 9% received blood products (Quinn and Mann, 1989; Quinn et al., 1986). In 1981 only 4% of prostitutes in Nairobi tested positive for HIV antibody, but in 1985 that number had risen to a startling 61% (Kreiss et al., 1986).

Perinatal transmission also characterizes the spread of the HIV type 1 (HIV-1) in sub-Saharan Africa. It has been estimated that 1-2% of all infants born in Kinshasa are infected with HIV. One study found that 3.6% of mothers tested positive for antibody to HIV-1 and 45.9% of their infants showed IgM antibodies to the virus (Ryder et al., 1987). In Kampala, 13% of mothers test seropositive.

B. The Americas

Not until the early to mid-1980s was AIDS reported from Latin America and the Caribbean: Brazil, Haiti, Mexico, Honduras, and the Dominican Republic lead the list. Initially the disease appeared in the gay community, but was spread rapidly by male prostitutes, many of whom did not view themselves as homosexual (C.S.G.A.H.A., 1987). Today bisexual men account for only 11-25% of all patients (Pape et al., 1985); the disease is primarily heterosexually transmitted. Perinatal transmission is uncommon, but unlikely to remain so. Transfusion-related AIDS is undocumented since blood donors are rarely screened due to economic constraints.

In Haiti, it is estimated that 8-12% of people living in urban areas and 1-5% of people from rural areas have been infected with HIV. Fifty-three percent of prostitutes living in Port-au-Prince are seropositive and prostitute contact is reported by 61% of male patients with AIDS. Injections, given by medical and nonmedical personnel with nondisposable needles, were reported by 85% of patients (Pape and Johnson, 1989).

A study of high-risk individuals in Brazil found 28% of homosexual and bisexual men to be seropositive, with 45% of male prostitutes and 9% of female prostitutes showing antibody to HIV. (Pan American Health Organization, 1987; Cortes et al., 1989). Bisexual men and female prostitutes may be the primary reservoir of transmission to the heterosexual community.

III. Virology

HIV is a retrovirus, which binds to the CD4 receptor on lymphocytes, macrophages, some B cells, colorectal mucosa, and neurons within the central nervous system (Weber, 1989). The virus destroys the helper T lymphocyte, producing a severe cell-mediated immune defect. Although the monocyte is not affected, it seems to transmit virus to other cells, particularly helper T cells. Central nervous system invasion, especially to deep brain structures (thalmus and basal ganglia), may lead to dementia. Invasion of B lymphocytes leads to the production of defective antibody, resulting in hypergammaglobulinemia and a humoral immune defect.

The virus is transmitted sexually and by blood. Although virus can be isolated from saliva, urine, and tears, these body fluids do not seem to spread virus. Rectal and vaginal mucosa seem particularly vulnerable to viral invasion (Fultz et al., 1986; Detels et al., 1989; Gordert et al., 1984). Thus, receptive rectal intercourse is a major risk factor. Transmission from men to women and women to men seems equally likely. Penile contact with infected menstrual blood and the presence of genital ulcers, secondary to other sexually transmitted diseases, may increase the likelihood of spread from female to male patients (Piot et al., 1987; Simonsen et al., 1988). All studies clearly indicate that exposure to multiple partners constitutes a major risk (Piot et al., 1988).

Seroconversion occurs 6-12 weeks after exposure, often with an associated flulike illness. There is a transient rise in antibody to viral envelope and core proteins. As HIV core antibody levels rise, there is a decline in detectable p24 antigen. A latent period then ensues and lasts a variable length of time, with 36% of patients progressing to AIDS in the first 6 years and then 7% advancing each subsequent year. Following this latent period, p24 core antibody levels decline and there is once again a rise in p24 antigen, indicating viral replication. A cause and effect relationship has not been established but is presumed. General lymphadenopathy may develop during this period. With viral replication, there is a decline in helper T cells and the syndrome we recognize as AIDS develops (Kaslow and Francis, 1989).

Although there is more genetic variability among African isolates, most HIV isolates resemble isolates from the United States in genetic structure and envelope proteins. These various strains do seem to differ in virulence. A virus with 50-60% genetic homology to HIV-1 has been isolated from patients in Western Africa and has been named HIV-2 (HTLV-IV) (Albert et al., 1987; Clavel et al., 1986). Cortes et al. reported antibody to HIV-2 in 3% of male AIDS patients in Brazil (1989). HIV-2 appears to be less virulent in vitro and in vivo than HIV-1, but, while the natural history of HIV-2 infection is not presently known, it clearly can cause AIDS (Piot et al., 1984; Clavel, 1987).

IV. Clinical Experience of Disease

The major manifestations of AIDS in these tropical areas are weight loss and chronic diarrhea, primarily due to *Cryptosporidium* and *Isospora belli*

(50% of the time no cause for the diarrhea can be determined; Colebunders et al., 1987). In Kinshasa, patients presented with weight loss (99%), fever (81%), diarrhea (68%), cough (37%), dysphagia (35%), and dyspnea (23%) (Mann et al., 1986a). Twenty-two percent of patients develop a generalized pruritic macular rash. These hyperpigmented lesions occur symetrically, particularly over the arms and legs, but may spread to the trunk and face. These represent a dermal hypersensitivity reaction, but the exact cause has not been determined (James et al., 1986). Generalized lymphadenopathy occurred in 11%.

Table 2 WHO Clinical Case Definition for AIDS

Adults: two major and one minor criteria in absence of another immunosuppressive disease; or the presence of generalized KS or cryptococcal meningitis alone.

Major criteria

1. Weight loss > 10% ideal body weight
2. Diarrhea > 1 month duration
3. Fever > 1 month duration

Minor criteria

1. Persistent cough > 1 month
2. Generalized pruritic dermatitis
3. Recurrent herpes zoster infection
4. Oropharyngeal candidiasis
5. Disseminated herpes simplex (HSV) infection
6. Generalized lymphadenopathy

Children: two major criteria and two minor criteria in the absence of another immunosuppressive disease

Major criteria

1. Weight loss or failure to thrive
2. Diarrhea > 1 month duration
3. Fever > 1 month duration

Minor criteria

1. Persistent cough > 1 month duration
2. Generalized pruritic dermatitis
3. Recurrent bacterial infections such as otitis, pharyngitis
4. Oropharyngeal candidiasis
5. Generalized lymphadenopathy
6. Confirmed HIV seropositivity of mother

The profound weight loss seen in African patients with AIDS has lead to the term "slim disease," which is the clinical presentation of approximately 80% of patients. Oroesophageal candidiasis, central nervous system cryptococcosis, toxoplasmosis, *Mycobacterium tuberculosis*, and cryptosporidiosis are the major infectious complications. Disseminated histoplasmosis, salmonellosis, and *Strongyloides* also cause major morbidity and mortality. Fifty-six percent of AIDS patients present with tuberculosis (Lesbordes, 1988) and 33% of all patients hospitalized at one hospital in Kinshasa with tuberculosis were HIV antibody-positive (Mann et al., 1986b). *Pneumocystis carinii* pneumonia occurred in only 25% of AIDS patients from central Africa (Clumeck et al., 1987, 1984). An aggressive form of KS was first noted in Zambia in 1983. AIDS patients develop KS lesions over the trunk, face, and genitals. Oral, gastrointestinal, and pulmonary lesions are common.

In Haiti, AIDS is called "maladi mor" ("illness of death"). Again the presentation is with oroesophageal candidiasis (68%), diarrhea due to gastrointestinal coccidioidomycosis (64%), cryptosporidiosis (48%), and *Mycobacterium tuberculosis* (31%) (Dehovits et al., 1986). *Pneumocystis* pneumonia only occurs in 7% of patients, as opposed to about 70% of U.S. AIDS patients (Pape and Johnson, 1989).

V. Pulmonary Involvement

A. *Pneumocystis carinii*

The pulmonary complications associated with AIDS can be infectious, neoplastic, or inflammatory. The infectious complications include *Pneumocystis carinii*, fungi, mycobacteria, and viruses. *Pneumocystis carinii* is a unicellular organism, which some believe to be a fungus, but is classifed as a protozoan. The organism reproduces on the surface of type 1 pneumocytes, destroying these cells. The cysts of *P. carinii* can be identified in bronchial secretions, bronchoalveolar lavage (BAL) fluid, or biopsy material by Giemsa or methenamine silver staining. Diffuse alveolar damage is combined with foamy, eosinophilic alveolar exudates. Epithelioid granulomas and multinucleated giant cells may occur.

Treatment is either with trimethoprim-sulfamethoxazole (15 mg/kg/day) or pentamidine isothionate (4 mg/kg/day). Current data suggest that these drugs are equally efficacious. The side effects of trimethoprim-sulfamethoxazole are rash, neutropenia, thrombocytopenia, fever, azotemia, and mild hepatitis. Pentamidine is associated with hypotension, hypoglycemia, neutropenia, and hepatitis. Aerosolized pentamidine may provide more selective delivery with fewer systemic side effects in patients with mild to moderate disease and may be useful as adjuvant therapy in patients with severe pneumocystosis. Dapsone, DFMO, clindamycin and praziqualtal, and trimetrexate are other drugs being studied. *Toxoplasma gondii* and cryptosporidia have also been found in the lung.

B. Fungi

Cryptococcus neoformans may cause an isolated pulmonary infection, but most commonly it is disseminated, particularly to the meninges, brain, and other vital organs. Clinically, patients may present with lobar or diffuse infiltrates or simply intrathoracic lymphadenopathy on the chest roentgenogram. The organism induces an inflammatory infiltrate with intra-alveolar macrophages. A diagnosis may be made by identifying organisms or antigen in serum (or cerebrospinal fluid). *Coccidioides immitis* is a soil-based fungus that is inhaled by patients. The disease is usually disseminated and causes nodular lung infiltrates. Patients frequently have minimal symptoms in the face of widespread disease. *Histoplasma capsulatum* produces interstitial inflammation with focal areas of abundant histiocytes. The organism can usually be recovered from blood or a bone marrow or lung biopsy. This budding yeast can be demonstrated with methenamine silver. Patients with AIDS generally do not form well-organized granulomas in response to these organisms. *Candida albicans* produces abscesses with yeast and pseudohyphae and invades vasculature. Patients with AIDS commonly develop oroesophageal candidiasis but, unlike other immunocompromised hosts, infrequently develop fungal lung infections. When they do, the disease is usually disseminated. Treatment is with amphotericin 0.6 mg/kg daily or 1 mg/kg every other day. The initial response to therapy is usually encouraging, but a persistent immune defect results in a high relapse rate and necessitates some form of maintenance therapy. This is accomplished with oral ketoconazole 400-800 mg daily or weekly amphotericin B.

C. Mycobacteria

Unlike in U.S. AIDS patients, *Mycobacterium tuberculosis* is the predominant mycobacterial pathogen found in patients from tropical areas. In Kinshasa, 56% of all AIDS patients present with tuberculosis, as opposed to 4-21% of U.S. patients. The incidence of tuberculosis (TB) in Haitian patients with AIDS has been reported to be as high as 69% (Pitchenik et al., 1984). In this patient population, skin tests are rarely positive and there is a high incidence of extrapulmonary TB (57-73%) (Sunderham et al., 1986; Chaisson et al., 1988). Of those presenting with TB, 43% have pulmonary TB, 23% have miliary disease, and 34% have tuberculosis lymphadenitis. The pulmonary involvement is diffuse or localized to the lower lobes. Pathological specimens show caseating granulomas 47% of the time, noncaseating granulomas in 35% of cases, and no granuloma in 18% (Chaisson et al., 1986). Although these organisms are usually sensitive to conventional drugs (Isoniazid, rifampin, and pyrazinamide or ethambutol), relapse is not uncommon after therapy is discontinued. Isoniazid prophylaxis is now recommended for all HIV antibody-positive patients with a postive tuberculin skin test.

Mycobacterium avium-intracellulare (MAI) and other atypicals resemble *M. tuberculosis* clinically, but are almost always disseminated. Blood cultures will usually identify the organism (96%) (Wong et al., 1985). Patients will present with fever, weight loss, and malaise, sometimes abdominal pain, and diarrhea. Lung pathological examination shows an organizing pneumonia, and occasionally granuloma formation. Although numerous organisms are typically seen, histological examination may fail to detect organisms. The diagnosis of MAI is often made at autopsy. The response to therapy is generally disappointing. Various regimens containing combinations of isoniazid, rifampin, ethambutol, clofazimine, pyrazinamide, cycloserine, ciprofoloxacin, ethionamide, and amikacin have been tried. The vast majority of patients (90%) die within 2 years with evidence of persistent disease, usually from other opportunistic infections or neoplasia (Snider et al., 1987).

D. Viral

Cytomegalovirus (CMV) and herpes simplex virus may produce pneumonitis in AIDS patients. Pulmonary involvement with CMV can be detected at autopsy in 90% of cases, but is frequently missed on transbronchial biopsy because of the focal nature of the disease. Nonspecific inflammatory changes, intra-alveolar hemorrhage, and typical inclusion bodies are seen histologically. Pleuritis occurs in 25% of patients. CMV pneumonitis is generally a manifestation of disseminated disease. Other manifestations include retinitis, encephalitis, esophagitis, colitis, and hepatitis. DHPG has been shown to have some efficacy in treating retinitis (91%), enterocolitis (69%), and pneumonitis (47%) in AIDS patients, but since the drug only inhibits viral replication relapse is common (Collaborative DHPG Treatment Study Group, 1986). The major toxicity with DHPG is bone marrow suppression. Foscarnet may also be of value in treating CMV pneumonitis. Pneumonitis secondary to herpes simplex occurs, but is surprisingly rare.

E. Neoplastic Diseases

KS and lymphomas are the major neoplastic processes that involve the lung. An aggressive form of KS is found in these patients. Presenting symptoms associated with pulmonary KS include cough and dyspnea. Pleural involvement may lead to pleuritis chest pain and a hemorrhagic pleural effusion.

Violaceous endobronchial lesions are usually evident at bronchoscopy. The presence of hemosiderin-laden macrophages in BAL fluid may suggest pulmonary KS in this setting. Chemotherapeutic regimens containing bleomycin and vincristine improve KS lesions in 40-60% of patients with pleuropulmonary involvement (Lewis et al., 1983).

Malignant lymphomas are also common in patient with AIDS. These tumors may infiltrate the interstitial space, following the lymphatics. Chest radiographs reveal interstitial disease with some degree of nodularity. Pleural involvement may be present.

F. Inflammatory Diseases

Lymphoid interstitial pneumonitis (LIP) is an idiopathic disease and is considered by the Centers for Disease Control as diagnostic of AIDS in children who are HIV seropositive. Predominantly reported in pediatric patients, LIP has been described in Haitian adults with AIDS. These patients present with nonspecific pulmonary symptoms and interstitial disease on chest radiographs. Pathologically, there is peribronchial and perivascular infiltration with small lymphocytes and plasma cells. Fibrosis and focal capillary hyperplasia are evident in the bronchial submucosa.

VI. Conclusion

As in previous epidemics, AIDS represents a major challenge to the medical profession and to modern society. In many parts of the Third World, the incidence of HIV-1 infection has been estimated at 10% of the population. In these parts of the world, the transmission of HIV is primarily by sexual activity among heterosexual partners. Since AIDS is predominantly a heterosexual disease, perinatal transmission of HIV from seropositive mothers is not unexpected. The high incidence of HIV infection, combined with inadequate financial resources to support blood donor screening, means that transfusion-related AIDS is likely to remain a problem in these areas of the world.

The clinical presentation of patients with AIDS in many developing areas is substantially different from that in the United States. The major manifestation is of a wasting illness, complicated by chronic diarrhea. Tuberculosis is the major pulmonary complication in these patients. Pneumocystis, which is common in U.S. AIDS patients, occurs in only a minority of Third World patients.

The cost of this epidemic to these nations is enormous, economically and socially, stressing the very fabric of society. The loss of young productive people robs these countries of a precious resource. These countries must organize in a cooperative manner to control the spread of this disease, the World Health Organization has been a leader in this regard.

References

Albert, J., Bredberg, U., Chiodi, F., Bottiger, B., Fenyo, E. M., Norrby, E., and Biberfeld, G. (1987). A new human retrovirus isolate of West African origin (SBL-6669) and its relationship to HTLV-IV, Lav II and HTLV IIB. *AIDS Res. Hum. Retroviruses* **3**:3-10.

Biggar, R. J., Bouvet, E., Ebbesen, P., Faber, V., Koch, M., Melbye, M., and Velimirovic, B. (1984). Clinical features of AIDS in Europe. *Eur. J. Cancer Clin. Oncol.* **20**:165-167.

Centers for Disease Control (1981). Pneumocystis pneumonia—Los Angeles. *MMWR* **30**:250.

Chaisson, R. E., Theuer, C. P., and Scheder, G. F. (1986). Clinical aspects of TB in AIDS patients: a population based study. II International Conference on AIDS, Paris: poster #304.

Clavel, F. (1987). HIV-2, the West African AIDS virus. *AIDS* **1**:135-140.

Clavel, F., Guetard, D., Brun-Vezinet, F., Chamaret, S., Rey, M. A., Santos-Ferreira, M. O., Laurent, A. G., Dauguet, C., Katlama, C., Rouzioux, C., Klatzmann, D., Champalimaund, J. L., and Montagnier, L. (1986). Isolation of a new human retrovirus from West African patients with AIDS. *Science* **233**:343-346.

Clumeck, N., Sonnet, J., Taelman, H., Mascart-Lemone, F., De-Bruyers, M., Van de Perre, P., Dasnoy, J., Marcelis, L., Lamy, M., Jonas, C., Robert-Guroff, M., Eyckmans, L., Noel, H., Vanhaeverbeek, M., and Butzler, J. P. (1984). Acquired immunodeficiency syndrome in African patients. *N. Engl. J. Med.* **310**:492-497.

Clumeck, N., Hermans, P., and Dewit, S. (1987). Some epidemiological and clinical characteristics of African AIDS. *Antibiotics Chemother* **38**:41-51.

Colebunders, R., Francis, H., Mann, J., Bita, K., Izaley, L., Kimputu, L., Behets, F., Van der Groen, G., Quinn, T., Curran, J., and Piot, P. (1987). Persistent diarrhea strongly associated with HIV infection in kinshasa, Zaire. *Am. J. Gastroenterol.* **82**:859-864.

Collaborative DHPG Treatment Study Group (1986). Treatment of serious cytomegalovirus infection with 9-(1,3, dihydroxy-2-prooxymethyl) guanine in patients with AIDS and other immunodeficiencies. *N. Engl. J. Med.* **314**:801-805.

Collaborative Study Group of AIDS in Haitian Americans (1987). Risk factors for AIDS among Haitians residing in the United States—evidence of heterosexual transmission. *J.A.M.A.* **257**:635-639.

Cortes, E., Detels, R., Aboulafia, D., Li, X. L., Moudgil, T., Alam, M., Bonecker, C., Gonzaga, A., Oyafuso, L., Tondo, M., Boite, C., Hammershlak, N., Capitani, C., Slamon, D. J., and Ho, D. D. (1989). HIV-1, HIV-2 and HTLV-I infection in high risk groups in Brazil. *N. Engl. J. Med.* **320**:953-958.

Dehovits, J. A., Pape, J. W., Boncy, M., and Johnson, W. D. J. (1986). Clinical manifestations and therapy of *Isospora belli* infection in patients with the acquired immunodeficiency syndrome. *N. Engl. J. Med.* **315**:87.

Detels, R., English, P., Visscher, B. R., Kingsley, L. A., Jacobson, L., Chmiel, J. S., Dudley, J. P., Eldred, L. J., and Ginzberg, H. M. (1989). Seroconversion, sexual activity and condom use among 2915 HIV seronegative men followed for up to 2 years. *J. AIDS.* **2**:77-83.

Fultz, P. N., McClure, H. M., Daugharty, H., Brodie, A., McGrath, C. R., Swenson, B., and Francis, D. P. (1986). Vaginal transmission of human immunodeficiency virus (HIV) to a chimpanzee. *J. Infect. Dis.* **154**: 896-900.

Gordert, J. J., Sarangadharan, M. G., Biggar, R. J., Weiss, S. H., Winn, D., Grossman, R. J., Greene, M. H., Bodner, A., Mann, D. L., Strong, D. M., Gallo, R. C., and Blattner, W. A. (1984). Determinants of retrovirus (HTLV-III) antibody and immunodeficiency conditions in homosexual men. *Lancet* **2**:711-715.

James, W. D., Redfield, R. R., and Lypton, G. P. (1986). A papular eruption associated with HTLV III disease. *J. Am. Acad. Dermatol.* **13**: 563-566.

Kaslow, R. A., and Francis, D. P. (1989). Epidemiology: general considerations. In *The Epidemiology of AIDS.* Edited by R. A. Kaslow and D. P. Francis. New York, Oxford University Press, pp. 87-116.

Kreiss, J. K., Koeck, D., Plummer, F. A., Holmes, K. K., Lightfoot, M., Piot, P., Ronald, A. R., Ndinya-Achola, J. O., D'Costa, L., Roberts, P., Ngugi, E., and Quinn, T. (1986). AIDS virus infection in Nairobi prostitutes—spread of the epidemic to East Africa. *N. Engl. J. Med.* **314**:414-418.

Lesbordes, J. L. (1988). [Clinical aspects of human immunodeficiency virus (HIV) infection in Central Africa: 6 years experience at a hospital in an endemic area.] *Med. Trop.* (Mars) **48**:351-357.

Lewis, B., Abrams, D., and Ziegler, J. (1983). Single agent or combination chemotherapy of Kaposi's sarcoma in acquired immune deficiency syndrome. *Am. Soc. Clin. Oncol.* **2**:59.

Mann, J. M., Francis, H., Quinn, T. C., Pangu, K. A., Ngaly, B., Nzila, N., Kapita, B., Muymbe, T., Kalisa, R., Piot, P., McCormick, J., and Curran, J. W. (1986a). Surveillance for AIDS in a central African city. *J.A.M.A.* **255**:3255-3259.

Mann, J. M., Snider, D. E., Francis, H., Quinn, T. C., Colebunders, R. L., Piot, P., Curran, J. W., Nzilambi, N., and Bagola, N. (1986b). Association between HTLV III and TB in Zaire. *J.A.M.A.* **256**:346.

Pan American Health Organization (1987). Acquired immunodeficiency syndrome (AIDS) in the Americas. *Bull. Pan. Am. Health Org.* **21**:422-429.

Pape, J. W., and Johnson, W. D. Jr. (1989). HIV-1 infection and AIDS in Haiti. In *The Epidemiology of AIDS.* Edited by R. A. Kaslow and D. P. Francis. New York, Oxford University Press, pp. 221-230.

Pape, J. W., Liautaud, B., Thomas, F., Mathurin, J.-R., St. Amand, M.-M., Boncy, M., Pean, V., Pamphile, M., Laroche, C., Dehovits, J., and Johnson, W. (1985). The acquired immunodeficiency syndrome in Haiti. *Ann. Intern. Med.* **103**:674-678.

Piot, P., Quinn, T. C., Taelman, H., Feinsod, F. M., Minlango, K. B., Wobin, O., Mbendi, N., Mazebo, P., Ndangik, K., Stevens, W., Kayembe, K., Mithcell, S., Bridts, C., and McCormick, J. B. (1984). Acquired immunodeficiency syndrome in a heterosexual population in Zaire. *Lancet* **2**: 65-69.

Piot, P., Kreiss, J. K., Ndinya-Achola, J. O., Ngugi, E. N., Simonsen, J. N., Cameron, D. W., Taelman, H., and Plummer, F. A. (1987). Heterosexual transmission of HIV. *AIDS* **1**:199-206.

Piot, P., Plummer, F. A., Mhalu, F. S., Lamboray, J. L., Chin, J., Mann, J. M. (1988). AIDS: an international perspective. *Science* **239**:573-579.

Pitchenik, A. E., Cole, C., Russell, B. W., Fischl, M., Spira, T., and Snider, D. E. (1984). Tuberculosis, atypical mycobacteriosis and AIDS among Haitian and non-Haitian patients in South Florida. *Ann. Intern. Med.* **101**:641-645.

Quinn, T. C., and Mann, J. (1989). HIV-1 infection and AIDS in Africa. In *The Epidemiology of AIDS.* Edited by R. A. Kaslow and D. P. Francis. New York, Oxford University Press, pp. 194-220.

Quinn, T. C., Mann, J. M., Curran, J. W., and Piot, P. (1986). AIDS in Africa: an epidemiological paradigm. *Science* **234**:955-963.

Ryder, R., Francis, H., and Matela, D. (1987). Congenital HIV transmission in a large urban hospital in Kinshasa. II International Symposium on AIDS and Associated Centers in Africa, Naples: 121.

Serwadda, D., Murgerwa, R. D., Sewankambo, N. K., Lwegaba, A., Carswell, J. W., Kirya, G. B., and Bayley, A. C. (1985). Slim disease: a new disease in Uganda and its association with HTLV-III infection. *Lancet* **2**:849-852.

Simonsen, J. N., Cameron, D. W., Gakinya, M. N., Ndiny-Achola, J. O., D'Costa, L. J., Karasira, P., Cheang, M., Ronald, A. R., Piot, P., and Plummer, F. A. (1988). Human immunodeficiency virus infection among men with sexually transmitted diseases. Experience from a center in Africa. *N. Engl. J. Med.* **319**:274-278.

Snider, D., Hopewell, P., Mills, J., and Reichman, L. (1987). Position paper: American Thoracic Society. Mycobacterioses and the acquired immunodeficiency syndrome. *Am. Rev. Respir. Dis.* **136**:492-496.

Sunderham, G., McDonald, R. J., Maniatis, T., Oleske, J., Kapila, R., and Reichman, L. (1986). Tuberculosis as a manifestation of AIDS. *J.A.M.A.* **256**:362-366.

Taylor, J. F., Templeton, A. C., Vogel, C. C. (1971). Kaposi's sarcoma in Uganda: a clinicopathological study. *Int. J. Cancer* **8**:122-135.

Van De Perre, P., Rourroy, D., Lepage, P., Bogaerts, J., Kestelyn, P., Kayihigi, J., Hekker, A. C., Butzler, J. P., and Clumeck, N. (1984). Acquired immunodeficiency syndrome in Rwanda. *Lancet* **2**:62-65.

Weber, J. (1989). The biology and epidemiology of HIV infections. In *AIDS and AIDS Related Infections: Current Strategies for Prevention and Therapy.* Edited by A. J. Bint and J. Oxford. San Diego, Academic Press, p. 4.

Wong, B., Edwards, F. E., Kiehn, T. E., Whimbey, E., Donnelly, H., Bernard, E., Gold, J. W., and Armstrong, D. (1985). Continuous high-grade mycobacteria in patients with AIDS. *Am. J. Med.* **78**:35-40.

World Health Organization (1989). Acquired immunodeficiency syndrome (AIDS). *WHO Wkly Epidemiol Rec.*

12

Pulmonary Schistosomiasis

ARMENIO GUIMARAES and ISABEL GUIMARAES

University of Bahia Medical School and
Hospital Edgard Santos
Bahia, Brazil

I. Introduction

Pulmonary involvement in schistosomiasis was first reported a long time ago (1885), when Belleli observed schistosomal eggs in the lungs of patients coming to necropsy in Alexandria. Thereafter, several reports described the presence of ova in the lungs, the presence of innumerable small fibrous tubercular nodules, or the presence of an endarteritis obliterans that could be diffuse or localized (Sorour, 1974). However, the first detailed description of the main pathological aspects of pulmonary schistosomiasis and its relation to cor pulmonale may be credited to Shaw and Ghareeb (1938). These authors found pulmonary lesions due to ova in 33% of 282 autopsies of patients with this parasitic disease, but in only 2.1% of them did they report widespread obliterative arteriolar lesions associated with right ventricular hypertrophy and systemic venous congestion, and called these cases of "Ayerza's disease of bilharzial origin."

From a clinical standpoint, chronic cor pulmonale secondary to diffuse arteriolar disease represents the most important type of schistosomal pulmonary complication. Very infrequently, however, the clinical picture of pulmonary schistosomal disease may be that of a "cyanotic syndrome," with universal cyanosis and clubbing, which was very well characterized by Faria et al. (1959). Other infrequent and less important clinical presentations may include acute and chronic bronchitis, pneumonia, or bronchopneumonia (Meira, 1942; Neves et al., 1966).

It is noteworthy, however, that when hemodynamic and pulmonary function studies have been carried out in patients with schistosomosal portal hypertension, the frequency of abnormal findings leads to the impression of a systemic rather than of a localized disease, which, eventually, may show manifestations in other areas than the portal system (Souza and Guimarães, 1977; Guimarães, 1982). Mechanical disturbances of pulmonary function have also been documented in patients either with isolated intestinal or hepatosplenic schistosomiasis. These abnormalities have included increased airways resistance, V/Q disturbances, decreased exercise diffusing capacity, restrictive ventilatory disturbances, and an increase in physiological dead space (Abdel-Latif et al., 1965; Frayser and Alonso, 1967; Fulahian and Abboud, 1968; Zaky et al., 1968; Souza and Guimarães, 1977). From a clinical point of view, however, the importance of these disturbances has been difficult to evaluate, since the majority of patients are asymptomatic or, when symptoms are present, they are usually associated with pulmonary hypertension.

The pulmonary disease has been reported in connection with *Schistosoma mansoni, S. haematobium,* and *S. japonicum* (Shaw and Ghareeb, 1938; Sorour, 1974). Ova of *S. haematobium* may be found more commonly in the lungs, but *S. mansoni* produces vascular lesions more often than *S. haematobium* (Shaw and Ghareeb, 1938), while these changes have been rarely observed with *S. japonicum* (Inokuchi, 1979).

II. Epidemiology

The epidemiological data on pulmonary schistosomiasis are scanty and related primarily to the manifestations of pulmonary hypertension. Its geographical distribution follows that of schistosomiasis, specially where *S. mansoni* is endemic.

Badran et al. (1961), studying three different populations in Egypt, found a prevalence of chronic cor pulmonale of 2.45% in a rural population of 5,042 individuals compared with a rate of 0.6% in an urban population of 2,536 individuals. These patients were screened by chest x-ray and then underwent clinical examination and electrocardiogram (ECG).

When selected hospital populations in endemic areas were studied, between 2 and 4% of the total cardiac population were diagnosed as having schistosomal chronic cor pulmonale (Barbato et al., 1962). If only patients with hepatosplenic schistosomiasis were studied, the frequency may be higher: 6.5% according to Kenawy (1950).

In necropsy studies the frequency rate has varied between 2.1 and 26.9%, again revealing the heterogeneous criteria used to select the populations under study (Shaw and Ghareeb, 1938; Faria, 1954; Andrade and Andrade, 1970).

As expected, the direct measurement of arterial pulmonary pressure by heart catheterization of patients with schistosomiasis reveals a substantially higher frequency of pulmonary hypertension than is shown by clinical methods: 21.6% by Bertrand et al. (1978) and 13.0% by Guimarães (1982). The higher figures noted by Bertrand may be explained by two basic methodological differences in sampling: the size of the sample—Bertrand et al. studied 37 patients while Guimarães studied 141 patients; and the origin of the sample—Bertrand's sample was a hospital population while that of Guimarães was a rural population who came to the hospital specifically to be studied.

Data on the incidence of pulmonary hypertension in schistosomiasis are almost nonexistent, except for those recently obtained by Godinho, Guimarães, and Guimarães (unpublished observations). They evaluated 51 patients with schistosomal portal hypertension for 15 years, and detected an increase in the mean pulmonary artery pressure to abnormal levels in 5 (9.8%): 16.2 ± 2.0 mmHg to 35.0 ± 13.5 mmHg. These figures will give an annual incidence rate of pulmonary hypertension of 0.6%.

As already mentioned, a "cyanotic syndrome" has been reported as a manifestation of pulmonary disease in patients with hepatosplenic schistosomiasis by Faria et al. (1959). However, this clinical presentation of schistosomiasis seems to occur very infrequently, with only a few cases being reported. Indeed, in Guimarães et al.'s (1977) series of 134 patients with *S. mansoni* portal hypertension, only 2 patients (1.5%) showed this type of clinical presentation. Nevertheless, similarly to when heart catheterization was used to detect pulmonary hypertension, blood gas studies showed an oxygen disturbance in 28.3% of these cases (38 of 134).

The prevalence of mechanical respiratory disturbances in a large population of patients with schistosomiasis is still unknown. The literature on this subject is restricted mainly to reports of small series of patients, ranging between 10 and 37 patients. In these series the prevalence of abnormalities in the pulmonary function tests is high, varying from 100% in three series (Frayser and Alonso, 1967; Zaky et al., 1968; Souza and Guimarães, 1977) to 63.6% in a fourth series (Fulehian and Abboud, 1968).

III. Pathological Findings

At necropsy of patients with schistosomiasis, light microscopic examination may reveal apparently normal lungs, as documented in 67.0% of the patients studied by Shaw and Ghareed (1938) and in 28.6% of the patients studied by Andrade and Andrade (1970). The striking differences in these percentages certainly reflect diverse criteria in sampling: 80% of the cases necropsied by Shaw and Ghareeb died of causes other than schistosomiasis and also included cases of *S. haematobium*, while Andrade and Andrade studied patients in whom hepatosplenic *S. mansoni* infection was the main cause of death.

Pulmonary injury may start during the invasive stage of the disease, when schistosomal cercariae circulate through the lungs, and may cause patchy congestion of these organs. This may be associated with clinical manifestations of tracheobronchitis, the so-called "larval pneumonitis" (Coura et al., 1963; Sorour, 1974). Thereafter, lung embolization by the adult worm may occur, but this is harmless unless the worm dies, which may happen after specific therapy. The product of the dead worm then may produce an acute necrotizing type of pneumonitis, which is characterized by small areas of consolidation heavily infiltrated with eosinophils and macrophages. Foreign giant cells may attack the dead worms leading to the formation of large granulomata; some of these lesions may undergo calcification.

The more important pulmonary lesions, however, are caused by embolized ova from the normal habitat of the worms which reach the pulmonary arterioles and produce a specific acute necrotizing arteriolitis. They then destroy the intima and the media of the arteriolar wall and reach the extravascular space where parenchymatous tubercles are formed, with the ovum surrounded by eosinophils, lymphocytes, macrophages, and giant cells. When the ovum dies it undergoes calcification and there is a proliferation of fibroblasts into the tubercle. Healing of the acute vascular lesion is followed by an obliterative arteritis, with the canalization of the occluded vessels by new capillaries (Fig. 1). These capillaries may sometimes hypertrophy, producing an angiomatoid lesion that may enlarge to cavernous dimensions (Fig. 2). These angiomatoid lesions may form communications among themselves or with branches of the pulmonary veins involved in the process, giving origin to micropulmonary arteriovenous fistulae (Shaw and Ghareeb, 1938; Faria et al., 1959; Marchand et al., 1962; Santiago et al., 1965a; Andrade and Andrade, 1970).

In patients with widespread obstructive arteriolar lesions caused by schistosomal eggs, the arterioles and small pulmonary arteries usually show diffuse medial hyperplasia and fibroelastic intimal thickening with marked narrowing of the vascular lumen (Fig. 1). The larger pulmonary arteries are dilated and commonly exhibit intimal atherosclerosis. The right ventricle shows concentric hypertrophy, but may also be dilated in more severe cases.

Nevertheless, in young patients widespread arteriolar lesions caused by schistosomal eggs may be associated with right ventricular hypertrophy in-

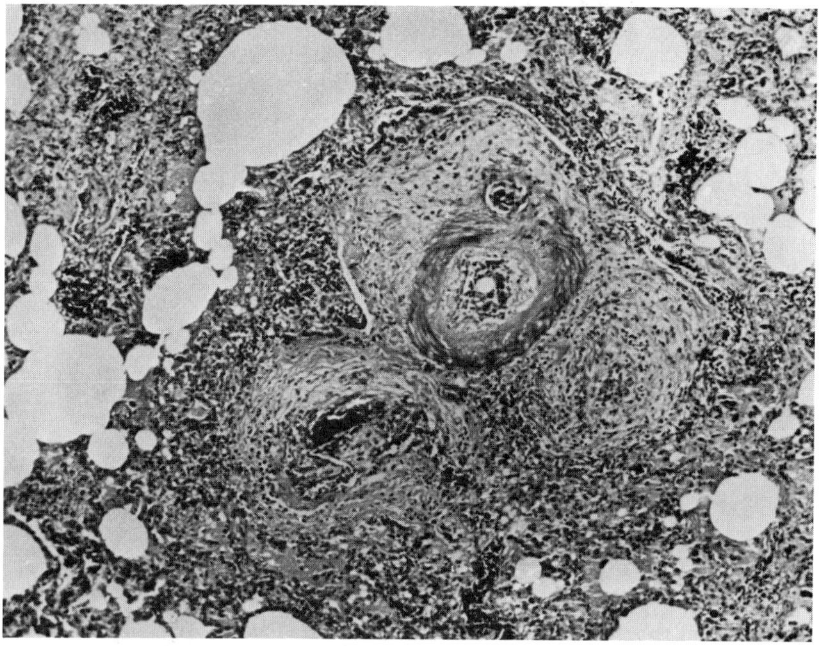

Figure 1 Advanced arteriolar lesion with intimal fibrosis and medial hypertrophy; around the central arteriole, periovular granulomata and other periarteriolar inflammatory and fibrotic changes can be seen, representing different stages of the pulmonary schistosomal lesion (hematoxylin and eosin, × 120; courtesy of Prof. Zilton Andrade, Fiocruz, Salvador, Bahia, Brazil).

dicative of pulmonary hypertension in the absence of hypertensive pulmonary arteriolar and arterial lesions (Andrade and Andrade, 1970).

Mixed with these vascular lesions, the lungs in schistosomiasis show bronchiolar and interstitial lesions (Andrade and Andrade, 1970) that also may lead to ventilatory disturbances (Souza and Guimarães, 1977).

IV. Pathogenesis and Pathophysiology

A. Pulmonary Hypertension

The presence of pathological findings indicative of pulmonary hypertension has been always connected with numerous egg granulomata, which suggests that massive pulmonary egg embolization must be an important requirement for the development of pulmonary hypertension. As Andrade and Andrade (1970) have pointed out, this massive infection should occur in the early

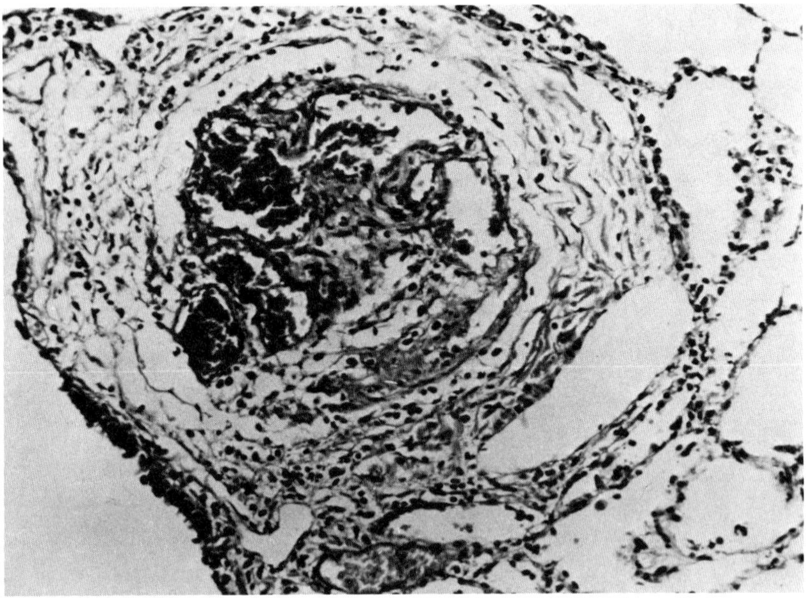

(a)

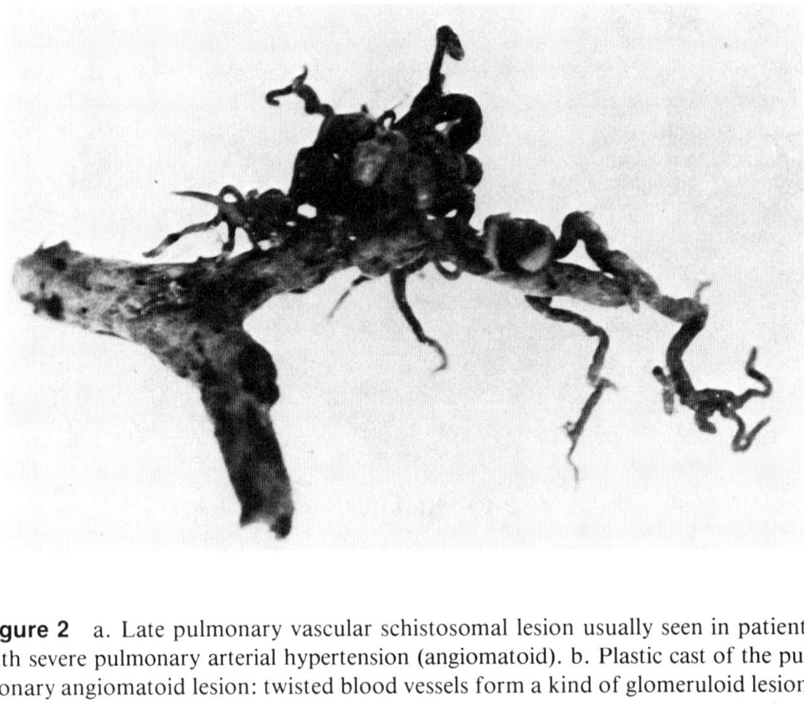

(b)

Figure 2 a. Late pulmonary vascular schistosomal lesion usually seen in patients with severe pulmonary arterial hypertension (angiomatoid). b. Plastic cast of the pulmonary angiomatoid lesion: twisted blood vessels form a kind of glomeruloid lesion; note that the lesion is entirely arteriolar (approximately $\times$ 5; courtesy of Prof. Zilton Andrade, Fiocruz, Salvador, Bahia, Brazil).

developmental stages of the disease, while worms and eggs are still abundant and the host resistance is low. Repeated but not massive pulmonary egg embolization tends to match increased host resistance, leading to the formation of small and discrete granulomata. Some authors, however, advocate the gradual development of pulmonary arteriolar lesions as a consequence of repeated egg embolization during the clinical evolution of the disease (Erfan et al., 1949; Kenawy, 1950; Girgis, 1952; Coura et al., 1963).

If massive pulmonary egg embolization is fundamental for the development of pulmonary hypertension, we must discuss the conditions that allow such massive embolization. The egg emboli come from the natural habitat of the schistosoma worms, the portal system in the case of *S. japonicum* and *S. mansoni* and the prostatic, uterine, vesical, and ureteric plexus in the case of *S. haematobium*. The eggs of the former parasites must bypass the liver to reach the lungs, which requires the formation of collaterals between the portal and systemic veins. Early and rapid development of portal hypertension should therefore be a prerequisite to massive pulmonary egg embolization. This rapid progression of an acute infection to the hepatosplenic form of the disease has already been demonstrated. This infection, in endemic areas, tends to occur mainly in the first two decades of life (Santiago et al., 1965b). These assumptions are in accord with the fact that the majority of the patients reported with schistosomosal cor pulmonale also have hepatosplenomegaly, except for patients with *S. haematobium* infection (Shaw and Ghareeb, 1938). Indeed, in patients infected with *S. mansoni* a relationship seems to exist between the degree of hypertension in the portal and pulmonary systems (El-Garen et al., 1970). Only rarely have patients with pulmonary hypertension in endemic areas for *S. mansoni* been reported without associated evidence of portal hypertension. The postulated mechanisms in such cases have been the occurrence of severe arteriolar lesions during the acute stage of the disease; eggs from the portal system reaching the caval system through the vertebral veins; the possibility of the development of metacercariae in the lungs; or the early passage of eggs through the injured hepatic sinus, before the full development of the hepatosplenic form of the disease (Cavalcanti et al., 1962; Marques, 1964). However, it should be pointed out that none of these postulated mechanisms have been documented, and some investigators stressed that they have never observed any such cases (Andrade and Andrade, 1970).

Some investigators, however, also postulate that gradual development of an increased pulmonary arteriolar resistance due to repeated pulmonary egg embolization along the clinical course of the disease may occur (Shaw and Ghareeb, 1938; Erfan et al., 1949; Kenawy, 1950; Girgis, 1952; Chaves, 1960; Coura et al., 1963). This hypothesis may be a good pathogenetic explanation for patients with schistosomal pulmonary hypertension occurring after the fourth decade of life, and seems to be backed by some clinical-epidemiological data. As shown by Guimarães (1982), when the age distribution of a subpopulation of patients with pulmonary hypertension is compared with that of the population of patients with portal hypertension from which it was selected, one can observe that the former is bimodal while the latter shows a left-skewed bell-shaped curve (Fig. 3). Although the mortality rate of patients with uncomplicated portal hypertension seems to increase progressively with age, that of patients with pulmonary hypertension peaked at the third and sixth decades of life. This finding can be interpreted as an evidence of two distinct subpopulations of patients with pulmonary hypertension: the first develops pulmonary hypertension at an earlier age due to massive pulmonary egg embolization, as proposed by Andrade and Andrade 1970); while in the older patients, after the third decade, the pulmonary hypertension may have been the result of a more gradual process due to repeated

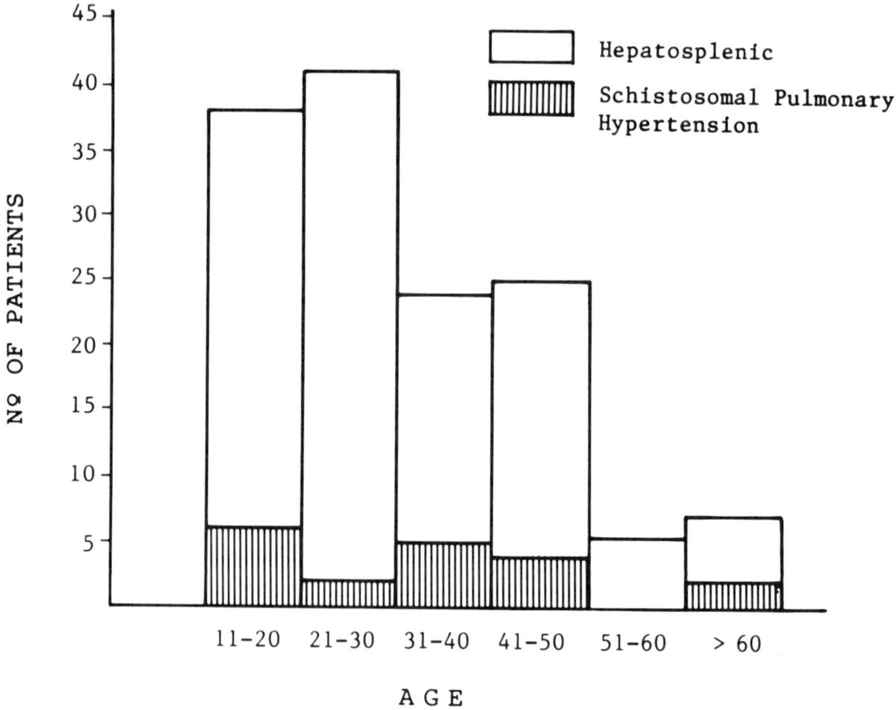

Figure 3 Age distribution of 141 patients with schistosomal portal hypertension compared with that of 19 patients with pulmonary hypertension derived from the former population (reprinted with permission of the *Arquivos Brasileiros de Cardiologia* from Guimarães, 1982).

egg embolization. This suggestion is supported by the fact that both subpopulations are exposed to infection since the first decade of life, almost ruling out the possibility that these findings can be the consequence of heavy infection at different ages instead of representing some variance in the pathogenetic mechanism.

These two ways of developing pulmonary hypertension seem more clear when this type of comparison is made by sex. While findings in male patients reproduce the distribution curves discussed above, findings in female patients are different: the main population with portal hypertension shows a bimodal distribution while the subpopulation with pulmonary hypertension shows a right-skewed bell shaped curve, Guimarães (1982) (Fig. 4). This bimodal type of distribution curve for female subjects with portal hypertension is suggestive of a progressive mortality, until the fourth decade, of female

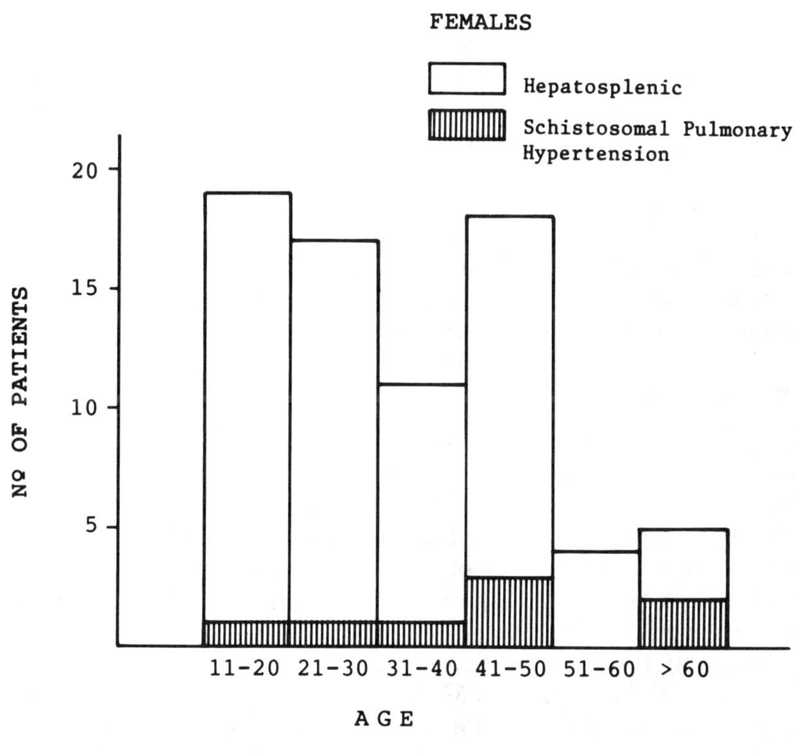

Figure 4 Age distribution of 74 female patients with schistosomal portal hypertension compared with that of 8 patients with pulmonary hypertension derived from the former population (reprinted with permission of the *Arquivos Brasileiros de Cardiologia* from Guimarães, 1982).

patients who have acquired the disease early in their lives. This is followed by an increase in frequency due to the appearance of another subpopulation of female patients who acquired the disease later on, despite having similar chances of infection to those of the younger subpopulation. The former subpopulation would represent the result of a massive infection with the early development of portal hypertension, while the latter the result of a gradual development of the disease. Regarding pulmonary hypertension, the age distribution curve of female subjects differs strikingly from that of the male patients. Female patients seem more prone to develop pulmonary hypertension after the fourth decade, suggesting that they are more susceptible to the gradual type of pathogenetic mechanism. The reason for that is not clear, but sex-related differences in immunology and/or hormone protection cannot be ruled out.

Beyond the mechanical obstruction, vasospasm seems to represent a contributory mechanism for elevation of the pulmonary arteriolar resistance in these patients. Indeed, the administration of 100% oxygen for 20 min or of intravenous reserpine was followed by a significant drop in the pulmonary arteriolar resistance of a group of patients with schistosomal pulmonary hypertension (Fig. 5) (Guimarães, 1982). This vasospasm, however, probably represents an unspecific reaction to the already decreased compliance of the pulmonary vascular bed, as has been noticed in pulmonary hypertension due to other causes (Harris, 1957).

Pulmonary hypertension in schistosomiasis is usually mild or moderate in degree. Therefore, in the series of Guimarães (1982) the pulmonary artery pressure was less than 35 mmHg in 73.7%, and equal to or higher than 40 mmHg in only 10.5% of the patients studied.

B. Hypoxemia

Hypoxemia is another type of disturbance due to the pulmonary injury of schistosomiasis. Cyanosis represents the most severe end of the spectrum of this complication, which occurs infrequently.

Similarly to pulmonary hypertension, when more sensitive methods of study were used, the frequency of subclinical hypoxemia was quite high: 38 of 134 (28.3%) patients with portal hypertension who had their PaO_2 and pulmonary shunt (Qs/Qt) determined (Guimarães et al., 1977). In 68% of them (26 of 38), there was only a decreased PaO_2, in 58% (22 of 38) an increased Qs/Qt, and in 26% (10 of 38) both abnormalities were present. These findings are indicative of two distinct pathophysiological mechanisms responsible for arterial desaturation. The increased pulmonary venous shunt may be the consequence of micropulmonary arteriovenous (AV) fistulae or of portopulmonary communications, which have been demonstrated both anatomically (Faria et al., 1959; Calabresi and Abelmann, 1957; Santiago

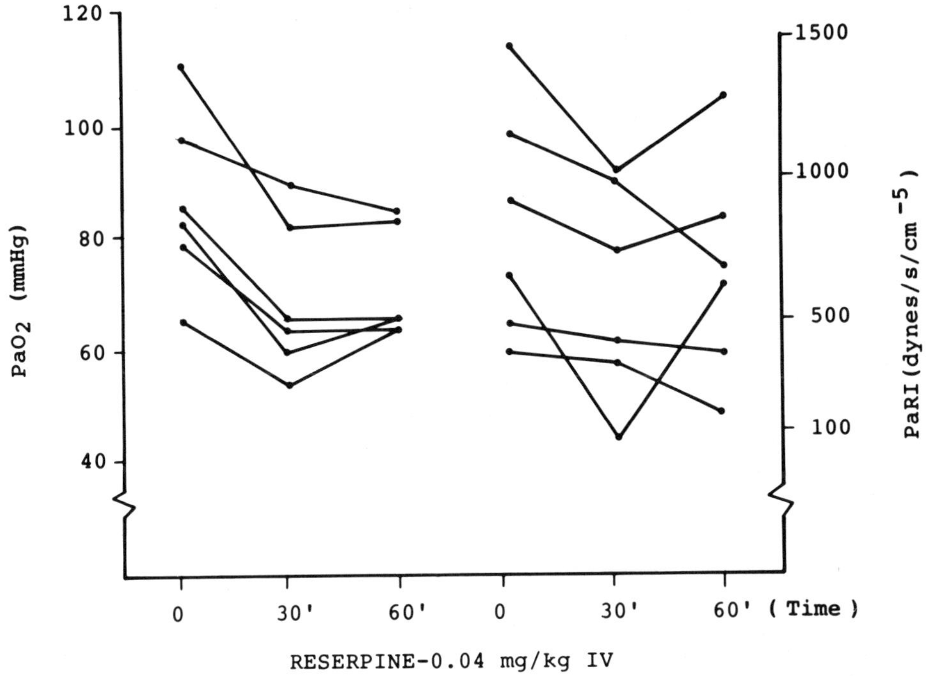

Figure 5 Effect on the PaO_2 and the pulmonary arteriolar resistance index (PaRI) of the intrapulmonary arterial injection of reserpine in six patients with schistosomal pulmonary hypertension (Guimarães, A. C., unpublished data, 1973).

et al., 1965a) and physiologically (Zaky et al., 1964). Indeed, radioisotopic studies with ^{85}Kr in 15 patients with schistosomal portal hypertension have suggested the presence of portal-pulmonary communications in 13 of them and of micropulmonary AV fistulae in 2 others.

That the degree of portopulmonary shunting is related to the severity of the portal hypertension is suggested by the significant correlation between the decrease in portal pressure and the increase in PaO_2, when breathing room air, and the decrease in the Qs/Qt when breathing 100% oxygen, following an intravenous infusion of vasopressin (Alves, 1975) (Fig. 6). Furthermore, the presence of an increased Qs/Qt was significantly higher in patients with esophageal varices, as demonstrated by x-ray, and/or suggested by episodes of esophageal bleeding (Guimarães et al., 1977).

Decreased PaO_2 in the absence of an increased Qs/Qt may be secondary to a V/Q disturbance. This is suggested by the significant drop in PaO_2 that occurred after the infusion of reserpine (0.04 mg/kg) into the pulmonary

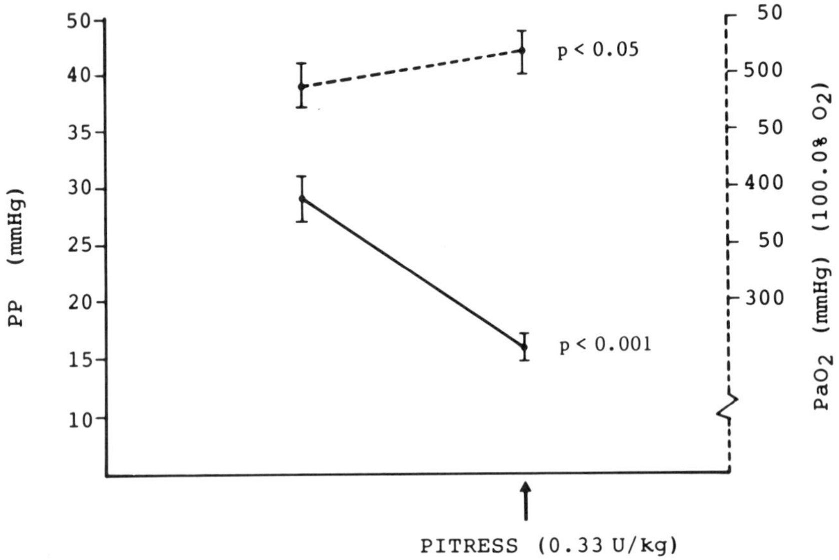

Figure 6 Effect on the portal pressure (PP) and the PaO_2 of the intravenous injection of vasopressin in 20 patients with schistosomal portal hypertension (derived from Alves, 1975).

artery (Guimarães, 1982) (Fig. 5). This drop was associated with a decrease in pulmonary arteriolar resistance and with an unchanged $PaCO_2$, which ruled out a drug-induced depression of the respiratory center as its main cause. This reserpine-induced hypoxemia is certainly the result of the widespread vasodilatory effect of the drug upon the pulmonary arterioles, which results in increased perfusion of hypoventilated areas in the lung.

C. Ventilatory Disturbances

These disturbances may occur independently of pulmonary hypertension (Frayser and Alonso, 1967). In a group of 36 patients with portal hypertension studied by Souza and Guimarães (1977), an increased minute ventilatory volume was found in all, an increased ventilatory equivalent in 96%, a decreased $PaCO_2$ in 42%, a decreased vital capacity in 28%, and signs of moderate to severe obstructive bronchial disease in 17%.

Zaky and co-workers (1964) found an inverse correlation between the degree of reduction of the vital capacity and the level of the mean pulmonary artery pressure in patients with pulmonary hypertension. Nevertheless, Souza and Guimarães (1977) found normal vital capacity in four patients with pulmonary hypertension of moderate to severe degree (mean pressure in the range of 36.0-50.7 mmHg).

The clinical importance of these abnormalities is still unknown and requires further studies in this field. From a pathophysiological standpoint, however, it is one more piece of evidence favoring schistosomiasis as a systemic disease with clinical manifestations that differ according to its severity.

V. Clinical Presentation

A. Pulmonary Hypertension

Clinical Picture

Pulmonary hypertension in schistosomiasis has been found in patients of a wide age range, varying between the first and the eight decades of life, with mean age between 26 and 31 years old (Turner, 1964; Bertrand et al., 1978; Guimarães, 1982). Some authors speak of a definitive male preponderance (Sorour, 1974), but some major series show that this preponderance is only slight (Vinhaes, 1977; Guimarães, 1982).

Clinical manifestations are related to the severity of the hypertension and are indistinguishable from those of other types of obstructive pulmonary arteriolar disease. Before symptoms and signs of right ventricular failure supervene, episodes of syncope and/or of dizzy spells may occur; these symptoms may be aggravated by anemia secondary to hypersplenism and/or gastrointestinal bleeding from esophageal varices.

Right ventricular failure may occur in patients at any age, but is more common in the youngest age group (between 10 and 35 years old). Cyanosis may appear rarely, at the end stage of decompensation, in patients with a patent foramen ovale or when there is association with the "cyanotic syndrome," which rarely occurs. Associated with severe systemic venous hypertension, severe jaundice may also be observed secondary to liver congestion.

At the asymptomatic phase, the diagnosis can be made based on the physical signs of pulmonary hypertension and concomitant portal hypertension. The diagnostic signs of pulmonary hypertension will include the presence of a right ventricular heave, and a narrow split-second sound with a loud P2. Nevertheless, a mild right ventricular heave and a soft ejection systolic murmur at the left sternal border may be also found in patients with hepatosplenomegaly without pulmonary hypertension, but in the absence of a loud P2. This certainly represents the effect of heart displacement by the hepatosplenomegaly.

Electrocardiographic Findings

The ECG may show signs of right atrial and ventricular hypertrophy, and usually reflects the degree of severity and duration of the pulmonary hyper-

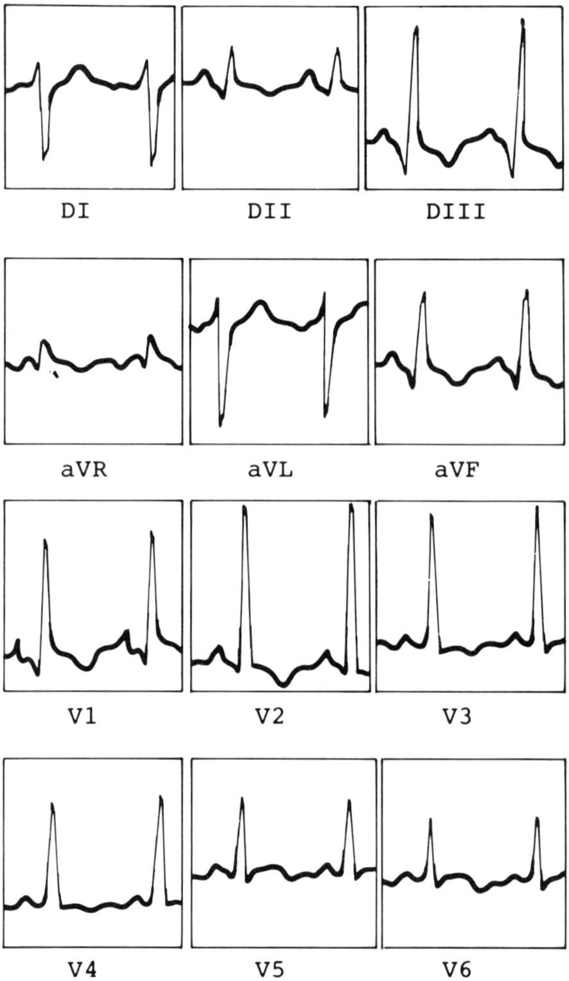

Figure 7 Twelve-lead ECG of a patient with severe schistosomal pulmonary hypertension exhibits right ventricular hypertrophy with strain (Guimarães, A. C., unpublished data, 1972).

tension (Fig. 7). Thus, in 19 patients in our series, the ECG showed evidence of right ventricular hypertrophy in only 3 (16.0%). The mean PA pressure in these 3 patients was 37.5, 39.1, and 40.0 mmHg, respectively; all but 1 of the other 16 patients, with normal ECGs, had PA mean pressures in the range of 20.0-35.8 mmHg, with a mean of 24.4 mmHg (Guimarães, 1982). Eventually, however, the ECG may be normal even in the presence of severe pulmonary hypertension. This is well illustrated by the remaining patient of this group, a 60-year-old woman, who had the highest PA pressure (62.7 mmHg). This finding may have been a reflection of the short duration of the hypertension and/or of associated lung parenchymal disease, a common event at this age, which may distort the ECG picture.

Radiologic Findings

The chest x-ray of patients with schistosomal pulmonary hypertension may vary from completely normal to one showing lung and heart abnormalities. As occurs with the ECG, these changes seem to be dependent on the intensity and duration of the hypertension, except for some parenchymatous changes that are probably correlated with the intensity of lung aggression by the schistosomal eggs.

In the most severe cases the cardiac silhouette is enlarged due to right atrial and ventricular dilatation, showing a rounded cardiac apex and a small aortic knob. The pulmonary arch and the main branches of the pulmonary artery are severely dilated while the secondary pulmonary arteries are narrowed, making the clear peripheral lung fields contrast with the dense hilar vascular shadows (Fig. 8).

In mild to moderate pulmonary hypertension or in cases with severe hypertension of short duration, the cardiac silhouette is usually normal. A mild degree of dilatation of the pulmonary arch may be found in patients with normal pulmonary artery pressure and so cannot be considered a definitive diagnostic sign of pulmonary hypertension. In this regard, some reference parameters can be taken into consideration: for instance, a diameter of the right pulmonary artery between 14.1 and 17.0 mm has a high statistical probability of belonging to a patient with pulmonary hypertension. If the diameter is greater than 17 mm it is always found in association with this pathological condition. For the pulmonary arch chord, the respective values are between 36.1 and 46.0 mm and greater than 46 mm, and for the arrow they are between 5.5 and 6.9 mm and greater than 6.9 mm (Vinhaes et al., 1977).

Hemodynamics

As already discussed, pulmonary hypertension in schistosomiasis is obstructive in type and secondary to a diffuse arteriolitis caused by schistosomal eggs. As a consequence, the hemodynamic picture shows increased pulmonary artery mean pressure, normal pulmonary capillary wedge pressure, and elevated pulmonary arteriolar resistance. In the more severe cases, complicated with right heart failure, the right ventricular end-diastolic and right atrial mean pressures are also elevated (Sorour, 1974; Bertrand et al., 1978; Guimarães, 1982). As expected, left ventricular pressures are normal (Guimarães, 1982).

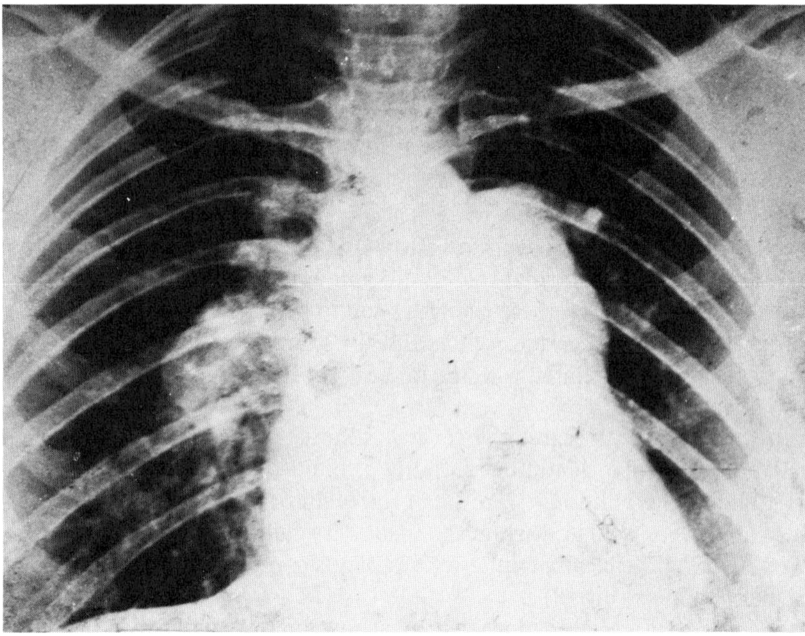

Figure 8 Chest x-ray of a patient with severe and long-standing schistosomal pulmonary hypertension: observe the huge dilatation of the pulmonary trunk and of the right main pulmonary artery, contrasting with the very narrow peripheral pulmonary arteries; the cardiac silhouette shows moderate to severe dilatation (Guimarães, A. C., unpublished data, 1972).

Elevation of the mean pulmonary artery pressure is mild to moderate in the majority of cases. Thus, of 19 patients studied, in 17 (84.9%) it was below 40 mmHg, and below 30 mmHg in 12 of them (70.5%) (Guimarães, 1982). It should be pointed out that these patients were randomly selected to undergo hemodynamic studies from a rural population of 141 patients with schistosomal portal hypertension. When a hospital-based population is studied, however, the chances for a higher frequency of more severe cases are greater. In a group of 37 patients with portal hypertension studied by Bertrand et al. (1978), pulmonary hypertension was found in 8 (21.6%) of them: mean pulmonary artery pressure was below 40 mmHg in 5 (62.5%) and below 30 mmHg in 4 (50.0%). In addition, from the clinical standpoint, six of them complained of effort dyspnea, and in four the cardiothoracic ratio (CTR) was higher than 50%, pointing to more severe disease than in the former series.

B. Cyanotic Syndrome

As already stated, the "cyanotic syndrome" is an infrequent manifestation of schistosomiasis, and does not always accompany pulmonary hypertension. Based on their clinical appearance, in areas endemic for schistosomiasis, these patients, when young, may be taken easily for patients with congenital cyanotic heart disease. In addition to universal cyanosis and clubbing, they present with a very active precordium, sometimes associated with a left ventricular heave, and a soft systolic murmur at the left sternal border. However, the presence of signs of portal hypertension, a normal ECG, and characteristic pulmonary densities, especially in the right lower lung lobe (Fig. 9),

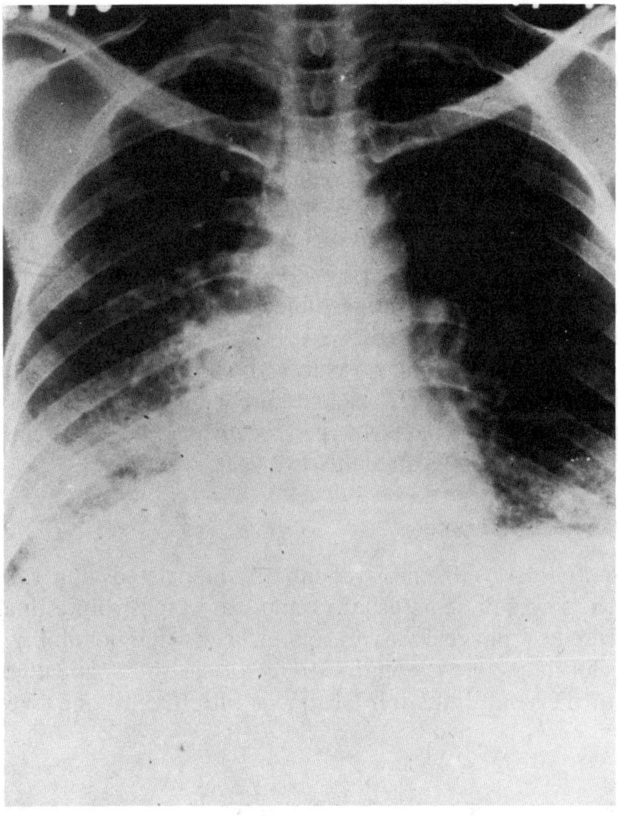

Figure 9 Confluent micronodular pulmonary densities at the lower lung lobes, more prominent on the right, in a patient with the schistosomal "cyanotic syndrome" (Guimarães, A. C., unpublished data, 1972).

favors the diagnosis of the "cyanotic syndrome" (Guimarães, unpublished observations, 1973).

VI. Natural History

A. Pulmonary Hypertension

The natural history of schistosomal pulmonary hypertension is still not well known. Indeed, the majority of reports included patients with clinical cor pulmonale, a great proportion of whom have right ventricular failure (Erfan et al., 1949; Kenawy, 1950; Barbato et al., 1962; Cavalcanti et al., 1962). At this stage the disease is usually fatal quickly.

However, when less advanced cases are studied prospectively, the clinical course is quite variable and unpredictable, but the mortality rate is still high. Of the 15 patients reported by Silva (1984), who belonged to the population initially studied by Guimarães (1982), 5 (33%) died during a 10 year follow-up period. The most probable cause of death was heart failure in four, and liver failure in the other. On the other hand, that the condition may remain stable for this length of time was revealed by the mean pulmonary artery pressure of the eight patients who were recatheterized: 30.4 ± 7.1 mmHg for the first value compared with 30.0 ± 11.0 mmHg for the second value. Further data recently were obtained by Godinho, Guimarães, and Guimarães (unpublished observations), who restudied five more patients from the same series of Silva (1984), 13-15 years afterwards. The following values were found for the first and second measurements: 32.2 ± 6.8 mmHg and 32.4 ± 10.1 mmHg, respectively. These data are in accord with previous report by Cavalcanti and Tompson (1964), who documented the stable clinical course of some of their patients evaluated for 7 years.

B. Cyanotic Syndrome

When present, this syndrome is commonly associated with severe portal hypertension. These patients usually die of major gastrointestinal bleeding due to ruptured esophageal varices. Nevertheless, the possibility of regression of the clinical picture is exemplified by the case of a patient who showed regression of the syndrome after treatment with hycanthone (Wessel et al., 1965).

VII. Final Remarks and Conclusions

Schistosomiasis was initially seen mainly as an intestinal disease with involvement of the portal system in more severe cases. Later on, pathologists identified lung lesions that indicated the systemic character of the condition, at least in some stage of its evolution. In a small proportion of these patients there was also evidence of right ventricular hypertrophy, with or without signs of systemic venous congestion, characterizing different evolutionary stages of the chronic cor pulmonale. Thereafter, the few existing epidemiological studies showed that only a small number of the patients with schistosomiasis had this clinical presentation. Hemodynamic studies, however, in patients with schistosomal portal hypertension, revealed a prevalence rate of pulmonary hypertension around 13%, indicating that the majority of these cases are clinically silent.

The consequences of the lung involvement are not restricted to the increase in pulmonary arteriolar resistance. Indeed, when gasometric and ventilatory studies were also carried out, they document variable degrees of hypoxemia and several ventilatory disturbances. In the great majority of them, however, their clinical importance still awaits proper evaluation.

It is fortunate that the few existing prospective data on patients with portal hypertension show a low incidence of pulmonary hypertension. A great proportion of those patients who are already hypertensive may remain stable for a long period of time without disability, as occurs in agricultural workers. Nevertheless, the mortality rate is high, and there is no present way to identify the patients at risk. If, however, one consider that the age of the patients who develop pulmonary hypertension was 34 ± 8.6 years, it should not be difficult to prevent this complication by the early treatment of schistosomiasis. This goal, and better sanitary conditions to prevent primary infection, must represent the main efforts against the development of schistosomal portal hypertension, since the treatment of the hypertension itself is still very frustrating and not well tolerated (Guimarães, unpublished observations, 1984).

References

Abdel-Latif, E. A., Atta, A. A., El-Garem, A., Fahmy, S., Abdel-Wahab, M. F., and El-Hawy, A. M. (1965). Clinical and physiological studies in broncho-pulmonary schistosomiasis. *J. Egypt. Med. Assoc.* **43**:452-466.

Alves, C. A. P. A. (1975). Contribuição ao estudo do "shunt" anatômico pulmonar na síndrome de hipertensão portal esquistossomótica. Thesis. Salvador, Bahia, Brasil, Medical School.

Andrade, Z. A., and Andrade, S. G. (1970). Pathogenesis of schistosomal pulmonary arteritis. *Am. J. Trop. Med. Hyg.* **19**:305-310.

Badran, A., El-Nagah, A., Abdalla, A., and Halawani, A. (1961). Radiological survey for the incidence of bilharzial cor pulmonale in Egypt. *J. Egypt. Med. Assoc.* **44**:967-975.

Barbato, E. C. D., Haebish, H., Fujioka, T., Pileggi, F., and Decourt, L. V. (1962). Schistosomal cor pulmonale. *Postgrad. Med. J.* **32**:246-252.

Bertrand, E., Dalger, J., Ramiara, J. P., Renambot, J., and Attia, Y. (1978). L'hypertension arterielle pulmonare bilharzienne. Etude clinique et hemodinamique chez 37 malades. *Arch. Mal. Coeur* **71**:216-221.

Calabresi, P., and Abelmann, W. H. (1957). Porto-caval and porto-pulmonary anastomosis in Laennec's cirrhosis and in heart failure. *J. Clin. Invest.* **362**:1257-1265.

Cavalcanti, I. L., and Tompson, G. (1964). História natural e diagnóstico diferencial da hipertensão arterial pulmonar esquistossomótica. *J. Bras. Med.* **8**:335-338.

Cavalcanti, I. L., Tompson, G., Souza, N., and Barbosa, F. S. (1962). Pulmonary hypertension in schistosomiasis. *Br. Heart J.* **24**:363-371.

Chaves, E. (1960). Cor pulmonale Esquistossomótico. I. Estudo das lesões vasculares associadas à hipertensão pulmonar. *Rev. Inst. Med. Trop. São Paulo* **2**:78-89.

Coura, J. R., Coutinho, S. G., Moraes, H. M., Dias, L. B., Rodrigues, N. P., and Silva, J. R. (1963). Esquistossomose pulmonar. *O Hospital* **63**: 993-1012.

El-Garen, A. A., El-Hawey, A. M., and Mousa, A. H. (1970). Study of the portal and the cardiopulmonary haemodynamic interelationship in schistosomal cases. *J. Egypt. Med. Assoc.* **53**:99-107.

Erfan, M., Erfan, H., Mousa, A. M., and Deeb, A. A. (1949). Chronic pulmonary schistosomiasis. A clinical and radiological study. *Trans. R. Soc. Trop. Med. Hyg.* **42**:477-485.

Faria, J. L. (1954). Cor pulmonale in manson's schistosomiasis. I — Frequency in necropsy material; pulmonary vascular changes caused by schistosoma ova. *Am. J. Pathol.* **30**:167-193.

Faria, J. L., Barbas, J. V., Fujioka, T., Lion, M. F., Silva, U. A., and Decourt, L. V. (1959). Pulmonary schistosomotic arteriovenous fistulas producing a new cyanotic syndrome in Manson's schistosomiasis. *Am. Heart J.* **58**:556-567.

Frayser, R., and Alonso, A. E. (1967). Studies of pulmonary function in patients with schistosomiasis. *Am. Rev. Respir. Dis.* **95**:1036-1040.

Fulehian, F. J. D., and Abboud, R. T. (1968). Pulmonary function in patients with early asymptomatic schistosomiasis before and after treatment with sodium antimony dimerceptosuccinate (Astiban). *Am. J. Trop. Med. Hyg.* **17**:372-377.

Girgis, B. (1952). Pulmonary heart disease due to bilharzia: The bilharzial cor pulmonale. *Am. Heart J.* **43**:606-611.

Guimarães, A. C. (1982). Situação atual dos conhecimentos sobre o envolvimento cardiopulmonar na esquistossomose mansônica. *Arq. Bras. Cardiol.* **38**:301-309.

Guimarães, A. C., Alves Junior, A. R., Santos Filho, A., Esteves, J. P., Vinhaes, L. S. A., Abreu, W. N., Souza, J. A. A., Bina, J. C., and Prata, A. R. (1977). Blood gas changes and pulmonary hemodynamics in portal hypertension due to schistosomiasis mansoni. *Rev. Inst. Med. Trop. São Paulo* **19**:80-93.

Harris, P. (1957). Influence of acetylcholine on the pulmonary arterial pressure. *Br. Heart J.* **19**:272-278.

Inokuchi, T. (1979). Pulmonary lesions in schistosomiasis japonica. I. Human autopsy cases. *J. Kurume Med. Assoc.* **42**:1082-1100.

Kenawy, M. R. (1950). The syndrome of cardiopulmonary schistosomiasis. *Am. Heart J.* **39**:678-696.

Marchand, E. J., Jesus, M., and Biascoechea, Z. A. R. (1962). Cyanotic syndrome of portal hypertension in hepatosplenic schistosomiasis and portal cirrhosis. Report of four cases. *Am. J. Cardiol.* **10**:496-506.

Marques, J. R. (1964). Esquistossomose mansônica. Aspectos semiológicos da forma cardiopulmonar. *J. Bras. Med.* **8**:325-333.

Meira, J. A. (1942). Estudo clínico das formas pulmonares da esquistossomose mansônica: doença de Manson-Pirajá da Silva. *Arq. Cirurg. Clin. Exp.* **6**:3-136.

Neves, J., Tonelli, E., and Carvalho, S. M. (1966). Estudo das manifestações pulmonares da forma toxêmica da esquistossomose mansoni. *Rev. Inst. Med. Trop. S. Paulo* **8**:22-29.

Santiago, J. M., Raick, A. N., and Maletta, C. A. (1965a). Contribuição ao conhecimento da esquistossomose pulmonar crônica com cianose universal (fístulas pulmonares artério-venosas). *Rev. Inst. Med. Trop. São Paulo* **7**:103-109.

Santiago, J. M., Neves, J., and Ratton, J. L. A. (1965b). Evolução da forma toxêmica da esquistossomose mansônica para o cor pulmonale. *Rev. Inst. Med. Trop. São Paulo* **7**:295-304.

Shaw, A. F. B., and Ghareeb, A. A. (1938). The pathogenesis of pulmonary schistosomiasis in Egypt with special reference to Ayerza's disease. *J. Pathol. Bacteriol.* **46**:401-424.

Silva, E. A. (1984). Aspectos clínico-epidemiológicos e evolutivos da hipertensão pulmonar esquistossomótica. Thesis. Brasília, Brasil, Medical School.

Sorour, A. H. (1974). Schistosomal cor pulmonale. In *Cardiovascular Disease in the Tropics*. Edited by A. G. Shaper, M. S. R. Hutt, and Z. Fejfar. London, British Medical Association, pp. 297-305.

Souza, L. S. F., and Guimarães, A. C. (1977). Estudo da função pulmonar de portadores da síndrome de hipertensão portal esquistossomótica. *Rev. Med. Bahia* **23**:11-25.

Turner, P. P. (1964). Schistosomal pulmonary arterial hypertension in east Africa. *Br. Heart J.* **26**:821-831.

Vinhaes, L. S. A., Guimarães, A. C., Santos Filho, A., Abreu, W. N., Esteves, J. P. Bina, J. C., and Prata, A. R. (1977). A circulação pulmonar na síndrome de hipertensão portal esquistossomótica. Interrelações radiológico-hemodinâmicas. *Arq. Bras. Cardiol.* **30**:13-18.

Wessel, H. U., Sommers, H. M., Gugell, D. W., and Paul, M. H. (1965). Variants of cardiopulmonary manifestations of manson's schistosomiasis. *Ann. Intern. Med.* **62**:757-766.

Zaky, H. A., El-Heneidy, A. R., and Kalil, M. (1964). Use of Krypton-85 in the study of hipoxia in porto-pulmonary bilharziasis (schistosomiasis). *Br. Med. J.* **1**:1021-1024.

Zaky, H. A., El-Heneidy, A. R., and El-Maksoud Tarabeih, A. A. (1968). Hyperventilation and effort dyspnea in porto-pulmonary bilharziasis. *Dis. Chest.* **53**:162-171.

13

Pulmonary Complications of Sickle Cell Disease

HARVEY EISENBERG

Lincoln Medical Center
Bronx, New York

The broad group of diseases in the lung that have come to be known as pneumonias of sickle cell anemia has attracted increasing recognition over the past several decades. Patients with sickle cell anemia (SS hemoglobin) are subject to painful and hematological crises; pulmonary, bone, or cerebral infarctions; and multiple infections, to name only the most serious consequences of the disease. In reviewing the course of patients with sickle cell anemia, Barrett-Conner (1971) noted that acute pulmonary disease was the most common reason for hospitalization.

I. Incidence

The sickle cell syndromes are particularly prevalent in black persons of African or Afro-American ancestry. However, the gene is also found at a lower frequency in persons of Mediterranean ancestry, southern Italians, Sicilians, and Greeks, in Saudi Arabia, and in India. The highest gene frequencies occur in equatorial Africa, in the so called "malaria belt." The heterogeneous state for HbS (sickle cell trait) probably confers a biological advantage against infection with *Falciparum malaria* and for this reason the gene frequency for HbS has achieved high levels through natural selection in geographic areas of endemic malaria. In the United States the frequency of the sickle cell gene in blacks is 8-10% and the number of homozygous persons approaches 50,000, or 1:400 births. In certain areas of western Africa (Ghana and Nigeria) the gene frequency can reach 25-30% (Forget, 1982).

II. Causes

The acute chest syndromes make up a group of disorders with multiple causes and more than one pathogenesis. Hemoglobinopathy plays a central role in the development of pulmonary disease associated with SS anemia. Disorders of its structure and function are responsible for several major manifestations of SS anemia.

The sickle cell syndromes are due to the inheritance of a gene for a structurally abnormal B globulin chain subunit of adult hemoglobin, the B_2 chain of the HbS ($2B_2{}^a$). The structural abnormality of the B_2 globulin chain consists of a single amino acid substitution or replacement: valine instead of the normal glutamic acid at position 6 of the B polypeptide chain. HbS can be found in the heterozygous state (HbSA or sickle cell trait), in the homozygous state (HbSS, sickle cell anemia), or in association with other structural hemoglobin variants (Forget, 1982).

The abnormalities of sickle cell disease are a consequence of these molecular changes, which result in vaso-occlusive or painful crises of varying severity and frequency, affecting different parts of the body. The pain is attributed to the occlusion of small vessels by cells containing polymerized HbS.

Organ damage is the consequence of multiple vaso-occlusive events and of chronic anemia. Organ damage is cumulative to some extent and adults with severe sickle cell anemia may have impairment of a number of organ systems as well as the lung (Bunn and Forget, 1986).

III. Pathological Findings

The sickling phenomenon resulting from aggregation or polymerization of HbS molecules causes a chronic hemolytic anemia and vaso-occlusive crises resulting in pain and tissue damage caused by infarction. These two phenomena are directly related to the physiochemical properties of the HbS molecule and result from alterations in red cell metabolism and red cell rheology, which are a consequence of the sickling phenomenon (Forget, 1982).

The sickling phenomenon occurs only when the HbS molecule is in the deoxy conformation. When HbS is in the oxyconformation it has essentially normal physiochemical properties. In the deoxyconformation, HbS molecules can aggregate with one another into long polymers and are aligned to form a gel of liquid crystals that are also called tactoids. The end result of the polymerization process is the transformation of the intracellular contents of the red cell from a fluid liquid to a viscous gel. In cell-free and membrane-free solutions, deoxygenated HbS, when examined under the microscope, may form crystals or tactoids and can assume the typical sickle shape. The abnormal shape (Forget, 1982) of sickled red cells is therefore conferred by the shape of the HbS crystals; the red cell membrane stretches and deforms to accommodate the abnormal shape of the intracellular gel (Fig. 1). The sickling phenomena is reversible with reoxygenation of the HbS molecule: the aggregate molecules dissociate, the gel becomes liquid, and the red cell shape can turn to normal if the red cell membrane has not become secondarily affected.

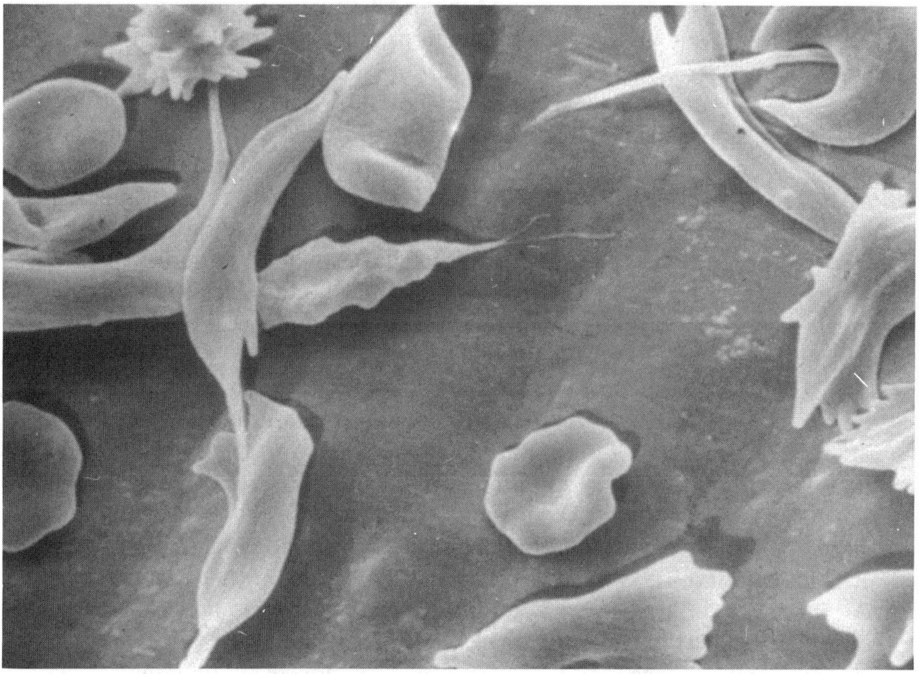

Figure 1 The abnormal shape of sickled red cells is conferred by the shape of the HbS crystals, as seen on scanning electron microscopic examination (courtesy of W. Jensen, M.D.).

IV. Clinical Features

Pulmonary infections are among the most serious infectious disease problems that a practicing physician will commonly encounter in patients with sickle cell disease. Of the causative agents identified by sputum culture on admission to the hospital in one large study of community-acquired pneumonia in patients with HbS, *Streptococcus pneumonia*, better known as *Diplococcus pneumoniae* or "*Pneumococcus*," was by far the most common cause of pneumonia. *Staphylococcus aureus*, other bacteria, and *Mycoplasma pneumoniae* were much less frequent causes.

The severity of the illness and precise manner of presentation vary considerably. There is almost always malaise, fever, and cough. The symptoms of headache and prostration that frequently precede the onset of the shaking chill suggest bacterial pneumonia. There is commonly pleural pain and sometimes cyanosis. There may be signs of consolidation (inspiration lag), impaired percussion, and bronchial breathing with rales sometimes associated with rhonchi. In severe pneumonia there may be severe prostration, delirium, jaundice, oliguria, and peripheral circulatory failure.

The following laboratory investigations may be extremely helpful. The extent and pattern of the changes in the chest radiograph are variable. It may reveal important evidence of related disease such as pulmonary tuberculosis or heart disease. A fresh specimen of sputum should be examined by Gram's stain to differentiate gram-positive organisms from gram-negative organisms. A Ziehl-Neelsen smear should be examined to rule out tuberculosis, since both diseases can coexist. For rapid identification of *Pneumococcus,* an opsonin test should be performed if available. A loopful of fresh sputum is placed on a slide treated with a loopful of antiserum. If capsular swelling is observed under light microscope, pneumococcal organisms are present.

Culture of the sputum is desirable and should be done before antibiotic therapy is started. However, therapy should not be withheld if the criteria described are present. Interpretation of the results of sputum culture demands some caution since the organisms identified may not be causative, but may be contaminants from the nasophaynx. An initial blood culture should be part of the work-up for the suspected bacterial pneumonia. Positive blood cultures may be the only clue to the nature of the lung infection.

The outlook in pneumococcal pneumonia occuring in the healthy individual is excellent. In patients with sickle cell anemia, the mortality rate from pneumococcal disease may be significant. The mortality rate remains high unless diagnosis is made within a few days of the onset of infection.

Patients with sickle cell anemia are at increased risk of pneumococcal infection, bacteremia, and meningitis. Some of these patients present with fever, cough, shortness of breath, and roentgenographic evidence of acute pulmonary infiltrate. In such cases there is little reason to doubt the diagnosis of pneumococcal pneumonia. However, another common presentation is seen in more than one-third of a bacteremic febrile episodes with a pulmonary infiltrate. Although considered to be pneumonia, these cases lack bacterial confirmation and the patients have prolonged fever despite administration of antibiotics.

Such disease diagnosed as "pneumonia" in adults with sickle cell anemia is probably pulmonary infarction. A number of articles have dealt with the sickling disorders. Although guidelines have been set to aid in differentiating between the two types of disorders, diagnosis usually remains in doubt. "Acute chest syndrome" has been suggested as a description for the combination of chest pain, fever, increased leukocytosis, and the appearance of a new shadow on chest roentgenograph.

The acute chest syndrome is a common cause of hospital admission in patients with sickle cell disease (Onwubalili, V. K. 1983). The illness is frequently self-limited, but it can rapidly progress and become massive and fatal. It is an acute illness characterized by chest pain, fever, prostration, and pneumonia-like pulmonary infiltrates. It frequently cannot be differentiated clinically from pneumonia.

The syndrome usually results from pulmonary infarction due to obstruction in the pulmonary vessels. Other causative factors included in situ sickling, thromboembolism, or embolization with aggregates of sickle cells, bone marrow, or marrow fat (Carache et al., 1985).

The chest syndrome can develop during the course of a painful sickle cell crisis, or it can precipitate a painful crises. Pleuritic chest pain is the dominant symptom. Involvement of the diaphragmatic pleura can result in abdominal pain. True lung pathological conditions must be differentiated from rib infarction or cholecystites. Depending on the extent of the pulmonary involvement, physical examination usually shows tachypnea, and there can be signs of pulmonary consolidation, pleural effusion, or occasionally a pleural friction rub.

The chest radiograph (Fig. 2) shows infiltrates in one or more lobes with or without pleural effusion. Films may be normal or diagnostic during the first 2 or 3 days, especially if the patient is dehydrated. Blood cultures and sputum culture occasionally reveal a bacterial pathogen. Measurement of arterial blood gases is necessary for initial assessment of the severity of the illness and for subsequent clinical management. Initial samples should be taken while the patient is breathing room air. Because patients with sickle cell disease may have a low PaO_2 during steady state, the interpretation of low oxygen tension can be difficult unless baseline arterial gases have been obtained previously.

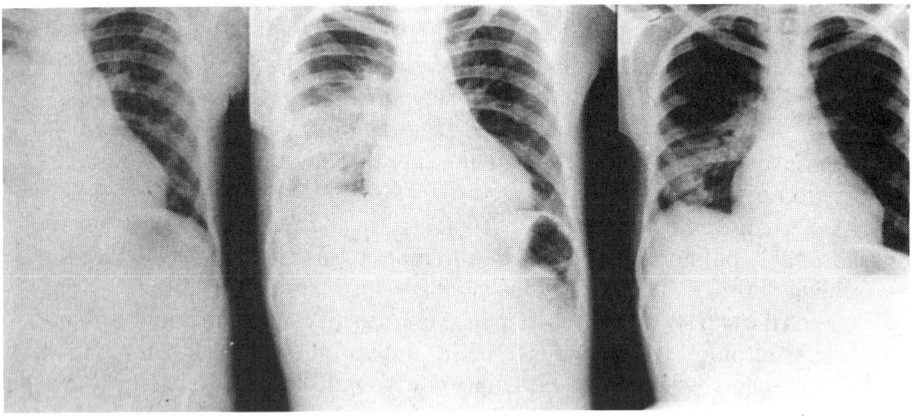

Figure 2 Chest posteroanterior roentgenogram in a 25-year-old man with pneumonia in axillary region of left lower lobe (courtesy of W. Jensen, M.D.).

Complete blood counts, including reticulocyte counts and differential, should be obtained serially. An increased count and shift to the left may indicate a bacterial infection.

Mycoplasma antibody titers and cold agglutinin titers may point to a mycoplasma pneumonia. The titers, however, may not become diagnostic until later in the course of disease.

Most experts consider that lung scans are not useful in diagnosing the chest syndrome. This view is due in part to the inability to be certain that abnormalities are recent if no steady-state lung scan is available for comparison.

Pulmonary angiography raises the theoretical risk of increasing sickling in these patients. Therefore, the procedure is rarely indicated, particularly since the chest syndrome is often self-limited (Carache, 1985).

Numerous writers have proposed that patients with SS hemoglobinopathy are unduly susceptible to infection (Barret-Connor, 1971; Margolies, 1951). The most frequent infection noted in several clinical series (Durant and Cortes, 1966; Carache, 1979) was a rapidly spreading and slowly resolving pneumonia, usually with no specific etiologic agent demonstrated. Barret-Connor's 1971 study confirmed that an acute, febrile pulmonary event is the most common cause of hospitalization in patients with sickle cell anemia. The illness is similar to bacterial pneumonia in patients without hemoglobinopathy, except for some of the following attributes. This "acute chest syndrome" seemed to have an increased incidence of multiple lobe involvement and multiple occurrences (Diggs, Barreras, 1967). It is uncommon to isolate *Pneumococcus* from the respiratory tract. The failure of bacteriological diagnosis increases the propensity for the diagnosis of pulmonary infarction. Pulmonary infarction is much more common in adults than in young children, even when hemoglobinopathy is present. It is frequently associated with a clinical crisis, either because generalized sickling also produces thrombosis in situ or because of pulmonary emboli from infarcted bone.

A comparison of patients with bacteremic pneumonia with those who had pulmonary infarction showed similar increases and ranges in temperatures and normal to increased leukocyte counts in both groups. Bloody sputum or the presence of migratory infiltrates occurs with similar frequency in both diseases. There is no difference in the seasonal distribution; one-third of the proved bacterial pneumonias and one-third of the pulmonary infarctions occurred in the summer months.

Pulmonary infarction has not been documented in patients under the age of 12 (Margolies, 1951; Marfat et al., 1978). Pregnancy apparently accentuates the risk of pulmonary infarction in SS anemia. A preceding sickle cell crisis suggests pulmonary infarction. In SS anemia, pulmonary infarction usually follows thrombosis in situ or bone marrow emboli and is unrelated to thrombophlebitis (Barrett-Connor, 1973).

Jaundice can complicate lobar pneumonia or pulmonary infarction in persons without hemoglobinopathies. In SS anemia, jaundice greater than the usual low-grade icterus suggests a diagnosis of pulmonary infarction. In Barrett-Connor's 1973 series, a total serum bilirubin level greater than 5 mg/100 ml was seen more commonly in patients with pulmonary infarction. Barreras et al. (1986) demonstrated the presence of blister cells in the peripheral blood of SS anemia patients with pulmonary infarction, but not in SS anemia patients with pneumonia (Barrett-Connor, 1973).

The young age of most of the patients, the frequency of involvement of the upper and middle lobes, the lack of association with clinical crises, and the known propensity for pneumococcal disease in this population suggest that the events represent pneumonia rather than pulmonary infarction. Pneumonia is probably many times more common in patients with SS anemia. In these patients, fluid-filled alveoli and congestion afford an excellent focus for bacterial multiplication and at the same time impair surface phagocytosis. Intrapulmonary shunting and reduced oxygen tension can impair phagocytosis of bacteria by alveolar macrophages. Deficient heat-labile serum opsonizing activity for *Pneumonoccus* has been shown in these patients (Winkelstein and Drachman, 1968). These patients also have functional autosplenectomy and show an increased risk of pneumococcal infection (Carache et al., 1979).

It is apparent that although a constellation of signs and symptoms is strongly suggestive of either pneumonia or infarction, in individual patients diagnosis may be impossible. Half of the features thought to be helpful for a differential diagnosis in patients without hemoglobinopathy have little value in patients with SS anemia. In such cases, definite diagnosis is possible only based on lung scanning or pulmonary angiography.

V. Pulmonary Function Tests

During the past 20 years a wide variety of pulmonary function studies have been carried out on patients with SS anemia. A restrictive ventilatory defect is characteristic of the pulmonary function pattern associated with SS lung disease. On spirometry, the vital capacity (VC) is reduced and the forced expired volume in 1 s (FEV_1) and other flow rates are normal or decreased in proportion to, or even to a lesser extent than, the reduction in vital capacity; thus the FEV_1/FVC ratio is normal or even high.

One may ask why the forced expiratory flow rates are often relatively high in SS lung disease. These flows are determined principally by the elastic recoil pressure of the lung and the resistance to air flow. In sickle cell lung disease the lung tissue is stiffened, probably due to infarcts or collagen deposition in the interstitium. Since the stiffened lung has a greater elastic recoil, it tends to return to the resting position with more force, thereby tending to increase the expiratory flow rates. In addition, the intrapulmonary airways may be held more widely open by the greater tethering action of the stiffened lung parenchyma, thereby reducing resistance and augmenting air flow.

Lung volumes determined by the helium dilution or nitrogen washout technique confirm the presence of a restrictive ventilatory abnormality. Total lung capacity is decreased and, in the later stages of the disease, all the subdivisions of the total lung capacity, including the functional residual capacity and residual volume, may be decreased.

Increased lung stiffness, manifested by decreased lung compliance, is the functional hallmark of this disease. Because of the decreased compliance the lung reaches its limit of extension at a relatively small lung volume, resulting in a restrictive ventilatory defect (i.e., both a diminished vital capacity and a decreased total lung capacity).

Patients with sickle cell anemia frequently have a lower vital capacity (VC) and total lung capacity (TLC) than that predicted for normal subjects. This may be related to repeated pulmonary infections and subsequent changing anatomical characteristics of the lung. In addition, previous episodes of pulmonary infarction may lead to the development of restrictive respiratory functional impairment (Moser and Shea, 1957). Since we do not have supportive evidence of these possibilities, the cause of reduced VC and TLC in these patients remains obscure.

The breathing rate is often increased while the tidal volume is decreased, resulting in an abnormally high minute ventilation at rest. The cause of the increased minute ventilation might be related to excessive stimulation of afferent receptors (probably J receptors) in the lung tissue by interstitial fibrosis or inflammation, resulting in vagally mediated stimulation of the respiratory center. Other causes of the increased minute ventilation are hypoxemia and increased dead space.

Asymptomatic persons with SS disease can demonstrate a decreased carbon monoxide diffusing capacity as well as restrictive disease and a decreased vital capacity during symptom-free intervals. The diffusing capacity of the lung for carbon monoxide (D_LCO) is generally reduced even before a restrictive ventilatory abnormality or decrease in lung compliance is evident (Powars et al., 1988). Therefore, the reduction in D_LCO is a sensitive and useful diagnostic test. The cause of the reduced D_LCO is probably a reduction in membrane-diffusing capacity and pulmonary capillary blood volume in SS anemia. The impaired diffusing capacity probably does not contribute significantly to hypoxemia at rest, but may do so during exercise.

The effect of anemia on pulmonary diffusing capacity DL and pulmonary capillary volume (Vc) has been studied by a number of investigators (Burrows and Niden, 1962; Rankin et al., 1961; Jouasset-Streider et al., 1965; Kilburn, 1960). Chronic anemia caused by sickle cell disease manifests strikingly different pathophysiological changes from those observed in other types of anemia (Bromberg and Jensen, 1965; Carache et al., 1964; Durant and Cortes, 1966; Moser and Shea, 1957; Sproule et al., 1958). These changes may include blood viscosity, thromboembolism, and hypoxia resulting in augmentation of pulmonary vascular resistance and right ventricular work.

Deje Femi-Pearse and co-workers (1970) found the D_LCO value disproportionately high in the presence of a reduced hemoglobin level. The mean membrane-diffusing capacity (DM) was significantly decreased in both SS and SC hemoglobin groups. There was a significant increase in the Vc in patients with SS hemoglobin disease although no appreciable change in Vc was observed in those with SC-hemoglobin disease.

Sproule et al. (1958) and Elegbelege (1978) suggested that the mechanism that produces hemodynamic changes may be operative to a greater extent in sickle cell patients than with other types of anemia because of a more profoundly decreased peripheral resistance.

It is well known that the pulmonary capillary bed has a remarkable capacity for expansion in various cardiopulmonary disorders and that an increase in D_LCO is caused by an increase in VC.

Arterial blood gas levels provide useful information in patients with SS anemia. A respiratory alkalosis (decreased arterial PCO_2, increased pH) is often present as a result of alveolar overventilation. At other times the PCO_2 may be normal or increased. An increased PCO_2, however, is unlikely unless severe restriction is present (vital capacity of less than 1 L). The arterial oxygen tension (PaO_2 may be normal or decreased at rest, but the alveolar-arterial oxygen difference (A-a) is generally abnormally widened at rest and especially during exercise. The PaO_2 is calculated from the alveolar gas equation. The alveolar-arterial oxygen difference is normally less than 10 mmHg at age 20, less than 20 mmHg at age 50, and less than 30 mmHg at age 70. In patients with SS anemia, the abnormally widened alveolar-arterial oxygen difference at rest is due mainly to maldistribution of ventilation in relation to blood flow, that is, a decreased ventilation/perfusion (V/Q) ratio. The maldistribution of ventilation results from a nonuniform decrease in compliance in different regions of the lung. During exercise, the PO_2 frequently drops and the alveolar-arterial oxygen difference widens still further as a result of the reduced diffusing capacity and/or a further reduction in regional V/Q. The alveolar-arterial oxygen difference during exercise has been found to correlate with the amount of parenchymal disease found histologically.

There is general consensus that there is a restrictive functional pattern in this disease, although the type and degree of lung function abnormality can relate to the location and extent of the pathological changes as well as the type of hemoglobinopathy and age of the patient.

The assessment of lung function in sickle cell hemoglobinopathies is confounded by a number of variables. Studies comparing results in adults with sickle cell anemia with average normal values for healthy subjects of the same stature may be invalidated by failure to account for a number of factors (Miller et al., 1978). In most of these studies, the lung volumes of black subjects with HbSS were compared to reference standards from predominantly white populations. However, because normal black persons have lung volumes 10-15% smaller than those of height-matched white persons (Rossiter and Weill, 1974; Binder et al., 1976), the use of race-specific control subjects is imperative for proper interpretation of the results of lung volume measurements in HbSS subjects. Using such control subjects, Miller and Sergent (1971) found that the lung volumes of adults with HbSS were only slightly smaller than those of normal black subjects and attributed this to small difference between HbSS adults and normal persons.

VI. Lung Function in Children with HbSS Anemia

Wall et al. (1979) investigated pulmonary function in children with HbSS and a group of normal black children as control subjects. There was no significant difference in lung volumes between HbSS patients and control subjects. The expiratory flows and FEV_1/FVC of the patients was the same as that of normal white children, whereas the FEV_1, $FEF_{25\text{-}75}$, and Vsmax were smaller than those of normal height-matched white subjects.

The mean uncorrected D_LCO of HbSS patients was normal when compared to normal values for white subjects with the same TLC. After being corrected for anemia, D_LCO was greater than normal in all cases. Mean values for Vc and DM were both increased.

When breathing room air, all patients had a PO_2 below the lower limits of normal for their age group (87 mmHg) and an abnormally high $(A\text{-}a)O_2$ (16 mmHg), while breathing 100% O_2. Their PO_2 failed to increase into the normal range (550 mmHg) and the (A-a) PO_2 was increased (86 mmHg) and was in all cases consistent with abnormal Qs/Qt (7%).

The study showed that the lung volumes and the expiratory flows of children with HbSS were not different from those of healthy black control subjects (Wall et al., 1979).

The heterozygous sickle cell trait (hemoglobin AS) occasionally manifests itself in acute clinical events related to vascular occlusion that most commonly involve the spleen. Sproule and co-workers (1958) studied patients with sickle cell trait (HbSA) and found FVC and arterial oxyhemoglobin saturation each to be reduced while subjects were breathing room air. Goodman and colleagues (1974) reported reduced FVC of patients with HbAS and reduced steady-state diffusing capacity for carbon monoxide during exercise at sea level. Neither of these studies included a race-matched group or considered race as a variable in predicted values. Data obtained by Dillard et al. (1987) seem to indicate that young healthy men with hemoglobin AS typically do not develop abnormalities in pulmonary function at rest. The finding of abnormal pulmonary function in persons with hemoglobin AS should lead to the consideration of additional diagnoses such as a coexisting hemoglobinopathy or pulmonary disease unrelated to the sickle cell trait.

Dillard et al. (1987) watched for pulmonary function abnormalities in patients with sickle cell trait by intensifying the hypoxic stimulus for the systemic formation of sickle cells using a hypobaric chamber to simulate high altitude. The generation of sickle-shaped erythocytes within the pulmonary circulation might be induced because of the relatively desaturated condition of normal mixed venous blood, which would desaturate further at altitude. If lung function became abnormal as a result of hypoxemia (formation of sickle cells), disturbances of gas exchange could then worsen arterial hypoxemia beyond the degree produced by altitude alone, thereby further promoting sickle cell formation in the systemic circulation.

They found no clinically significant acute or cumulative declines in spirometric values or D_LCO after altitude exposures from 5000 up to 25,000 feet.

There was no difference in oxyhemoglobin saturation between cases and controls before or during altitude exposure.

The effect of altitude on pilots, crews, or passengers with sickle cell trait in an important concern. Many persons have hemoglobin AS and may be exposed to high altitudes in the course of air travel. For example, pressurized civilian aircraft normally maintain cabin conditions equivalent to those present at altitudes of 7500 feet during flights at altitudes of 40,000 feet. The results of Dillard et al. (1987) indicate the cumulative effects of transient altitude exposures did not alter DL_{CO} or sperometric values in patients with SA trait.

VII. Treatment

All patients with acute chest syndrome should be admitted to the hospital. Depending on the patient's extent of lung involvement and respiratory distress, the intensive care unit may be required for appropriate monitoring of a rapidly changing clinical state. Analgesics should be administered and intravenous hydration should be given during painful crises. Oxygen is indicated for hypoxemia, tachycardia, and tachypnea.

Many patients with acute chest syndrome will recover with no more than modest supportive care. If the reticular count rises or remains high, and the patient is not dyspneic at bed rest, transfusions need not be carried out solely because of a fall in hemoglobin concentration (Carache et al., 1979).

Because it is often impossible to make a reliable, a priori differentiation between pulmonary infarction and bacterial pneumonia, strong recommendations have been made for penicillin to be used empirically in all sickle cell patients with lung infiltrates. This is especially true in young children who have particularly severe pneumococcal pneumonia. Carache et al. (1979) have suggested that adults with acute chest syndrome have a much less fulminant course than children. If normal-appearing flora are seen on a Gram's-stained sputum smear from a patient who is not seriously ill, no antibiotics should be used. Choice of antibiotics should take into consideration local patterns of bacterial antibiotic resistance. If gram-positive cocci in clumps predominate, one of the penicillinase-resistant penicillin analogues should be used. Predominance of gram-negative coccobacillary forms suggests the use of ampicillin or tetracycline in the severely ill patient. Adjustment of the antibiotic regimen will depend on the results of the bacterial cultures.

Partial exchange transfusions should be considered in patients with multiple lobe involvement, rapidly progressive disease, or signs of respiratory insufficiency (PO_2 below 60 mmHg in a adult). Patients in whom there is chronic hypoxemia, as determined by baseline studies, should be considered for exchange transfusion when there is greater than a 25% drop in their steady-state PO_2. A second indication for transfusion is severe anemia in a patient with borderline abnormal pulmonary function, in which case packed red cells are given instead of an exchange (Carache et al., 1985).

A polyvalent pneumococcal vaccine is now available for the immunization of patients with sickle cell anemia. The vaccine provokes antibody production in children over the age of 2 years. Its efficacy in patients with sickling disorders is not yet proven (Akinyanju and Johnson, 1987), but preliminary data suggest that it can prevent life-threatening infection in children.

Warley et al.'s (1968) studies in Uganda and the Congo concluded that treatment with benzathine penicillin and chloroquine protected homozygous sicklers against infection, reduced rate of dactylic crisis, and resulted in a higher average hemoglobin value.

References

Akinyanju, O., and Johnson, A. O. (1987). Acute illness in Nigerian children with sickle cell anemia. *Ann. Trop. Paediatr.* **7**(3):181-186.

Barrett-Connor, E. (1971). Acute pulmonary disease and sickle cell anemia. *Am. Rev. Respir. Dis.* **104**:159-165.

Barrett-Connor, E. (1973). Pneumonia and pulmonary infarction in sickle cell anemia. *J.A.M.A.* **224**:997-1000.

Binder, R. E., Mitchell, C. A., Schoenberg, J. B., and Bouhuys (1976). Lung function among black and white children. *Am. Rev. Respir. Dis.* **114**: 955-959.

Bromberg, P. A., and Jensen, W. A. (1965). A possible mechanism for decreased oxygen affinity of SS blood. *J. Clin. Invest.* **44**:1031.

Bunn, H. F., and Forget, B. G. (1986). Sickle cell disease—clinical and epidemiological aspects. In *Hemoglobin: Molecular, Genetic and Clinical Aspects.* Philadelphia, W.B. Saunders.

Burrows, B., and Niden, A. H. (1962). Effect of anemia on CO diffusion in the perfused dog lung. *Fed. Proc.* **21**:443.

Carache, S., and Conley, C. L. (1964). Rate of sickling of red cells during deoxygenation of blood from persons with various sickling disorders. *Blood* **24**:25-49.

Carache, S., Scott, J. C., and Carache, P. (1979). Acute chest syndrome in adults with sickle cell anemia. *Arch. Intern. Med.* **139**:67-69.

Carache, S., Lubin, B., and Reid, C. D. (1985). Management and therapy of sickle cell disease. US Department of Health and Human Services, Public Health Service, INH. Publication No. 85-2117.

Deji Femi-Pearse, Gazinglu, K. M., and Yu, P. N. (1970). Pulmonary function studies in sickle cell disease. *J. Ap.* **280**:574-577.

Diggs, L. W. (1967). *Mephis Med. J.* **42**:375.

Dillard, T. A., Kark, J. A., Rojagopal, K. R., Keg, J. A., Conik, J. J., and Ruehle, C. J. (1987). Pulmonary function in sickle cell trait. *Ann. Intern. Med.* **106**:191-196.

Durant, J. R., and Cortes, F. M. (1966). Occlusive pulmonary vascular disease associated with hemoglobin S-C disease. *Am. Heart J.* **71**:100-107.

Elegbelege, O. O. (1978). Pulmonary function studies in sickle cell anemia. *Trop. Geogr. Med.* **30**(4):473-476.

Forget, B. G. (1982). Sickle cell anemia and associated hemoglobinopathies. In *Textbook of Medicine*, Section 110, vol. 1. Edited by V. B. Wyngaarden and L. H. Smith, Jr. Philadelphia, W.B. Saunders.

Goodman, R. L., Hazlett, D. R., Bergin, J. J., Flannerg, E. P., and Schwartz, M. (1974). Sickle cell trait and loss of pulmonary function at 5,280 feet and sea level. *Thromb. Diath. Haemorrh.* **53**:91-94.

Green, G. M. (1988). Pulmonary clearing of infectious agents. *Annu. Rev. Med.* **19**:315.

Jouasset-Strieder, D., Cahill, J. M., Byrne, J. M., and Gaensler, E. A. (1965). Pulmonary diffusing capacity and capillar blood volume in normal and anemic dogs. *J. Appl. Physiol.* **20**:113-117.

Kilburn, K. H. (1960). Ventilation, dead space and hemoglobin level as modifiers of steady state method for diffusing capacity for carbon monoxide. *Am. Rev. Respir. Dis.* **81**:945-948.

Marfat, Y., Pieron, R., Rethers, C., and Lesborne, B. (1978). Pulmonaires de la dreponocytose:acquisitions recentes. *Med. Trop.* **38**(2):175-182.

Margolies, M. P. (1951). Sickle cell anemia, a composite study and survely. *Medicine* **30**:357-443.

Miller, G. J., Sergeant, G. R., Saunders, M. J., Richardson, C., and Gilson, R. J. C. (1978). Interpretation of lung function tests in the sickle-cell hemoglobinopathies. *Thorax* **33**:85-88.

Miller, G. J. and Serjeant G. R. (1971). *Thorax J.* **26**:309.

Moser, K. M., and Shea, J. G. (1957). The relationship between pulmonary infarction, cor pulmonale and the sickle cell states. *Am. J. Med.* **22**:561-580.

Onwubalili, V. K. (1983). Sickle cell disease and infection. *J. Infect.* **7**(1):2-20.

Powars, D., Weidman, J. A., Tamara, O. M., Niland, V. C., and Johnson, C. (1988). Sickle cell chronic lung disease. Prior morbidity and the risk of pulmonary failure. *Medicine* **67**:66-76.

Rankin, J. R., McNeil, R. S., and Forster, R. E. (1961). The effect of anemia on the alveolar capillary exchange of carbon monoxide in man. *J. Clin. Invest.* **40**:1323-1330.

Rossiter, C. E., and Weill, H. (1974). Ethnic differences in lung function: evidence for proportional differences. *Int. J. Epidemiol.* **3**:55-61.

Sproule, B. J., Halden, E. R., and Miller, W. F. (1958). A study of cardiopulmonary alterations in patients with sickle cell disease and its variants. *J. Clin. Invest.* **37**:486-496.

Wall, M. A., Platt, O. S., and Sheeider, D. J. (1979). Lung function in children with sickle cell anemia. *Am. Rev. Respir. Dis.* **130**:210-214.

Warley, M. A., Hamilton, P. J. S., Marsdes, P. D., Brown, R. E., Merselis, J. G., and Wilks, N. (1968). Chemoprophylaxis of homozygous sicklers with antimalarials and long acting penicillin. *Br. Med. J.* **2**:86-88.

Winkelstein, J. A., and Drachman, R. H. (1968). Defeciency of serum opsonizing activity in sickle-cell disease. *N. Engl. J. Med.* **279**:459-466.

14

Paragonimiasis: Clinical, Radiological, and Therapeutic Consideration
An African Profile

C. NWOKOLO

University of Nigeria
Enugu, Nigeria

I. Introduction

Paragonimiasis is a parasitic disease caused by the trematode lung fluke *Paragonimus*. The lungs and sometimes other organs in humans and other mammals are affected when suitable ecological conditions, including available appropriate intermediate hosts, are present. Human disease has so far been recorded in Asia, some Pacific islands, Africa, and Central and South America. Each continent seems to have its own group of specific parasite species and hosts. The main Asian foci are in Korea, Thailand, the Philippines, China, and Japan.

In Africa endemic foci exist in Nigeria (Nwokolo, 1972a,b, 1974), Cameroon (Kum and Nchinda, 1982; Zahra, 1952), and Liberia (Sachs et al., 1986). It is extremely likely that the disease exists in its zoonotic form over a much wider area than indicated above, since the appropriate hosts exist in most of the nonarid areas of Africa. Sporadic cases have been recorded in Zaire (Van Hoff, 1933), Gambia (Bowesman, 1960), and Gabon (Sachs et al., 1983), the Ivory Coast (Coulibaly et al., 1976), and Natal, South Africa (Goldsmid, 1975).

In South and Central America, human paragonimiasis has been recorded in Peru, Ecuador, Brazil, Panama, Mexico, and Honduras (Yokogawa, 1969).

There are no known geographical or geological links between the Asian and the African foci. However, the continental drift and plate tectonics theories (Wegener, 1912; Hallam, 1973) offer a reasonable explanation for the similarities in geophysical and ecological features between the areas in West Africa and South America where the disease has been found.

The theories postulate a period of antedeluvian physical contiguity between West Africa and parts of South America. The steadily increasing separation of the two continents led to the formation of the Atlantic Ocean. The process is still continuing. The theories have obtained support from isotopic dating of fossils and various rock types of the same ages found on opposite sides of the Atlantic.

II. Parasitological Characteristics

For the cycle of the *Paragonimus* parasite to be completed, it must utilize not only the definitive hosts, but also the two different intermediate hosts: a mollusc and a crustacean host. The definitive host may be humans, but they are more frequently reservoir hosts such as wild felines, civet cats, crab-eating mongooses, rodents, monkeys, pigs, and dogs.

In West Africa, civet cats, monkeys, and mongooses have been identified as important reservoir hosts (Sachs et al., 1986; Voelker and Sachs, 1977). Rodents are strongly suspected as participants in the cycle, especially in areas where land crabs are active.

The crustacean intermediate host is classically a freshwater crab or crayfish. Crabs of the *Sudanonautes* species are the dominant hosts in Africa. In West Africa, *Sudanonautes africanus, Sudanonautes aubryii,* and *Sudanonautes pelii* are the crabs most often involved. *Liberonautes latidactylus* has also been found to be a vector in Liberia (Voelker, 1973). In some areas of eastern Nigeria, *S. aubryii* behaves like a land crab, and in the rainy season may be caught in farms up to 1 km from the nearest stream.

No crayfishes have been incriminated so far in West Africa. The snail intermediate host has also not yet been identified in Africa despite intensive search.

The dominant *Paragonimus* parasite, which has now been identified in the five West African countries of Nigeria, Cameroon, Liberia, Guinea, and Gabon, is *Paragonimus uterobilateralis*, but *Paragonimus africanus* has also been found in Cameroon (Voelker and Vogel, 1965; Sachs and Voelker, 1982).

The different species of *Paragonimus* parasites are identified by their anatomical features, especially the detailed anatomy of the ovaries and testes, the relative position of the suckers, and sometimes the shape and size of the eggs and the cuticular spines (Yokogawa M, personal communication, 1974).

The best known parasite of the *Paragonimus* species is *P. westermani*, which is widespread in Asia and has been most intensively studied. Fortunately it shares important immunological characteristics with most other members of the group and most of them also respond to similar chemotherapeutic agents.

III. Pathological Findings and Pathogenesis

The work of Yokogawa on laboratory animals (personal communication, 1974) shows that on ingestion into the alimentary tract *Paragonimus metacercariae* soon leave the bowel, enter the peritoneal cavity, and move towards the liver. Ultimately they pierce the diaphragm and pleura and enter the lungs. They encyst in the bronchioles, often in pairs, and mature.

Occasionally the migrating metacercarcae may lose their way and end up in the liver, subcutaneous tissues, or central nervous system.

The encysted adults provoke a granulomatous tissue response and are surrounded by macrophages, polymorphonuclear leukocytes, eosinophils, and fibrous tissue. In the lungs they live in the caverns so created but keep open their communication with the bronchi, through which the eggs produced by the adult worms find their way into the sputum.

The adult Paragonimus parasite is a small, fleshy fluke about 6-12 mm × 4-6 mm × 3-5 mm (Fig. 1).

The eggs, which measure about 68 × 40 μm, can be recovered in sputum or feces (Fig. 2).

IV. Human Acquisition of *Paragonimus* Infestation

Human infection is usually acquired by the consumption of infected crabs in a raw or inadequately cooked form. Careful dissection of infected crabs shows that the limb muscles are usually the most heavily parasitized parts, but sometimes the other soft tissues or the liver may be involved.

After the metacercariae have been swallowed, they ultimately reach the lungs and mature into adult worms in 5-6 weeks. The total incubation period in humans varies from 3 to 24 months. Heavy infections have a shorter incubation period. The adult parasites often encyst in pairs and produce eggs that are coughed up or swallowed. The eggs are passed out in the sputum or feces.

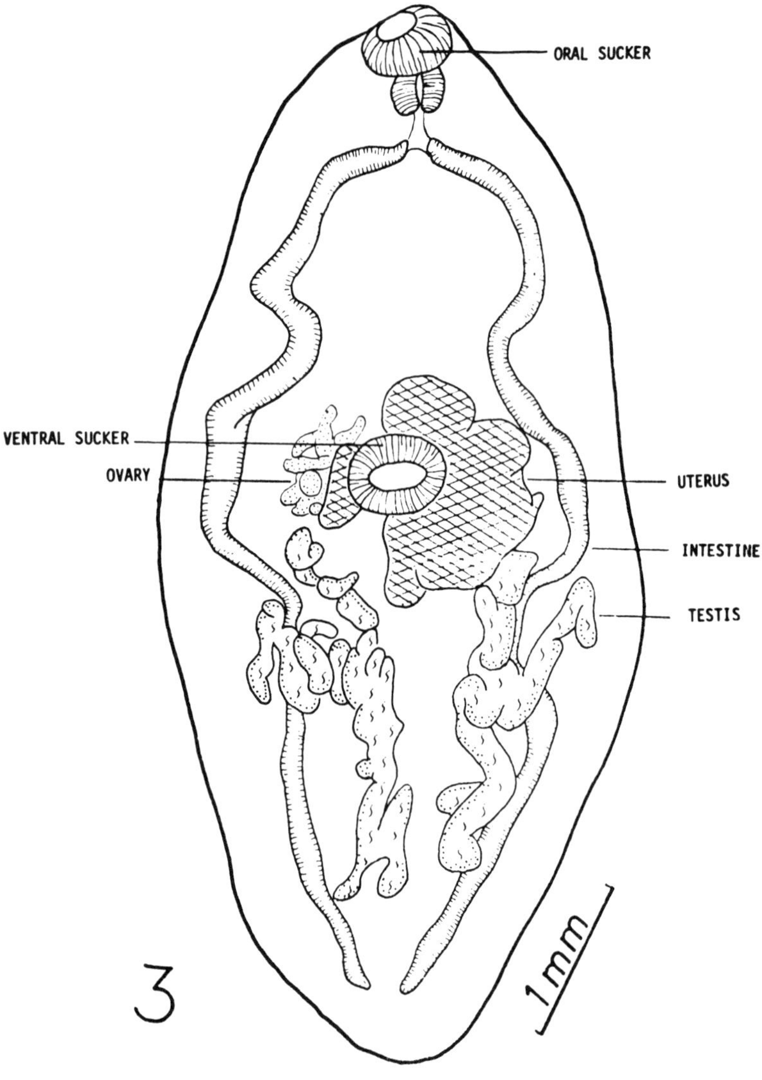

Figure 1 *Paragonimus uterobilateralis* (adapted from Voelker and Nwokolo, 1973).

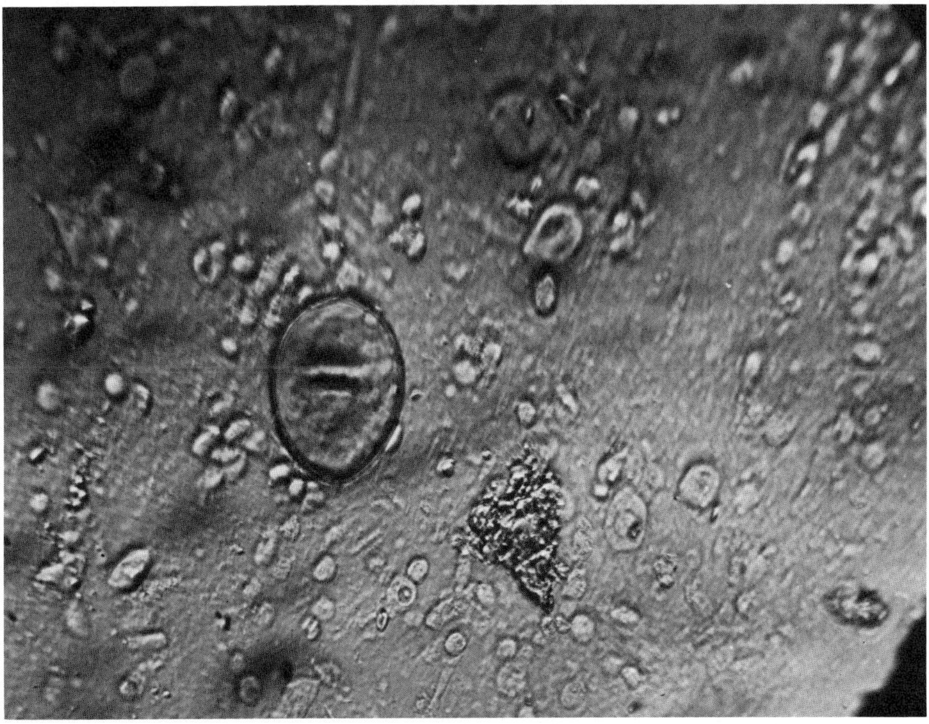

Figure 2 *Paragonimus* egg surrounded by red blood cells in a sputum specimen (× 350).

V. The Organism's Cycle

The eggs hatch into miracidia that swim in water and ultimately enter a suitable snail. Within 8 weeks the miracidia develop into two generations of rediae. The rediae develop further into cercariae. These cercariae are released from the snails and swim about, ultimately entering the muscles and soft tissues of the appropriate crab or crayfish. There they develop into metacercariae that are the forms that infect the definitive hosts when eaten (Fig. 3).

Apart from the existence of the *Paragonimus* parasite, the factors that determine whether human paragonimiasis will occur are:

1. The availability of the molluscan and crustacean intermediate hosts.
2. The cultural factor, which determines whether or not edible crabs or crayfishes are acceptable in a raw or semicooked form.

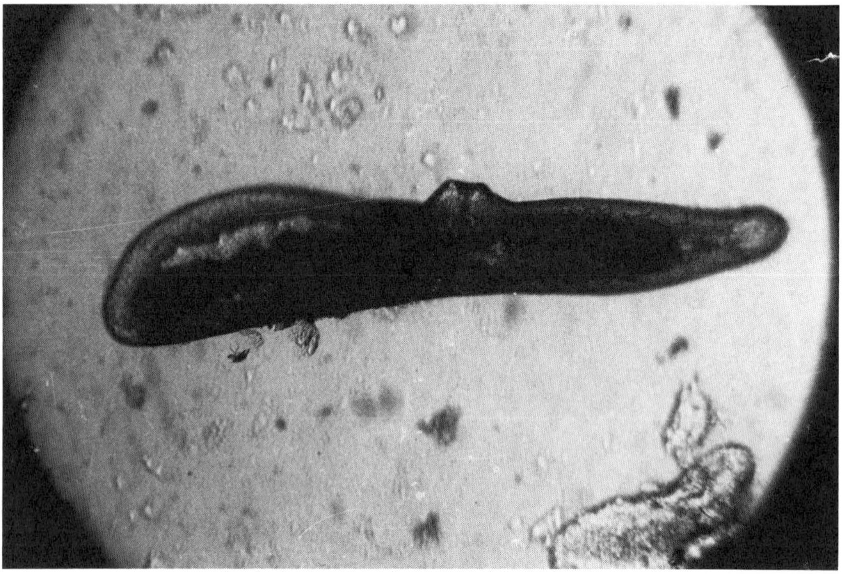

Figure 3 Metacercaria of *Paragonimus uterobilateralis* (× 100).

3. The availability of the definitive reservoir type of host (e.g., wild cats), whose infection ensures a constant pool of viable *Paragonimus* eggs to maintain the cycle. The reservoir and intermediate hosts thrive best in wet forests in the neighborhood of large rivers and their tributaries. They do not thrive in arid geographical areas. For example, paragonimiasis occurs in southeastern Nigeria in the neighborhood of the Cross and Imo rivers, but not in the dry northernmost parts of the country, which is close to the Sahara desert.

VI. Clinical Features

Like other infections and parasitic infestations in Africa, human paragonimiasis is mainly a disease of the young. The relatively short lifespan in developing countries is partly responsible for this (Fig. 4).

In a personal series of nearly 1000 cases seen over a period of about 30 years, about 95% were under the age of 40 years and the male/female ratio was about 3:2. Most of them were seen within a few years of onset, during and after the Nigerian civil war, which had facilitated the spread of the disease by encouraging the widespread consumption of crabs and other lower sources of animal protein.

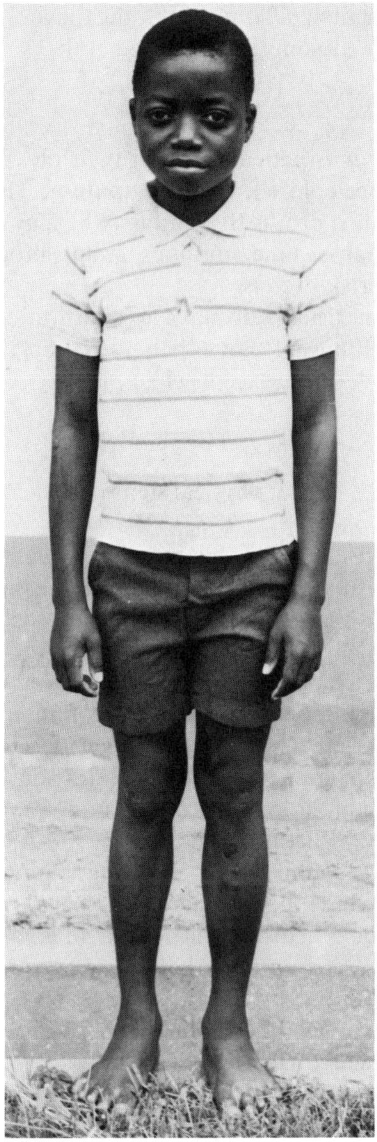

Figure 4 A healthy-looking 13-year-old Nigerian boy who has paragonimiasis.

Nearly all the patients (98%) in whom the diagnosis of paragonimiasis was ultimately confirmed admitted to eating crabs.

A. Symptoms

Over 90% of *Paragonimus* patients consult their physicians for evaluation of blood-stained, coffee-colored, or rusty sputum. The hemoptysis is not usually massive. Cough is productive and may or may not be troublesome. Sputum is usually available in the mornings, and its production can be facilitated at any time by brisk exercise.

The average patient usually displays no constitutional symptoms; fever and loss of weight are unusual. Some patients complain of an aching pain in the chest that is ill-defined, except when pleurisy is present.

B. Signs

There are usually few abnormal physical signs in patients with African paragonimiasis.

This may be because most of those studied in detail have been of relatively recent onset. A small number (about 5%) of the patients have mild clubbing of the fingers that cannot be explained otherwise. There may be patchy crackles or rhonchi over the lungs. On the rare occasions when pneumothorax, pleurisy, or empyema is present, the appropriate physical signs are also present. Extrapulmonary disease is uncommon in Africa, but unexplained hemiparesis, paraplegia, or focal convulsive episodes in young persons in endemic areas should arouse suspicion. Sometimes subcutaneous nodules resembling lymphoid or *Onchocerca* nodules prove to be the result of *Paragonimus* infection in endemic areas.

Very rarely it is the complications of paragonimiasis that bring the patient to the physician. These, in my experience, include pneumothorax, massive hemoptysis, or focal neurological lesions (e.g., hemiplegia). Because paragonimiasis produces symptoms that cause alarm, most patients seek medical treatment relatively early, and we have not seen many chronic or long-standing cases, but a few cases of proven bronchiectasis have been noted after successful treatment for paragonimiasis.

VII. Diagnosis

The diagnosis of paragonimiasis relies on careful history, microscopic examination of sputum and feces, immunodiagnostic procedures, and radiological examination.

Clinical awareness or a raised index of suspicion is the most important factor in making a provisional diagnosis of paragonimiasis. Knowledge of areas of the world where the disease has been reported is also of great value in developing clinical awareness. The repeated occurrence of mild hemoptysis in patients from parts of the world where crabs are eaten should alert the physician about the need to acquire and frequently exercise at his or her clinic the skill of simple microscopic examination of unstained sputum. This is required for the precise diagnosis of paragonimiasis.

Early morning sputum or sputum produced after exercise is often rich in eggs. Once the telltale operculated eggs are seen under the low power of the microscope, the diagnosis is made. The eggs are relatively large, golden brown, ovoid, and 7 to 10 times the length of red blood cells that usually surround them (Fig. 2). If the eggs are not found in the sputum, a careful examination of the feces will be required. Both sputum and faeces can also concentrated and reexamined when necessary. Since paragonimiasis may coexist with pulmonary tuberculosis, the standard investigations for hemoptysis, even in endemic areas, should always include a test of stained sputum for acid-fast bacilli and other microbes.

Next in value for precise diagnosis is the use of intradermal skin test with special *Paragonimus* extracts. I have used *P. westermani* extracts supplied by Professor M. Yokogawa of Chiba University, Chiba, Japan, and by the Medical Research Institute in Tokyo. In this test, 0.1 ml of the antigen is injected intradermally, producing a wheal the diameter of which is recorded immediately. Twenty minutes later, the diameter is measured again; in positive cases the wheal has increased by 5 mm or more in diameter. A positive response means that the patient has, or has had, paragonimiasis.

Our experience in Nigeria (Nwokolo, 1974) suggests that *Paragonimus westermani* shares similar antigens with other *Paragonimus* species. We found no evidence of cross-reactions with other (non-*Paragonimus*) parasites that exist in Nigeria.

The intradermal test is thus of great value in epidemiological studies. It remains positive after treatment and therefore cannot be used as a test of successful therapy. It is, however, useful at the bedside in the diagnosis of extrapulmonary disease; for example, when cerebral paragonimiasis must be differentiated from other space-occupying intracranial disorders in a patient from an endemic area.

One serological test, the indirect hemagglutination test, is also of value at the clinic (Yokogawa, 1969; Oerelich and Nwokolo, 1974). Its major advantage is that it becomes negative after successful chemotherapy.

According to Yokogawa, some other serodiagnostic tests that are useful in the diagnosis of paragonimiasis and in differentiating one species of paragonimiasis from others are the double gel Ouchterlony test, which is highly accurate, and the complement fixation test. This is not as consistently reliable as the other tests because false-positive results are common in areas where other parasites such as *Schistosoma* are common.

VIII. Radiological Diagnosis

The radiological appearances in pulmonary paragonimiasis are not pathognomonic. Their importance lies in the frequency with which they can be mistaken for other shadows, such as pulmonary tuberculosis and tumors and other infections of the lung.

A positive diagnosis (with *Paragonimus* eggs in the sputum) could begin with a good account of the patient's places of domicile in recent years, a previous history of hemoptysis, and consumption of crabs. These hints may alert the radiologist who, in turn, may suggest sputum examination to the clinician.

Even the absence of any significant shadows in a patient with hemoptysis need not put off the radiologist if the history is right, because about 21% of patients with proven paragonimiasis exhibit no significant shadows (Ogakwu and Nwokolo, 1973).

When shadows are present, they show no particular pattern of distribution. An analysis of the shadows in 100 cases of proven paragonimiasis showed that the lung often contained one or more shadows, each 10-40 mm across. About one-third of the shadows were of a hazy, low-density, "cotton wool" type. Another third consisted of more discrete and dense lesions. About one-quarter consisted of linear streaks, and the remainder consisted of bubblelike cystic shadows often within areas of consolidation. There is often a distinct predilection for the mid zones (64%), while the upper zones harbor 20% of the lesions, leaving the balance (16%) in the lower zones.

Lobular perihilar shadows resembling lymph node enlargement were observed occasionally.

The radiological shadows of pulmonary paragonimiasis may be indistinguishable from those of early pulmonary tuberculosis. The presence of *Paragonimus* eggs in the sputum or feces is the only sure proof of paragonimiasis.

IX. Treatment

Until 1961, there was no specific treatment for paragonimiasis. Emetine and chloroquine were often suggested but they were of no real value, and most cases relapsed after treatment. In 1961, Yokogawa and colleagues introduced bithionol, which revolutionized the treatment and for nearly two decades remained the standard treatment.

Menichlopholan (Bilevon), a biphenyl compound, was examined in the 1970s for its value in the treatment of paragonimiasis. In 1977, Nwokolo and Volkmer presented a report of a clinical trial carried out in two centers in eastern Nigeria, and recommended it as a possible single-dose treatment of the future. However, it was not put on the market, having been superseded by praziquantel, which, because of its lower toxicity, is now the drug of choice for the treatment of paragonimiasis.

In the treatment of African paragonimiasis, we obtained good results with Bithionol orally in a dosage of 50 mg/kg on alternate days for 10 doses. About 75-80% of patients respond well to a single course of treatment and most of the rest are cured after a second course. About one-third of patients treated with Bithionol complain of diarrhea and, less commonly, vomiting, which are easily controlled.

With menichlopholan, we used a single dose of 2 mg/kg body weight (Nwokolo and Volkmer, 1977). The cure rate was 73-90%.

We have also used praziquantel successfully in Nigeria in the treatment of several cases of pulmonary paragonimiasis. The dosage we use in 40 mg/kg daily for 2 days.

Both praziquantel and menichlopholan are manufactured by the same company, but only praziquantel is on the market at present because of its broad-spectrum anthelminthic qualities. It is equally effective in the treatment of paragonimiasis, schistosomiasis, and taeniasis.

X. Control

Adequate cooking of crabs before consumption is the obvious preventive measure in paragonimiasis. In some endemic areas where crabs are avoided for superstitious reasons, human paragonimiasis does not occur. Normally, the spread of paragonimiasis is slow and the habit of eating raw crabs or crayfish is uncommon in Africa. It required the social upheavel of the Nigerian civil war to modify traditional eating habits and produce an outbreak (Nwokolo, 1972a). Even then only a few patients admitted eating raw crabs. The majority ate them roasted and this gave some metacercariae a chance to survive and infect them.

In eastern Nigeria, there has been a substantial reduction in the prevalence of human paragonimiasis, partly because of the health education campaign against the eating of improperly cooked crabs, and also because of the vast improvement in other sources of edible protein since the end of the Nigerian civil war.

XI. Summary

Paragonimiasis is second only to schistosomiasis among clinically important trematode parasitic diseases in Africa.

The mammalian definitive and reservoir hosts as well as the molluscan and crustacean intermediate hosts exist around most major river basins and nonarid areas of Africa. Human disease probably exists among all crab-eating peoples, but endemic areas for human disease have been identified only in eastern Nigeria, Cameroon, and Liberia. The dominant parasite in West Africa is *Paragonimus uterobilateralis*; but *P. africanus* also exists in Cameroon. Blood-stained sputum is the major symptom of the disease. There are few physical signs, and radiological shadows resembling the early lesions of pulmonary tuberculosis are present in over three-quarters of cases of paragonimiasis. The disease responds well to treatment with bithionol, menichlopholan and praziquantel.

References

Bowesman, A. (1960). *Surgical and Clinical Pathology in the Tropics*. Edinburgh, Churchill-Livingstone.

Coulibaly, N., Cornet, L., Doucet, J., and Loubiere, R. (1975). Paragonimose pulmonaire associee a une bilharziose en Cote-d'Ivoire. *Nouv. Presse Med.* **4**:886.

Goldsmid, J. M. (1975). Ecological and cultural aspects of human trematodiasis (excluding schistosomiasis) in Africa. *Cent. Afr. J. Med.* **21**(3):49-53.

Hallam, A. (1973). *A Revolution in the Earth Sciences*. Oxford, Clarendon Press.

Kum, P. N., and Nchinda, T. C. (1982). Pulmonary paragonimiasis in Cameroon. *Trans. R. Soc. Trop. Med. Hyg.* **76**(6):768-771.

Nwokolo, C. (1972a). Outbreak of paragonimiasis in eastern Nigeria. *Lancet* **1**:32-33.

Nwokolo, C. (1972b). Endemic paragonimiasis in eastern Nigeria. *Trop. Geogr. Med.* **24**:138-147.

Nwokolo, C. (1974). Endemic paragonimiasis in Africa. *Bull. W.H.O.* **50**: 569-571.

Nwokolo, C., and Volkmer, K. J. (1977). Single dose therapy of paragonimiasis with menichlopholan. *Am. J. Trop. Med. Hyg.* **26**(4):688-692.

Oelerich, S., and Nwokolo, C. (1974). Serologische Untersuchungen mit Paragonimus uterobilateralis und anderen Trematoden- Antigenen an seren von Paragonimiasis patienten aus Nigeria. *Tropenmed. Parasitol.* **25**(2):137-146.

Ogakwu, M., and Nwokolo, C. (1974). Radiological findings in pulmonary paragonimiasis as seen in Nigeria: a review based on 100 cases. *Br. J. Radiol.* **46**:699-705.

Sachs, R., Albiez, E. J., and Voelker, J. (1986). Prevalence of *Paragonimus uterobilateralis* infection in children in a Liberian village. *Trans. R. Soc. Trop. Med. Hyg.* **80**:800-801.

Sachs, R., Kern, P., and Voelker, J. (1983). Le paragonimus uterobilateralis comme cause de trois cas de paragonimose humain Gabon. *Tropenmed. Parasitol.* **34**:105-108.

Sachs, R., and Voelker, J. (1982). Human paragonimiasis caused by *Paragonimus uterobilateralis* in Liberia and Guinea West Africa. *Tropenmed. Parasitol.* **33**:15-16.

Van Hoof, L. (1933). Un cas de diastomase au Congo Belge. *Ann. Soc. Belg. Med. Trop.* **13**:473-474.

Voelker, J. (1973). Morphological-taxonomical studies on *P. uterobilateralis* as well as observations of life cycle and spread of parasites of life cycle and spread of parasites in Liberia. *Tropenmed. Parasitol.* **24**(1):4-20.

Voelker, J., and Nwokolo, C. (1973). Human paragonimiasis in Eastern Nigeria caused by *Paragonimus uterobilateralis. Tropenmed. Parasitol.* **24**:323-328.

Voelker, J., and Sachs, R. (1977). Monkeys and lower primates as natural and experimental hosts of African lung flukes. *Tropenmed. Parasitol.* **28**(2):137-144.

Voelker, J., and Vogel, H. Z. (1965). Zwei neue Paragonimus- Arten aus West African. *Tropenmed. Parasitol.* **33**:15-16.

Wegner, A. (1912). Cited in Hallam, 1973.

Yokogawa, M. (1969). Paragonimus and paragonimiasis. *Adv. Parasitol.* **7**:375-387.

Yokogawa, M., Yoshimura, H., Okura, T., Sano, M., Iwasaki, M., and Hirose, H. (1961). Chemotherapy of paragonimiasis with bithionol. *Jpn. J. Parasitol.* **10**:317-327.

Zahra, A. (1951). Paragonimiasis in southern Cameroons. *West Afr. Med. J.* **1**:72.

15

Cryptic Miliary Tuberculosis in the Tropics

Y. L. YU and W. K. LAM

University of Hong Kong
Queen Mary Hospital
Hong Kong

I. Introduction

Cryptic miliary tuberculosis (CMTB) is a term introduced by Proudfoot et al. (1969) to describe a form of disseminated tuberculosis that does not exhibit the classic clinical and radiological features of miliary tuberculosis. Since there are no specific clues, the diagnosis is often made late or missed, resulting in delayed treatment and, consequently, high mortality and morbidity rates.

The tropics refers to the geographical area between the Tropics of Cancer and Capricorn. Compared with the temperate zones, not only is the climate hotter, but countries in the tropics are also in general underdeveloped. The gross national product is low and medical and health services are therefore underfunded. The per capita expenditure on health alone in the most affluent countries is about 200 times that in the least developed ones. Moreover, nutrition, living conditions, and education are generally substandard in developing countries (Aquinas and Todd, 1987).

These factors contribute to a high prevalence and incidence of tuberculosis in developing countries. It is estimated that about 10 million new cases develop annually (Aquinas and Todd, 1987). In addition, more children are affected and the disease manifests in more severe forms than in developed countries (Miller, 1984). This relative lack of success in controlling tuberculosis is directly or indirectly related to scarce resources (Shimao, 1986), resulting in a delay in case-finding, shortage of medical facilities and drugs, underdevelopment of primary health care, and failure to comply by patients.

In the tropics, CMTB is probably more prevalent because of the higher incidence of tuberculosis, although this is not reflected by reports on CMTB. Of about 300 cases obtained from a survey of the English literature (Chapman and Whorton, 1946; Ball et al., 1951; Treip and Meyers, 1959; Petersdorf and Beeson, 1961; Böttiger et al., 1962; Linell and Östberg, 1966; Proudfoot et al., 1969; Jacques and Sloan, 1970; Beerman et al., 1971; Ashba and Boyce, 1972; Grieco and Chmel, 1974; Rosenthal et al., 1975; Edlin, 1978; Enarson et al., 1978; Prout and Benatar, 1980; Slavin et al., 1980; Bobrowitz, 1982; Monie et al., 1983; Yu et al., 1986), only 15 reported from Hong Kong (latitude 22°20′N, longitude 114°12′E) were from the tropics. Thus, there can be no claim to wide experience of CMTB in the tropics. However, apart from the difference in socioeconomic conditions and the provision of medical service between the tropical and temperate regions, the medical aspects of CMTB are similar.

II. Pathogenesis

In primary tuberculosis infection, most commonly acquired by airborne infection and usually in children, a nonspecific inflammatory reaction occurs as soon as the mycobacteria reach the alveoli, and phagocytosis and intracellular replication take place. A bacteremia is thought to occur with dissemination throughout the body. The vast majority of the primary lesions heal, and reactivation as a result of decreased body defenses owing to various causes is the mechanism by which tuberculosis in the adult usually develops, whether in the lungs or the disseminated form.

Disseminated or miliary tuberculosis may therefore result from the hematogenous spread of tubercle bacilli directly from a primary infection, from the reactivation of an old focus with resulting spread into the blood stream or lymphatics, or as a terminal event in a patient with extensive organ tuberculosis. The interplay between bacilli multiplication and host defense determines the form of disease progression and dissemination clinically and pathologically (Dannenberg and Tomashefski, 1988). In classic miliary tuberculosis, there is marked cellular response with well-formed tubercles. On the other hand, when numerous bacilli are discharged into the bloodstream of a severely immunocompromised host, an acute nonreactive form of disseminated tuberculosis occurs with abundant caseation and tissue necrosis and a large number of bacilli but little or no encapsulation or granulomatous reaction (Rosenthal et al., 1975; Dannenberg and Tomashefski, 1988). These cases are the ones most likely to be missed in life because of the absence of the miliary chest radiograph and the nonspecific clinical picture; hence the term CMTB is used. Autopsies of these patients show that the lungs, liver, spleen, bone marrow, and lymph nodes are the sites frequently involved (Chapman and Whorton, 1946; Grieco and Chmel, 1974; Rosenthal et al., 1975; Slavin et al., 1980; Yu et al., 1986), but data on the brain, spinal cord, and meninges are not available, since the nervous system is usually not examined at autopsy.

III. Clinical Picture

A. Sex and Age of Patients

In the reported cases, there were approximately equal numbers of male and female patients. However, in most series the elderly were predominantly affected. This is in keeping with the current trend that disseminated tuberculosis occurs more commonly in the elderly than in children (Jacques and Sloan, 1970). Moreover, this age group is at particular risk of death from tuberculosis (Mackay and Cole, 1984). Hence, in elderly patients, a high index of suspicion for CMTB is indicated (Treip and Meyers, 1959; Enarson et al., 1978; Yu et al., 1986).

B. Risk Factors and Underlying Medical Conditions

Immunocompromised subjects, especially those associated with impaired cellular immunity, have a greater propensity to develop active tuberculosis. In series with adequate data (Treip and Meyers, 1959; Böttinger et al., 1962; Proudfoot et al., 1969; Beerman et al., 1971; Grieco and Chmel, 1974; Rosenthal et al., 1975; Slavin et al., 1980; Bobrowitz, 1982; Monie et al., 1983; Yu et al., 1986), 30-60% of patients had concomitant diseases or received treatment that compromised host defense. Alcoholism with or without cirrhosis, diabetes mellitus, hematological or other malignancies, collagen diseases, poor nutrition, and end-stage renal disease are the commonly documented conditions. A previous history of tuberculosis or close contact with patients having active tuberculosis is also relevant (Chapman and Whorton, 1946). Immunosuppressive therapy either with steroids or cytotoxic drugs is being used with increasing frequency in various diseases and it is salutary to remember that these patients have a high risk of disseminated or pulmonary tuberculosis (Sahn and Lakshminarayan, 1976; Millar and Horne, 1979).

C. Presenting Symptoms and Clinical Features

The symptoms of CMTB are, by definition, nonspecific. Pyrexia of unknown origin, malaise, anorexia, and weight loss are the most common presenting symptoms. Other symptoms include cough, dyspnea, hemoptysis, abdominal pain or distention. In general, these symptoms are present for a variable period, from just a few days to as long as months. The common abnormal physical signs, in descending order of frequency, are fever, pallor, hepatomegaly, splenomegaly, and abnormal chest signs (Yu et al., 1986). In a patient with a combination of two or more of these features, the clinician should be alerted to the possibility of disseminated tuberculosis. Choroidal tubercles, when present, are a pathognomonic sign (Chapman and Whorton, 1946). However, choroidal tubercles are known to be uncommon in nonwhite patients with tuberculous meningitis or miliary tuberculosis (Tandon, 1978).

IV. Laboratory Investigations and Diagnosis

A. Chest Radiograph

Classic miliary shadows are absent in the lung fields of chest radiographs, which is a major reason for the elusiveness of CMTB. One report (Berger and Samortin, 1970) has suggested that careful inspection of an underpenetrated film with special attention to the intercostal spaces may reveal miliary shadows in such patients. Another short communication described miliary shadows detected on computed tomographic scans in one case (Amos et al., 1987). Abnormalities more commonly seen in other lung pathological conditions may be present. Patchy shadowing suggestive of bronchopneumonia may cause delay in the diagnosis. However, the presence of pleural effusion, fibrosis, and calcification at the apices and hilum should alert the clinician to the possibility of tuberculosis. Nevertheless, there remains a group of patients in whom the chest x-ray is entirely normal (Böttinger et al., 1962; Proudfoot et al., 1969; Monie et al., 1983; Yu et al., 1986), and hence a normal chest x-ray can by no means exclude disseminated tuberculosis.

B. Hematological Indices

A wide range of hematological abnormalities, many of which reflect tuberculosis in the bone marrow, have been described in patients with disseminated tuberculosis (Ball et al., 1951; Oswald, 1963). These include leukemoid reaction, pancytopenia, agranulocytosis, aplastic anemia, thrombocytopenia, leukoerythroblastic anemia, polycythemia, and eosinophilia. While these findings are nonspecific and certainly not diagnostic, their presence in the appropriate clinical setting should alert the clinician to the possibility of CMTB. A bone marrow aspirate and biopsy should be performed and are often positive for tubercle bacilli (Ball et al., 1951; Oswald, 1963). On the other hand, one must be suspicious of an underlying primary hematological dyscrasia in patients with tuberculosis who show a pancytopenia or leukemoid reaction (Munt, 1972).

C. Biochemical Profiles

Because of liver involvement, abnormalities in liver functin tests including raised levels of alkaline phosphatase and γ-glutamic pyruvate transferase and hypoalbuminemia are often encountered (Grieco and Chmel, 1974; Prout and Benatar, 1980; Yu et al., 1986). Hyponatremia in tuberculosis was first described in 1938 by Winkler and Crankshaw, and subsequently reported in about one-third of patients with disseminated tuberculosis (Munt, 1972; Yu et al., 1986). This phenomenon may be due to inappropriate secretion of antidiuretic hormone induced by pulmonary and/or cranial tuberculosis, or adrenal insufficiency. Yu et al. (1986) for instance, found adrenal involvement at autopsy in two of three patients with CMTB who had hyponatremia during life.

D. Investigations Specific for Tuberculosis

Largely because the diagnosis is not suspected during life and because some patients were frail and very ill, relevant investigations are either not performed or delayed. However, the tuberculin test was negative in most cases tested (Böttinger et al., 1962; Bobrowitz, 1982; Yu et al., 1986), which probably reflects the host's compromised defenses. Grieco and Chmel (1974) have also stressed the association between cutaneous anergy and advancing age. The yield of Ziehl-Neelsen stain for tubercle bacilli in sputum, urine, and cerebrospinal fluid is low, and while culture has an improved yield, management decisions cannot be based on such results because of a time lag of 4-6 weeks in receiving results.

Histological and bacteriological examination of liver and bone marrow biopsies is much more helpful (Yu et al., 1986). The classic tuberculosis granuloma with Langhans' giant cell, caseation, and positive stain for tubercle bacilli is diagnostic but by no means always present. In some cases, only microgranulomas (Fig. 1) are detected. Although this is a nonspecific finding observed in a large variety of diseases, tuberculosis and sarcoidosis are leading causes (Klatskin, 1977). It should be noted that sarcoidosis, which is already an uncommon condition in white patients, is rarely reported in Asian patients, except in Japanese. Hence, in the appropriate clinical setting, the presence of microgranulomas is a strong indication for a therapeutic trial of antituberculous treatment; a good clinical response would indicate a correct diagnosis.

Mycobacteria are rich in antigens that stimulate the production of antibodies and lymphokines, but serological methods based on enzyme-linked immunosorbent assays (ELISA) and radioimmunoassay for the diagnosis of tuberculosis have been studied with disappointing results (Good, 1989). Information obtained would be more useful for population surveys than for

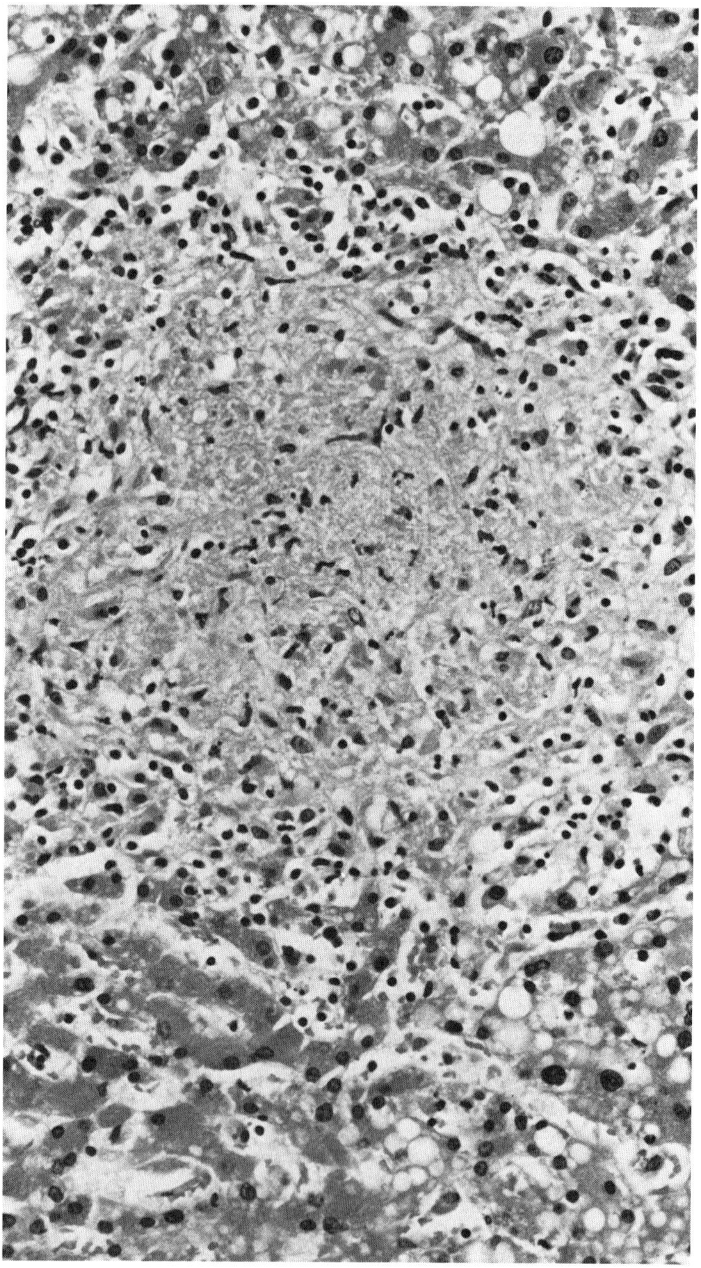

Figure 1 Photomicrograph of a hepatic micrograuloma composed of epithelioid and inflammatory cells (H&E × 100).

clinical diagnosis. Chau and co-workers (1987) in Hong Kong found that the ELISA method yielded a positive result only if the disease was chronic or extensive. It would be of interest to have the method further tested in patients with suspected miliary tuberculosis.

E. Diagnosis

The diagnosis of CMTB is often difficult because of the nonspecific symptoms and the absence of typical radiological findings. In over half of the reported cases, the diagnosis was not made during life. In this regard, a high index of suspicion for CMTB is essential, particularly in the elderly and in those with preexisting disease or who are receiving immunosuppressive therapy. Once the possibility is considered, appropriate investigations should be performed promptly.

V. Treatment

Therapy should be started early as soon as CMTB is suspected, even in the absence of any microbiological or histological proof of the disease (Petersdorf and Beeson, 1961; Proudfoot et al., 1969; Beerman et al., 1971; Grieco and Chmel, 1974; Yu et al., 1986). Even with treatment, early mortality rates (within 2 weeks) due to advanced disease in moribund, elderly patients are high. In one series (Proudfoot et al., 1969) in which antituberculous therapy (p-aminosalicylic acid and isoniazid, with or without streptomycin) was initiated before death in 14 cases, the mortality rate was 14% (2 of 14). If the patient survives the first 2-3 weeks after initiating therapy, the outlook for cure is good. The improvement may, however, be delayed for several weeks, and an adequate trial of at least 6 weeks may be needed.

Adequate controlled trials of treatment have not been conducted for disseminated tuberculosis, but increasing clinical experience with treatment of extrapulmonary tuberculosis indicates that 9-12 months duration of therapy should be sufficient (American Thoracic Society, 1986). In Hong Kong, where there is a high level of initial drug resistance (about 15-20%) to one or more of the drugs isoniazid (INH), streptomycin (SM), and rifampicin (RIF), selection of four drugs—INH, RIF, pyrazinamide (PZA), and SM or ethambutol (EMB)—for initial therapy is indicated (Hong Kong Chest Service/British Medical Research Council, 1981; Aquinas, 1982). Our recommended daily dosages are INH 300 mg, RIF 450 mg or 600 mg, PZA 1.5 g or 2.0 g, SM 0.75 g, and EMB 25 mg/kg for 2 months, and then 15 mg/kg. The higher dosages of RIF and PZA are given to patients weighing 50 kg or more. In America, the recommended daily dosage would be 5 mg/kg for INH (maximum 300 mg), 10 mg/kg for RIF (maximum 600 mg), 15-30 mg/kg for PZA (maximum 2 g), 15-25 mg/kg for EMB (maximum 1.5 g), and 15 mg/kg for SM (maximum 1 g; in persons older than 60 years of age, 10 mg/kg with maximum 750 mg; American Thoracic Society, 1986). Isoniazid and RIF should be given throughout whereas PZA plus EMB or SM may be given in the initial 2-4 months according to clinical response. Isoniazid, RIF, and PZA are all well absorbed orally, with good tissue penetration for all sites (Ellard, 1969; Furesz, 1970; Bailey, 1988; Steel and Des Pres, 1988). Hence, regimens containing these three drugs are very effective in eliminating tubercle bacilli populations in pulmonary and extrapulmonary sites.

The role of corticosteroids is controversial, and no controlled study has addressed this issue in the treatment of disseminated tuberculosis. However, steroids have been widely prescribed for extremely ill patients in an attempt to improve their sense of well-being and food intake to reduce the risk of immediate mortality. We would give steroids for moribund and extremely toxic patients in the first 2 months of antituberculous therapy, except when the intestine is involved by disease, with the potential risk of perforation with steroid therapy. Corticosteroid therapy is, of course, necessary when the adrenal glands have been destroyed by disseminated tuberculosis.

VI. Acquired Immunodeficiency Syndrome

Because of the T-helper cell defects in patients with acquired immunodeficiency syndrome (AIDS), mycobacterial infection, along with other opportunistic infections, is common and may be due to *M. tuberculosis* or atypical mycobacteria such as *M. avium-intracellulare.* The AIDS epidemic has had a profound impact on tuberculosis morbidity, particularly in those demographic groups that already have a high incidence of tuberculosis, such as in central African countries. Separate consideration of the special characteristics of the infection in these patients is warranted.

Tuberculosis in AIDS patients is characterized by a high proportion of the lymphatic and disseminated forms. Also, unusual clinical presentations occur frequently (Pitchenik et al., 1988): generalized lymphadenopathy, retroperitoneal lymphadenopathy presenting as abdominal masses, mediastinal lymph node-esophageal fistula, pericardial-cutaneous fistula, small intestinal fistula, abscesses in the brain, spinal cord, rectum, testis, and soft tissues.

Since the diagnosis may be elusive, the physician must have a high index of suspicion for disseminated tuberculosis in AIDS patients, particularly in populations with a high prevalence of tuberculosis. As expected in the setting of severe T-helper cell defects, tubercle bacilli abound in the body; therefore, sputum, urine, stool, and blood specimens should be taken for smear and/or culture (Pitchenik et al., 1988). Moreover, tuberculin skin test would be positive only in a minority of patients (about 30%), and granulomas would tend to be poorly formed or nonexistent, and caseation necrosis uncommon.

Most AIDS patients with tuberculosis respond to standard antituberculous drugs, although side effects tend to be more frequent (Chaisoon et al., 1987), and the appropriate duration of treatment is not yet established. The American Thoracic Society and the Centers for Disease Control (1987) have recommended a regimen of INH plus RIF, supplemented by PZA for the first 2 months of therapy. Ethambutol is also recommended to supplement the initial treatment regimen in patients with disseminated disease. Treatment should continue for a minimum of 9 months and for at least 6 months after documented culture conversion. Some experts recommend continuing INH and RIF therapy for 12 months and for at least 9 months after documented culture conversion (Pitchenik et al., 1988).

References

American Thoracic Society (1986). Treatment of tuberculosis and tuberculosis infection in adults and children. *Am. Rev. Respir. Dis.* **134**:355-363.

American Thoracic Society/Centers for Disease Control (1987). Mycobacterioses and the acquired immunodeficiency syndrome. *Am. Rev. Respir. Dis.* **136**:492-496.

Amos, A., Denning, D., Katz, D., and Smith, H. (1987). Computed tomography of chest in diagnosis of miliary tuberculosis. *Lancet* **2**:1269-1270.

Aquinas, M. (1982). Short-course therapy for tuberculosis. *Drugs* **24**:118-132.

Aquinas, M., and Todd, D. (1987). Particular problems of tuberculosis in developing countries. In *Oxford Textbook of Medicine*, 2nd ed. Edited by D. J. Weatherall, J. G. G. Ledingham, and D. A. Warrell. Oxford, Oxford University Press, pp. 5.299-5.303.

Ashba, J. K., and Boyce, J. M. (1972). Undiagnosed tuberculosis in a general hospital. *Chest* **61**:447-451.

Baily, W. C. (1988). Chemotherapy of tuberculosis. In *Tuberculosis*, vol. 2. Edited by D. Schlossberg, New York, Praeger, pp. 39-53.

Ball, K., Joules, H., and Pagel, W. (1951). Acute tuberculous septicaemia with leucopenia. *Br. Med. J.* **2**:869-873.

Beerman, B., Engström, J., Hellström, K., Holm, G., and Lönnqvist, B. (1971). Disseminated tuberculosis in elderly patients. *Acta Med. Scand.* **190**:45-48.

Berger, H. W., and Samortin, T. G. (1970). Miliary tuberculosis: diagnostic methods with emphasis on the chest roentgenogram. *Chest* **58**:586-589.

Bobrowitz, I. D. (1982). Active tuberculosis undiagnosed until autopsy. *Am. J. Med.* **72**:650-658.

Böttiger, L. E., Nordenstrom, H. H., and Weston, P. L. (1962). Disseminated tuberculosis as a cause of fever of obscure origin. *Lancet* **1**:19-20.

Chaisoon, R. E., Schecter, G. F., Theuer, C. P., Rutherford, G. W., Echenberg, D. F., and Hopewell, P. C. (1987). Tuberculosis in patients with the acquired immunodeficiency syndrome. *Am. Rev. Respir. Dis.* **136**: 570-574.

Chapman, C. B., and Whorton, C. M. (1946). Acute generalized miliary tuberculosis in adults. A clinicopathological study based on sixty-three cases diagnosed at autopsy. *N. Engl. J. Med.* **235**:239-248.

Chau, P. Y., Wan, K. C., Ng, W. S., So, S. Y., Lau, W. Y., Fan, S. T., and Lee, D. K. Y. (1987). Enzyme-linked immunosorbent assay (ELISA) in the diagnosis of active tuberculosis: evaluation of its potential and limitation in a high prevalence area. *Trop. Geogr. Med.* **39**:228-232.

Dannenberg, A. M., and Tomashefski, J. F. (1988). Pathogenesis of pulmonary tuberculosis. In *Pulmonary Diseases and Disorders.* Edited by A. P. Fishman. New York, McGraw-Hill, pp. 1821-1842.

Edlin, G. P. (1978). Active tuberculosis unrecognized until necropsy. *Lancet* **1**:650-652.

Ellard, G. A. (1969). Absorption, metabolism and excretion of pyrazinamide in man. *Tubercle* **50**:144-158.

Enarson, D. A., Grzybowski, S., and Dorken, E. (1978). Failure of diagnosis as a factor in tuberculosis mortality. *Can. Med. Assoc. J.* **118**:1520-1522.

Furesz, S. (1970). Chemical and biochemical properties of rifampicin. *Antibiot. Chemother.* **16**:316-351.

Good, R. C. (1989). Serologic methods for diagnosing tuberculosis (Editorial). *Ann. Intern. Med.* **110**:97-98.

Grieco, M. H., and Chmel, H. (1974). Acute disseminated tuberculosis as a diagnostic problem: a clinical study based on twenty-eight cases. *Am. Rev. Respir. Dis.* **109**:554-560.

Hong Kong Chest Service/British Medical Research Council (1981). Controlled trial of 4 thrice-weekly regimens and a daily regimen all given for 6 months for pulmonary tuberculosis. *Lancet* **1**:171-174.

Jacques, J., and Sloan, J. M. (1970). The changing pattern of miliary tuberculosis. *Thorax* **25**:237-240.

Klatskin, G. (1977). Hepatic granulomata: problems in interpretation. *J. Mt. Sinai. Hosp.* **44**:798-812.

Linell, F., and Östberg, G. (1966). Tuberculosis in an autopsy material. *Scand. J. Respir. Dis.* **47**:200-208.

Mackay, A. D., and Cole, R. B. (1984). The problems of tuberculosis in the elderly. *Q. J. Med.* **53**:491-510.

Millar, J. W., and Horne, N. W. (1979). Tuberculosis in immunosuppressed patients. *Lancet* **1**:1176-1178.

Miller, F. J. W. (1984). The natural history of primary tuberculosis. *W.H.O. Tech. Bull.* 84.**144**:9.

Monie, R. D. H., Hunter, A. M., Rocchiccioli, K. M. S., White, J. P., Campbell, I. A., and Kilpatrick, G. S. (1983). Retrospective survey of the management of miliary tuberculosis in South and West Wales 1976-8. *Thorax* **38**:369-372.

Munt, P. W. (1972). Miliary tuberculosis in the chemotherapy era: with a clinical review in 69 American adults. *Medicine* (*Baltimore*) **51**:139-155.

Oswald, N. C. (1963). Active tuberculosis and granulocytic disorder. *Br. Med. J.* **2**:1489-1495.

Petersdorf, R. G., and Beeson, P. B. (1961). Fever of unexplained origin: report on 100 cases. *Medicine* (*Baltimore*) **40**:1-30.

Pitchenik, A. E., Fertel, D., and Bloch, A. B. (1988). Pulmonary effects of AIDS: mycobacterial disease—epidemiology, diagnosis, treatment, and prevention. *Clin. Chest Med.* **9**:425-441.

Proudfoot, A. T., Akhtar, A. J., Douglas, A. C., and Horne, N. W. (1969). Miliary tuberculosis in adults. *Br. Med. J.* **2**:273-276.

Prout, S., and Benatar, S. R. (1980). Disseminated tuberculosis—a study of 62 cases. *S. Afr. Med. J.* **58**:835-842.

Rosenthal, T., Pitliks, S., and Michaels, D. (1975). Fatal undiagnosed tuberculosis in hospitalized patients. *J. Infect. Dis.* **131**:S51-S56.

Sahn, S. A., and Lakshminarayan, S. (1976). Tuberculosis after corticosteroid therapy. *Br. J. Dis. Chest.* **70**:195-205.

Shimao, T. (1986). Review of tuberculosis control programmes in the Far East Region of the IUAT. *Bull. IUAT* **61**:7-27.

Slavin, R. E., Welsh, T. J., and Pollack, A. D. (1980). Late generalized tuberculosis: a clinical pathological analysis and comparison of 100 cases in the preantibiotic and antibiotic eras. *Medicine* (*Baltimore*) **59**:352-366.

Steel, M. A., and Des Pres, R. M. (1988). The role of pyrazinamide in tuberculosis chemotherapy. *Chest* **94**:845-850.

Tandon, P. N. (1978). Tuberculous meningitis (cranial and spinal). In *Handbook of Clinical Neurology*, vol. 33, *Infections of the Nervous System*, Part I. Edited by P. J. Vinken and G. W. Bruyn. Amsterdam, North Holland Publishing, pp. 195-262.

Treip, C., and Meyers, D. (1959). Fatal tuberculosis in a general hospital. A diagnostic problem. *Lancet* **1**:164-167.

Winkler, A. W., and Crankshaw, O. F. (1938). Chloride depletion in conditions other than Addison's disease. *J. Clin. Invest.* **17**:1-6.

Yu, Y. L., Chow, W. H., Humphries, M. J., Wong, R. W. S., and Gabriel, M. (1986). Cryptic miliary tuberculosis. *Q.J. Med.* **59**:421-428.

16

Common Pulmonary Allergic Disorders in Southeast Asia

SOMCHAI BOVORNKITTI, RUNGSUN PUSHPAKOM, NANTA MARANETRA and SUCHAI CHAROENRATANAKUL

Siriraj Hospital, Mahidol University
Bangkok, Thailand

I. Background

To the present authors, the terms *allergy* and *hypersensitivity* denote an immunological state acquired by a host as a consequence of contact with and sensitization by allergens or antigens, and in whom subsequent interaction between the antigen and its specific humoral antibodies or specifically sensitized host cells may give rise to various clinical manifestations.

Aeroallergens are the principal causes of respiratory allergic conditions through the route of inhalation, whereas a variety of allergens can also sensitize and/or provoke reactions via other routes, namely ingestion, injection, and mere skin contact.

Although most of the pulmonary allergic disorders listed in Table 1 (Tharavanij, 1971) are distributed worldwide, only bronchial asthma is prevalent in Southeast Asian countries. Certain types of allergic or hypersensitivity pneumonitis and insect allergies are relatively less common.

Table 1 Known Pulmonary Allergic Disorders

Disorders of Type I hypersensitivity
Anaphylactic reaction: penicillins, antiserum, toxoids, insect allergy, intravenous contrast media
Sudden death in infancy owing to hypersensitivity to milk
Allergic bronchial asthma
Disorders of Type III hypersensitivity
Bronchopulmonary aspergillosis
Hypersensitivity pneumonitis: Farmer's lung and related disoders (bagassosis, maple bark disease, bird fancier's disease, etc.)
Serum sickness
Chronic pneumonia owing to allergy to cow milk
Polyarteritis nodosa
Disorders of Type IV hypersensitivity
Silicosis
Berylliosis
Disorders of hypersensitivity of unknown mechanisms
Rheumatic lung
Pulmonary eosinophilia: Loffler's syndrome, and Tropical pulmonary eosinophilia

II. Bronchial Asthma

A. Definition

Bronchial asthma is characterized by an abnormality of the airways expressed by a variable degree of persistent hyperresponsiveness to a wide variety of provoking stimuli, specific and nonspecific, which cause them to narrow easily and excessively.

B. Pathological Features

The basic pathological features of bronchial asthma are increased wall thickness of the airways associated with a chronic inflammatory process that compromises cellular infiltration (including eosinophils and mast cells), deposition of connective tissue, hypertrophy of smooth muscles and mucous glands, goblet cell metaplasia, epithelial damage, distention of blood vessels, and an inflammatory exudate containing mucus in the airway lumen (Hogg et al., 1988; Reed, 1988).

C. Pathogenesis

The causes and the induction of bronchial asthma remain poorly understood even after extensive studies over many years. However, among the several hypotheses proposed, allergy is considered to be the most important of the likely causes (Tuchinda et al., 1987; Miyamoto et al., 1988; Tan, 1988). The majority of asthmatics are atopic, that is, they show positive skin test reactivity and increase of IgE in the blood circulation. It is evident that patients with an atopic constitution are more easily sensitized by allergens than those without atopy (Frankland, 1953). Pollens from tropical grasses, weeds, and trees seem to be potential inducers of asthma in Southeast Asia (Cau-Lim et al., 1978; Tuchinda et al., 1983; Tan, 1988). There is well-documented evidence of a strong association between asthma and house dust mites (especially *Dermatophagoides pteronyssinus* and *D. farinae*), which suggests that they may be inducers of asthma (Choovivathanavanich et al., 1971a, b; Wongsathuaythong et al., 1972; Thomas et al., 1978; Hsieh, 1984).

There is accumulated evidence that bronchial hyperreactivity is the genetic localization factor that, apart from the hereditary factor causing atopic sensitization, is the hallmark of bronchial asthma (Longo et al., 1987). However, the manner in which bronchial hyperreactivity develops is not yet fully understood. A number of airborne agents (viruses, irritative gases, etc.) probably cause mucosal damage, which may increase the sensitivity of the irritant receptors, thereby lowering the nonspecific irritative threshold and paving the way for nonimmunological bronchial hyperresponsiveness. Nonetheless, at present, no single mechanism can be identified that would explain, in a unifying fashion, how those agents cause asthma.

The historic triad of bronchial asthma, nasal polyposis, and intolerance to aspirin and related chemicals, which recently has been designated Samter's syndrome, is a condition of unknown cause and pathogenesis (Zeitz, 1988). Intolerance to aspirin is a manifestation, not a cause, of the disease. Viral infection probably plays a significant role, and hereditary factors are important in some patients. There is evidence suggesting a possible association between Samter's syndrome and the DR and/or DQ loci of the major histocompatibility complex (Jones et al., 1984; Mullarkey et al., 1986).

There are still unanswered questions in the field of occupational asthma. The pathogenic mechanisms of many causes of occupational asthma are unknown (Chan-Yeung, 1988). Some sensitizing agents found in the workplace (Table 2) clearly cause (occupational) asthma in some workers (Belin, 1983). Only some of them become sensitized and subsequently an airway response may be provoked that may be immediate, late, or dual. The late reaction usually results in more severe asthma. In many workers, continuing exposure to sensitizing agents leads to persistent asthma, which continues even after the agent has been removed. By far the greatest number of occupational agents causing asthma have been known or suspected to possess allergic properties; some agents cause sensitization via IgE antibodies, whereas the mechanism of sensitization by others remains unknown.

Table 2 Sensitizing Agents in the Work Place

Work place/occupation	Agent
Bakery	Flour (wheat, rye, etc.), moulds
Mill workers	Insect allergen from flour weevil (*Sitophilus gran.*)
Food handlers	Soya flour, spice dust (pepper), egg and flour products, papain, etc.
Laboratory personnel, veterinary surgeons	Animal dander, laboratory animals-urinary protein
Gardeners	Pollens
Pharmaceutical personnel, health service personnel	Ispaghula powder, trypsin wound-dressing powder, penicillin, lycopodium, etc.
Detergent factory	*B. subtilis* enzymes: amylases, proteases
Coffee-roasters	Raw coffee dust
Typographers	Gum arabic, humidifier microbes
Carpenters	Sawdust, moulds

Asthmatic attacks (bronchoconstrictive reaction) may be induced through different trigger mechanisms, for example, by exposure to irritative nonimmunological stimuli such as smoke, dust, and cold air, as well as by exercise and even stress, in addition to specific allergens. This means that the airways are hyperreactive, either specifically through an immunological amplification mechanism mediated by IgE antibodies, or simply expressed through a biochemical or neurogenic interference with or imbalance of the mediator and receptor systems controlling the bronchial structure.

D. Prevalence

There are considerable worldwide variations in the prevalence of bronchial asthma, the occurrence of which has shown an increase over time (Hsieh and Shen, 1988; Miyamoto et al., 1988; Tan, 1988). The reported prevalence rates vary from lows of 0.06% in Finland and 1.4% in Sweden, to 6.6% in the United States, and a high of 11.4% of Australian children at the age of 10 years (Tuchinda et al., 1987). In Southeast Asian countries, the disease is regarded as one of the most common problems after respiratory infection (Tuchinda, 1983; Mangunnegoro and Manuhutu, 1988; Tan, 1988; Lam, 1989) and the rates are generally comparable to those of Western countries (Hsieh and Shen, 1988); however, the true prevalence is not known. Available documents from Papua New Guinea indicate a prevalence rate of at least 7.3% in adults and 0.6% in children (Woolcock et al., 1983); from the

Philippines, of 3.9% during the period 1983-1987 (de Guia, 1988); from Indonesia, of 7.45% in 1987 (Mangunnegoro and Manuhutu, 1988); from Taiwan, of 5.07% in 1985 (Hsieh and Shen, 1988); from Singapore, of 13.7% in 1987 (Tan, 1988); and from Hong Kong, of 5% or more (Lam, 1989). Although the rate for Thailand was recorded as 2.39% for adults in 1975 and 4.30% for children in 1987 (Tuchinda, 1978; Tuchinda et al., 1987), the actual prevalence rate among Thais is unknown. Ethnic differences in the prevalence of asthma were found to be as follows: prevalence among Chinese was 13.1%; among Malays, 19.1%; and among Indians 15.1% (Tan, 1988).

The disease may occur at any age, but is common in children and young adults. The onset of asthma is mainly in children, mostly before the age of 10 years; late onset beyond the age of 40 is uncommon. In children under 10 years of age, asthma is more prevalent among boys. However, there are no sex differences in children over 10 years of age or in asthmatic adults. The preponderance among males has been attributed to higher vulnerability to respiratory infections among boys (Tan, 1988).

The prevalence rate of occupational allergic asthma has not yet been determined in Southeast Asia, although from time to time one encounters isolated cases with a history suggestive of occupational linkage, such as among painters, carpenters, and laboratory technicians. Studies either on particular patients (except for one report by So et al., 1981) or on a wide epidemiological scale have not been carried out.

Aspirin-induced asthma has been noted primarily among whites, although blacks and Asians also are affected. Prevalence has been reported to vary between 2 and 3% in asthma patients in general, and up to 20% in patients with severe asthma (Zeitz, 1988). Incidence is uncommon in Southeast Asian countries, especially Thailand (Tuchinda, 1983).

E. Clinical Signs

Symptoms and signs of bronchial asthma are the same all over the world. The classic symptoms are intermittent, reversible episodes of bronchospasm manifested by cough, wheezing, and dyspnea. In allergic patients, there may be an association with rhinitis and conjunctivitis. Early cases often include a vague, heavy feeling of tightness in the chest. The cough is initially nonproductive, and may progress to expectoration of a profuse, viscous, mucoid, or purulent and discolored sputum. Some patients' asthma is characterized solely by distressing cough without overt wheezing.

Patients with allergic asthma usually exhibit seasonal exacerbations and/or experience clearly recognized allergen-triggering events, related to exposure to pollens, house dust, animal danders, feathers, mold spores, occupational dust, or insects, and, especially among children, certain foods. However, the association may not be clear, and in a number of cases the provocation is due to nonallergic conditions, such as exposure to cigarette smoke, noxious fumes, upper respiratory tract infections, or weather conditions. In extraordinarily rare circumstances, the asthmatic attacks are regularly brought on during lovemaking (due to the inhalation of allergens in the bedclothes that are released during the movements of lovemaking, as well as exertion, or sweat allergy), or after the male's ejaculation as a result of semen allergy. Acute gastroesophageal reflux, induced by an overweight partner on top of the patient while assuming the missionary position may be another cause of asthma occurring during intercourse (Riley, 1989).

Physical examination plays a vital role in assessing the severity of asthma. With an acute exacerbation, the patient is restless, agitated, breathing with accessory muscles of respiration, audibly wheezing, diaphoretic, orthopneic, and tachypneic. Cyanosis (due to profound arterial oxygen desaturation) together with marked tachypnea, a widened pulse pressure, and a pulsus paradoxicus are reliable indicators of acute severe asthma. Examination of the chest will often show signs of lung hyperinflation and different degrees of bronchospasm. In a completely asymptomatic patient, results of physical examination will be normal.

The clinical characteristics of allergic occupational asthma are those of an IgE-mediated type I reaction, manifested similarly to those of allergic asthmatics in general. The onset of respiratory symptoms during exposure is usually rapid and this can be registered objectively by spirometry performed before and after the patient's work shift. Occupational allergy often starts after a patient has worked for about 10 years with cereals, for example, but occurs after a considerably shorter exposure time among workers handling detergents and those exposed to enzymes, raw coffee dust, and laboratory animals. The symptoms of the late-type reaction, which appear after the end of the working day, are almost always a nonspecific bronchial hyperreactivity that can be verified by means of a standardized bronchial provocation test.

F. Management

For patients with mild asthma, the administration of bronchodilators such as procaterol, hexoprenaline, and salbutamol (by inhalation or orally) is all that is necessary. For children with minimal symptoms, a long-acting bronchodilator preparation (e.g., procaterol) given just before the child goes to bed, with postural drainage in the morning, usually is sufficient treatment. A prophylactic regimen of steroid or cromoglycate inhaler may be required in addition to inhaled or oral bronchodilators in some moderately severe cases.

In more severe cases the beta-2-adrenoceptor drugs, theophylline and sodium cromoglycate may not totally control frequent attacks, which would necessitate occasional hospitalization. Such cases require the use of inhaled steroids at higher doses for maintenance therapy in addition to the use of bronchodilators. Children and a few adults who have difficulty using a conventional metered-dose inhaler can obtain the benefits of inhaled medication via a bulb-spacer that is breath-activated and therefore precludes the need for coordination. Oral steroids are prescribed for immediate use only during exacerbations and in certain cases requiring maintenance oral therapy at low concentrations sufficient to control symptoms.

In cases of acute severe attack ("status asthmaticus"), hospitalization is imperative, preferably in a critical respiratory care unit. Most patients can be treated successfully with oxygen, intravenous fluids, intravenous aminophylline, beta-2-agonist nebulizer, and intravenous hydrocortisone. When there is no improvement over time, or when the initial situation is considered to be serious (e.g., silent chest, Pco_2 above mmHg, or marked cyanosis), endotracheal intubation and the use of a respirator are mandatory steps that must be taken urgently.

As with all allergic diseases, the cornerstone of treatment is environmental control, involving avoidance of respiratory irritants and specific provoking allergens.

III. Allergic Bronchopulmonary Aspergillosis

A. Definition

Allergic bronchopulmonary aspergillosis (ABPA) affects only patients with previously existing asthma, characterized by chest roentgenographic infiltrates with peripheral eosinophilia and an array of immunological reactions such as elevated total serum IgE levels, immediate cutaneous reactivity to *Aspergillus fumigatus* (AF), serum precipitins to AF, and proximal bronchiectasis with normal tapering of distant bronchi (Greenberger, 1988).

B. Pathogenesis

Aspergillus organisms, particularly AF, when present in the bronchial tree, act as potent allergens although they do not invade the bronchial wall or lung tissue. Exacerbations of ABPA occur during periods of highest mold counts in the environment. Both IgE and IgG are implicated in the intense immunological response to intrabronchial growth of the fungus. *Aspergillus*-specific IgE is released by peripheral blood lymphocytes during exacerbation of the illness. The specific IgEs trigger mast cell degranulation and mediator-induced bronchial spasm. Although most allergic bronchopulmonary syndromes are attributable to AF or other species of the genus *Aspergillus*, other noninvasive fungi have been incriminated.

C. Histopathological Findings

Bronchial plugs seen in ABPA are composed of degenerating eosinophils intermixed with the hyphae of the fungus. The proximal bronchi are dilated, producing saccular bronchiectasis, but the distal bronchi are normal.

D. Prevalence

Fungi of the genus *Aspergillus* are uniquely ubiquitous in the environment, and their reproductive spores are airborne and widely distributed (Bunnag et al., 1982; Lim et al., 1983). It is noteworthy that the incidence of skin reaction to *Aspergillus* in asthmatic patients in Singapore was rather low compared to findings in temperate countries (Lim et al., 1983). Their finding has been correlated with the negligible incidence of ABPA in this part of the world (Lam, 1989).

E. Clinical Features

The patient may have dyspnea, pleuritic chest pain, fever, and typically coughs up tenacious plugs of brown mucus during attacks. Acute asthma does not always accompany these episodes. Repeated attacks can lead to a characteristic proximal bronchiectasis.

F. Diagnosis

In Western countries, when asthma is associated with transient lung infiltrates and eosinophilia of greater than 1,000 cells/mm^3, it is likely that the cause is a fungus, but in Southeast Asian countries such pictures are usually seen in cases with parasitic migration. Since a large number of asthmatic patients without ABPA have roentgenographic abnormalities, a positive immediate skin test reaction, and serum precipitins to AF antigen, the sensitive and specific means of differentiating ABPA from asthma is the demonstration of high levels of specific IgE by radioallergosorbent tests (RAST), radioimmunoassay (RIA), or enzyme immunoassay (EIA) techniques.

G. Treatment

Corticosteroid administration hastens recovery from acute exacerbation and may prevent permanent residual damage.

IV. Insect Allergy

In tropical countries, various kinds of insects are prevalent, some of which cause annoying skin lesions among residents; however, from time to time,

Table 3 Some Severe Allergic Airway Reactions to Insects and Mites

Families/species	Clinical manifestations
Hymenoptera: bees, wasps, yellow-jackets, hornets, fire ants	Anaphylaxis, asthma
Mites: House-dust mites, storage mites	Asthma
Others: Cockroaches, crickets, locusts	Asthma

rarely dangerous and even fatal reactions occur (Schenken et al., 1953; Tuchinda, 1976). Table 3 lists common clinical allergic disorders induced by insects and mites.

Some workers in insect-breeding operations can develop occupational asthma from allergens inhaled from insects (especially crickets, locusts, and cockroaches). Hypersensitivity to bee sting is caused by a protein antigen that is part of the stinger mechanism of the bee. Usually a person must be stung at least once previously before allergic reactions occur. Cross-sensitization can exist between protein antigens of the bee, wasp, and ant.

A. Anaphylaxis

The severity of the allergic manifestations depends on the degree of hypersensitivity, and death may occur as a result of anaphylactic shock. Respiratory difficulties with bronchial spasm or laryngeal edema occur: the shorter the time interval between the sting(s) and the onset of symptoms, the more severe the reactions. In fatal cases symptoms of cyanosis, shock, and respiratory difficulty usually last for about 30 min. Autopsy usually reveals laryngeal edema with obstruction, acute pulmonary emphysema, and acute pulmonary and cerebral edema.

The mechanism of anaphylaxis production is IgE-mediated immediate hypersensitivity in most, but not all, instances. The majority of patients have positive skin-test reactions to venom, and venom-specific IgE antibodies are detected. However, in a minority of patients the result of these tests is negative and there is no evidence of IgE involvement. The reaction may be provoked by the direct effect of some venom constituents on mast cells or possibly by the histamine content of the venom itself, the level of which may rise following multiple stings.

B. Diagnosis

The patient's history is most important to the diagnosis. Tests to demonstrate IgE-mediated sensitivity and to identify the insect's species are skin tests and RAST assay or related enzyme-linked immunosorbent assay (ELISA). Correlations between skin test and RAST results are good, but the latter has the advantage that patients need not be exposed to venom in vivo for the purpose of a skin test, thus preventing the skin test from enhancing the patient's sensitivity. RAST disks are available for different species of stinging insects.

C. Management

Active treatment of rapidly developing allergic manifestations may be lifesaving. Epinephrine (1:1000) should be given slowly in doses of 0.5 ml intravenously as often as necessary to prevent progression of the reaction. Oxygen should be given to combat anoxia. Tracheostomy may be useful in the event of obstruction from laryngeal edema, but difficulty may be encountered if associated bronchospasm and tenacious mucus are present. Fluids and corticosteroids are given intravenously to help counteract the shock.

D. Desensitization

A number of different regimens have been used to hyposensitize patients with venom. These range from a very slow increase in the venom dose over a 20 week period to rapid protocols, in which patients receive three or four doses each day until they reach a maximum dose of 100 μg within a few days. The rapid schedule is more convenient because it requires fewer injections; it also produces higher antivenin IgG levels. Patients who are able to tolerate 100 μg of venom are in effect clinically desensitized, since a single sting contains about 50 μg of venom. However, the higher the level of IgG antibodies, the safer the patient in case he or she is exposed to multiple stings.

V. Hypersensitivity Pneumonitis

Hypersensitivity pneumonitis, also known as extrinsic allergic alveolitis, refers to a group of immunological lung diseases that result from the inhalation of organic dusts by sensitized persons (Bernado et al., 1979).

A. Causes and Pathogenesis

Table 4 lists some of the occupational causes of hypersensitivity pneumonitis (Kazantzis, 1987). Common allergens are fungi, actinomycetes, and

Table 4 Occupational Causes of Hypersensitivity Pneumonitis

Condition	Source of allergen
Farmers' lung	Mouldy hay
Pigeon breeders' lung	Pigeon droppings
Bird fanciers' lung	Budgerigar droppings
Mushroom pickers' lung	Mushroom compost
Malt workers' lung	Mouldy barley/malt
Wheat weevil disease	Infested wheat flour
Cheese washers' lung	Mouldy cheese
Bagassosis	Mouldy bagasse
Suberosis	Mouldy cork dust
Maple bark strippers' lung	Mouldy maple-bark
Woodpulp workers' lung	Woodpulp
Sequoisis	Mouldy sawdust
New Guinea lung	Mouldy dust from thatched roof

Source: Modified from Occupational diseases by G. Kazantzis, 1987.

bacteria. Regardless of the antigens involved, the similarity of the symptoms and pathophysiology suggests that the pathogenesis is due to common mechanisms (Kurup, 1983).

B. Prevalence

Owing to the scarcity of documentation, it may be concluded that hypersensitivity pneumonitis is uncommon in Southeast Asian countries. Cases of bagassosis, resulting from the inhalation of thermophilic actinomycetes (*Thermoactinomyces sacchari, I. candidus, T. vulgaris*) growing in moldy bagasse, were reported in Thailand during the period 1973-1974 (Boonpucknavig et al., 1973; Kamtorn et al., 1974), but there have been no further publications since then.

C. Clinical Features

Acute Form

Following a sensitizing period of exposure that may vary from weeks to years, the patient experiences repeated episodes of an influenza-like illness accompanied by cough and undue breathlessness 3-9 h after inhalation of the relevant antigen, and the symptoms may persist for up to 24 h. Most subjects recover from each acute exacerbation. However, repeated acute exacerbations will eventually be associated with permanent impairment of lung function.

Respiratory distress at rest with fever and gravity-dependent crackles are the major physical signs; chest roentgenograms show a diffuse alveolar filling pattern.

Chronic Form

There is a slowly increasing loss of exercise tolerance due to shortness of breath, but no systemic upset occurs apart from an occasional prominent loss of weight. This is the result of diffuse pulmonary fibrosis that has been progressing for sometime before the patient seeks advice. Eventually, hypoxia and pulmonary hypertension and right-sided heart failure may supervene.

D. Diagnosis

Establishing a diagnosis of hypersensitivity pneumonitis is made based on occupational and medical histories, clinical findings, chest roentgenograms, and respiratory function tests, which show a fall in transfer factor and possibly a restrictive defect, and on the presence of precipitating antibody.

E. Management

Ideally, the patient must change completely the relevant environment, but this is often impossible. Management, therefore, should be aimed at reducing to a minimum further exposure to the offending agent. Modifications must always be made in the environment to lessen the level of exposure and minimize the risk it poses to other.

VI. Conclusion

Pulmonary allergic disorders are the result of hypersensitive or pathological immunological reactions to environmental factors or substances. With an increase in awareness, knowledge, and understanding of the immune system and, specifically, of IgE-mediated reactions, more cases of previously rare or unknown diseases are now being recognized and managed properly. At this point, the authors conclude that among the varieties of pulmonary allergic disorders worldwide, only bronchial asthma is relatively prevalent in the Southeast Asian region; other illnesses pertaining to respiratory allergy are not problems in this part of the world.

References

Belin, L. (1983). *Occupational Asthma*. Sandoz Pub., Asthma series 8. Basle, Sandoz Ltd., pp. 3-11.

Bernardo, J., Hunninghake, G. W., Gadek, J. E., Ferrans, V. J., and Crystal, R. G. (1979). Acute hypersensitivity pneumonitis: serial changes in lung lymphocyte subpopulations after exposure to antigen. *Am. Rev. Respir. Dis.* **120**:985-994.

Boonpucknavig, V., Bhamarapravati, N., Kamtorn, P., and Sukumalchandra, Y. (1973). Bagassosis: a histopathologic study of pulmonary biopsies from six cases. *Am. J. Clin. Pathol.* **59**:461-472.

Bunnag, C., Dhorranintra, B., and Plangpatananichya, A. (1982). A comparative study of the incidence of indoor and outdoor mold spores in Bangkok, Thailand. *Ann. Allergy* **48**:333-339.

Cau-Lim, F., Payawal, P., and Laserna, G. (1978). Studies on atmospheric pollens in the Philippines. *Ann. Allergy* **40**:117-123.

Chan-Yeung, M. (1988). Occupational asthma update. *Chest* **93**:407-411.

Choovivathanavanich, P., Suwanprateep, P., and Kanthavichitra, N. (1971a). House-dust mite and house dust. *Siriraj Hosp. Gaz.* **23**:931-936.

Choovivathanavanich, P., Oshima, S., Miyamoto, T., Kanthanvichitra, N., and Suwanprateep, P. (1971b). Mite sensitivity studies on *Dermatophagoides farinae* an house-dust allergy in Thai subjects. *J. Med. Assoc. Thai.* **54**:826-835.

de Guia, T. S. (1988). Bronchial asthma in the Philippines. Proceedings, 1st Congress Asian Pacific Society of Respirology, Tokyo, Japan, pp. 86-88.

Frankland, A. W. (1953). Locust sensitivity. *Ann. Allergy* **11**:445-453.

Greenberger, P. A. (1988). Allergic bronchopulmonary aspergillosis and fungosis. *Clin. Chest Med.* **9**:599-608.

Hogg, J. C., James, A. L., and Pare, P. D. (1988). Pathology of bronchial asthma. Proceedings, 1st Congress Asian Pacific Society of Respirology, Tokyo, Japan, pp. 76-81.

Hsieh, K. H. (1984). A study of intracutaneous skin tests and radioallergosorbent tests on 1000 asthmatic children in Taiwan. *Asian Pac. J. Allergy Immunol.* **2**:56-60.

Hsieh, K. H., and Shen, J. J. (1988). Prevalence of childhood asthma in Taipei, Taiwan, and other Asian Pacific countries. *J. Asthma* **25**:73-82.

Jones, D. H., May, A. G., and Condemi, J. J. (1984). HLA DR typing of aspirin-sensitive asthmatics. *Ann. Allergy* **52**:87-89.

Kamtorn, P., Charoenpan, P., Sukumalchantra, Y., Boonpucknavig, V., Kitiyakara, K., Suchato, C., and Nuchprayoon, C. (1974). Bagassosis: a report of 8 cases. *J. Med. Assoc. Thai.* **57**:468-474.

Kazantzis, G. (1987). Occupational diseases. In: Weatherall, D. J., Ledingham, J. G. G., and Warrell, D. A., eds. *Oxford Textbook of Medicine*, 2nd Ed. Oxford, Oxford University Press, pp. 143-161.

Kurup, V. P. (1983). Farmer's lung and related hypersensitivity pneumonitides. *Indian J. Chest Dis. Allergy Sci.* **26**:242-255.

Lam, W. K. (1989). Hong Kong, personal communication.

Lim, T. K., Chan, T. B., Tan, W. C., and Teoh, P. C. (1983). The prevalence of skin sensitization to *Apergillus* antigens among asthmatic patients in Singapore. *Asian Pac. J. Allergy Immunol.* **1**:123-124.

Longo, G., Strinati, R., Poli, F., and Fumi, F. (1987). Genetic factors in non-specific bronchial hyperreactivity. *Am. J. Dis. Child.* **141**:331-4.

Mangunnegoro, H., and Manuhutu, E. J. (1988). The problem of asthma in Indonesia. Proceedings, 1st Congress Asian Pacific Society of Respirology, Tokyo, Japan, pp. 89-93.

Miyamoto, T., Okudaira, H., and Ohta, K. (1988). Issues in immunology. Proceedings, 1st Congress Asian Pacific Society of Respirology, Tokyo, Japan, pp. 67-70.

Mullarkey, M. D., Thomas, P. S., Hansen, J. A., Webb, D. R., and Nisperos, B. (1986). Association of aspirin-sensitive asthma with HLA-DQw. *Am. Rev. Respir. Dis.* **133**:261-263.

Reed, C. E. (1988). Basic mechanisms of asthma; role of inflammation. *Chest* **94**:175-190.

Riley, A. J. (1989). Asthma, allergy and sex. *Asian Med. News* 25 April, p. 14.

Schenken, J. R., Tamisiea, J., and Winter, F. D. (1953). Hypersensitivity to bee sting. Report of fatal case and review of literature. *Am. J. Clin. Pathol.* **23**:1216-1221.

So, S. Y., Lam, W. K., and Yu, D. (1981). Colophony-induced asthma in a poultry vender. *Clin. Allergy* **11**:395-399.

Tan, W. C. (1988). Bronchial asthma in Singapore—prevalence and diagnostic patterns. Proceedings, 1st Congress Asian Pacific Society of Respirology, Tokyo, Japan, pp. 95-98.

Tharavanij, S. (1971). Allergic diseases of the respiratory system. *Siriraj Hosp. Gaz.* **23**:741-780.

Thomas, V., Tan, B. H. A., and Rajapaksa, A. C. P. (1978). House dust allergy in West Malaysia. *Ann. Allergy* **40**:114-116.

Tuchinda, M. (1976). Insect allergy. *Siriraj Hosp. Gaz.* **28**:1876-1879.

Tuchinda, M. (1978). Prevalence of allergic diseases in Mahidol University students. *Siriraj Hosp. Gaz.* **30**:1285-1298.

Tuchinda, M. (1983). Allergic disorders in Southeast Asia: viewpoint from Thailand. *Med. Prog.* Special Issue, pp. 7-14.

Tuchinda, M., Theptaranon, Y., and Limsartayourat, N. (1983). A 10 year surveillance of atmospheric pollens and moulds in the Bangkok area. *Asian Pac. J. Allergy Immunol.* **1**:7-9.

Tuchinda, M., Habananda, S., Vareenil, J., Srimaruta, N., and Piromrat, K. (1987). Asthma in Thai children: a study of 2000 cases. *Ann. Allergy* **59**:207-211.

Wongsathuaythong, S., and Lakshana, P. (1972). House-dust mite survey in Bangkok and other provinces in Thailand. *J. Med. Assoc. Thai.* **55**: 272-286.

Woolcock, A. J., Dowse, G. K., Temple, K., Stanley, H., and Turner, K. J. (1983). The prevalence of asthma in the South-Fore people of Papua New Guinea. A method for field studies of bronchial reactivity. *Eur. J. Respir. Dis.* **64**:571-581.

Zeitz, H. J. (1988). Bronchial asthma, nasal polyps, and aspirin sensitivity: Samter's syndrome. *Clin. Chest Med.* **9**: 567-576.

17

Chronic Obstructive Pulmonary Disease
An Indian Perspective

SUDHAKAR R. KAMAT

K.E.M. Hospital
Bombay, India

Along with its rapid industrialization, India is developing a modern medical system capable of diagnosing and treating common and uncommon disease. Epidemiological data on the prevalence of chronic disease are becoming precise and easily available. Diseases due to infection, poor nutrition, and lack of sanitation are declining, and chronic diseases related to environmental pollution, unhealthy dietary habits, smoking, allergies, stress, and other factors are gaining ground.

India has wide climatic variations. It is believed that chronic obstructive lung disease (COPD) is more common in northern India because of the long cold winters, small houses, and high levels of indoor pollution due to cooking or heating stoves. The widespread tobacco smoking habit in the Himalayan belt aggravates the situation for both sexes. The population studies from Nepal, a region similar to northern mountainous India, (Pandey, 1984; Pandey et al., 1988) showed a COPD prevalence of 11.2% in mountainous cities, 11.9% in villages on the plains, 17.6% in hills, and 30.9% in mountainous villages. The disease was more common in women; tobacco smoking and indoor pollution were thought to have synergistically contributed to the disease. Furthermore, the period spent near the fireplace increased the clinical

Table 1 Prevalences of Chronic Bronchitis

					Prevalence (%)		
Site	Yr.	Source	Population	No.	Male	Female	Total
Delhi	1964	Wig, 1973	Campus	656	7	5	6
Delhi	1964	Malik, 1986	Campus	2366	1.2	0.6	1.0
U.P. city	1966	Malik, 1986	Cotton workers	900	11	-	11
Punjab town	1975	Joshi et al., 1975	Cycle workers	473	12.5	-	12.5
Dehli	1976		Residents	993	8	4.3	6.3
Bihar city	1966		Residents	14910	2.1	1.3	1.7
Madras city	1977		Residents	817	1.4	2.7	1.6
Orissa village	1988	Behera and Malik, 1988a	Residents	105	-	2.9	-
Himachal: town/village	1984	Malik, 1986	Adults	446	21.7	8.5	20.8
Rajasthan village	1974		Old (60 +)	10325	85.9	50	70
M.P. city	1982		Residents	1424	8.1	4.5	6.5

Bombay	1981	Kamat et al., 1981a	Cotton workers		20	-	-
M.P. city	1980		Residents		16.5		
U.P. village	1975	Bhattacharya et al., 1975	Adult residents	1140	6.7	4.5	5.7
Punjab: city	1986	Malik, 1986	Adults	1006			-
			Male NSM/SM	444	0.9/9.9		
			Female	1366		1.6	
Village			Adults	1569	4.1/10.4	5.0	
City			Hospital families	3046	5.2/20	4.1	
City			Teachers	743	0.6/8.2	1.2	-
Nepal: hill village	1984	Pandey, 1984	Adult residents	2826	17.6	18.9	18.3
City	1984	Pandey, 1984	Adult residents	576	11.2	11.4	11.3
Plains village	1984	Pandey et al., 1988	Adult residents	652	11.9	14.3	13.1
Mountainous village	1984	Pandey et al., 1988	Adult residents	641	33.9	28.3	30.9
U.P.	1986	Gupta and Gupta, 1986	Cotton workers	330	43.7	-	43.7
Bombay: city	1980	Kamat et al., 1984b		4129	-	-	4.5
Village							5.0

morbidity, which was significantly higher in both smokers and exsmokers. Most of the individuals with chest symptoms showed evidence of COPD; 1.0-1.5% had cor pulmonale.

Many workers have studied the incidence of COPD in India (Table 1). The early pioneers in the field were Wig (1973), Viswanathan (1964), and Malik (1986). Some studies consisted of hospital campus residents. Two such studies showed the prevalence rate ranging from 1 to 7%. The study in the general population revealed 1.7% prevalence in the northeast, 1.6% in the south, 6.3% in Delhi, and 20.8% in the mountainous north. In older subjects, prevalence rates were higher. Several recent population studies reveal a prevalence rate of 0.9-1.6% in nonsmokers and levels 2-10 times higher in smokers. In the 1980s in Bombay the prevalence of COPD was 4.5% in polluted areas, 2.3% in less polluted sites, and 5% in a nearby rural area (Kamat et al., 1984b). There is evidence of a much higher COPD distribution in industrial workers, 11-12.5% in the north, which increases to 20-43% in cotton workers (Kamat et al., 1981a). It is possible that the lower prevalence of COPD in southern states is partially due not only to semantic differences but also to a reduced need for heating fuel during the winter months. It appears that, in general, throughout most of India, the prevalence of COPD is 5-8%. It is slightly higher in mountainous areas in the north and among certain occupational groups.

I. Cor Pulmonale

If the prevalence of COPD can be judged precisely, the estimation of cor pulmonale can be fallacious. Table 2 summarizes the important published data. Depending on the source, the prevalences in indoor hospital population can be misleading. However, it seems that clinical prevalences in the medical patient population may reflect that in the general population. Thus, the former may include 2-3% of all cardiac admissions and the latter about 1.5%. It should be stressed, however, that this prevalence applies to the clinical stage of cor pulmonale (Kamat et al., 1971). The polycythemia seen in 50-60% of the patients is related to blood oxygen saturation (Agarwal et al., 1974a). Malnutrition and infection may dampen the response, with resulting hypochromia. Cor pulmonale can be diagnosed in early stages if multiple methods, including electrocardiography (ECG), radiographs, clinical examination, and hemodynamic monitoring, are used. Although, tall P waves are frequently seen in most of the ECG tracings, changes of right ventricular hypertrophy are present in only 20.8% of the patients. The clockwise rotation occurs in 70-75%; it may yield to ischemic changes seen in one-half of patients. Frequent ventricular arrhythmias are uncommon (Kamat et al., 1984a). These

Table 2 Cor Pulmonale: Prevalences in India

		Hospital Admissions (%)		
		Cardiac Ward	Medical Ward	Approx. Prevalence (%)
Bombay	1949-54[a]	9.3-21.8	0.6	—
	1958-62	5.2-6.0	—	—
	1965	13.0	—	—
Delhi	1958-64[a]	16.6-19.2	0.3-5.0	1.2
	1969	15.1-26.3	0.7	2.1
Punjab	1951-61[a]	1.0-10.8	—	2.2
U.P.	1958-63[a]	15.8-19.0	1.5	—
Himachal	1956	4.0	0.4	—
M.P.	1969	19-24.5	4.5	3.1
Rajasthan	1960[a]	18.0	—	3.1
M.P.	1967[a]	40.2	2.4	2.1
Bihar	1968	18.9	2.1	
Bengal	1966	4.8-16	—	4.1
Karnataka	1964-67	3.8-16.0	0.4-1.2	—
Nepal	1980-88[b,c]	—	—	1.0-1.5
Madras	1974	—	—	1.5

[a]Kamat et al., 1971.
[b]Pandey, 1984.
[c]Pandey et al., 1988.

patients may have shorter life expectancy with a lower basal lung function unless the precipitation of cor pulmonale is due to acute infective exacerbation. COPD is the cause of cor pulmonale in 40-80% of cases (Kamat et al., 1971).

Like COPD, the prevalence of cor pulmonale goes up after the age of 30 and the prognosis is not very good after age 60. It is higher in ex-smokers (due to people stopping smoking late in India). Poor people with a history of heavy smoking, impaired lung function, and severe grades of dyspnea and ECG changes tend to die sooner. Of the 258 patients reported from Bombay, 85.7% had both cough and dyspnea (Kamat et al., 1984a). Women experienced milder dyspnea, but developed cor pulmonale more often. Cor pulmonale developed in 31.8% of all patients. Those with severe dyspnea had a greater degree of expiratory obstruction. Those with moderate airway obstruction demonstrated a larger improvement in forced expiratory volume in 1s (FEV1) after bronchodilator treatment. Low FEV1 was associated with low PO_2 and high PCO_2 ($p<0.01$) (Kamat et al., 1984a). The relation of PO_2 to FEV1 was linear, while that for PCO_2 was curvilinear. The patients who were regularly evaluated and treated maintained a better functional and clinical status (Kamat et al., 1984a; Rupwate et al., 1989a).

II. Causative Factors

Although several studies lend strength to the concept that northern India has a higher prevalence of COPD and associated cor pulmonale, it appears now that the disease prevalence is not much lower in the rest of India. Tobacco smoking, indoor fuel, ambient air pollution, and occupational dust exposure are some of the reasons for such a high prevalence. Kamat has shown that in Bombay and other cities chronic obstructive lung disease and recurrent upper respiratory symptoms are closely correlated to fluctuations in daily ambient sulfur dioxide (SO_2), suspended particulate matter (SPM), and nitrogen dioxide (NO_2) levels (Kamat and Doshi, 1987). The relation to occupation, tobacco smoking, and undernutrition was obscure and that of fuel, housing, sanitation, age, and sex was of a small significance. The effect of fuel on COPD has been assessed as LPG 1.6%; paraffin 1.4%: paraffin mixed with coal 2.6%; and cow dung/wood 5.0% (Kishore et al., 1982) (Table 3).

The relationship of alpha-1 antitrypsin levels and COPD has also been investigated extensively (Table 4) (Vishwanathan et al., 1976; Malik et al., 1977; Kulpati et al., 1979; Parvez et al., 1979; Kishore et al., 1982; Tyagi et al., 1981; Kulkarni et al., 1982; Talib et al., 1982; Nath et al., 1986; Agarwal et al., 1974b; Bhambure et al., 1988; N.I.O.H., 1982). These may give the impression that in comparison to controls, COPD patients may show lower alpha-1 antitrypsin levels. There were higher alpha-1 antitrypsin values in patients with diabetes, but there was no relation to smoking, sex, changes in chest radiographs, lung function, or ECG. However the homozgous deficient subjects were more symptomatic. The family members of COPD also showed more abnormalities (Kishore et al., 1982). However fewer or no deficiencies were found in controls (Vishwanathan et al., 1976; Malik et al., 1977; Kulkarni et al., 1982; Nath et al., 1986; Bhambure et al., 1988). In the clinical presentation of COPD in India, alpha-1 antitrypsin deficiency does not seem to play a large role (Malik et al., 1977) and the measurement of alpha-1 antitrypsin does not seem to be a helpful diagnostic procedure (Bhambure et al., 1988).

Table 3 Assessment of Indoor Pollution (μg/m–) Due to Kitchen Fuel[a]

Type	No. Studied	SO_2	NO_2	SPM
LPG	22	201 ± 266	422 ± 375	943 ± 1371
Coal	15	1583 ± 2028[xx]	170 ± 1886	25795 ± 31637[xx]
Wood	22	164 ± 186	318 ± 458	15801 ± 18325[xx]
Wood + coal	10	86[xx] ± 50	75[xx] ± 42	5474[x] ± 5389
Wood + cow dung	22	269 ± 306	326 ± 486	18378 ± 15082
Cowdung	32	242 ± 275	144 ± 330	18256 ± 19417
Other (kerosene)	7	274 ± 197	249 ± 288	22435 ± 22491[x]

Cooking Fuel and Chronic Bronchitis[b]

Fuel Type	No. of Subjects	COPD (%)
LPG	388	1.6
Paraffin oil	542	1.3
Coal + paraffin	352	2.6
Cowdung + wood	898	5.0

SO_2, sulfur dioxide; NO_2, nitrogen dioxide; SPM, suspended particulate matter.
[a]N.I.O.H., 1982.
[b]Malik, 1986.

The role of cooking/heating fuel in generating significant indoor pollution has been studied by the National Institute of Occupational Health. Coal and kerosene produced high levels of suspended particulate matter (SPM) (followed by wood); coal produced high SO_2 levels (followed by cow dung). In Nepal, it was shown that burning of wood liberated 8800/μg SPM, 21 parts per million (PPM) CO, and 368 parts per billion (PPb) NO. The levels are lower when improved stoves were used (Pandey, 1984; Pandey et al., 1988). In experimental animals, cow dung produces bronchiolitis. In a study of 85 patients with COPD and respiratory failure, 30% showed abnormal sella turcica. This was related to a chronic rise in intracranial tension due to CO_2 retention. Several of these patients showed chronic renal glomerular changes (Gilhotra et al., 1986).

The clinical presentation of COPD in India is similar to that in Europe. Patients who lose weight get more breathless with an overinflated chest and

Table 4 Trends in Alpha-1 Antitrypsin Deficiency in COPD

		Material			COPD		
Site	Source	COPD	Control	Values C	% Heterozygous	% Homozygous	Remarks
Western India	Vishwanathan et al., 1976	33	43	All normal	18	12	
Punjab	Malik et al., 1977	70	60	All normal	11.4	2.8	Not important
Delhi	Kulpati et al., 1979	58	32	2.66 ± 80	22	34	Higher values in patients with diabetes
U.P.	Parvez et al., 1979	50	50	All normal mean 106 (5 ± 7.7)	4	24	95 ± 9 Similar
U.P.	Kishore et al., 1982	300	300	223.6 ± 30 2.7% abnormal (0.7% homozygous)	21.3	10	192.2 ± 79.5 More abnormalities in family
U.P.	Tyagi et al., 1981	100	50	238 ± 20 6% heterozygous	12	23	No relation to smoking, x-ray, ECG, or function. More symptomatic
Western India	Kulkarni et al., 1982	50		All normal	14	2	More in smokers
Western India	Talib et al., 1982	38	101	1% heterozygous	9	0	More symptomatic No difference by sex or function
U.P.	Nath et al., 1986	44	31	All normal	2.3	19.3	More dyspnea No other relation
U.P.	Agarwal et al., 1974[b]	29	35	3 Heterozygous	21	6	—
Western India	Bhambure et al., 1988	50	23	All normal	4	—	Not helpful

eventually exhibit low lung function. Only a small proportion of patients in India develop severe CO_2 retention. However, in the stage of acute infection and cardiac failure, about 30% present with CO_2 retention varying from 55 to 85 mmHg. In comparison, only 4% of asthmatics in acute status asthmaticus show a P_{CO_2} level higher than 45 mmHg.

III. Clinical Pattern

We analyzed 750 cases of obstructive airway disease (Table 5). Dyspnea was present in 68% of 22 patients with chronic nasal syndrome (N) paroxysmal dyspnea was present in 36%, intermittent dry cough in 46%, and productive cough in 22%. In contrast, of 266 patients with an asthmatic-type (A) history, 98% had paroxysmal dyspnea and 8% exertional dyspnea; 79% had some cough: dry (70%) or productive (9%). In 407 cases with chronic bronchitis

Table 5 Clinical and Functional Pattern in Obstructive Lung Disease

	Nasal	Asthma	Bronchitis	Emphysema	P
	22	236	407	55	
Age (%)					
15-24 years	14	37	16	4	
25-44 years	45	45	41	26	
45 + years	41	18	42	71	<0.001
Symptoms					
Paroxysmal dyspnea (%)	36	98	42	42	<0.001
Chronic cough + sputum	22	9	94	55	<0.001
Chest x-ray	47	24	54	57	
Parenchymal scars (%)					
Lung function					
Reduction Normal (%)	27	17	7	4	
Obstruction reversible (%)	46	37	19	7	
Partially reversible (%)	18	30	37	38	
Mixed (%)	0	7	28	49	Significant ridit trend
FVC/predicted (%)	74.4	71.3	65.6	59.4	
FEV_1/FVC%	72.4	62.6	56.3	48.1	
Bronchodilator improvement % (FEV_1)	23.0	34.2	22.5	25.9	

(B) only 2% did not have dyspnea (exertional in 76% and paroxysmal in 42%) and all had some cough (mostly dry in 6%). In 55 cases with emphysema (E) on exertion dyspnea was predominant in 85%; 42% had paroxysmal dyspnea, 24% had no chronic cough. Blood eosinophilia was not a significant feature. A history of seasonal exacerbation was elicited in 25%. A history of chest problems in childhood was present more often (20%) in the asthmatic group than the other three categories (7%:$p<0.05$). The latter three groups were also made up of more older people. Forty-four percent of patients gave a history of frequent (eight or more per year) colds, with insignificant intergroup differences. The incidence of finger clubbing varied from 1% (A) to 9% (B) and 11% (E), which were significant differences; and a clinically deformed chest cage was seen in 7, 10, and 20% of cases, respectively, ($p<0.05$). Hemoptysis occurred in 3% in A and 12% in B and E categories; clinical cyanosis was seen in 1 and 4% cases, respectively. Only 2% patients had a hemoglobin concentration below 11 g/100 ml and in 44% the erythrocyte sedimentation rate (ESR) was above 20 mm. In 44% of chest radiographs there were nonspecific parenchymal scars; these occurred more often in group E (57%) than group A (24%). The common radiographic changes were overinflation (46%) and pulmonary hypertension (28%). These were seen somewhat more frequently in the B and E groups ($p<0.05$).

Asthmatics showed positive cutaneous reactivity to various agents more often than bronchitics; and also an increased reactivity to the graded histamine aerosol test.

IV. Functional Impairment

Of our patients in the nasal group 27% had normal lung function and 64% showed some airway obstruction. In group A, 17% had normal lung function, 37% had reversible obstruction, and 30% showed partially reversible obstruction. In group B, obstruction was seen in 56% (reversible in 19%), while there was a mixed picture in 28%. In group E, 45% showed obstruction (reversible in 7%) and 49% showed a mixed picture. Thus there was a continuous trend of increasing functional disability in four groups with a higher tendency for a mixed functional change. If bronchodilator-treatment-related improvement in FEV_1 is compared, it is only insignificantly higher in the A group of patients.

A detailed study of 85 COPD patients over 5-10 years (Table 6) showed that 9 died, 26 were lost to follow-up, and 50 were regularly treated (Kamat et al., 1984a). Of the total, only 23 (27%) men were smokers. Congestive cardiac failure was present in 22% of regularly treated patients as opposed to 45% in other patients ($p<0.05$). The spirometric function declined minimally

Table 6 COPD Patterns on Follow Up

Smokers: 23 (27%)

	Regular treatment	Default/Death
No.	50	31
CCF%	22	45
Decline/yr(ml)		
FEV_1	− 9.3	− 26
FVC	+ 0.7	− 1.2

Pattern of decline (113) in asthma, bronchitis, & emphysema

	A (44)	B (49)	E (20)	Difference
Initial FEV_1 (L)	1.73 ± 0.56	1.18 ± 0.40	0.68 ± 0.56	+ $p<0.01$
FEV_1 decline/yr	-46 ± 342	-21 ± 247	-23 ± 227	NS
Age and bronchoreversibility (%) (FEV_1)				
10-44	$31.6^{\bigcirc x}$	27.2	$20.2^{\bigcirc}$	○ $p<0.05$
45 +	21.2^{x}	27.0*	15.5*	x $p<0.05$
				* $p<0.05$
Decline ml/yr. Initial FEV_1 % of predicted				
<40	+ 387	− 63	− 36	
40-65	− 7	+ 93	+ 51	
>65	− 114	− 116	—	

in this group. We analyzed for annual spirometric decline in 113 patients classified as having asthma (44), bronchitis (49), and emphysema (20). The initial mean FEV_1 was significantly different in these three groups ($p<0.05$), but the declines in FEV_1 or forced vital capacity (FVC) (due to large scatter) were not statistically different. When bronchoreversibility (FEV_1) was related to age, it was higher in young group A patients, but smaller in group E patients at all ages. In the B group it was intermediate at all ages. When yearly declines in FEV_1 were related to initial FEV_1 (percentage of predicted), it was seen that mean declines were large in those with higher FEV_1 values.

The bronchoreversibility and the annual decline in a selected group of asthmatic (25) and COPD (23) patients evaluated over 10 years were compared (Table 7). The mean ages, FVC, and bronchoreversibility were similar, but FEV_1 and FEV_1/FVC% were significantly higher in group A. The annual decline in both groups by sexes were similar. In the patients with COPD,

Table 7 Clinical and Functional Patterns in Selected Matched Pairs of Patients with Bronchial Asthma and COPD with Long Followup

	A (25)	B (23)	
Males (No)	11	18	
Mean age (yr)	42.8	47.5	
Initial FEV_1 (L)	1.79^+	1.39^+	$P<0.05$
FVC (L)	2.15	2.13	NS
FEV_1/FVC (%)	83.7	66.6	$P<0.01$
Bronchoreversibility (FEV_1, %)	33.4	32.2	NS

	M	F	M	F
Annual decline by gender (ml/yr) FEV_1	90.8	90.4	101	109 NS
FVC	144	136	238	179 NS
COPD	—		Sm (13)	NSm (12)
Smoking Initial FEV_1			1.36	1.42
Decline/yr			96	110
Initial FVC			2.22	2.04
Decline/yr.			234	219
Bronchoreversibility (%)			22.8	42.4
CCF COPD			Present (9)	Absent (14)
Initial FEV_1 (L)	—		1.19	1.52
Decline/yr (ml)			68	125
Bronchoreversibility (%)			36	29

	A	B	
ECG changes (no)			
Normal	22	11	
Ischemia	1	2	
RV/RA change	2	12+	+ $p<0.02$

	A	B	
FEV_1 < 1500 ml	77	86	
1500 ml Decline/yr.	98	134	NS

Asthma				
Pearson's coefficient Decline/yr.	FEV_1	FVC	Initial FEV_1	
Initial FVC	0.07	0.11	—	
Initial FEV_1	0.20	—	—	
Bronchoreversibility	0.34	0.28	0.21	
	COPD			
Initial FVC	0.21	0.65+	—	
Initial FEV_1	0.38	— —	—	
Bronchoreversibility (%)	0.42^x	0.06	0.28	x $P<0.05$ + $P<0.001$

while nonsmokers had a larger bronchoreversibility there were no other differences from smokers. In those without cor pulmonale, FEV_1 was higher, but in both categories declines were insignificantly different. To correlate bronchoreversibility and annual declines (FEV_1 and FVC), multifactorial analyses were performed. These indicated that in asthmatics only bronchoreversibility showed a slight relation to the declines. In the patients with COPD, the decline in FVC was related to the initial FVC ($p<0.01$) and, to a lesser degree, the decline in FEV_1 was related to the initial FEV_1. However, the bronchoreversibility was again closely correlated with the decline in FEV_1.

In most of our patients with COPD, blood gas values are normal. Bronchoreversibility differs in three categories of obstructive airways disease (Pande et al., 1970). When COPD progresses, FVC and FEV_1 decline concomitantly with DCO (Jain et al., 1972; Guleria et al., 1969).

V. Physiological Mechanisms in COPD

These have been studied extensively at our institute. Diurnal variations were studied in normals (10) and patients with asthma (20) and COPD (20) for 2 days over 16 h daily and over 3 mornings every week (Patil et al., 1989). The normal controls display a variation of up to 1.6% (51 ml) for FVC, 1.5% (51 ml) for FEV_1, and 34 L (3.4%) for PEF (Peak expiratory flow). The values for patients with asthma were 25% for FVC, 39% for FEV_1, 43% for PEF, and 65% for MEFR (Mid expiratory flow rate) 0.25-0.75%. For patients with bronchitis, these variations were 22, 33, 29, and 52% respectively. Similar trends were observed for the weekly variations in which the asthmatic patients showed 15-39% variations and bronchitis a variation from 15 to 23%. Thus this may be a good way of differentiating among these three categories.

When graded histamine aerosol sensitivity was tested in 15 normals, and patients with asthma (52) and chronic bronchitis (107), it was found that mean PC_{20} FEV_1 was 8.2 ± 1.5, 0.4 ± 0.5, and 0.65 ± 0.85 mg/ml, respectively (Rupwate et al., 1990a). There was a significant tendency for higher reactivity in those with lower FEV_1 ($p<0.05$) and greater obstruction (as indicated by FEV_1/FVC%). There were no significant differences in the two patient groups, but percentage PC_{20} may be affected by low FEV_1 in bronchitic patients. There was no significant relation to bronchoreversibility, but the asthmatic group showed a significantly greater ($p<0.05$) prevalence of cutaneous atopy (67.3% A vs. 21.6% B).

When looking at allergic markers in clinically diagnosed (as per Ciba Symposium criteria) patients with asthma (25) and bronchitis (16), asthmatics were younger, often nonsmokers, and had higher FEV_1 and greater bronchoreversibility ($p<0.05$) (Rupwate et al., 1990b). For sputum eosinophilia (2.12

$\pm$ 1.8 and 0.8 $\pm$ 1.0), serum IgE (852 $\pm$ 467 and 379 $\pm$ 237), and cutaneous allergy (4.9 $\pm$ 2.5 and 0.9 $\pm$ 0.9), the former had significantly higher scores ($p<0.05$).

In study of 125 patients with stable COPD, PO_2 was related ($r = 0.43$) to FEV_1 but PCO_2 was poorly related ($r = 0.23$) (Rupwate et al., 1989a). Both PO_2 and PCO_2 showed a good interrelationship ($r = 0.70$). There was no relation to residual volume/total lung capacity percent (RV/TLC%), FEV_1/FVC%, or pH. If FEV_1 is above 1.25 L, blood gases are likely to be in the normal range. Only below FEV_1 levels of 750 ml will PCO_2 start rising. Thus, FEV_1 may be a useful test for assessing progression of COPD and development of respiratory failure.

In a study of responses to graded hypoxia and hypercapnia by inhalation in normals (10) and patients with COPD (11), differences in response were detected (Shah et al., 1988). In normals, the reaction to hypoxia was curvilinear, to hypercapnia it was linear. In nine patients with COPD, the response was smaller but similar to that of normals. In 2 patients with COPD, smaller but linear responses were noted. These results may indicate the mechanism by which some patients show a greater propensity to develop respiratory failure.

We have already shown that 3 weeks of oxygen therapy in stable COPD patients with chronic respiratory failure did not result in spirometric functional improvement (Taskar et al., 1990). However, right descending posteroanterior diameter and cardiothoracic ratio decreased ($p<0.05$) along with the height of the P wave in the ECG. There were significant serial improvements in basal PO_2 and PCO_2 levels after 3 weeks of oxygen therapy (2-3 L/min), along with a reduction in PA pressure ($p<0.01$). The initial and 3 week PO_2 level correlated significantly with right descending PA diameter and to the P wave height on ECG. The change in PO_2 levels also correlated with PVR.

VI. Pathological Findings

Whether COPD results in different pathological changes in India has been investigated (Singh et al., 1980; Kinare et al., 1981). In Delhi, contrilobular emphysema was more common (often in upper zones); in Bombay it was seen only in 19.6% patients. Panacinar emphysema was observed in 65.7% in Bombay. In Delhi, data on necropsy material (100 cases) showed the highest prevalence of emphysema in patients aged 51-60 years (Fig. 1). However, most of the patients had only mild changes; in 9% of necropsies there were advanced changes of emphysema (Singh et al., 1980). In Bombay, the prevalence in 163 autopsies was similar in both sexes and advanced changes were rare (Kinare et al., 1981). A total of 70.8% (in Delhi, 39%) showed emphysema. In a detailed study of three lung autopsies in cotton mill workers (Kamat et al., 1981a) with byssinosis, history of severe (grade IV-V) dyspnea and productive cough, and chronic respiratory failure with recurrent infective exacerbations, anthracotic deposits and severe focal emphysema with bullae were seen (Fig. 2). There were extensive bronchiolar dilatations without peribronchial fibrosis (Fig. 3). There was panacinar emphysema in two cases with mucus gland hyperplasia. These data may indicate that although the type of emphysematous changes is similar to those seen in western countries, the prevalence in an industrial city like Bombay is higher, and in an occupational lung disease (byssinosis) there seem to be the additional changes of bronchial dilatation.

Although the bronchial mucosa is similar in patients with asthma, bronchitis, and emphysema, asthmatic airways show a thickened basement membrane and eosinophilic infiltrates (Wig, 1973).

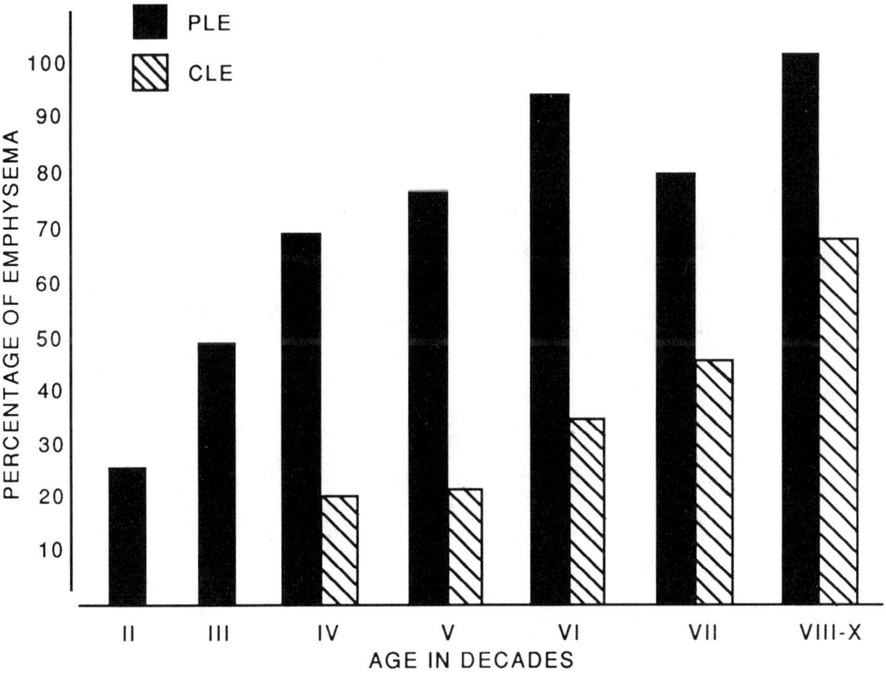

Figure 1 Bar diagram shows prevalence of panlobular (PLE) and centrilobular (CLE) emphysema in 10-year age groups from 11-20 (II) to 80+ (VIII). CLE appears only after age 30 and increases gradually, while the prevalence of PLE rises after 40 years and seems stable later.

VII. Dermal Changes

In patients with advanced emphysema, cutaneous thickness was measured in the interscapular area and dorsum of left hand. There were significantly lower values in these patients emphysema (8.5 and 1.91 mm vs. 11.7 and 2.24 mm in normals). The dermis was normal in all controls and in 21 patients. In 4 patients, loose collagen with thinner fibrils were seen. It has been shown elsewhere that these changes are due to wasting and weight loss associated with advanced lung disease. These changes occur in 33% of patients with COPD, 25% with bronchiectasis, 40% with chronic tuberculosis, and 89% with cor pulmonale (Saha and Damodaran, 1972).

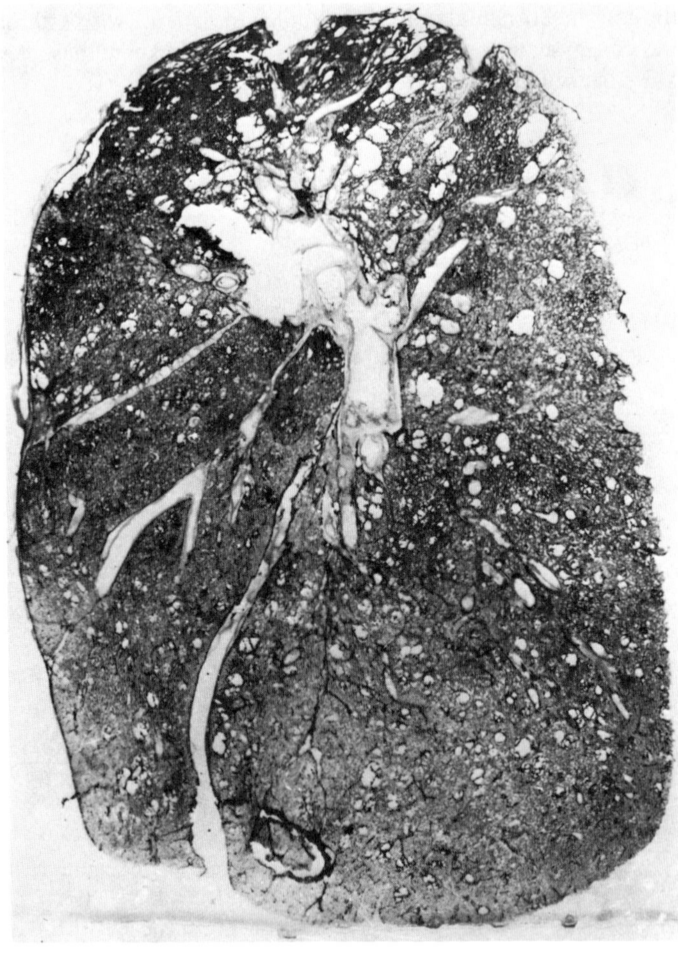

Figure 2 Full lung section shows asymmetrical distribution of panlobular emphysema with some anthracosis.

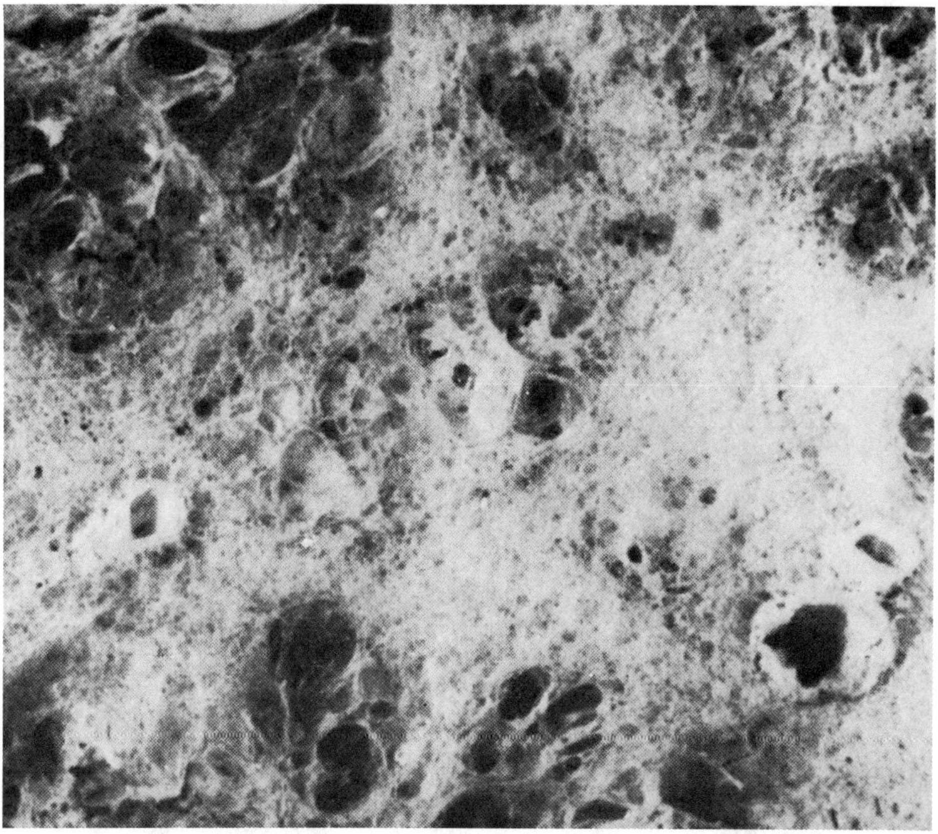

Figure 3 Photograph of inflated lung shows focal emphysema and dilated bronchioli.

VIII. Management

Over the last 20 years, there has been definite trend of change from the use of combination drugs, consisting of ephedrine, phenobarbitone, theophylline, and others, to oral beta stimulants and plain theophylline (Kamat et al., 1976; Sanghavi et al., 1988). Several workers have reported fewer side effects with the former and equally good results with the latter used alone. The role of steroids in COPD seems small, and uncommon except during acute bronchospastic crises. Administration of beta stimulants by gas flow-powered nebulizers has been shown to be superior to the use of metered-dose aerosols (Gupta et al., 1978). However, the latter mode is more convenient and safer than the use of oral beta stimulants (Behera and Malik, 1988b; Srivastava et al., 1973). In similar fashion, except for bromhexine (Misra et al., 1984), no other mucolytics have found common use. In India, the mainstay for treatment of

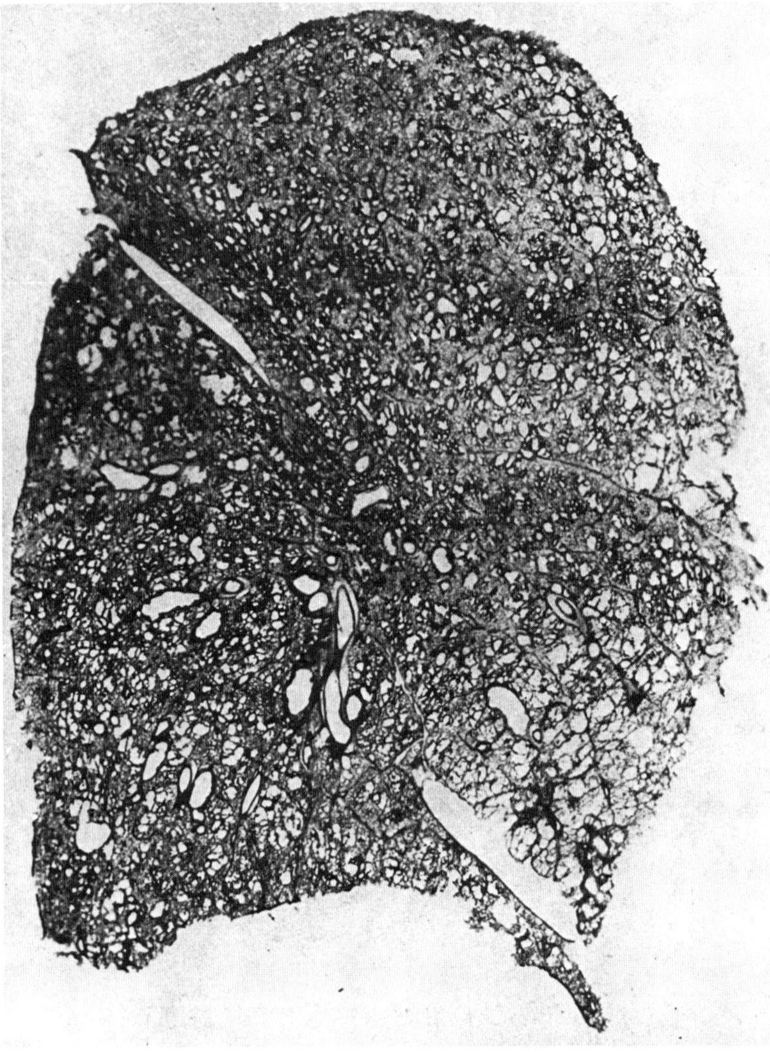

Figure 4 Full lung section shows gross generalized panlobular emphysema.

acute bronchospasm remains parenteral theophylline and beta stimulants except epinephrine. Perhaps the fear of arrhythmias has delayed the acceptance of beta stimulants in general management. The Indian data show that terbutaline is slightly superior and results in more prolonged benefit; otherwise, very little difference exists between various beta stimulants. Ipratropium

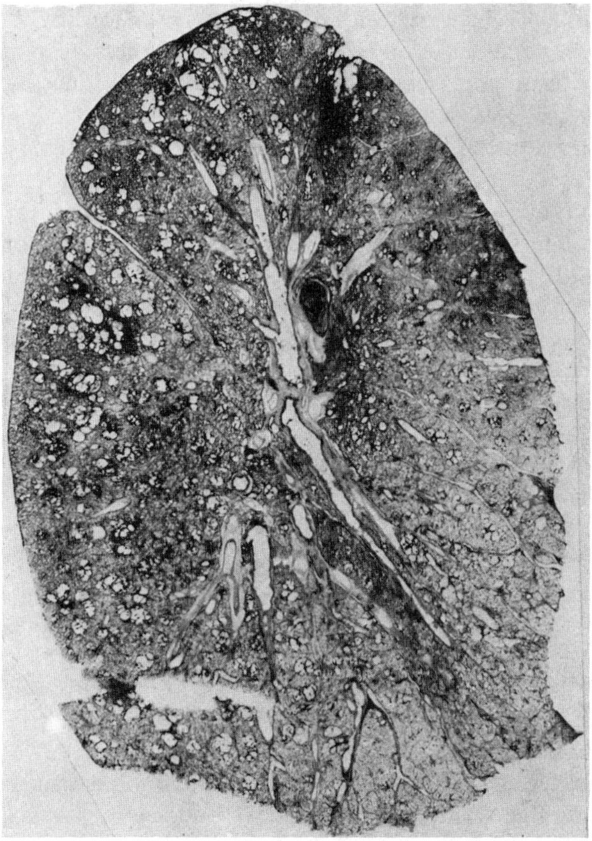

Figure 5 Full lung section shows centrilobular emphysema.

has not yet been introduced in India. Anhydrous sustained theophylline plays a major role.

In a recent study of various oral theophylline and standard bronchodilators (Rupwate et al., 1989b), anhydrous theophylline gave the best blood levels, with a peak between 1.7 and 2.0 h; aminophylline was the next most effective. The former gave the best improvement in area under the curve for FEV_1. There was no added benefit in giving ephedrine (30 mg), phenobarbitone (15 mg), or prednisolone (2.5 mg) over a period of 4-6 h.

In a study of 246 lower respiratory infections (34% with COPD), common pathogens isolated were staphylococci, streptococci, *Klebsiella,* and *Pseudomonas. H. influenzae* was also isolated but *Streptococcus* pneumoniae (3-4%) or anaerobes (6-8%) seem uncommon (Kamat et al., 1981b).

In a study of 85 patients with COPD, 41% were lost to follow-up (10% had died). The defaulting group has a shorter history, less frequent paroxysmal and milder exertional dyspnea, and a slower progress of disease. Those with higher initial FEV_1 showed a significant decline; those with lower FEV_1 initially did not show much decline. There were many fluctuations, particularly in female patients, but declines in FVC or FEV_1/FVC% were less clear. In 258 patients over 12 years over 31.8% developed cor pulmonale (23.1% in 5 years, 31.2% in 6-10 years, and 39.3% in those evaluated longer than 10 years). Usually this complication developed more often in female patients. In 38-41% of cases, parenchymal scars were seen radiographically. There was a greater evidence of expiratory obstruction with a higher grade of exertional dyspnea (Kamat et al., 1984a).

The role of chest physiotherapy, postural drainage, and breathing exercises is well understood in most major institutes. However, in addition, yoga-type exercises are used in several units. A comparison between the use of bronchodilator drugs, physiotherapy, or "Yogasana" in 3 groups of 75 patients (COPD) matched for FEV1/FVC% for 12 weeks has been reported (Kulpati and Kamath, 1982). Thus postural drainage, pursed lip, and segmental and diaphragm training (as physiotherapy) were compared with 11 types of yogic postures given for 30 min twice daily. With the latter usage, improvement in heart rate, respiratory rate, and well-being was significantly better. In another study of 30 asthmatics for 2-½ months, PEF and FVC improved significantly (but not FEV_1/FVC%) along with the symptoms and need for drugs over the control period (Murthy et al., 1984). In a similar study in bronchitis (26), as well as FEV_1 and FVC, flow rates and FEV_1/FVC% also showed a significant improvement. This change was associated with an increased O_2 uptake during exercise, increased breath-holding time, and creatine phosphokinase (CPK) levels; female patients showed a lesser improvement. In an earlier study of yoga used for 9 months in 11 patients with COPD matched with 11 controls, maximum work load increased by 60.6 kg/min but there was no improvement in function (Anil Kumar et al., 1985). There was also clinical improvement in dyspnea, exercise tolerance, and a quicker recovery. Thus, unlike chest physiotherapy and muscle training, which leads to better fitness, yoga may help to improve objective functional parameters at rest or during exercise.

IX. Summary

The clinical spectrum of chronic obstructive airway disease in India is similar to that observed in western countries. There are many differences between clinical and functional asthma and COPD; there are, however, also many areas where these two syndromes overlap. Thus while differentiation of asthma from chronic obstructive airway disease may serve a clinically useful purpose, in terms of progress, the disorders may behave similarly.

References

Agarwal, K. N., Gupta, G. D., and Khosla, K. (1974a). Blood volume and hematological studies in chronic cor pulmonale. *J. Assoc. Physicians India* **22**:377-380.

Agarwal, S. S., Tandon, V. K., and Farooqui, J. Z., and Misra, R. N. (1974b). Alpha-1 antitrypsin deficiency in pulmonary disease. *J. Assoc. Physicians India* **22**: 789-796.

Anil Kumar, K., Gnana, Kumari, K., Girija Kumari, D., Sahay, B. K., and Murthy, K. J. R. (1985). Immediate effects of Pranayama in airways obstruction. *Lung India* **3**:77-81.

Behera, D., and Malik, S. K. (1988a). Chronic respiratory disease and PEFR in rural Oriya females. *Lung India* **6**:127-128.

Behera, D., and Malik, S. K. (1988b). A comparative study of fenoterol and ipratropium bromide aerosols in Indian bronchial asthmatics. *Lung India* **6**:5-11.

Bhambure, N. M., Rupwate, R. U., Prabhakaran, L. C., Taskar, S. D., Potdar, P. V., and Kamat, S. R. (1988). Serum alpha-1 antitrypsin levels. *J. Assoc. Physicians India* **36**:742.

Bhattacharya, S. N., Bhatnagar, J. K., Kumar, S., and Jain, P. C. (1975). Chronic bronchitis in rural population. *Indian J. Chest Dis.* **17**:1-7.

Gilhotra, R., Malik, S. K., and Kataria, S. (1986). Radiological changes in sella turcica in COPD. *Lung India* **4**:119-122.

Guleria, J. S., Pande, J. N., and Gupta, R. G. (1969). Chronic obstructive lung disease in Northern India. *Am. Rev. Respir. Dis.* **100**:490-498.

Gupta, S., and Gupta, B. K. (1986). A study of byssinosis and associated respiratory disorders in cotton mill workers. *Indian J. Chest Dis.* **28**: 183-188.

Gupta, S., Poddar, S. P., and Nath, S. (1978). Aerosolized bronchodilator therapy with and without IPPR in bronchial asthma: a comparative evaluation. *Indian J. Chest Dis.* **20**:118-125.

Jain, B. P., Pande, J. N., and Guleria, J. S. (1972). Membrane diffusion capacity and pulmonary capillary blood volume in COPD. *Am. Rev. Respir. Dis.* **105**:900-907.

Joshi, R. C., Madan, R. N., and Brash, A. A. (1975). Prevalence of chronic bronchitis in an industrial population in North India. *Thorax* **30**:61-67.

Kamat, S. R., and Doshi, V. B. (1987). Sequential health study in relation to air pollution in Bombay, India. *Eur. J. Epidemiol.* **3**:265-277.

Kamat, S. R., Warrier, N. V. U., Panandikar, S. G., and Store, S. D. (1971). Cor pulmonale in India. *Cardiovasc. Rev.* p. 82-95.

Kamat, S. R., Panandikar, S. G., Purohit, S. D., Jagasia, R. S., and Kulkarni, S. T. (1976). Experiences with various preparations of ephedrine-theophylline combinations in COPD. *Indian J. Chest Dis.* **18**:25-35.

Kamat, S. R., Kamat, G. R., Salpekar, V. Y., and Lobo, E. (1981a). Distinguishing byssinosis from COPD: results of a prospective 5 year study of cotton mill workers in India. *Am. Rev. Respir. Dis.* **124**:31-40.

Kamat, S. R., Mehta, A. P., Doshi, V. B., Walimbe, S., Jayakar, V. V., and Mahashur, A. A. (1981b). A comparative study of various antibacterial drugs in lower respiratory tract infections and pneumoniae in adults. *J. Assoc. Physicians India* **31**:209-215.

Kamat, S. R., Doshi, V. B., Mahashur, A. A., et al. (1984a). Behavior on follow-up in COPD. *Lung India* **2**:76-83.

Kamat, S. R., Godkhindi, K. D., Shah, V. N., et al. (1984b). Prospective 3 year study of health morbidity in relation to air pollution in Bombay, India: methodology and early results up to 2 years. *Lung India* **2**:120.

Kinare, S. G., Dave, K. M., and Sheth, R. A. (1981). Incidence of emphysema in Bombay. *Indian J. Med. Res.* **74**:273-282.

Kishore, B., Agarwal, Y. B., Hazra, D. K., Pandey, D. N., and Kishore, N. (1982). Hereditary alpha-1 antitrypsin deficiency in cases of chronic obstructive disease. *J. Assoc. Physicians India* **30**:579-583.

Kulkarni, V. R., Pradhan, M. G., Bharaswadkar, M. S., and Sengupta, S. R. (1982). Alpha-1 antitrypsin deficiency in COPD. *J. Assoc. Physicians India* **30**:281-282.

Kulpati, D. D. S., and Kamath, R. K. (1982). The influence of physical conditioning by Yogasanas and breathing exercises in patients of COPD. *Lung India* **1**:35-38.

Kulpati, D. D., Batra, A. K., and Gupta, P. S. (1979). Interrelationship of COPD, diabetes mellitus and serum alpha-1 antitrypsin. *Indian J. Chest Dis.* **21**:24-30.

Malik, S. K. (1986). Profile of chronic bronchitis in North India: the P.G.I. experience 1972-85: *Lung India* **4**:89-100.

Malik, S. K., Khatri, G. K., and Sehgal, S. (1977). Alpha-1 antitrypsin deficiency in chronic lung disease. *Indian J. Chest Dis.* **19**:188-191.

Misra, M. P., Tiwari, U. C., Chaubal, C. C., and Gilhotra, R. (1984). Double blind cross-over randomized study of bromhexine in COPD. *J. Assoc. Physicians India* **32**:423-425.

Murthy, K. J. R., Sahay, B. K., Sitarama Jaju, P., et al. (1984). Effect of Pranayama (Rechaka, Puraka and Kumbhaka) on bronchial asthma: an open study. *Lung India* **2**:187-91.

Nath, J., Garg, R. K., Mehrotra, R., Mukerji, P. K., Prasad, R., and Nath, P. (1986). Alpha-1 antitrypsin in COPD. *Indian J. Chest Dis.* **28**:11-17.

National Institute of Occupational Health, Ahmedabad, India (1982). Domestic source of air pollution and its effect on respiratory system of housewives in Ahmedabad. Annual report, p. 32-42.

Pande, J. N., Jain, B. P., and Guleria, J. S. (1970). Reversibility of airway obstruction in chronic obstructive lung disease. *Am. Rev. Respir. Dis.* **101**:371-376.

Pandey, M. R. (1984). Prevalences of chronic bronchitis in a rural community of the hill region of Nepal. *Thorax* **39**:331-6.

Pandey, M. R., Basnyat, B., and Neupane, R. P. (1988). Chronic bronchitis and cor pulmonale in Nepal. Monograph, Mrigendra Medical Trust, Kathmandu, pp. 1-182.

Parvez, M., Sharda, D. P., Mittal, V. K., and Misra, S. N. (1979). A study of alpha-1 antitrypsin deficiency in pulmonary emphysema. *Indian J. Chest Dis.* **21**:134-139.

Patil, J. D., Rupwate, R. U., Kolhatkar, V. P., Potdar, P. V., and Kamat, S. R. (1989). Comparison of diurnal and circadian variations in normals, bronchial asthma and chronic bronchitis subjects. *Lung India* **7**:107-111.

Rupwate, R. U., Vaidya, P. R., Kolhatkar, V. P., and Kamat, S. R. (1989a). Intercorrelation of ventilatory tests and arterial blood gases in chronic bronchitis. *Lung India* **7**:23-25.

Rupwate, R. U., Kolhatkar, V. P., Parmar, D. M., Shah, S. V., Mahashur, A. A., and Kamat, S. R. (1990a). Significance of histamine sensitivity in normals and subjects with bronchial asthma and chronic bronchitis. *Lung India* **8**:15-18.

Rupwate, R. U., Potdar, P. V., and Kamat, S. R. (1990b). Comparison of allergic markers and airway hyperreactivity in bronchial asthma and chronic bronchitis. *Lung India* **8**:19-21.

Rupwate, R. U., Kolhatkar, V. P., Mahashur, A. A., Desai, N. K., Satoskar, R. S., and Kamat, S. R. (1989b). Clinical, physiological, and pharmacodynamic comparison with various theophylline preparations and combination bronchodilators. *Lung India* **7**:155-160.

Saha, N. C., and Damodaran, V. N. (1972). Dermal connective tissue in chronic respiratory disease. *Am. Rev. Respir. Dis.* **105**:118-120.

Sanghavi, N. G., Shah, J. J., Shah, C. R., and Batham, A. K. (1988). A clinical evaluation of a conventional bronchodilator combination against selective beta-adrenergic sympathomimetics. *Lung India* **6**:13-17.

Shah, S. V., Kolhatkar, V. P., Patel, M. H., and Kamat, S. R. (1988). A study of responses to graded hypoxia and hypercapnia in normal and obstructive pulmonary cases. *Lung India* **6**:91-95.

Singh, T., Chandra, K., and Kumar, B. (1980). A necropsy study of pulmonary emphysema in Delhi. *Indian J. Chest Dis.* **22**:230-235.

Srivastava, B. N., Shrivastava, V. K., Rao, V. S. C., Vyas, G. P., and Kochar, A. S. (1973). Beta-adrenergic stimulant aerosols in bronchial asthma. *Indian J. Chest Dis.* **15**:123-131.

Talib, S. H., Toshniwal, P. R., Deshpande, A. D., and Patil, S. D. (1982). Serum alpha-1 deficiency in COPD and normals. *J. Assoc. Physicians India* **30**:283-286.

Taskar, V. S., Rupwate, R. U., and Kamat, S. R. (1990). Effects of 3-week 02 therapy on clinical functional and hemodynamic parameter in COPD. *J. Assoc. Physicians India*

Tyagi, A. P., Mittal, H. S., Malhotra, T. N., Singh, V. S., Elhence, G. P., and Kumar, M. (1981). Serum alpha-1 antitrypsin in pulmonary emphysema. *J. Assoc. Physicians India* **29**:545-550.

Viswanathan, R. (1964). Chronic bronchitis-emphysema syndrome Incidence, aetiology and natural history. *Indian J. Chest Dis.* **6**:171-182.

Viswanathan, R., Sainani, G. S., and Mutalik, G. S. (1976). Alpha-1 antitrypsin deficiency and COPD. *Indian J. Chest Dis.* **18**:36-42.

Wig, K. L. (1973). Some aspects of chronic obstructive lung disease. *Indian J. Chest Dis.* **15**:331-348.

18

Pneumoconiosis in Developing Countries
Diagnosis and Management

YUTAKA HOSODA

Radiation Effects Research Foundation
Hiroshima, Japan

HISAO SHIDA

Rosai Hospital for Silicosis
Tochigi, Japan

YOHMEI HIRAGA

JR Sapporo Hospital
Sapporo, Japan

I. Introduction

Pneumoconioses are a group of pulmonary disorders caused by the accumulation of inhaled mineral or organic dusts. The term covers silicosis caused by free silica, asbestosis due to a silicate, asbestos, and berylliosis due to beryllium. Early in the 1900s, this disease was detected because of workers' complaints and it was graded according to a loss of work capacity. Almost all patients with pneumoconiosis at that time had tuberculosis and it was often difficult to differentiate pneumoconiosis from pulmonary tuberculosis.

In 1930, experts at an International Conference of Silicosis organized by the International Labour Office (ILO) recognized the importance of radiographic examination over worker's complaints in the classification of pneumoconiosis. Since 1950, the ILO International Classification of Radiographs of Pneumoconiosis (ICRP) has been widely used as the common scale for the diagnosis of pneumoconiosis. A recent study has revealed a higher prevalence of chronic bronchitis and pulmonary ventilatory abnormalities among workers with normal chest radiographs who had been occupationally exposed to dusts. These workers, if biopsied, might show "histopathological pneumoconiosis.'' However, clinical diagnosis is usually concerned with ''radiographic pneumoconiosis.'' These two should be clearly differentiated when pneumoconioses are discussed.

II. Radiographic Features of Pulmonary Parenchymal Changes

Note: The diagnostic scale of pneumoconioses is internationally based on the reading of a posteroanterior (PA) radiograph, although many other sophisticated means of diagnostic means are available. The 1980 ILO text did not mention these modern techniques, but the next version in preparation will probably refer to some of these techniques, as supplementary information. For readers' better understanding of the numerous small opacities distributed on a cross-section of the lung, computed tomographic scans (CT) are referred to in this section together with a PA radiograph constituted by the summation of abnormal opacities of the chest organs. In spite of CT's usefulness, CT is never recommended routinely because of the cost and radiation dose required. A PA radiograph will still be the basis of pneumoconiosis diagnosis.

The two-dimensional radiographic image on a PA radiograph is the summation of the pulmonary changes of the three-dimensional thorax. Consequently, the images do not mirror the histopathological changes. Pathological features of pneumoconiosis vary considerably with the nature of inhaled dusts. However, there are two principal types of pulmonary parenchyma changes. One is characterized by the formation of pneumoconiotic nodules; the other produces diffuse interstitial pulmonary fibrosis. The former is found in silica and coal miners' pneumoconiosis and the latter in asbestos pneumoconiosis. Small rounded opacities in free silica pneumoconiosis often coalesce to form a mass, or a large opacity. Hilar lymph nodes affected by silica are often enlarged and sometimes calcified, even when no small rounded opacities are clearly seen on the radiograph.

A. Small Opacities

For radiographic interpretation, no shadows are pathognomonic for pneumoconiosis, but two types of small opacities are basic components of pneumoconiotic changes of pulmonary parenchyma (Fig. 1). ''Small rounded opacities'' with discrete, roughly round shape often represent silicosis or coal miners' pneumoconiosis. ''Small irregular opacities,'' composed of a nonanatomical linar component often described as curvilinear, reticular, network, fibrotic, exaggerated markings, or small ring shape often represent asbestos pneumoconiosis. These small opacities are usually diffuse in nature;

however, rounded opacities are predominant in the upper lungs and irregular opacities in the lower lung fields. These two shapes may coexist on the same radiograph.

The dose-response relationship has been confirmed (Fletcher, 1955) between the profusion of small rounded opacities and the dust weight in autopsied lungs of patients with coal miners' pneumoconiosis. On the other hand, the

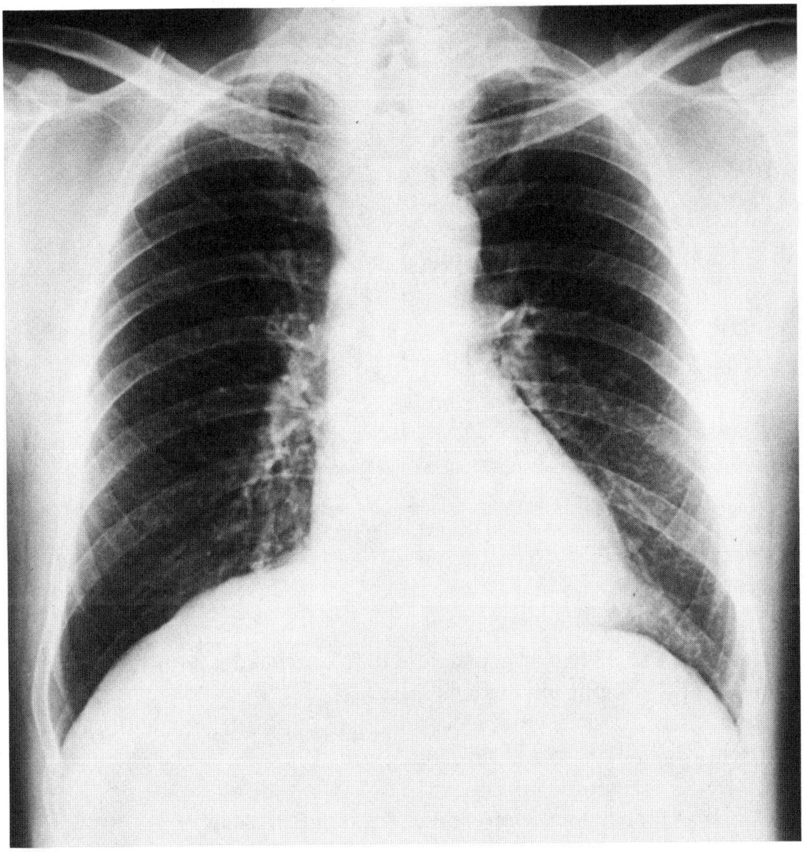

(a)

Figure 1 Small rounded opacities in a 55-year-old man engaged in drilling work for 10 years in a copper mine. Profusion 1/1 (a few). Shape/size p/p (less than 1.5 mm diameter). The CT (b) demonstrates much more numerous small opacities than a PA (a).

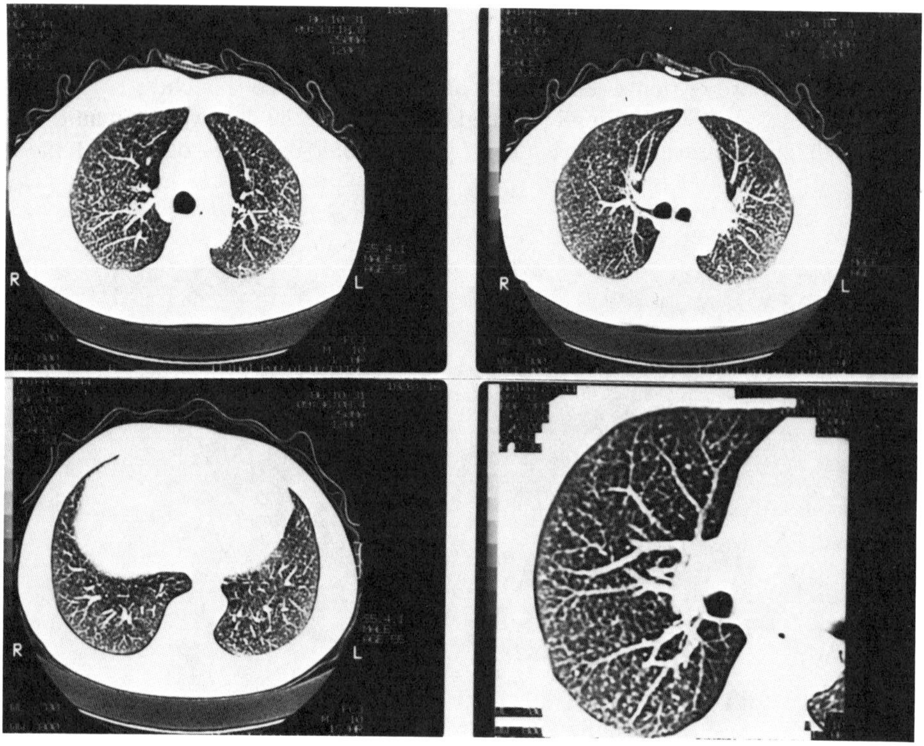

(b)

Figure 1 (continued)

development of small irregular opacities may be related not only to the amount of deposited dusts but also to host factors.

Pulmonary parenchymal changes other than small opacities are either coincidental or due to other diseases.

B. Large Opacities (Progressive Massive Fibrosis)

A large opacity is a consolidated mass resulting from the confluence of small rounded opacities caused by inhalation of a high concentration of free silica dust. Usually seen in upper lung fields, these opacities are unrelated to segmental anatomy and are accompanied by surrounding emphysematous areas. The margins of the large opacity are often ill-defined and sometimes mixed with tuberculous infection (silicotuberculosis) or lung cancer.

C. Hilar Lymph Node Changes

In silicosis, hilar lymph nodes are often enlarged and sometimes calcified, producing so-called "egg shell" calcification that also occurs in mediastinal, thoracic wall, and intraperitoneal lymph nodes. Calcifications are mostly "egg shell" type in silicosis, "central mass" in tuberculosis, and "coral" shape in sarcoidosis.

III. Radiographic Features of Pleural Changes

In addition to two types of small opacities mentioned above, the third basic component of pneumoconiosis is parietal pleural involvement. In general, two types of pleural changes are related to asbestos exposure: circumscribed and diffuse. Most frequent is the circumscribed pleural thickening, or pleural plaque, which occurs in the parietal layer of the pleura as a discrete, raised, gray-white lesion on the inner surface of the rib cage and on the diaphragm. Much less common is the diffuse pleural thickening involving both visceral and parietal layers, usually as a consequence of pleural effusion in patients with asbestos pneumoconiosis. Calcification often occurs in the pleural plaques, situated in the central zone of the plaque. On the PA radiograph, the profile (edge on) of the plaque has sharp contour unrelated to the anatomical structure, roughly paralleling the inner margin of the lateral thoracic walls or the ribs. The face on (en face) noncalcified manifestation gives a faint, veil-like opacity superimposed on the lung field. When the plaque is calcified, the shadows present a dense opacity with a holly-leaf-like shape, usually edged with the sharp margin. The diaphragmatic manifestation yields small localized protuberances on the diaphragm close to the central tendon. The only visible change in the visceral layer is the thickened interlobar fissure.

Pleural plaques on PA radiographs are commonly bilateral, but not always symmetrical. The profile noncalcified plaques are often found in the posterolateral aspect of the pleura in the region of the 5th-8th ribs, while the face on calcified lesions are frequently located in the anterolateral area. The costophrenic angles are commonly free from obliteration, except in cases of advanced pulmonary interstitial fibrosis with small irregular opacities or prior pleural effusion. The mediastinal pleural involvement may be radiographically detectable when calcification occurs.

IV. Reading

A. Quality

The technical quality of a radiograph is most important for accurate reading. Too black or too white radiographs may cause misdiagnosis. Before rendering an interpretation, the reader should always pay attention to the quality of radiographs and record the quality as graded below.

To compare with standard radiographs, the radiograph to be examined is preferably sandwiched on the bright viewing box by two standard radiographs whose images are closest to the radiograph to be examined. Even experienced readers refer to the ILO standard radiographs when interpreting radiographs. Trusting to a memorized image of standard radiographs is not recommended (Fig. 2).

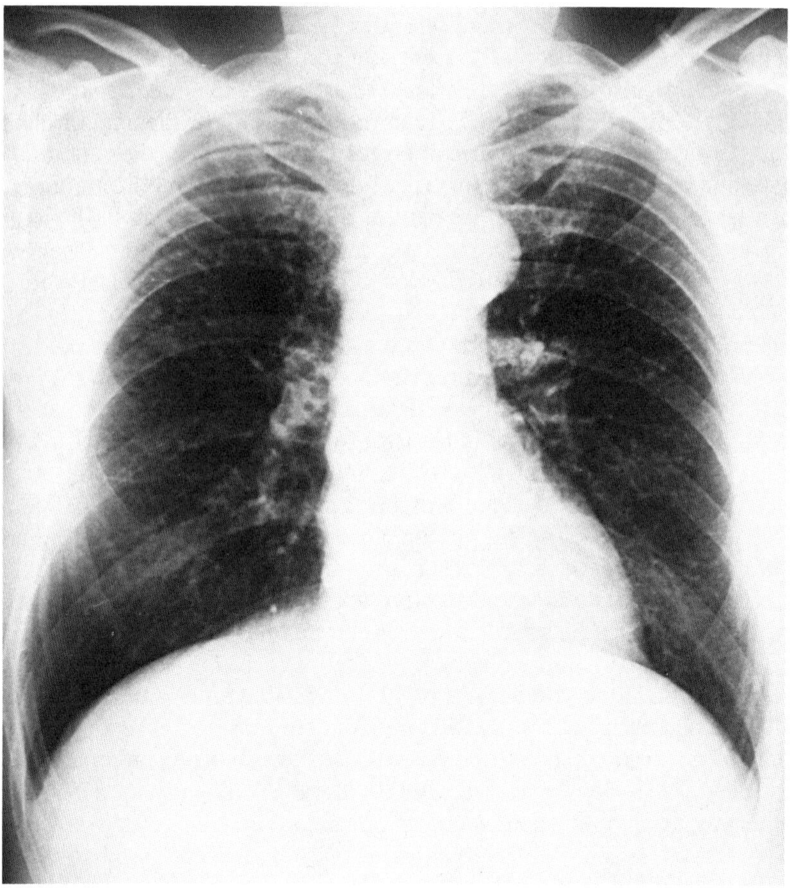

(a)

Figure 2 Small rounded opacities in a 63-year-old man engaged in drilling work for 21 years in a copper mine. Profusion 1/1 (a few). Shape/size q/q (1.5-3.0 mm in diameter). The CT (b) shows small blebs in the posterior subpleural regions.

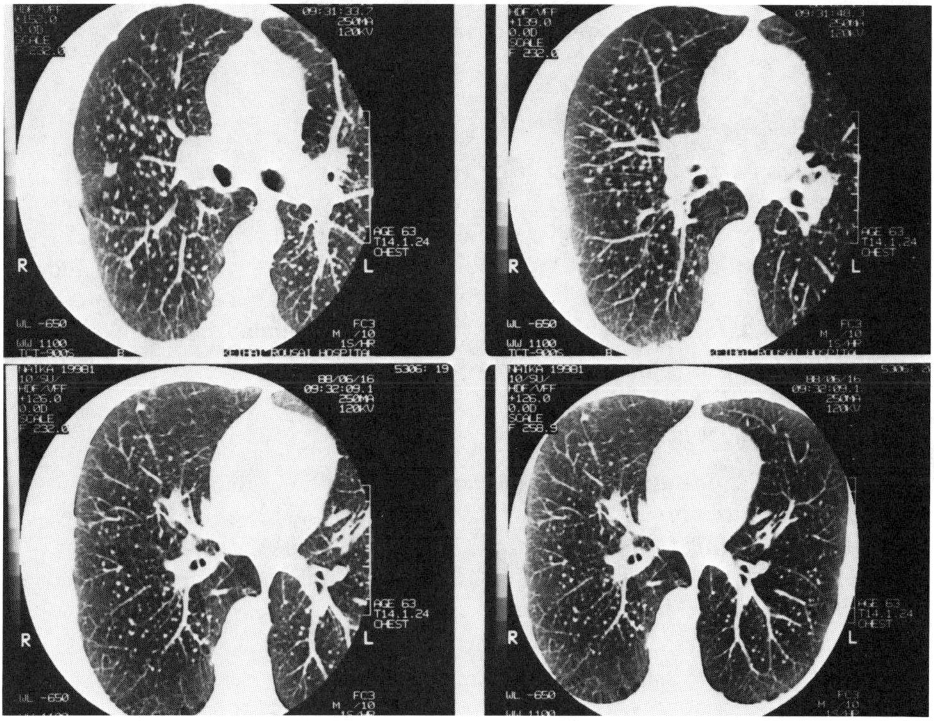

(b)

a. Good: excellent in quality
b. Acceptable: not excellent, but readable with no major technical defect
c. Poor: still readable with some technical defect
d. Unacceptable: not readable

Unacceptable radiographs should not be interpreted; a request should be made for another chest x-ray, with a comment made on the original's quality.

The most frequent causes of poor-quality chest x-ray films are overexposure, underexposure, unsatisfactory gross image contrast, poor screen-film contact, and fog (high background density). To improve the quality of a radiograph, one needs a well-trained technologist and a physician or a radiologist concerned with the quality who work closely together. The use of a pocket densitometer helps to ensure the appropriate blackness. In general, a higher kilovoltage radiograph usually provides more information than a low kv radiograph.

B. Reading Pulmonary Parenchymal Changes

Normal or Abnormal Radiograph?

Readers must develop their skill by reading many normal radiographs of young and old, skinny and fat patients, and of men and women. Although the ILO set provides two normal radiographs, it may be better for the reader to select intrainstitutional control radiographs (one of a young person and the other of an old person) so that a comparison can easily be made between normal radiographs and examinees' radiographs of similar quality taken in the same clinic.

Compatible with Pneumoconiosis?

If radiographic features are probably compatible with pneumoconiosis, which usually presents with diffuse small opacities distributed in both sides, proceed with the following ILO classification. If not, comments should be recorded, but the reader may proceed with the classification along the lines recommended by the American Thoracic Society.

Where are the Small Opacities Distributed?

For the diagnosis of pneumoconiosis, the ILO standard radiographs must be referred to as the international scale. Written texts may be of help in understanding the ILO system, but cannot replace the standard radiographs.

Put marks (x) on reading sheet indicating the zones where small opacities are distributed (Fig. 3). For this purpose, the lung fields are organized into three zones (upper, middle, and lower) on each side by horizontal lines drawn at one-third and two-thirds of the vertical distance between the lung apex and the dome of the diaphragm.

How Numerous are Small Opacities (Profusion)?

There are two ways of classifying the profusion of small opacities: the short (simplified) and the complete classifications. The short classification classifies the profusion as levels 0, 1, 2, and 3, from no opacities to very numerous opacities (major category). The complete classification further organizes each major category into 3 subcategories (minor category), making up a 12 point scale. Although the major category is sufficient, the 12 point scale system is useful if the reader wishes to know whether a category 1 radiograph is closer to a category 0 or category 2.

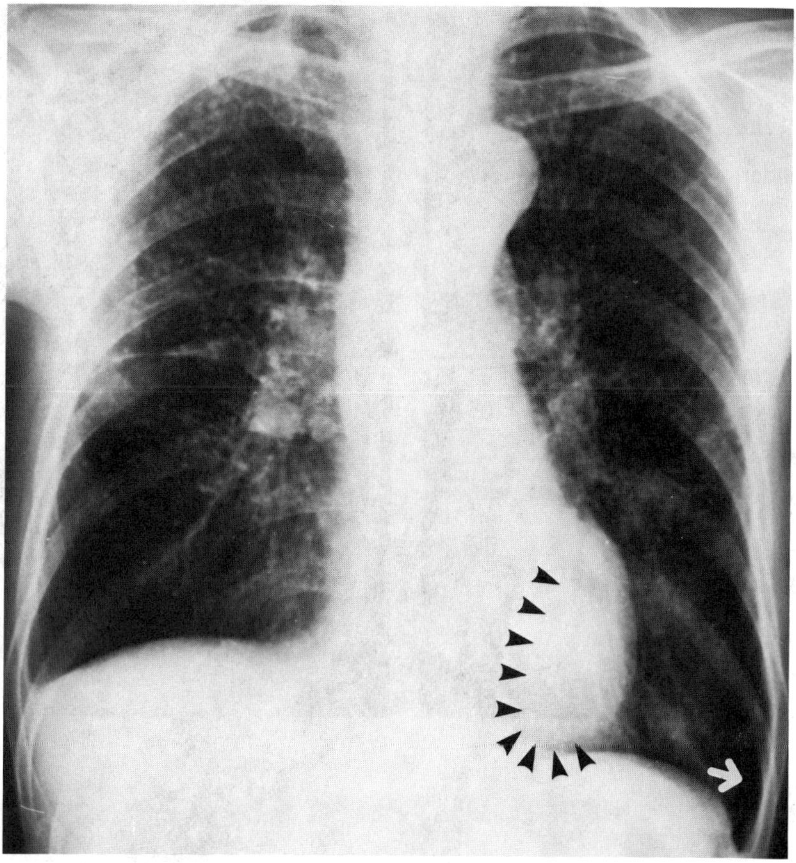

(a)

Figure 3 Small rounded opacities in a 67-year-old man who did carrying work for 23 years in a copper mine. Profusion 2/2 (numerous). Shape/size q/q:pi, interlobar fissure thickening; hi, hilar enlargement; px, pneumothorax (white arrow). Black arrows show collapsed lower lobe. The CT demonstrates these findings more affirmatively as well as blebs that are not visible on a PA.

Short Classification

Category 0: Small opacities absent or less profuse than the lower limit of category 1. The set provides a radiograph of the middle of category 1.

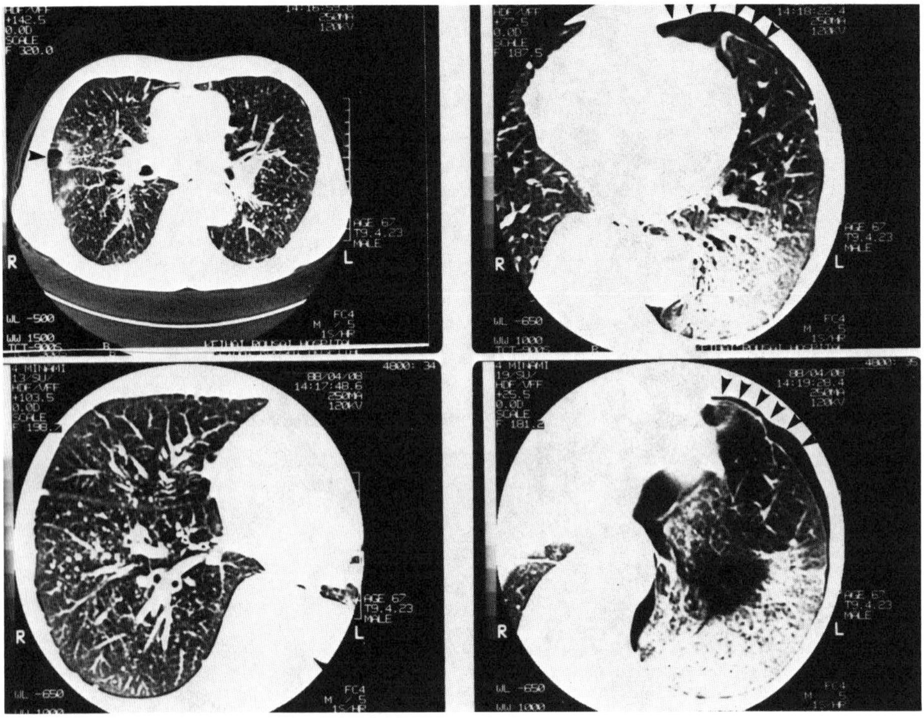

(b)

Figure 3 (continued)

Category 1: Small opacities definitely present, but few in number

Category 2: Small opacities numerous. The normal lung markings are usually still visible.

Category 3: Small opacities very numerous. The normal lung markings are partly or totally obscured.

The terms "few," "numerous," and "very numerous" should be understood by referring to standard radiographs. The terms cannot reproduce the true image.

The Complete Classification

This classification is based on the idea that there is a continuity of change from no small opacities to the most advanced category. When the profusion seems to be defined by major category 2, but category 1 is seriously considered as an alternative, the complete classification system allows us to describe it as 2/1 (minor category), the first numerical denoting the major category and the second one the alternative major category. Likewise 2/2 is the major category 2 but near the middle of category 2, and 2/3 is the major category 2, but near the major category 3. Thus, the 4 major categories in the short classification become the complete 12 point scale: 0/ – , 0/0, 0/1, 1/0, 1/1, 1/2, 2/1, 2/2, 2/3, 3/2, 3/3, and 3/ + . These 12 points can be scored from 1 to 12 when the results are analyzed.

Although 0/ – denotes a completely normal radiograph an 0/0 denotes no small opacities, but some nonpneumonic changes. Both 0/ – and 0/0 can be treated as the same. Now one can understand why standard radiographs have a description of 1/1 instead of short category 1, 2/2 instead of 2, and 3/3 instead of 3.

What Shapes are the Small Opacities?

The ILO system combines shape with size. However, for the sake of simplicity it should differentiate shape from size. Such separation was provided in the ILO 1980 draft, but this was deleted in the final text. If the reader wishes to mention shape only, the shape can be classified by coding rounded opacities as R and irregular ones as I. If the reader considers that all or virtually all opacities are of one shape R, this should be recorded as RR. If the other shape I is mixed, this "I" should be put as the second letter: RI. Thus, the system has four overall shape groups; RR, RI, IR, and II. If the size of small opacities foretells the prognosis, the size should obligatorily be added. However, this method does not, so far, elucidate the prognosis in relation to the size of small opacities.

How Large Are Small Opacities of Each Shape? (Shape and Size)

In each shape, rounded and irregular, three sizes are differentiated, as shown in standard radiographs.

Rounded:
- p: diameter up to about 1.5 mm (pinhead size)
- q: diameter exceeding 1.5 mm and up to about 3 mm (micronodular size)
- r: diameter exceeding about 3 mm and up to about 10 mm (nodular size)

Irregular:
- s: width up to about 1.5 mm (fine) (Figs. 5 and 6)
- t: width exceeding 1.5 mm and up to about 3 mm (medium)
- u: width exceeding 3 mm and up to 10 mm (coarse)

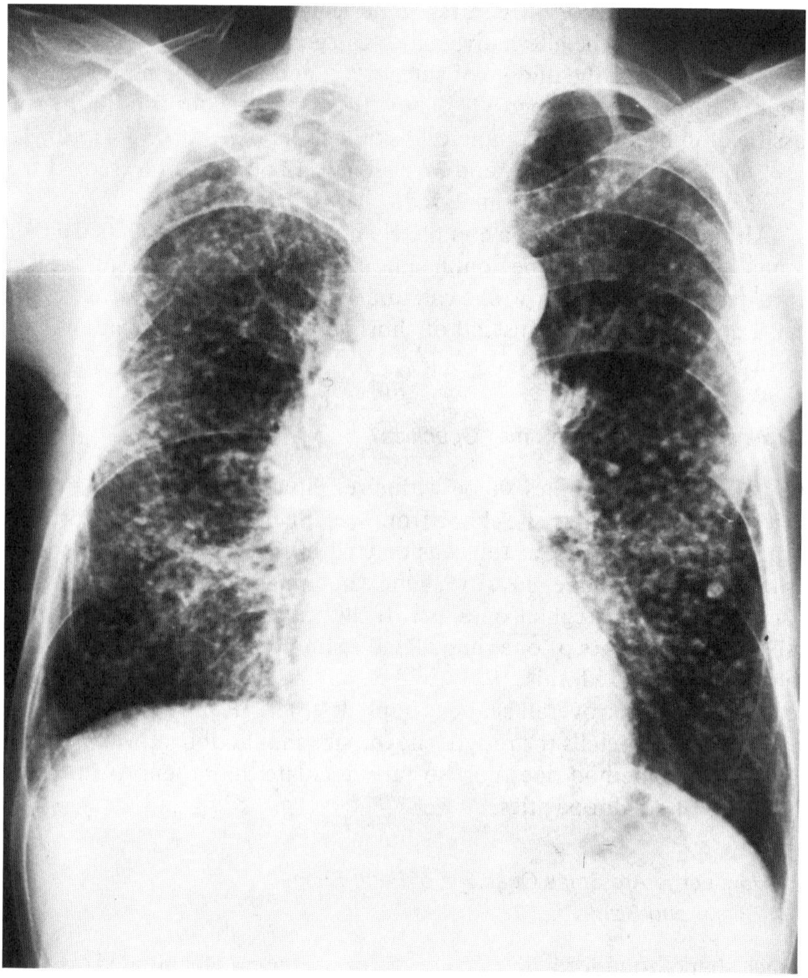

(a)

Figure 4 Small rounded opacities in a 62-year-old man engaged in drilling work for 28 years in a copper mine. Profusion 3/3 (very numerous). Shape/size r/r (3 mm up to 10 mm in diameter). Pleura; right costphrenic angle obliterated: es, Eggshall calcifications. (a) A PA reveals resected 5th and 6th ribs to to trauma resulting in diffuse pleural thickening on the chest wall on the right. (b) CT demonstrates small rounded opacities in the middle to the posterior areas with a tendency to confluence. Normal blood vessels are obscure.

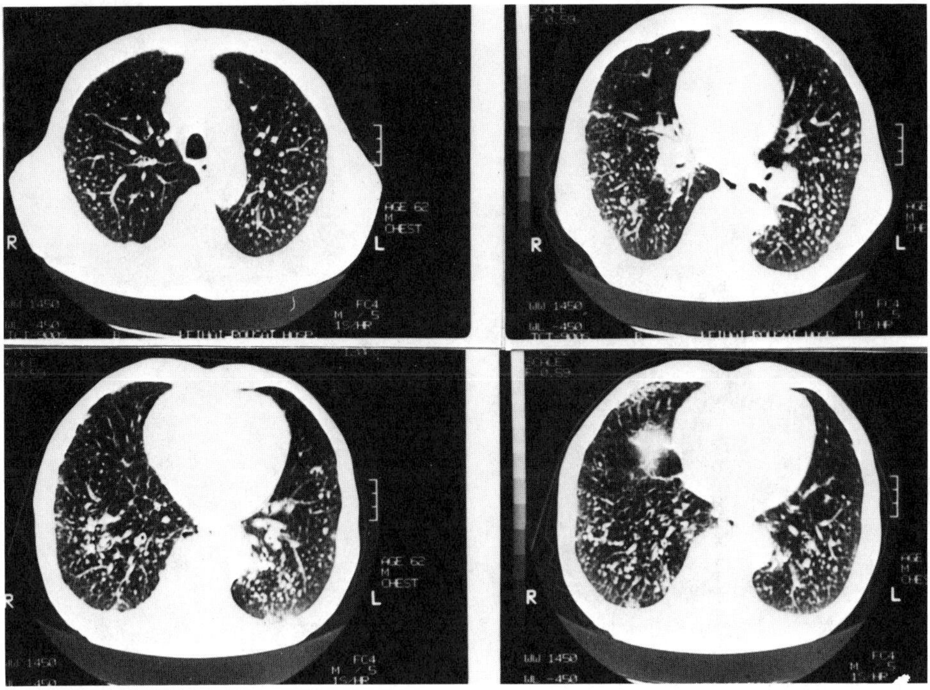

(b)

These pqr groups were originally termed pinhead, mixed, or nodular on radiographs (according to Fletcher). The stu categorization was produced later to match the pqr categorization. Therefore, standard radiographs should take precedence over written definitions such as 1.5 mm, 3 mm, or 10 mm.

To record shape and size, two letters must be used. If the reader considers that all or virtually all opacities are of one shape and size, (e.g., "q"), this should be recorded as q/q. If, however, another shape or size (e.g., "t"), is mixed, this should be recorded as q/t, which would denote predominant q opacities but mixed with a significant number rated as "t."

Large Opacities

Large opacities result from the conglomeration of the small opacities frequently seen in silicosis. A large opacity is defined as that greater than 10 mm

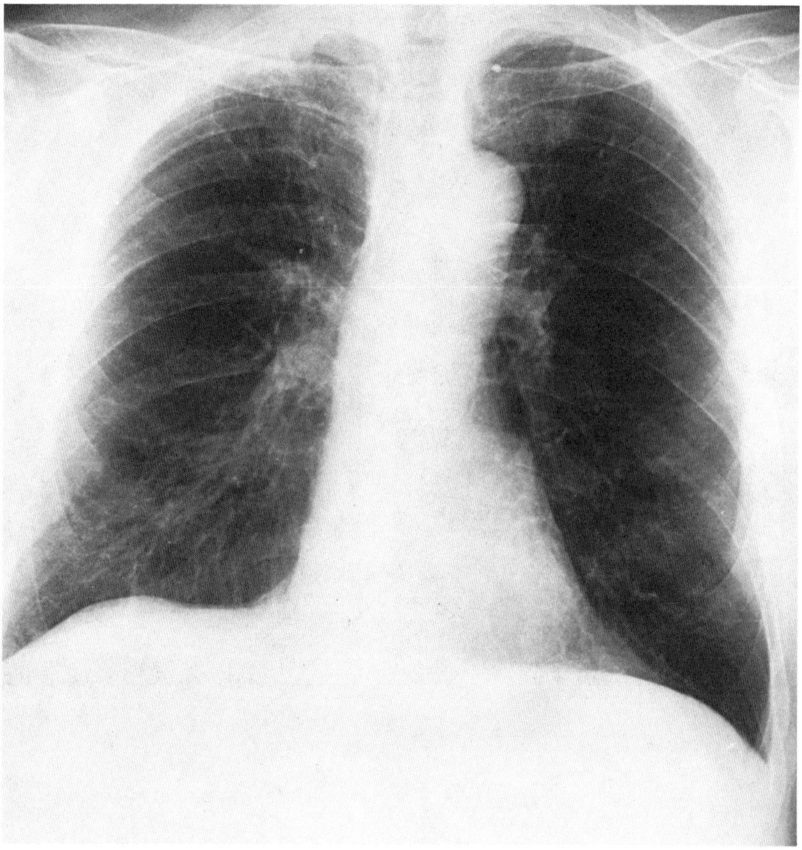

(a)

Figure 5 Small irregular opacities in a 59-year-old subject who was an arc welder for 15 years. Profusion 1/1 (a few). Shape/size s/p (irregular mixed with small rounded, less than 1.5 mm in diameter). (a) PA reveals a long opacity along the upper edge of the left 6th anterior rib, which later proved to be extrapleural fat by CT, although density resembles pleural plaques. (b) CT taken every 5 mm slice thickness demonstrates fine strand or streak, pulmonary emphysema, bullae, and honeycomb patterns compatible with interstitial fibrosis. The bullae are located in the posterior subpleural regions with predominance of the left side, which caused hyperlucency of a PA. The irregular patterns are dominant in this case.

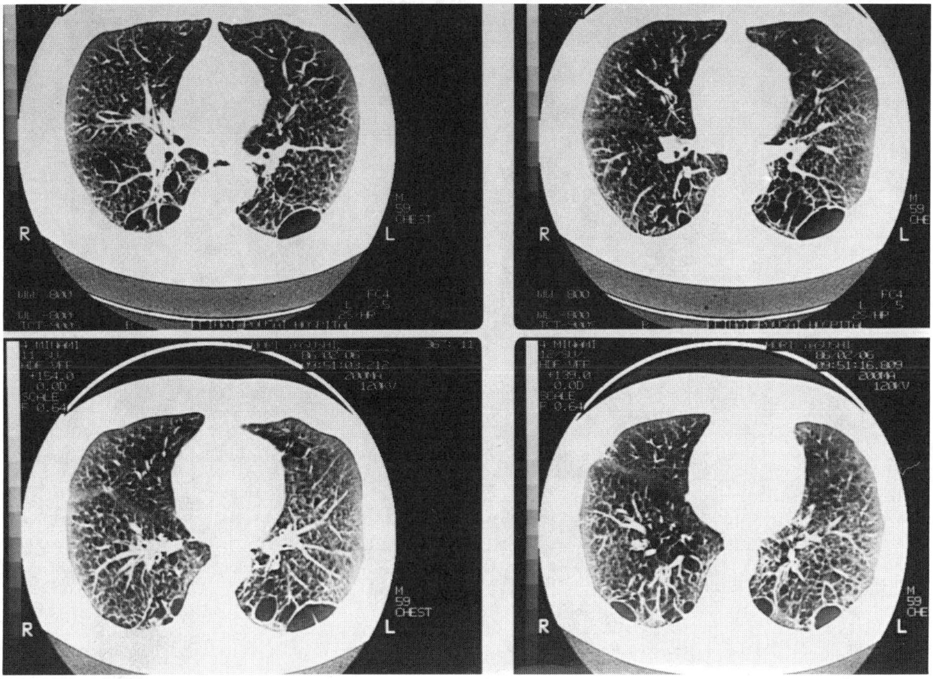

(b)

in diameter, although such opacities will become less frequent with the improvement in dust in the environment (Fig. 7).

Category A: The diameter of an opacity or the sum of several opacities exceeding about 10 mm and up to 50 mm inclusive

Category B: The diameter of an opacity or the sum of several opacities larger than category A and not exceeding the equivalent of the right upper zone.

Category C: The diameter of an opacity or the sum of several opacities exceeding the equivalent of the right upper zone.

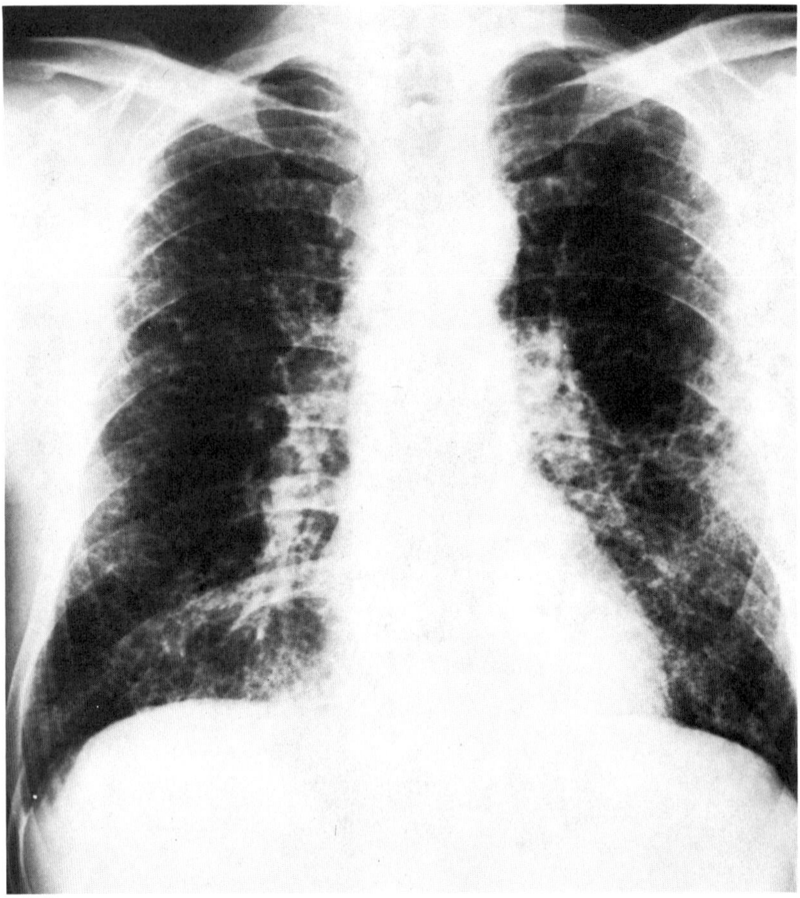

(a)

Figure 6 Small irregular opacities in a 42-year-old man who did foundry work for 10 years following occupational exposure to dust for many years. Profusion 2/2 (numerous) Shape/size t/t (coarse, 1.5-3.0 mm in diameter): bu, Bullae; hi, hilar enlargement; ho, honeycomb. (a) PA reveals hyperlucency in the left upper and middle lung zones. (b) CT demonstrates small irregular opacities of reticulolinear or complicated network patterns with pulmonary emphysema, compatible with interstitial fibrosis. Bullae are visible on the left anterior subpleural region (black arrows), causing the left-sided hyperlucency on the PA. Honeycomb patterns are also noted on the posterior areas.

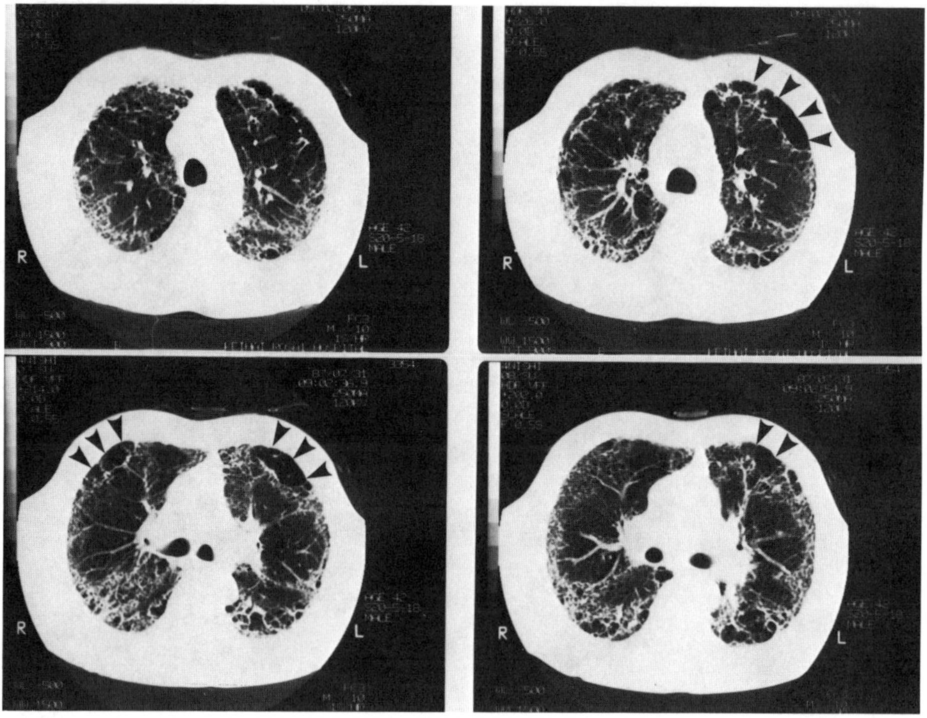

(b)

C. Reading Pleural Changes

Plaques

Noncalcified (hyaline) plaques are seen on chest walls, diaphragm, and mediastinum, although they are usually not visible en face on the chest walls and diaphragm. Calcified plaques are most often seen on the diaphragm, followed by en face on chest walls, mediastinum, and the profile chest walls (Figs. 8 and 9).

When plaques are seen on a radiograph, the side and site should first be recorded. Plaques in the profile chest walls should be measured for their width and extent. The calcification also should be measured as defined below.

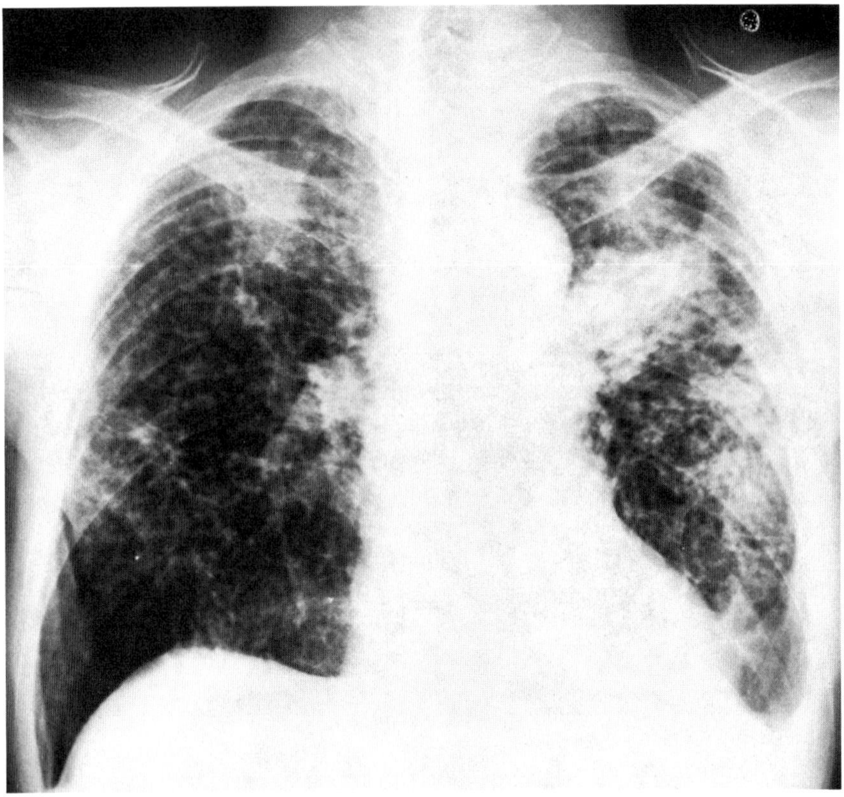

(a)

Figure 7 Large opacities: category C in a 71-year-old woman who had worked packing activated carbon powder for 10 years. Profusion 2/2 (numerous) Shape/size r/r. (a) PA shows several large opacities, the sum of which does not exceed the area equivalent to the right upper zone: category B. (b) CT demonstrates a more marked tendency of confluence than a PA. A cavity is found in a large opacity (upper left CT).

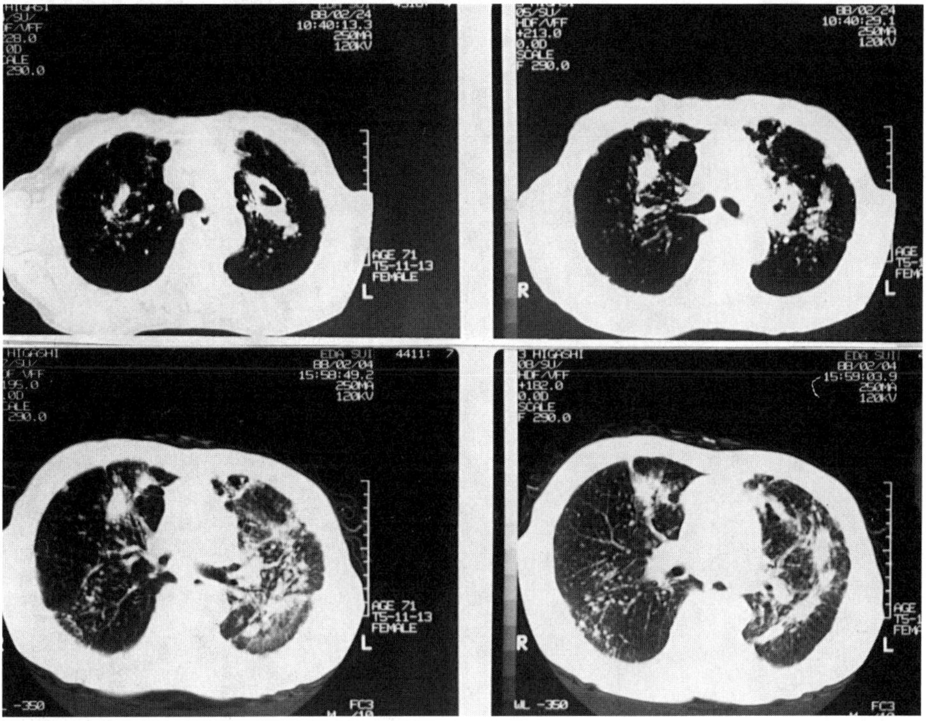

(b)

Side and site: Right and left. Chest walls (profile or face on), diaphragm, and mediastinum.

Maximum width and extent for the profile chest walls

Width: a: maximum width up to about 5 mm

b: maximum width over about 5 mm up to about 10 mm

c: maximum width over about 10 mm

Extent: 1: total length equivalent to up to one-quarter of the projection of the lateral chest wall

2. total length exceeding one-quarter but not one-half of the lateral chest wall

3. total length exceeding one-half of the lateral chest wall

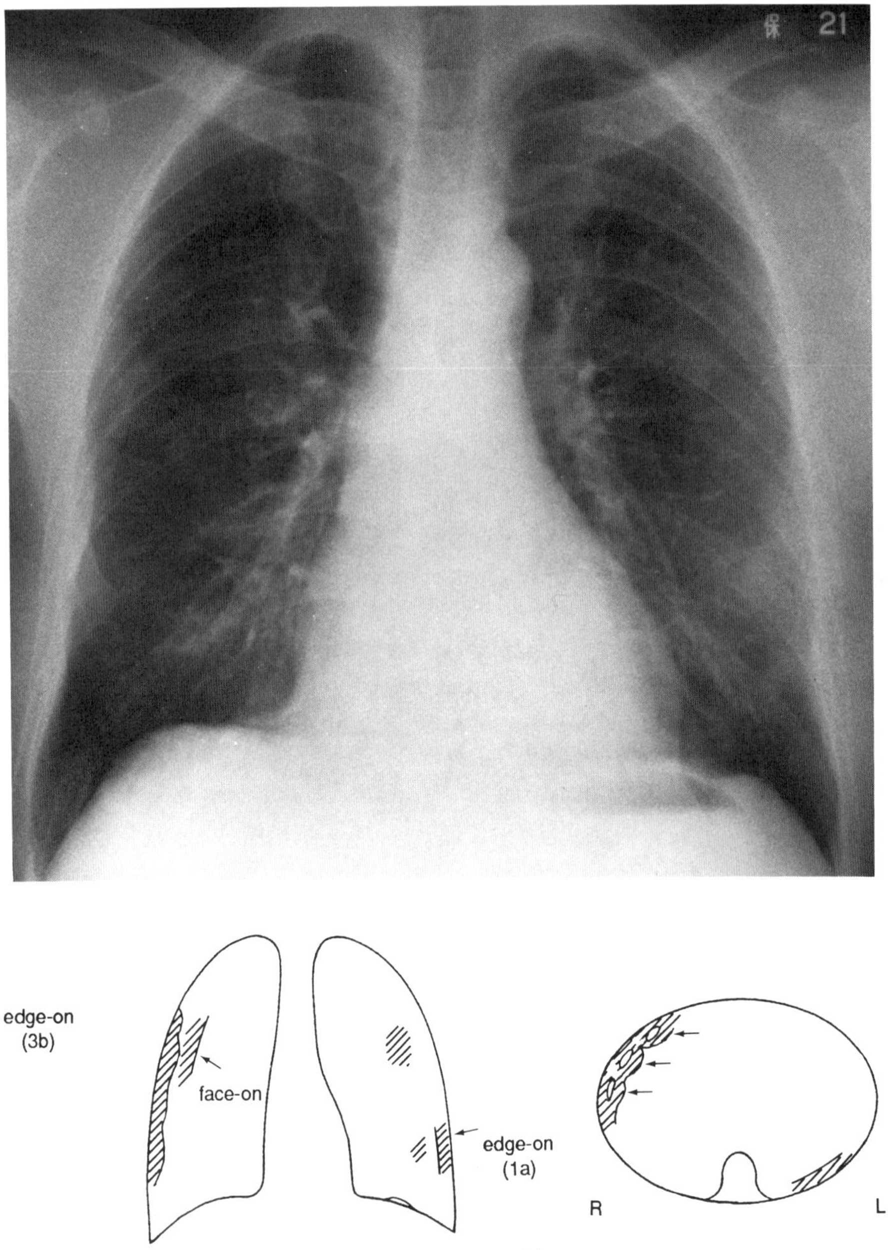

Figure 8 Pleural plaques in a 54-year-old man who was an insulation worker for 21 years while asbestos textile was used. (a) PA reveals noncalcified plaques on the right chest wall edge-on (3b) and face-on sites and also on the left chest wall edge-on (la) and face-on sites.

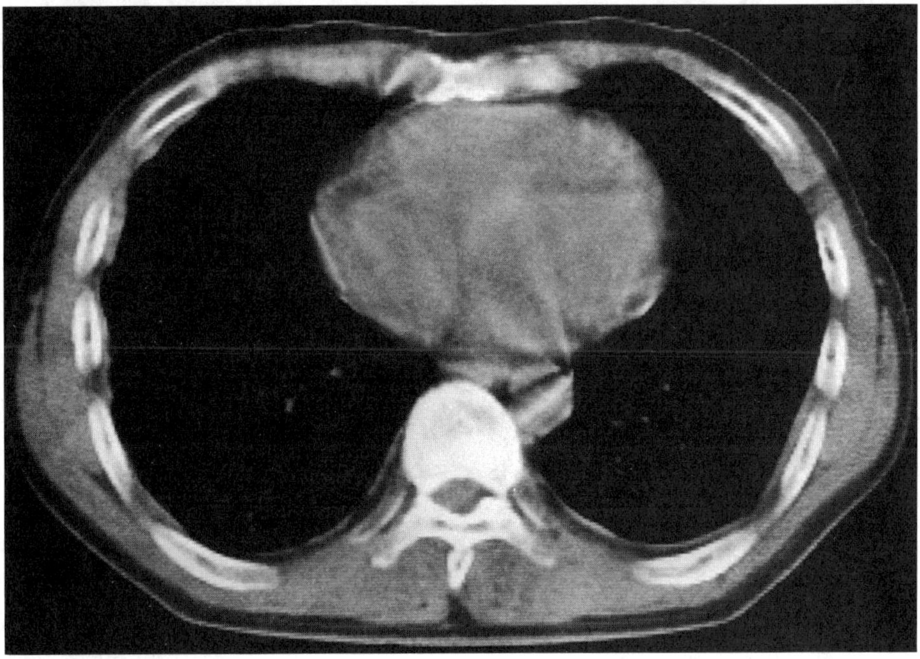

(b)

Figure 8 (continued). (b) CT demonstrates 10 cations of plaques.

Extent of calcified plaques

1: an area or the sum of the area of calcified pleura with the greatest diameter not exceeding about 20 mm

2: an area or the sum of the area of such exceeding about 20 mm and up to 100 mm

3: areas exceeding about 100 mg

Diffuse Pleural Thickening

Costophrenic Angle Obliteration

If the examinee inspires very deeply, a slightly rounded costophrenic angle is seen even in normal subjects. Minimal change in this condition is shown in a standard radiograph. Pleural thickening is often accompanied by costo-

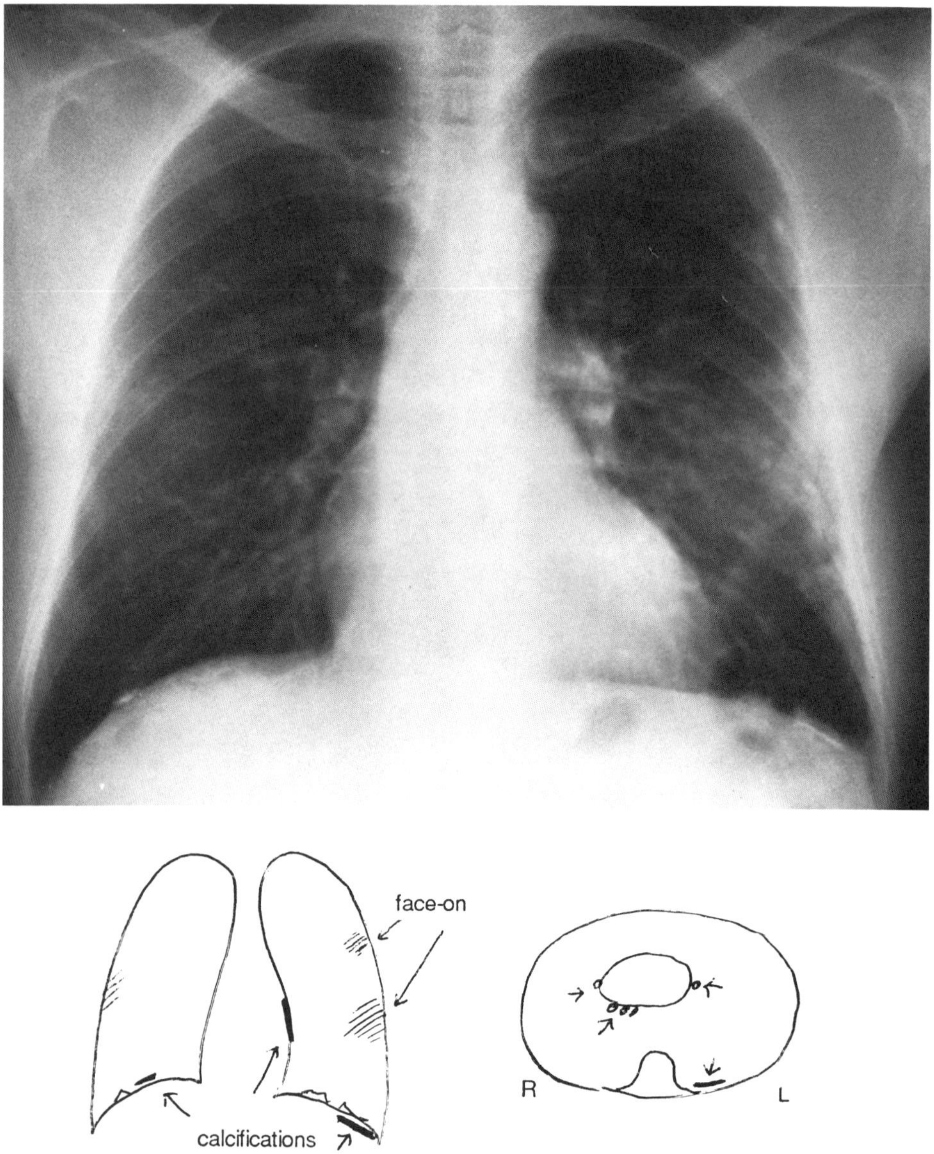

(a)

Figure 9 Pleural plaques. (a) PA reveal right: face-on chest wall with noncalcified plaques and the diaphragma with noncalcified and calcified plaques; left: the face-on chest wall with noncalcified plaques and the diaphragma with noncalcified and calcified plaques. (b) CT demonstrates calcified plaques on the diaphragm and in the pravertebral site that cannot be seen on PA.

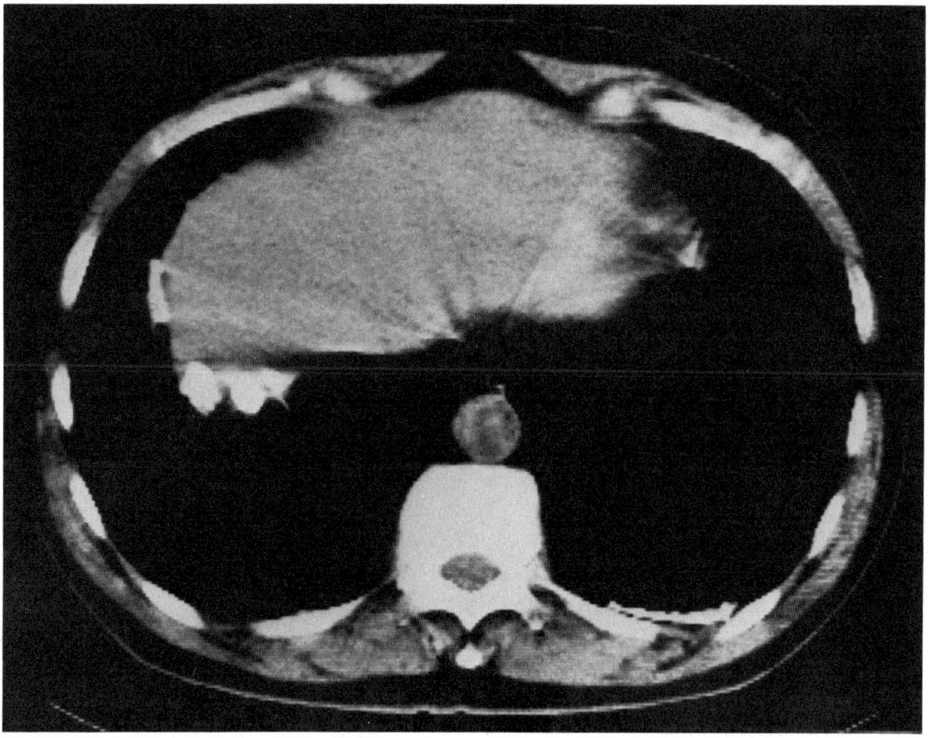

(b)

phrenic angle obliteration. In cases of costophrenic angle obliteration combined with continuous chest wall thickening in profile, the width and length should be added.

Chest Wall Face On

It is rather difficult to recognize noncalcified pleural thickening on the chest wall when viewed face on. If such thickening exists extensively, the image has a veiled appearance. If the thickening lasts for many years, there may be some distortion of the thoracic cage, such as asymmetry or narrowing of rib spaces on the affected side.

D. Reading Other Symbols

There are many symbols to help one describe the radiological findings. Symbols which are commonly used are listed here.

Coalescence of small pneumoconiotic opacities (ax)
Bulla(e) (bu)
Cancer of lung or pleura (ca)
Calcification in small pneumoconiotic opacities (cn)
Cavity (cv)
Marked distortion of the intrathoracic organs (di)
Effusion (ef)
Definite emphysema (em)
Eggshell calcification of hilar or mediastinal lymph nodes (es)
Enlargement of hilar or mediastinal lymph nodes (hi)
Honeycomb lung (ho)
Septal (Kerley's) line (kl)
Pleural thickening in the interlobar fissure or mediastinum (pi)
Pneumothorax (px)
Tuberculosis (tb)

E. Individual Diagnosis

Patients with the profusion category 1/0 or more are usually regarded as having pneumoconiosis. Those with 0/1 are considered to have suspected pneumoconiosis. For this reason, the distinction between 1/0 and 0/1 is thought to be more important than that between other profusion categories. This might be so in practice; however, logic dictates that every border between categories may have the same importance.

The diagnosis of pneumoconiosis is not difficult if the examinee (1) has a long-term occupational history of exposure to dusts of a high concentration; (2) has one of basic patterns of diffuse pulmonary parenchymal small opacities, either rounded or irregular, and plaques; and (3) is either asymptomatic or experiences the insidious appearance of symptoms.

The diffuse small opacities should be differentiated from many other diseases that present with similar patterns, such as miliary tuberculosis, fungus or parasite infection, malignancy (metastatic, alveolar carcinoma), histocytosis X, sarcoidosis, and amyloidosis, which present with small rounded opacities; and idiopathic interstitial fibrosis and rheumatic disease, which present with irregular small opacities.

Pulmonary function studies may be of help in judging the severity of the disease but are of no importance in making the diagnosis.

Pleural plaques should be differentiated from extrapleural fat in obese workers, whose shadows are usually symmetrical and look smoother than circumscribed plaques. Serratus muscles should be excluded by reading many radiographs from workers not exposed to dust. Some plaques are situated in a similar site to rib companion shadows, but plaques are much denser than these shadows.

V. Management

A. Individual Care

Once a worker is diagnosed as having pneumoconiosis, he or she should be reexamined at intervals of every 1-2 years, to check the progress of the disease. The ILO classification can be used to determine the severity. Pulmonary ventilatory function tests and diffusing capacity tests should be included in individual examinations.

B. Administrative Care

The only way to prevent the worker from developing advanced pneumoconiosis is to transfer him or her to a less dusty workplace. This is especially true for patients with asbestos pneumoconiosis, which often present more severe symptoms than those with nonsilicotic pneumoconiosis caused by long-term inhalation of the dust. The same is true for patients with berrylium or organic dust pneumoconiosis, which may involve immunological mechanisms. If there are national regulations on pneumoconiosis, a physician should treat the worker accordingly.

C. Malignancies

If the patient reaches the so-called cancer age, a physician should be aware a high risk of the development of malignancies: lung cancer, pleural or peritoneal mesothelioma.

Since pneumoconiotic shadows are complicated in the advanced stages of disease, it may be difficult to detect an early lung cancer developing on the preexisting pneumoconiotic disease. For early detection, physicians or radiologists should carefully compare the recent radiographs with previous ones. It is generally accepted that asbestos workers have a higher risk of malignancies than workers not exposed to asbestos.

D. Prevention

Since there is no radical treatment for pneumoconiosis, prevention is the best therapy. All dust workers should cease smoking, whether or not they have radiographically documented pneumoconiosis. Among asbestos workers, smoking has been proved to affect the occurrence of lung cancer synergistically, but not that of malignant mesothelioma.

VI. Case Reporting

The international scale for the diagnosis of pneumoconiosis is based on the reading of PA radiograph, although many other sophisticated means of diagnosis are available at present.

Reference

International Labour Office (1980). Guidelines for the use of ILO International Classification of Radiographs of Pneumoconioses, Revised edition 1980. Occupational Safety and Health Series, 22 (Rev. 80).

19

Summer-Type Hypersensitivity Pneumonitis

MASAYUKI ANDO

Kumamoto University Medical School
Kumamoto, Japan

I. Introduction

Hypersensitivity pneumonitis (HP), or extrinsic allergic alveolitis, is an interstitial lung disease resulting from an immunological reaction to inhaled organic or inorganic antigens (Pepys, 1969; Fink, 1984; Salvaggio, 1987). Symptoms, which develop 4-8 h after exposure, generally include fever, cough, dyspnea, and general malaise. Although farmer's lung, bird breeder's disease, and humidifier or air-conditioner lung are familiar types of the disease, it may present in a number of clinical types, depending on such factors as the immunological response of the patient, the duration and amount of exposure to the inhaled antigen, and the nature of that antigen.

Since 1973, HP with certain clinical characteristics has been reported in Japan. One characteristic is its seasonal nature: it occurs in the summer months and subsides spontaneously in midautumn, only to reappear in sensitized persons the following summer. Other characteristics are the provocation of symptoms when the affected patients are at their own home, and familial occurrence. The first detailed report was by Ochi et al. (1978) and the disease was named summer-type HP (Ochi et al., 1980). It was found to be the most prevalent type of HP in Japan (Kawai et al., 1984). Environmental factors, such as the muggy weather during the summer in Japan, and residence in old, wooden houses, were considered causes, but the offending antigen remained undefined because of the complexity of the home environments.

In 1984, we proposed *Trichosporon cutaneum*, an arthrospore-forming yeast, as a likely causative agent (Shimazu et al., 1984). Since then, we have been studying the causes and pathogenesis of the disease in human beings (Ando et al., 1986, 1988, 1989, 1990; Soda et al., 1986, 1988; Yoshida et al., 1988, 1989), and also experimental HP induced by *T. cutaneum* in rabbits (Sakata et al., 1988; Yamasaki et al., 1989). Our studies clearly indicate that a major causative agent of summer-type HP is *T. cutaneum*, and that the disease, a new type of HP, should be considered a house (building)-related illness. Although HP induced by *T. cutaneum* is peculiar to Japan at the present time, we suggest the possibility of this disease in other countries, especially in temperate and tropical regions since *T. cutaneum* is distributed in these areas.

This chapter describes the clinical and immunological features of summer-type HP, including case reports, with special respect to the causes, pathogenesis, diagnosis, and treatment of the disease.

II. Geographic Distribution and Epidemiology

Summer-type HP occurs in all areas of Japan except the north (Fig. 1). There is a hot and humid summer season following a rainy season from June to mid-July. The incidence of the disease is uncertain, but there may be more than 100 cases a year. During 1987 and 1988, 119 patients who consulted our laboratory for the serodiagnosis of anti-*T. cutaneum* antibody were diagnosed clinically and immunologically as having summer-type HP. These patients' place of residence was mostly in the western and southern parts of the country, with a distribution from Akita prefecture at a latitude of 40° degrees north to Okinawa prefecture at 27° degrees north (Fig. 1). Most of the patients lived in old wooden houses, although some lived in concrete buildings. Female patients were affected approximately twice as often as male patients, probably as a result of more exposure to offending antigens at home since most of them were homemakers without an outside occupation. The age of the patients at onset ranged from 11 to 78 years old, with a peak age incidence in the 40s. Almost all patients showed initial symptoms in the period from May to October, and their symptoms spontaneously subsided in November. Recurrence in the summer season for 2 years or more was seen in 38% of the patients. A familial accumulation was also seen in approximately 30% of the cases. Most of the patients had no history of atopy.

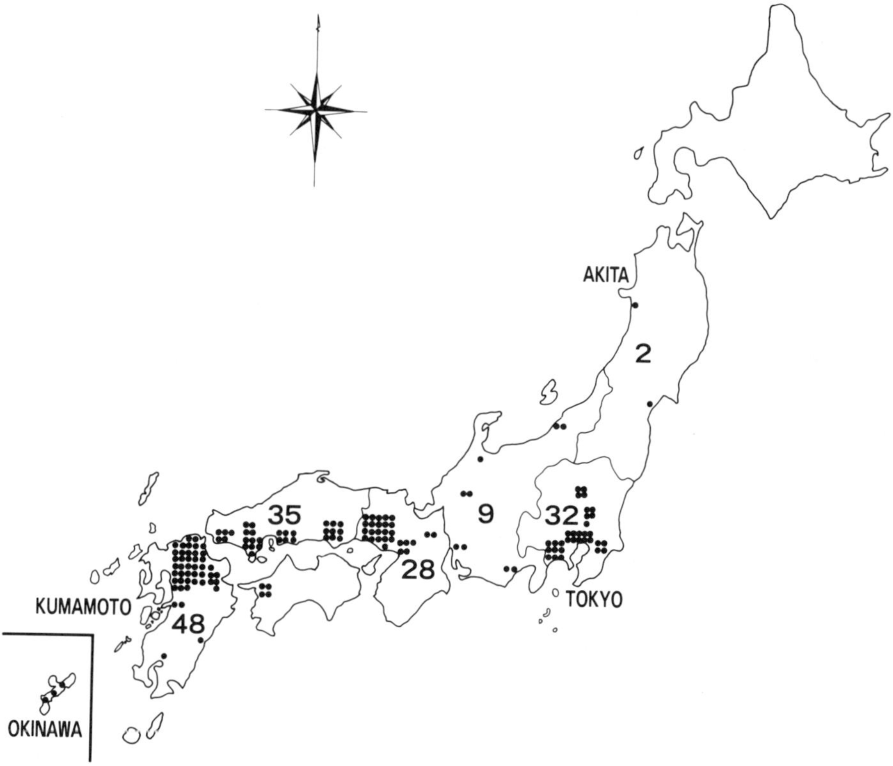

Figure 1 Geographic distribution of 119 cases of Japanese summer-type HP.

This epidemiological evidence indicates that the disease affects susceptible individuals of all ages, especially homemakers, in the summer months, which suggests that the offending antigen is present in the patient's home environment and is related to the hot and humid conditions.

III. Causes

A major causative agent of summer-type HP is *T. cutaneum*. This was determined in our recent studies with environmental and immunological surveys (Shimazu et al., 1984; Ando et al., 1986, 1988, 1990; Soda et al., 1986; Yoshida et al., 1988, 1989). Environmental studies are indispensable for investigating the unknown causative agents of HP. Such surveys have revealed the causative agents of other types of HP, such as farmer's lung, humidifier or air-conditioner lung, maple barker's lung, and cheese worker's

HP. Immunological studies, including the assay of specific antibody to the isolates and inhalation challenge with the antigen, are also necessary to determine the disease's causative agent.

In our cases of summer-type HP, all patients had recurrent episodes after returning home from the hospital during summer months. So we considered that the causative agents might be seasonal molds contaminating the home environments. We then did cultures of indoor sampling by open-plate culture, house dust culture, and swab culture. When the incidence of fungi in patients' homes was compared with that in homes of control subjects, extensive distribution of *T. cutaneum* was observed in the home environments of patients with summer-type HP but not in those of normal control subjects (Yoshida et al., 1988, 1989). Moreover, the fungus was observed only in summer months, not in winter months. The isolated *T. cutaneum* demonstrated high reactivity to all serum samples from patients with summer-type HP, but not to those from unexposed normal subjects or from patients with other pulmonary diseases as assessed by the indirect immunofluorescent antibody (IFA) method. Precipitating antibody to the culture filtrate antigen of the yeast was also observed in most cases (Shimazu et al., 1984; Ando et al., 1988; Yoshida et al., 1988). Inhalation challenge, which is the most reliable test to determine the causative antigen of HP, was done in the HP patients with culture filtrate antigens of the *T. cutaneum*, resulting in positive responses in nearly all patients with the disease. On the other hand, asymptomatic exposed family members, whose serum samples showed anti-*T. cutaneum* antibody activities, showed no response to the inhalation challenge (Ando et al., 1990). In other words, *T. cutaneum* is distributed in the patient's home environment, sensitizes the patients, and causes the disease.

The colonizing locations of *T. cutaneum* revealed by the swab method were damp and decayed wood, damp tatami mats, bedclothes that had not been exposed to direct sunlight, and budgerigar droppings. These seemed to be related to the high moisture and the nutrients of the places (see section on Treatment). Undoubtedly, atmospheric *T. cutaneum* is scattered in the air from colonizing places, since *T. cutaneum* was isolated by open plate culture in the home environment (Yoshida et al., 1988). The elimination of *T. cutaneum* from the home environment resulted in no recurrence the next summer (Yoshida et al., 1989). This evidence also supports our discovery that *T. cutaneum* is a major causative agent of summer-type HP. There are no reports on allergic diseases caused by this organism. In other words, summer-type HP induced by *T. cutaneum* is a new type of HP.

T. cutaneum, or *T. beigelii*, is well known as the cause of white piedra, a superficial mycosis involving hair, which has been found in temperate and tropical regions of Europe, Asia, South America, and, rarely, in the southern United States (Emmons et al., 1977). It is seldom isolated from respiratory and urine specimens, and only rarely causes opportunistic infection in immunocompromised patients (Yung et al., 1981). The prevalence in airborne molds of ordinary homes is extremely low (Saito, 1904; Richards and Wales, 1954; Morrow et al., 1964; Lumpkins et al., 1973; Yoshida et al., 1988). The reason the yeast grows in the patients' homes and induces the disease remains uncertain. A possible explanation is that *T. cutaneum* has a relatively high antigenic activity to human beings and therefore induces HP when once it grows in home environments (see section on Pathogenesis). High antigenic activity of *T. cutaneum* has been demonstrated in experimental HP in rabbits (Sakata et al., 1988; Yamasaki et al., 1989).

T. cutaneum grows rapidly at a temperature of 28°C, producing a cream-colored yeast-like colony, which, at the age of 2-4 weeks, becomes yellowish-gray and has a wrinkled or radially furrowed surface. The colony consists of hyphae and many arthrospores, 2-4 × 3.5-9 μm in size, and some blastospores (Fig. 2). It becomes powdery and is readily scattered in the air. The

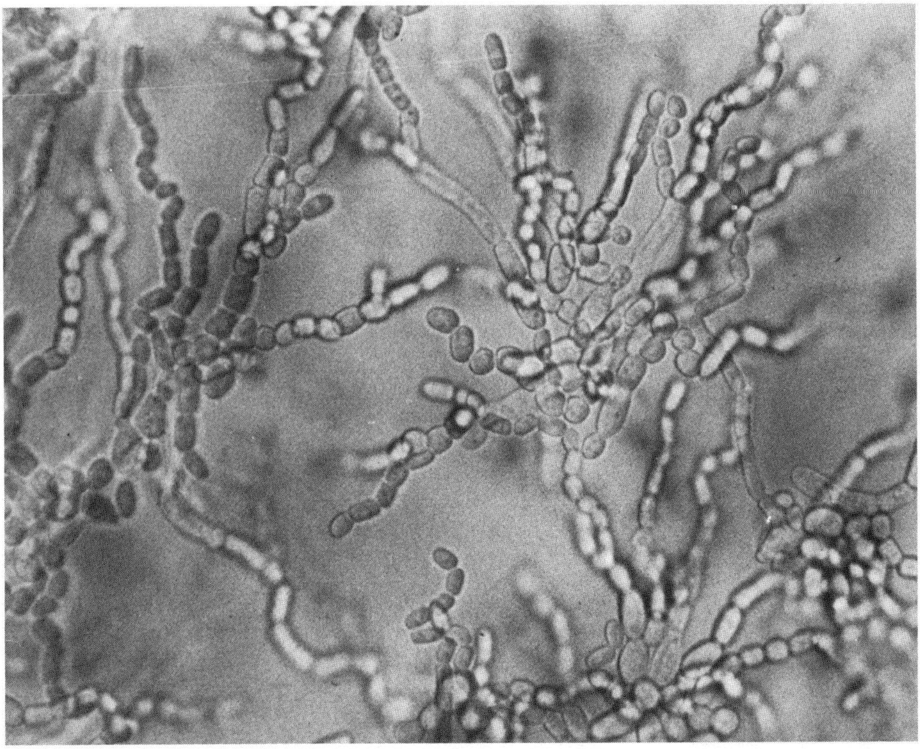

Figure 2 *Trichosporon cutaneum*; colonies grown on a slide culture (× 400).

yeast does not ferment carbohydrates but it assimilates glucose, galactose, sucrose, maltose, and lactose. It does not assimilate potassium nitrate (Emmons et al., 1977; Kreger-van Rij, 1984). There are at least two species of serotype: serotype I and serotype II (Ando et al., 1990). (More recently we found a new strain with an antigenic activity different from those of serotypes I and II.) The serotyping of the yeast is very important because the serotype-related polysaccharide-rich antigen is important in the induction of HP (see section on Pathogenesis).

Miyagawa et al. (1978) reported that all the sera from 41 patients tested had higher IFA titers to *Cryptococcus neoformans* and proposed that *C. neoformans* or an antigenically related *Cryptococcus* species may cause Japanese summer-type HP. However, they failed to find *C. neoformans* in the patients' houses, and the bronchial challenge test with the antigen was only slightly successful (Miyagawa et al., 1982). In our patients, we also found antibodies to both *T. cutaneum* and *C. neoformans*. This is not surprising because *T. cutaneum* belongs to the same family of Cryptococcaceae that *C. neoformans* and *Candida albicans* do, and serotype II *T. cutaneum* is serologically cross-reactive to *C. neoformans* (Seeliger and Schröter, 1963) (Fig. 3). We believe that *C. neoformans* could not be a main causative agent for the following reasons: (1) *C. neoformans* was not isolated from the patients' houses; (2) prevalence and titers of the anti-*C. neoformans* antibody were usually lower than those of *T. cutaneum*; and (3) all the antibody to serotype A-D *C. neoformans* was completely absorbed with serotype II *T. cutaneum*, whereas the antibody to *T. cutaneum* was only partly absorbed with the *C. neoformans* in most serum samples (Shimazu et al., 1984). There are several fungi cross-reactive to *T. cutaneum*: *Cryptococcus* species (*C. neoformans, C. diffluens, C. albidus*) and *Candida* species (*C. curvata, C. humicola*). A few of them were isolated from the patients' home environments, but they were only slightly reactive to the patient's serum samples, suggesting their weak antigenic activities (Yoshida et al., 1988, 1989).

Whether *T. cutaneum* is the sole antigen of the disease is uncertain. there is a report that summer-type HP might be due to *C. albicans* (Dobashi et al., 1980). However, *C. albicans* is detectable anywhere in the home environments of both patients and normal subjects, not only in summer months but also in winter months. The precipitating antibody to *C. albicans* is seen in high incidence not only in patients with summer-type HP but also in patients with other pulmonary diseases and in normal subjects (Shimazu et al., 1984). Thus, it is not reasonable to consider the fungus as a causative agent of the disease. Our environmental mycological study in the patients' homes revealed several fungi reactive to the patients' serum samples. However, these were each a different species, except *T. cutaneum* (Yoshida et al., 1988). All serum samples from the acute form of the disease, except those

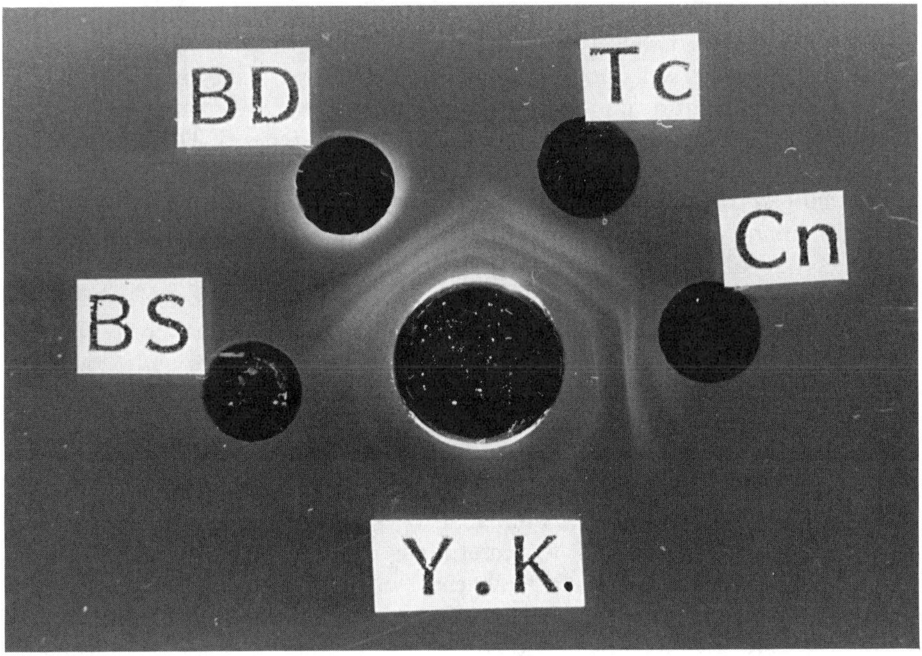

Figure 3 Serum precipitating antibody activities in a patient with summer-type HP. Tc, culture filtrate antigen of serotype II *T. cutaneum*; Cn, culture filtrate antigen of serotype A-D *C. neoformans*; BD, extract of budgerigar droppings where *T. cutaneum* was grown; BS, budgerigar's serum.

of steroid-treated cases, showed anti-*T. cutaneum* antibody activity. These results indicate that the causative agent of summer-type HP is *T. cutaneum* (or its antigenically related fungi).

IV. Pathogenesis

Pathogenesis of HP groups is multifactorial. In the pathogenesis of summer-type HP, there may be three important factors involved: immunological factors, host and genetic factors, and home environmental and climate factors.

A. Immunological Factors

Regardless of the type of HP and the causative agent, the clinical and pathological findings are strikingly similar in all HP groups, suggesting similar immunological mechanisms in the development of the pulmonary lesions of the disease. Although the importance of humoral (type III, immune complex) and cell-mediated (type IV, delayed type) hypersensitivity to the offending antigen is well known, the precise mechanisms of the immunopathogenesis remain poorly defined. One reason may be that the great majority of observations on the immunopathogenesis of other types of HP have used crude antigenic substances as offending antigen. Undoubtedly, the offending antigen of HP contains many antigenic substances, but only one or a small number of all the possible antigens is important in the pathological effects. Needless to say, to investigate the immunopathogenesis of the disease, only purified antigen(s) related to the induction of the disease should be used. Antigenic analysis of mold in HP has been done extensively in *Thermoactinomyces vulgaris* and *Micropolyspora faeni* (Roberts and Moore, 1977), the major causative antigens of farmer's lung. The exact nature of the antigenic composition inducing the disease, however, has not been fully defined. This is because molds contain many antigenic substances such as proteins, polysaccharides, and their complexes, and because there are no reliable tests to determine their antigenicity, except the bronchial inhalation challenge, which is difficult to perform routinely.

To investigate the immunopathogenesis of summer-type HP, we partially purified the antigenic substance(s) of *T. cutaneum* and investigated the antigenicity in relation to the induction of HP in human beings and experimental HP in rabbits. First, we performed the inhalation challenge with culture filtrate antigen of two strains of different serotypes of *T. cutaneum* (TIMM 1573, serotype I, and TIMM 1318, serotype II) in patients with summer-type HP. We found that the inhalation challenge was related to the serotype of the inhaled antigen, and that there was a good correlation between the serotype of the inhalation challenge positive antigen and that of *T. cutaneum* isolated from patients' homes (Ando et al., 1990). These results indicate that the most important antigen in the induction of the disease is the serotype-related antigen of the yeast. This was also confirmed by experimental HP in rabbits: the granulomatous alveolitis, the principal feature of HP, was induced only when the serotypes of the *T. cutaneum* used as the source of culture filtrate antigen for sensitization and challenge were identical.

We also tried to purify the serotype-related antigenic substances with column chromatography. The molecular weight of the partially purified antigenic substances was greater than 1,000,000 and the antigenic activity was sodium periodate-sensitive and pronase-insensitive, suggesting a polysaccharide nature. This antigen(s) induced both humoral and cellular immune responses, resulting in the induction of granulomatous alveolitis in experimental HP (Yamasaki et al., 1990). On the other hand, other antigens induced alveolitis in rabbits, but not granuloma formation. Furthermore, in our preliminary study, positive results were obtained in some patients with summer-type HP by inhalation challenge with the partially purified antigen(s). This indicates the importance of serotype-related polysaccharide-rich antigen of *T. cutaneum* in the induction of the disease. To gain insight into the immunopathogenesis, we are currently carrying out studies to determine the exact nature of specific antigens relating to the serotyping of *T. cutaneum*.

Recent investigations of other types of HP have given rise to questions on the importance of antibody activity in the disease's pathogenesis (Salvaggio, 1987). There are three reasons for this: (1) evidence of serum precipitating antibody activity to offending antigens was often encountered in asymptomatic exposed control subjects; (2) the results of the bronchial inhalation challenge failed to correlate with serum IgG antibody activities; and (3) vasculitis, the principal characteristic feature of immune complex disease, was rarely seen in the lesions. These observations might be the result of using crude antigenic substances of the offending antigen. If so, these problems could be solved by using purified antigen to induce the disease. It is reasonable to consider that immune complex resulting from the antigen-antibody reactions in the alveolar air spaces or in the interstitium may not necessarily induced vasculitis. In the pathogenic effect of HP, local immunological responses in the lung are more important than systemic immune responses in the peripheral blood.

In summer-type HP, high tiers of specific IgG, IgA, and secretory (S)-IgA antibodies to crude culture filtrate antigen of *T. cutaneum* were detected in the patients' serum and bronchoalveolar lavage (BALF) samples, while in asymptomatic family members, the specific IgG antibodies but not the IgA and S-IgA antibodies were detected (Ando et al., 1986; Soda et al., 1986). The BALF/serum ratios of IgA and S-IgA antibody activities were markedly increased locally in the respiratory tract in proportion to the intensity of the immune reaction. Moreover, we have shown the presence of Clq and C3 in the BALF of patients with summer-type HP and a good correlation between the increased level of Clq (as well as specific IgG and IgA antibody activities to *T. cutaneum*) and clinical symptoms and decreased diffusing capacity (Soda et al., 1988). These results suggest the involvement of immune complexes in the respiratory tract.

Of particular interest, our results in the experimental HP induced by *T. cutaneum* indicate that there is an apparent parallel between local IgA antibody activity and granuloma formation (Sakata et al., 1988; Yamasaki et al., 1990). Johnson et al. (1984, 1986) reported that the immune complexes containing IgA antibody had lung-damaging properties and that the nature of this effect was related to the requirement for complements but not for neutrophils. On pathological examination, lungs exposed to IgA immune complexes showed mononuclear cell infiltration but no neutrophils. If these results are correct, it is possible that humoral factors including IgA antibody might also be involved in the pathogenic process of HP. The mechanisms of IgA and S-IgA antibody production in our patients are unclear, but there seem to be at least three explanations: (1) *T. cutaneum* antigen may have some immunomodulating activity to induce IgA and S-IgA antibody production; (2) the elevated IgA and S-IgA antibody activity, which we observed in the patients but not in the asymptomatic family members, may have resulted merely from the inflammation of the respiratory tract; (3) genetic factors, with immune responses as yet undefined, might also be an explanation. Persons who are highly responsive to *T. cutaneum* antigen in the IgA and S-IgA antibody production might be susceptible to summer-type HP.

Bronchoalveolar lavage (BAL) studies on both humans and animals have demonstrated the importance of cell-mediated (type IV) hypersensitivity. Moore et al. (1980) and Keller et al. (1984) reported that BALF lymphocytes from symptomatic pigeon breeders showed a marked increase in proliferative response to pigeon antigen when compared with asymptomatic breeders, suggesting the presence of specifically activated T lymphocytes in the lung parenchyma. On the contrary, in farmer's lung, Solal-Celigny et al. (1982) reported that stimulation of peripheral blood and BALF lymphocytes with *M. faeni* antigen did not result in any significant proliferative response. In summer-type HP, the BALF lymphocytes from 6 of the 14 patients responded to the inhalation-challenge-positive antigens of *T. cutaneum*, but the responsiveness was very weak (not only to the antigen but also to phytohemagglutinin [PHA]) when compared with the reported data from subjects with pigeon breeder's disease (Ando et al., 1990). One possible explanation is the fact that the CD4/CD8 ratio was very low in our cases as compared with other reports. Reinherz et al. (1979) revealed that the $OKT4^+$ (helper/inducer) population in peripheral blood responded maximally to PHA and soluble antigen, whereas the $OKT4^-$ (suppressor/cytotoxic) population showed a diminished response. The other explanation is that HP induced by fungal antigen may have a slightly different immunopathological mechanism from that induced by avian protein. Although these results do not directly indicate that the lymphocyte proliferative response is due to the T-cell proliferation related to cell-mediated hypersensitivity, a correlation between the inhalation challenge test and the BALF cells' proliferative response test suggests the participation of cell-mediated hypersensitivity in the development of the disease. In accordance with this concept, the experimental HP in rabbits clearly showed that the antigen-induced lymphocyte proliferative response of regional lymph node cells correlated well with the granuloma formation (Sakata et al., 1988; Yamasaki et al., 1990). Thus, there is no doubt that cell-mediated hypersensitivity participates in the induction of the disease.

Recently, Cormier and colleagues (1986) reported that BAL lymphocytosis is a persistent phenomenon in a large number of asymptomatic dairy farmers, and that this finding is not related to significant disease, at least not in the time span studied. This is also true in most cases of asymptomatic exposed family members of subjects with summer-type HP (Ishihara et al., 1988). These results indicate that the role of lymphocytes in the development of the disease should be investigated from the viewpoint of immunoregulatory function.

More recently, several investigators have proposed that antigen-induced degranulation of mast cells present within the lung parenchyma has a central role in the pathogenesis of HP. Haslam et al. (1987) reported that the mast cell counts in patients with HP exceeded 0.5% in 12 of the 15 patients with HP, but in only 11 (7%) of the 153 patients in other groups, and that higher concentrations of histamine were demonstrated in HP BAL cell lysates. Soler et al. (1987) reported that the number of mast cells recovered by BAL from patients with HP was more than 1000 times greater than those recovered from normal individuals, and that discontinuation of antigen exposure resulted in an increase in the number of mast cells observed, consistent with the possibility that antigen exposure had induced mast cell degranulation. Whether the hypothesis is true in the immunopathogenesis of summer-type HP has not been investigated. To answer the question, BAL cell analysis should be done in the initial or early phase of the acute form. Our BAL findings in patients with summer-type HP, in which most BALs were carried out in the acute form but not in the early phase, demonstrated that very few mast cells were in the BALF.

In summary, the serotype-related polysaccharide-rich antigen of *T. cutaneum* is important in the induction of summer-type HP, and both type III (immune complex) and type IV (cell-mediated) hypersensitivity are involved in the pathological effect of the disease, especially in the lung parenchyma. Further immunological studies using purified antigen are needed for a better understanding of the precise mechanisms of the immunopathogenesis.

B. Host and Genetic Factors

A characteristic feature of HP is that although most people exposed to the common antigens develop an immune reaction to them, usually in the form of specific serum antibodies, a few people manifest overt respiratory disease. Obviously, a certain degree of unique host susceptibility or resistance may influence the individual response. In summer-type HP, there is no evidence that susceptibility is entirely related to the duration and intensity of antigen exposure, although there is a relatively high incidence in homemakers. Therefore, we investigated the possibility of genetic predisposition by identifying an association between summer-type HP induced by *T. cutaneum* and a particular HLA specificity. Our results showed an increase in the frequency of HLA-DQw3 antigen in the 67 patients (66% compared with 49% in the 475 normal healthy subjects; $X^2 = 5.48$, $p = 0.018$, rr = 1.92), suggesting the importance of host factors for generation of the disease (Ando et al., 1990). Sasazuki et al. (1983) have shown that HLA-DQw3 is an immunosuppressive gene. If so, the immune suppressive gene controls the resistance to HP by controlling the nonresponse to *T. cutaneum*, and HLA-DQw3 may be in negative linkage disequilibrium with the immune-suppressing gene for *T. cutaneum*. To our knowledge, there is only one report, by Rittner et al. (1983), on the DQ antigen in patients with pigeon breeder's disease in a Mexican population. They found no association between locus DQ and the disease. The reason for this may be the small number of alleles (1, 2, and 3) and/or the size of the studied samples (21 patients and 20 control subjects). In contrast, we could not demonstrate any association with HLA-DR3 or HLA-DR7 antigens, which have been associated with pigeon breeder's disease in a Mexican population (Rittner et al., 1983) and a non-Hispanic white population (Selman et al., 1987). This was because the frequencies of these antigens were very low in a Japanese population. Undoubtedly, the present knowledge of locus D is incomplete, necessitating further study. Needless to say, the pathogenesis of summer-type HP is multifocal, but the results of our HLA study suggest the importance of genetic predisposition in the development of the disease.

Cigarette smoking is known to have a suppressive effect in patients susceptible to HP (Warren, 1977). McSharry and co-workers (1985) reported that circulating IgG specific for pigeon antigen was found in 55% of nonsmoking and 4% of smoking pigeon breeders. Therefore, cigarette smoking may influence the development of summer-type HP. This is currently under study by our group.

C. Home Environmental and Climatic Factors

Summer-type HP is caused by seasonal mold contamination in the home environment. Among a number of indoor molds, *T. cutaneum* induces the disease. But how does the yeast reach the patients' homes? Why does it grow in these particular environments? And how does it survive competition, grow, sporulate, and persist there? Our indoor mycological studies reviewed that among all the environmental factors associated with the indoor growth of *T. cutaneum*, the existence of damp wood or moldy places had the most direct effect on the occurrence of the disease, and that the colonizing locations of *T. cutaneum* were damp and decayed wood, damp tatami mats, bedclothes that had not been exposed to direct sunlight, and budgerigar droppings (Yoshida et al., 1988). These indicate that *T. cutaneum* grows best in warm, humid, decaying matters. It is well known that indoor mold growth correlates with the age of the home, relative humidity, water problems, decayed wood, high shade, water-damaged carpets, used pillows and mattresses, and pets (Solomon, 1976; Gravesen et al., 1986). A high relative humidity promotes fungal growth indoors as well as out of doors. The muggy summer season following the rainy season in Japan is in perfect accord with this condition: for instance, the mean temperature and relative humidity of the summer season in Kumamoto city, located in the southern part of the country, are 27°C and 80%, respectively. As for the nutrients, *T. cutaneum* can thrive on the nutrients of decayed wood or on those released by the decaying fungi. Tatami mats, a floor fitting made of straw and peculiar to Japan, are not unsanitary in ordinary conditions. However, if their moisture content rises to about 20%, they become heavily contaminated by fungi, bacteria, and mites. We also identified nutrients for *T. cutaneum* in budgerigar droppings (Shimazu et al., 1984). Since *T. cutaneum* grows best at a temperature of 25-28°C with a relative humidity of 80% or more in the presence of damp wood or vegetation, HP by *T. cutaneum* is likely to occur in other countries with a similar climate and home environment.

V. Pathological Features

The histopathological appearance of pulmonary lesions in summer-type HP is similar to that of other types of HP (Kawanami et al., 1983). The lesions consist of a combination of bronchiolitis and alveolitis with granuloma. The alveolitis, seen in virtually all cases, consists predominantly of lymphocytes accompanied by variable numbers of macrophages, plasma cells, and polymorphonuclear leukocytes. The lymphocytes are mostly composed of T cells, with a relatively higher percentage of CD8 cells (suppressor/cytotoxic T cells) than CD4 cells (helper/inducer T cells) as assessed by immunohistological analysis with monoclonal antibodies against different lymphocyte subpopulations. The infiltrate is usually patchy in distribution with a tendency to more severe involvement of peripheral regions. Granulomas are characterized by being immature, loose, and noncaseating with giant cells (Fig. 4). Masson's body often coexists with other findings. In specimens obtained by transbronchial lung biopsy (TBLB), granuloma formation is observed in approximately 60% of acute and subacute forms of the disease (Yoneda, 1983).

VI. Clinical Features

The clinical presentation of summer-type HP is acute, subacute, or chronic, depending on frequency, intensity, and duration of inhalational exposure and perhaps on host or other factors that determine immunopathogenesis. The patient becomes sensitized to *T. cutaneum*, after a variable period of exposure, by inhalation at home. Both respiratory and systemic symptoms

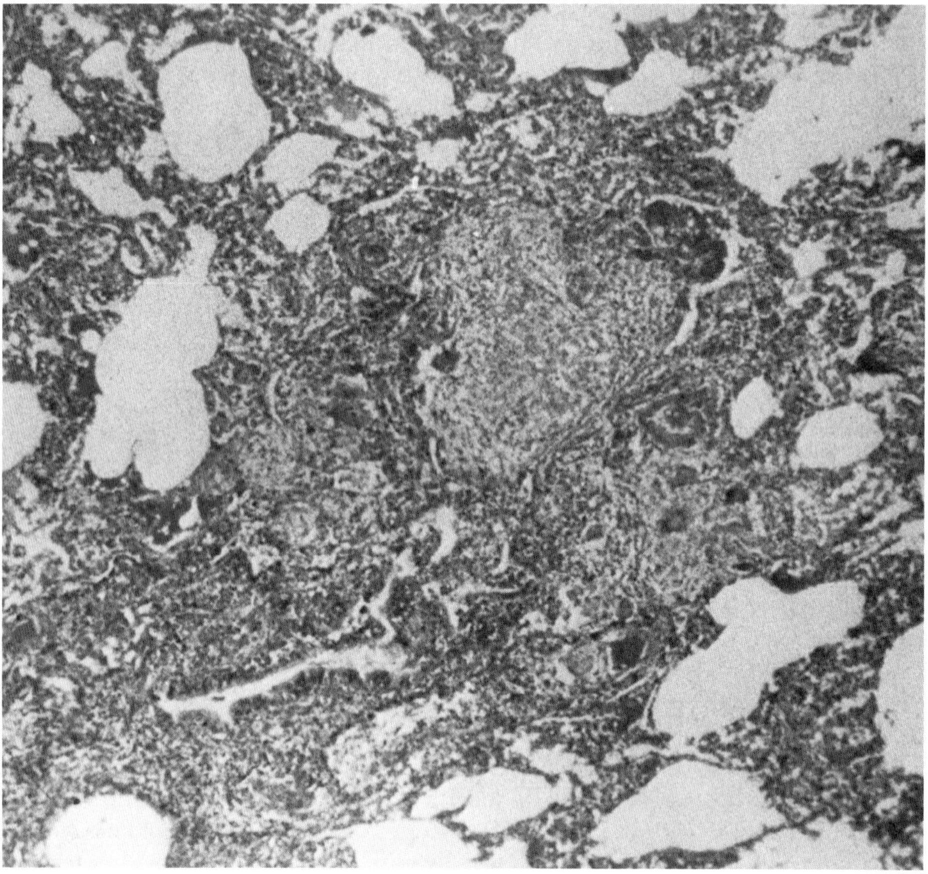

Figure 4 A lung specimen from a patient with summer-type HP; bronchiolitis and granulomatous alveolitis with an infiltrate of mononuclear cells (hematoxylin and eosin, × 200; courtesy of Dr. Ryousuke Ishihara, Kobe Central City Hospital).

consisting of fever, cough, sputum, and fatigue occur insidiously in most cases. Then cough, fever, and dyspnea gradually become prominent. Cough is most common but not universal. Fever of 37-40°C is seen in about 90% of patients. Exertional dyspnea is also seen in approximatley 80%. The most important diagnostic clue is that the symptoms only appear when the patient is at home during the summer season from May to October. After the patient is admitted to the hospital, the symptoms generally resolve spontaneously within several days or weeks. However, they recur 4 to 8 h after reexposure upon the patient's return home. During the winter season they spontaneously subside. Asthma is almost never a symptom. The chronic form of the disease is also occasionally reported. Its clinical symptoms also include exertional dyspnea similar to that of the chronic form of the groups of HP.

Physical examination shows bibasilar or more generalized crepitant end-inspiratory rales in any of the forms of presentation. Fever is common after acute exposure. Cyanosis may be seen in severe cases. Clubbing is not expected.

VII. Laboratory Findings

Laboratory studies are nonspecific except for anti-*T. cutaneum* antibody activity in patients' serum and BALF samples (see section on Diagnosis). A polymorphonuclear leukocytosis up to 15,000/mm^3 with a shift to young forms is detected in acute and subacute forms. Eosinophilia of up to 10% is occasionally observed. C-reactive protein (CRP) is positive in most cases. The erythrocyte sedimentation rate (ESR) is either slightly or moderately increased. The serum level of free interleukin-2 receptor rises, probably reflecting the activation of T lymphocytes in the lungs. Sometimes the tuberculin reaction is transiently negative, and levels of immunoglobulins, except for IgE, are mildly increased. Angiotensin-converting enzyme and adenosine deaminase activity in serum samples are usually normal.

Chest x-ray findings vary with the stage of the disease. They usually parallel the severity of the clinical symptoms and the impairment of pulmonary function. The fine nodular or ground-glass opacity is characteristic of the disease. The interstitial and alveolar nodular infiltrates are usually bilateral and equally distributed, but they frequently spare the apices (Fig. 5). Sometimes a diffuse, soft, patchy interstitial infiltrate occurs, with or without nodulation. No hilar lymph node enlargement is seen. The chest x-ray may be normal, even in symptomatic patients, in the early phase of the disease. In chronic cases, the chest x-ray findings may show the characteristics of diffuse interstitial fibrosis.

The pulmonary function test shows a restrictive impairment, reflecting the interstitial thickening seen histologically. During the acute attack, there is a decrease in lung volumes, particularly the vital capacity (VC). Diffusing capacity and lung compliance are also reduced. Airway resistance usually remains normal. Examination of blood gases shows arterial oxygen desaturation with a mild reduction in $PaCO_2$ due to chronic alveolar hyperventilation.

VIII. Diagnosis

The diagnostic criteria of summer-type HP are listed in Table 1. A history of recurrence of clinical and radiologic features suggestive of HP when the

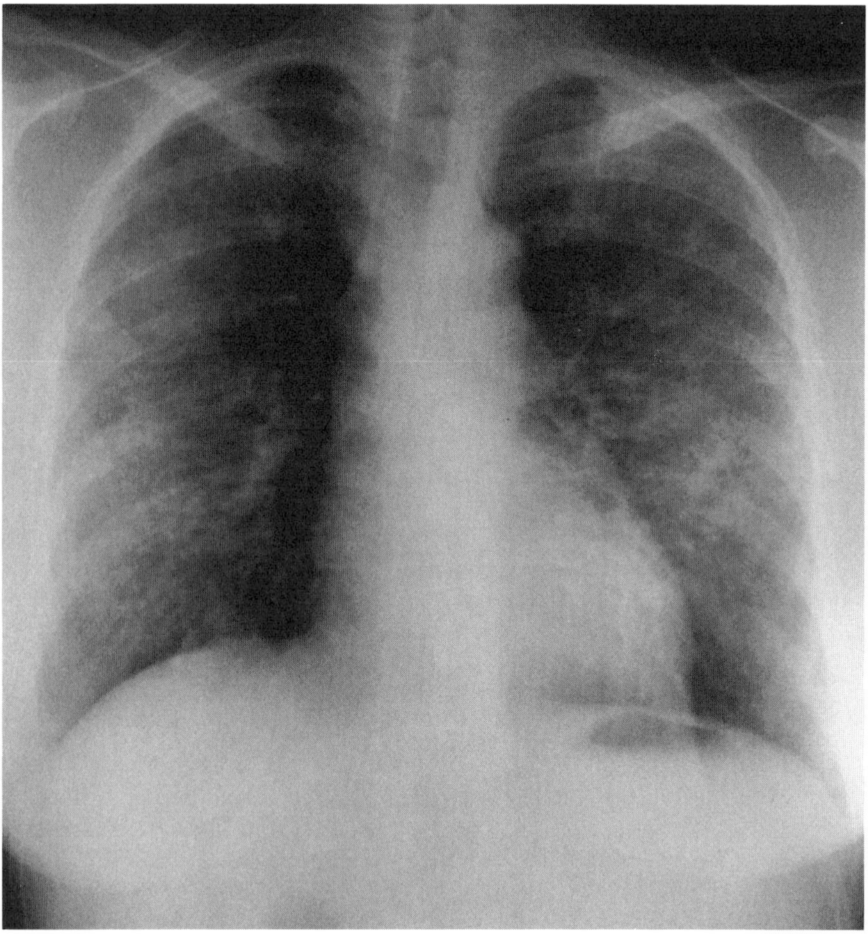

Figure 5 An acute form of summer-type HP shows diffuse fine nodular infiltrates.

Table 1 Diagnostic Criteria for Summer-Type HP

History of recurrent fever, cough, and dyspnea when at home during the summer
Laboratory, radiological, and functional respiratory records and morphological appearance compatible with those of the groups of HP
Presence of specific antibody activities to *T. cutaneum* in patient's serum and BALF samples
Positive inhalation challenge by natural exposure in the home environment or by bronchial exposure to *T. cutaneum* antigen
BALF findings with a predominance of T cells, especially with CD4/CD8 ratio of 1.0 or less

patient is at home should prompt immunological tests to establish the diagnosis of summer-type HP.

A. Anti-*T. cutaneum* Antibody

The assay of anti-*T. cutaneum* antibody activities in patients' serum and BALF samples is very useful to establish the diagnosis of summer-type HP, because the antibody activities are virtually positive in all cases of summer-type HP, but not in unexposed normal subjects (Shimazu et al., 1984; Soda et al., 1986). Details of the assay procedures are given below.

Test Samples

Both serum and BALF samples are available for assay of the antibody. These samples may be kept at −20°C until use.

Preparation of T. cutaneum *Antigen*

An isolate or preservative strain of the fungus may be used. We usually use two strains of different serotype: serotype I (TIMM 1573) and serotype II (TIMM 1318), which were originally taken from the homes of patients with summer-type HP, isolated in our laboratory, and preserved in Teikyo University Center for Medical Micology, Tokyo, Japan. The use of both strains is important because the antigen involving the pathological effects of the disease is the serotype-related polysaccharide-rich antigenic material, and because there is some difference between the prevalence of the antibody activities to the antigens of serotype I and II (see section on Pathogenesis).

Ethanol-Treated Antigen

Fungus grown in a Sabouraud agar or liquid medium with 1% yeast extract is treated with 100% ethanol for 24 h. The fungus was washed three times with distilled water (DW), suspended in phosphate buffered saline (PBS) (0.01 M, pH 7.4), and stored at −20°C until used. This antigen is used for the IFA method.

Culture-Filtrate Antigen

This antigen is prepared by the double dialysis method of Edwards (1972). Fungus is grown at 28 °C with intermittent aeration in a 5 L bottle containing 0.1 M glycine in 0.075 M NaCl (external phase, 1 L). The nutrient is composed of a double concentration of Sabouraud liquid medium (glucose 80 g and peptone 20 g, in 1 L of DW with 1% yeast extract. It is kept in Visking dialysis tubing (internal phase, 1 L). Fungus grown in an external phase is harvested after 28 days by centrifugation of the external phase at 6,000 *g* for 30 min, and may be used for ethanol-treated antigen. The supernatant was dialyzed against DW, passed through a 0.45 μm membrane filter, and freeze-dried. The lyophilized antigen is dissolved in saline at a concentration of 10 mg/ml. The stock solution is used, at appropriate dilutions, for the antigens in the gel double diffusion method, the enzyme-linked immunosorbent assay (ELISA) method, and the inhalation challenge test.

*Assay for Anti-*T. cutaneum *Antibody*

Three methods are available: the IFA method, the precipitating antibody method, and the ELISA method.

IFA Method

Ethanol-treated fungus is smeared on a glass slide and fixed by drying. The fungus smear is then covered with test serum and incubated at 37°C for 30 min. After removal with PBS, the smear is stained with fluorescent-labeled antiserum to human IgG, IgA, or gamma-globulin for 30 min, and then washed with three changes of PBS. After the smear is covered with a drop, it is examined using an ultraviolet microscope (Shimazu et al., 1984). This is a relatively simple and sensitive method, and is useful for screening isolates from the home environment.

Gel Double-Diffusion Method

The method of Gerber and Jones (1973) is performed using 1% agar in a veronal buffer (pH 8.6) containing 1% sodium citrate and 1% NaN_3. This is well known as a standard method in the detection of specific antibody activities in HP.

ELISA Method

Stock solution of the culture filtrate antigen is optimally diluted in carbonate-bicarbonate buffer (0.05 M, pH 9.6), and 0.1 ml of the antigen solution is placed in each well of a polystyrene plate at 4°C overnight. The plate has first been washed three times with PBS-Tween solution containing 0.05% Tween 20 (0.01 M, pH 7.4) for 5 min each time to remove any unbound antigen. Then, 0.1 ml of diluted serum in saline is added to the antigen-coated wells and incubated at 37°C for 1 h. After being washed three times in the same manner, 0.1 ml of substrate solution containing *p*-nitrophenyl-phosphate is added in 10% diethanolamine buffer (pH 9.8) at a concentration of 1 mg/ml. The wells are left for 30 min at room temperature. The reaction is stopped by adding 0.05 ml of NaOH (3M). The liberated yellow *P*-nitrophenolate is measured by a Titertek Multiskan (Soda et al., 1986). All data are shown by the absorbance at 492 nm obtained at appropriate sample dilutions. The ELISA method is a most sensitive method and is useful for the assay of BALF samples.

*Prevalence of Anti-*T. cutaneum *Antibody*

The prevalence of anti-*T. cutaneum* antibody assayed by the IFA method, the gel double diffusion method, and the ELISA method is listed in Table 2. When the antibody activity to *T. cutaneum* was assayed by the IFA method, 68 serum samples from acute and subacute cases were all positive, except in one case treated with corticosteroids. The IFA titers ranged from 1:32 to 1:1024. On the other hand, all control serum samples from the 100 normal subjects and the 100 patients with other pulmonary disease were less than 1:8, except for a level of 1:32 in a patient with sarcoidosis. The prevalence of the precipitating antibodies to *T. cutaneum* in serum from patients with summer-type HP and asymptomatic exposed family members was 89% and 13%, respectively. In contrast, the antibody activities were not detectable in 100 serum samples each from patients with other pulmonary disease and from unexposed normal subjects. The ELISA method was carried out on 68 serum samples, of which 68 (100%) samples were positive for IgG antibody activity and 55 (80%) samples were positive for IgA antibody activity. Measurement of the IgA antibody activity is especially helpful in differentiating between symptomatic and exposed asymptomatic family members (Ando et al., 1986; Soda et al., 1986).

B. Inhalation Challenge

Inhalation challenge is the only reliable test to determine the causative antigen of summer-type HP. There are two methods: natural inhalation challenge

Table 2 Prevalence of Anti-*T. cutaneum* Antibody in Serum Samples

	No. Tested	Precipitating Antibody (%)	IFA Titers (%)	ELISA Titers (%) IgG	ELISA Titers (%) IgA
Patients with summer-type HP	68	85	99	100	80
Asymptomatic family members	17	17	59	84	18
Patients with other pulmonary disease	100	0	0	ND	ND
Unexposed normal subjects	100	0	0	0	0

ND, not done.

in the patients' home environment and inhalation challenge with *T. cutaneum* antigen. Natural inhalation challenge is carried out by reexposing the patient to the suspected causative environment. Although it does not help in identifying the specific antigen responsible for the symptoms, it is very important for locating where the antigen is present. On the other hand, inhalation challenge with the suspected antigen is useful in determining the causative antigen. Our methods and results with use of the inhalation challenge are described below.

Natural Inhalation Challenge in the Home Environment

Patients are required to stay in the suspected places of their own home for several hours in conditions similar to when they had the symptoms at home previously. If the inhalation challenge is positive, the patient will have some of the symptoms and signs of cough, fever, dyspnea, and crepitant rales 4-8 h after exposure. Their symptoms and signs may disappear 12-24 h after they leave their home. One should give attention to the time of year: the result might be negative if the test is carried out after mid-autumn, since the dose of offending antigen may be reduced at that time.

All of our 40 cases showed positive results of the natural inhalation challenge in their home environment. The places where they had symptoms were generally shady, poorly ventilated, and poorly drained. In some cases, pet budgerigars were breeding in their rooms. These results indicate that the natural inhalation challenge in the patient's home environment is useful not only for the diagnosis of summer-type HP but also for detection of the offending antigen's colonizing places.

Inhalation Challenge with T. cutaneum *Antigen*

Six ml of culture filtrate antigen of *T. cutaneum* (2.5 mg/ml) is inhaled through an ultrasonic nebulizer without use of a nose clip. To avoid hyperventilation, a 1 min recess every 5 min may be given. During the next 24 h, two sets of data are recorded: (A) symptoms and signs (37°C or higher fever, appearance of dry cough, appearance of exertional dyspnea, appearance of crepitant rales) and (B) changes in laboratory data (increase of 30% or more in leukocytes, positive CRP, decrease of 10 mmHg or more in PaO2, decrease of 15% or more in VC, decrease of 20% or more in carbon monoxide diffusing capacity [DLCO]). Judgment is as follows: strongly positive, if all four of A, or two or more of both A and B are observed; mildly positive, if two or more of either A or B are observed; negative, if anything other than the above. The clinical features from inhalation challenge with *T. cutaneum* are identical to those of clinical illness. These appeared 4-8 h after exposure, and disappear after persisting for 6-12 h.

We performed the inhalation challenge with the culture filtrate antigens prepared from two strains of different serotypes of *T. cutaneum* (TIMM 1573, serotype I; TIMM 1318, serotype II) on patients with summer-type HP and asymptomatic exposed family members (Ando et al., 1990). Of the 17 patients with summer-type HP, 16 reacted to the inhalation challenge with either or both serotypes of culture filtrate antigen of *T. cutaneum*, while 2 asymptomatic exposed family members did not respond to either antigen. One patient who gave a negative reaction to both antigens of serotypes I and II showed a mild reaction to serotype III isolated from her home, as assessed by inhalation challenge in winter. The most interesting findings were that the reactivity was related to the serotype of the inhaled *T. cutaneum* antigen, and that there was a good correlation between the serotype of inhalation-challenge-positive antigens and that of *T. cutaneum* isolated from the patients' homes. In other words, inhalation challenge in patients with summer-type HP is provoked by the serotype-related antigen of *T. cutaneum*, reflecting the sensitization of these patients in their home. This finding should be noted when the causative antigen of HP induced by mold is determined by the inhalation challenge test.

C. Skin Test

In general, a skin test with appropriate antigen is very useful in the diagnostic evaluation of allergic disorders. For HP, however, the test is not useful because available antigens are crude, irritating, and nondiscriminatory. In summer-type HP, a skin test with crude culture filtrate antigen of *T. cutaneum* in patients with summer-type HP evoked a late or dual-phase reaction in all patients tested. The time course was identical to that of the symptoms and signs that appeared after inhalation challenge with the same antigen. However, 10% of unexposed normal controls also experienced a similar reaction. Thus, a skin test with the crude antigen is not helpful in the diagnosis of the disease at the present time. It is possible, however, that a skin test with a purified serotype-related polysaccharide antigen may become useful for diagnosis.

D. BAL

The utility of BAL in the diagnosis of summer-type HP is obvious. The BAL findings of acute and subacute forms of the disease are characterized by an increase of lymphocytes, particularly T cells (Nakayama et al., 1983). In contrast to sarcoidosis, in which the increased lymphocyte population is due to CD4 cells, the lymphocytes in the summer-type HP patients are predominantly CD8 cells, and the CD4/CD8 ratios drop to 1.0 or less (Ando et al., 1990). When symptoms subside, the BAL lymphocytes exhibit a recovery of

CD4 cells, a decrease in CD8 cells, and an increase in the CD4/CD8 ratio to the normal range (Ishihara et al., 1988). These findings are consistent with those in other types of HP reported (Costabel et al., 1986; Trentin et al., 1988). In the acute phase of the disease, neutrophils are also seen in a relatively higher percentage in the BAL cells, as in idiopathic pulmonary fibrosis. However, the increase of BAL neutrophils in idiopathic pulmonary fibrosis is not accompanied by a marked increase in lymphocytes (Reynolds, 1987). The assay of specific IgG and IgA antibody activities to *T. cutaneum* in BALF is very useful in the diagnosis of summer-type HP (Ando et al., 1986; Soda et al., 1988).

IX. Prognosis

The prognosis is good for patients whose disease is recognized in its early stages and who are removed from exposure to the antigen. However, if *T. cutaneum* is not eliminated from the patients' home, attacks usually recur. The recurrence rate the next summer is approximately 40%. The prevalence of the chronic form remains uncertain, but undoubtedly there are some patients who have developed chronic respiratory failure.

X. Treatment

A. Prevention and Management

Elimination of the antigen from the patient's environment is important in treating HP. In summer-type HP, most patients need hospitalization for the entire summer season because of recurrence of their disease on returning home. Since patients' conditions often fail to improve in their home environment, they are compelled to move into another house. We have succeeded, however, in discharging many patients to their own homes at summer season by intensively cleaning the colonizing places. Thus, to find and clean the colonizing places of the causative agent are very important for managing this disease. The usefulness of open-plate and house dust cultures for indoor sampling of causative agents of allergic pulmonary diseases has been proved by studies on bronchial asthma and HP. For summer-type HP, we stress the usefulness of the swab culture method to find the colonizing places of the causative agents. Undoubtedly, atmospheric *T. cutaneum* is scattered in the air from colonizing places, such as floor mats, bed clothes, and old damp wood, since most patients demonstrated extensive symptoms 4-8 h after sweeping. Accordingly, we stress the efficacy of cleaning the patient's home.

While the cleaning or sterilization of a hospital or factory has been fully demonstrated, that of a home has been little studied. In our preliminary examination, we tested the sensitivity of *T. cutaneum* to certain disinfectants. We found it was sterilized completely within 5 min by solutions of 5% sodium hypochlorite, 70% ethanol, 0.05% chlorohexidine gluconate, or a mixture of ethanol and chlorhexidine gluconate. But in practice, disinfecting with the disinfectants alone could not prevent recurrence. Therefore, we gave special attention to removal of the colonizing locations. This proved effective enough to prevent recurrence because it was based on thorough environmental studies. There is no home without molds, but in some homes the molds need to be controlled. Further studies of the efficacy and techniques of the cleaning and sterilization of homes are needed.

In the treatment of summer-type HP, we proved a cause and effect relationship. In other words, the colonization of *T. cutaneum* in a patient's home causes the outbreak of the disease, and the elimination of *T. cutaneum* from the home results in no recurrence the next summer. HP induced by indoor mold has been reported in other countries, but the causative antigens were not identified. We recommend assessment and cleaning of the home to prove, locate, and eliminate the causative agent.

B. Drug Therapy

Mildly acute episodes clear spontaneously if patients are removed from their homes. More severe attacks or progressive impairment require treatment with corticosteroids at dosages equivalent to prednisolone, 40-60 mg daily, and other routine supportive care such as oxygen treatment. The prednisolone should be continued until there is significant clinical improvement, clearing on the roentgenogram, and return of pulmonary function tests to normal. This may be continued for 1-2 weeks, depending upon the response, and tapered slowly unless a relapse occurs. Corticosteroid treatment is generally not effective in improving pulmonary function in patients with the chronic and fibrotic form.

XI. Case Reports

A. Case 1

A 75-year-old man had a fever of 38-39°C in July, 1987. Cough and sputum increased gradually. On August 24, he was admitted to a hospital. He was treated with antibiotics under the diagnosis of acute respiratory infection and discharged home 2 weeks after. On September 16, he was readmitted to the hospital because of recurrence of his symptoms and was treated again with antibiotics for 2 weeks. He was then well until the next summer season, when fever developed with cough and exertional dyspnea. In May, 1988, he was admitted to another hospital with severe dyspnea; he recovered with oxygen therapy. Based on a suspicion of summer-type HP, he was allowed to go home to see whether his illness would relapse. Eight hours after exposure, there was a recrudescence of symptoms with high fever of 39.8°C, cough, dyspnea, and general malaise.

He was then admitted to Kumamoto University hospital on June 13. On admission he was afebrile with a dry cough. Physical examination showed crepitation at both lung bases. The chest x-ray showed bilateral diffuse micronodular infiltration. The leukocyte count was $6100/mm^3$, with 13.4% eosinophils. The ESR was 108/h. The C-reactive protein (CRP) level was 1.31 mg/dl. Free interleukin-2 receptor level in the serum was elevated to 1036 U/ml (normal range, 80-300 U/ml). Pulmonary function test revealed a forced vital capacity (FVC) of 74.8% of predicted value and a forced expiratory volume in 1 s of 71.0% of FVC. The single-breath DLCO was 14.0 ml/min/mmHg, 104% of predicted value. PaO_2 was 68.4 mmHg and $PaCO_2$ was 34.1 mmHg. TBLB revealed a noncaseous granulomatous alveolitis. On June 20, BALF was performed with three aliquots of 50 ml physical saline instilled in the right anterior basal segmental bronchus. The recovery volume was 47% of the instilled amount and there was an increased total number of cells (59×10^4/ml) with 95% lymphocytes, 2% neutrophils, and 3% alveolar macrophages. Levels of CD3-positive (T) cells were 98% and the CD4/CD8 ratio was 0.41.

Serum IFA titers to serotype I (TIMM 1573) and serotype II (TIMM 1318) of *T. cutaneum* were each 1:128. Serum precipitating antibody to the culture filtrate antigen of serotype II was positive, while that to serotype I was negative. Inhalation challenge with the culture filtrate antigen of serotype II was strongly positive, but that with serotype I was weakly positive. A home environmental mycological survey was carried out on June 18. His home was shady, surrounded with a high fence and trees on every side, and there was a poorly drained place outside. Some strains of *T. cutaneum* were isolated from tatami mats in the living room and from decayed wood in the kitchen, where ventilation was poor and the humidity high. The isolates were found to be of both serotypes, I and II. His home was extensively disinfected. All tatami mats were replaced with new ones, and a broken drainpipe was repaired. After the elimination of *T. cutaneum* was confirmed, he was discharged home on August 2, and experienced no recrudescence.

B. Case 2

A patient with familial summer-type HP (three of four family members were symptomatic and one was asymptomatic) was admitted to Kumamoto University hospital on October 21, 1985. A 43-year-old married man noticed cough, sputum, dyspnea, fever, and weight loss of 10 kg at the end of June.

On July 20, he was admitted to a hospital with severe dyspnea. After admission he became well gradually, but recrudescence occurred upon returning home. His wife experienced general fatigue and intermittent fever, and his young daughter had exertional dyspnea. Their symptoms and signs and laboratory data on admission were compatible with those of patients with summer-type HP. The elder daughter, a smoker, was free from symptoms.

Results of mycological and immunological studies in this family case were as follows: serotype I of *T. cutaneum* was isolated from the moist and decayed floor near the kitchen. All three patients were reactive to the inhalation challenge with the crude culture filtrate antigen from the isolate but not to the culture filtrate antigen prepared from serotype II of *T. cutaneum* isolated from another patient's house. The elder daughter, an asymptomatic family member, did not show any response to either antigen, although her serum and BALF samples showed anti-*T. cutaneum* antibody activities to both antigens. BAL was examined 24 h after the inhalation challenge. All three patients showed a marked increase of polymorphonuclear leukocytes and lymphocytes, but the asymptomatic family member showed almost normal values. This was the first clinical report indicating the importance of serotype-related antigen in mold-induced HP. The reason the elder daughter, whose HLA-typing was the same as that of her father, was free from the disease is uncertain, but smoking might be a factor since none of the others smoked.

XII. Summary

Summer-type HP, the most prevalent type of HP in Japan, is caused by seasonal mold contamination in the home environment. The major causative agent of the disease is *T. cutaneum*, an athrospore-forming yeast. The fungus grows best in warm, moldy, decaying organic matter such as decayed wood, floor mats, used pillows, and budgerigar droppings. *T. cutaneum* is apt to scatter in the air from the colonizing places. The inhaled fungi sensitize susceptible patients intratracheally and induce the disease. Serotype-related polysaccharide-rich substance(s) of the fungus has a potent antigenicity that can induce granulomatous alveolitis. An assay of *T. cutaneum* antibody is very useful to establish the diagnosis of the disease because the antibody activity is virtually positive in all cases of the disease. Elimination of *T. cutaneum* from the colonizing places successfully prevents recrudescence. Summer-type HP, a new disease in the groups of HP, is peculiar to Japan at the present time. Soon, however, it is likely to be found in other countries, especially in temperate and tropical regions, where *T. cutaneum* is present.

References

Ando, M., Yoshida, K., Soda, K., and Araki, S. (1986). Specific bronchoalveolar lavage IgA antibody in patients with summer-type hypersensitivity pneumonitis induced by *Trichosporon cutaneum*. *Am. Rev. Respir. Dis.* **134**:177-179.

Ando, M., Yoshida, K., Sakata, T., Soda, K., Sugimoto, M., Suga, M., Nakashima, H., and Araki, S. (1988). Environmental and mycological studies on the causative agent of summer-type hypersensitivity pneumonitis. In *Proceedings of the XI World Congress on Sarcoidosis and Other Granulomatous Disorders*. Edited by C. Grassi, G. Rizzato, and E. Pozzi. Amsterdam, Excerpta Medica, pp. 681-684.

Ando, M., Hirayama, K., Soda, K., Okubo, R., Araki, S., and Sasazuki, T. (1989). HLA-DQw3 in Japanese summer-type hypersensitivity pneumonitis induced by *Trichosporon cutaneum*. *Am. Rev. Respir. Dis.* **140**:948-950.

Ando, M., Sakata, T., Yoshida, K., Yamasaki, H., Araki, S., Onoue, K., and Shinoda, T. (1990). Serotype-related antigen of *Trichosporon cutaneum* in the induction of summer-type hypersensitivity pneumonitis: correlation between serotype of inhalation-challenge positive antigen and that of the isolates from patients' homes. *J. Allergy Clin. Immunol.* **85**:36-44.

Cormier, Y., Bélanger, J., and Laviolette, M. (1986). Persistent bronchoalveolar lymphocytosis in asymptomatic farmers. *Am. Rev. Respir. Dis.* **133**:843-847.

Costabel, U., Bross, J. J., Rühle, K. H., Löhr, G. W., and Matthys, H. (1985). Ia-like antigens on T-cells and their subpopulations in pulmonary sarcoidosis and in hypersensitivity pneumonitis. *Am. Rev. Respir. Dis.* **131**:337-342.

Dobashi, K., Nakazawa, T., Nagasawa, T., Umegai, Y., Inazawa, M., Tomioka, S., Fueki, R., and Kobayashi, S. (1980). A case of hypersensitivity pneumonitis caused by *Candida albicans*. *Jpn. J. Intern. Med.* (in Japanese) **69**:574-579.

Edwards, J. H. (1972). The double dialysis method for producing farmer's lung antigens. *J. Lab. Clin. Med.* **79**:683-688.

Emmons, C. W., Binford, C. H., Utz, J. P., and Kwon-Chung, K. J. (1977). *Medical Mycology*, 3rd ed. Philadelphia, Lea & Febiger, pp. 181-184.

Fink, J. N. (1984). Hypersensitivity pneumonitis. *J. Allergy Clin. Immunol.* **74**:1-9.

Gerber, J. D., and Jones, R. D. (1973). Immunologic significance of Aspergillin antigens of six species of *Aspergillus* in the serodiagnosis of aspergillosis. *Am. Rev. Respir. Dis.* **108**:1124-1129.

Gravesen, S., Larsen, L., Gyntelberg, F., and Skov, P. (1986). Demonstration of microorganisms and dust in schools and offices: an observational study of non-industrial buildings. *Allergy* **41**:520-525.

Haslam, P. L., Dewar, A., Butchers, P., Primett, Z. S., Newman-Taylor, A., and Turner-Warwick, M. (1987). Mast cells, atypical lymphocytes, and neutrophils in bronchoalveolar lavage in extrinsic allergic alveolitis: comparison with other interstitial lung diseases. *Am. Rev. Respir. Dis.* **135**:35-47.

Ishihara, R., Hasegawa, M., Okazaki, M., Kataue, N., Sakamoto, M., Iwasaki, H., Umeda, B., and Nakai, H. (1988). Bronchoalveolar lavage findings in patients with summer-type hypersensitivity pneumonitis: comparison of symptomatic and asymptomatic summer seasons. *Jpn. J. Thorac. Dis.* (in Japanese) **26**:236 (abstract).

Johnson, K. J., Wilson, B. S., Till, G. O., and Ward, P. A. (1984). Acute lung injury in rat caused by immunoglobulin A immune complexes. *J. Clin. Invest.* **74**:358-369.

Johnson, K. J., Ward, P. A., Kunkel, R. G., and Wilson, B. S. (1986). Mediation of IgA induced lung injury in the rat: role of macrophages and reactive oxygen products. *Lab. Invest.* **54**:499-506.

Kawai, T., Tamura, M., and Murao, M. (1984). Summer-type hypersensitivity pneumonitis: a unique disease in Japan. *Chest* **85**:311-317.

Kawanami, O., Basset, F., Barrios, R., Lacronique, J. G., Ferrans, V. J., and Crystal, R. G. (1983). Hypersensitivity pneumonitis: light- and electron-microscopic studies of 18 lung biopsies. *Am. J. Pathol.* **110**: 275-289.

Keller, R. H., Swartz, S., Schlueter, D. P., Bar-Sela, S., and Fink, J. N. (1984). Immunoregulation in hypersensitivity pneumonitis: phenotypic and functional studies of bronchoalveolar lavage lymphocytes. *Am. Rev. Respir. Dis.* **130**:766-771.

Kreger-van Rij, N. J. W. (1984). Trichosporon Behrend. In *The Yeasts: A Taxonomic Study*, 3rd ed. Edited by N. J. W. Kreger-van Rij. Amsterdam, Elsevier Science Publishers, pp. 933-962.

Lumpkins, E. D., Corbit, S. L., and Tiedeman, G. M. (1973). Airborne fungi survey: culture-plate survey of the home environment. *Ann. Allergy* **31**:361-370.

McSharry, C., Banham, S. W., and Boyd, G. (1985). Effect of cigarette smoking on the antibody response to inhaled antigens and the prevalence of extrinsic allergic alveolitis among pigeon breeders. *Clin. Allergy* **15**: 487-494.

Miyagawa, T., Ochi, T., and Takahashi, H. (1978). Hypersensitivity pneumonitis with antibodies to *Cryptococcus neoformans*. *Clin. Allergy* **8**: 501-509.

Miyagawa, T., Hamagami, S., Ochi, T., Osugi, T., Kikui, M., and Takahashi, H. (1982). Japanese summer-type hypersensitivity pneumonitis: studies using *Cryptococcus* antigen. *Clin. Allergy* **12**:343-354.

Moore, V. L., Pedersen, G. M., Hauser, W. C., and Fink, J. N. (1980). A study of lung lavage materials in patients with hypersensitivity pneumonitis: in vitro response to mitogen and antigen in pigeon breeders' disease. *J. Allergy Clin. Immunol.* **65**:365-370.

Morrow, M. B., Meyer, G. H., and Prince, H. E. (1964). A summary of air-borne mold surveys. *Ann. Allergy* **22**:575-587.

Nakayama, T., Yasuoka, S., Nakayama, T., Mitsui, M., Kawano, T., Ozaki, T., and Tsubura, E. (1983). Characteristics of the cellular composition, especially the lymphocyte sub-populations of bronchoalveolar lavage fluid from patients with summer-type hypersensitivity pneumonitis. *Clin. Allergy* **13**:107-117.

Ochi, T., Miyagawa, T., Oosugi, T., Fujita, K., Yamamoto, H., Kikui, M., and Takahashi, H. (1978). Studies on forty-two cases of hypersensitivity pneumonitis. *Jpn. J. Thorac. Soc.* (in Japanese) **16**:320-328.

Ochi, T., Miyagawa, T., Kikui, M., Osugi, T., Takahashi, H., Izumi, T., Tachibana, M., Yamamoto, M., Iwai, K., Yamamoto, M., Kondo, A., Hosoda, Y., and Mikami, R. (1980). A new type of hypersensitivity pneumonitis in Japan. In *Proceedings of the VIIIth International Conference on Sarcoidosis and Other Granulomatous Diseases.* Edited by W. J. Williams and B. H. Davies. Cardiff, Wales, Alpha Omega, pp. 705-710.

Pepys, J. (1969). Hypersensitivity disease of the lungs due to fungi and other organic dusts. In *Monographs in Allergy.* Edited by P. Kallos. New York, Albert J. Phiebig, Inc., pp. 1-149.

Reinherz, E. L., Kung, P. C., Goldstein, G., and Schlossman, S. F. (1979). Separation of functional subsets of human T cells by a monoclonal antibody. *Proc. Natl. Acad. Sci. USA* **76**:4061-4065.

Reynolds, H. Y. (i987). Bronchoalveolar lavage. *Am. Rev. Respir. Dis.* **135**: 250-263.

Richards, M., and Wales, C. (1954). Atmospheric mold spores in and out of doors. *J. Allergy* **116**:429-439.

Rittner, C., Sennekamp, J., Mollenhauer, E., Rösinger, N., Niese, D., Lüttkenhorst, M., Baur, M. P., and Stroehmann, I. (1983). Pigeon breeder's lung: association with HLA-DR3. *Tissue Antigens* **21**:374-379.

Roberts, R. C., and Moore, V. L. (1977). Immunopathogenesis of hypersensitivity pneumonitis. *Am. Rev. Respir. Dis.* **116**:1075-1090.

Saito, K. (1904). Untersuchungen über die atmosphärischen pilzkeime. *J. Coll. Sci. Tokyo* **18**:1-58.

Sakata, T., Soda, K., Ando, M., Shimazu, K., and Araki, S. (1988). Experimental hypersensitivity pneumonitis in rabbits induced by *Trichosporon cutaneum*: role of local cellular and humoral immune responses. *J. Clin. Lab. Immunol.* **25**:191-199.

Salvaggio, J. E. (1987). Hypersensitivity pneumonitis. *J. Allergy Clin. Immunol.* **79**:558-571.

Sasazuki, T., Nishimura, Y., Muto, M., and Ohta, N. (1983). HLA-linked genes controlling immune response and disease susceptibility. *Immunol. Rev.* **70**:51-75.

Seeliger, H. P. R., and Schröter, R. (1963). A serological study on the antigenic relationships of the form genus *Trichosporon. Sabouraudia* **2**: 248-263.

Selman, M., Terán, L., Mendoza, A., Camarena, A., Martinéz-Cordero, E., Lezama, M., and Rubio, H. M. (1987). Increase of HLA-DR7 in pigeon breeder's lung in a Mexican population. *Clin. Immunol. Immunopathol.* **44**:63-70.

Shimazu, K., Ando, M., Sakata, T., Yoshida, K., and Araki, S. (1984). Hypersensitivity pneumonitis induced by *Trichosporon cutaneum. Am. Rev. Respir. Dis.* **130**:407-411.

Soda, K., Ando, M., Shimazu, K., Sakata, T., Yoshida, K., and Araki, S. (1986). Different classes of antibody activities to *Trichosporon cutaneum* antigen in summer-type hypersensitivity pneumonitis by enzyme-linked immunosorbent assay. *Am. Rev. Respir. Dis.* **133**:83-87.

Soda, K., Ando, M., Sakata, T., Sugimoto, M., Nakashima, H., and Araki, S. (1988). Clq and C3 in bronchoalveolar lavage fluid from patients with summer-type hypersensitivity pneumonitis. *Chest* **93**:76-80.

Solal-Céligny, P. H., Laviolette, M., Hébert, J., and Cormier, Y. (1982). Immune reactions in the lungs of asymptomatic dairy farmers. *Am. Rev. Respir. Dis.* **126**:964-967.

Soler, P., Nioche, S., Valeyre, D., Basset, F., Benveniste, J., Burtin, C., Battesti, J. P., Georges, R., and Hance, A. J. (1987). Role of mast cells in the pathogenesis of hypersensitivity pneumonitis. *Thorax* **42**:565-572.

Solomon, W. R. (1976). A volumetric study of winter fungus prevalence in the air of midwestern homes. *J. Allergy Clin. Immunol.* **57**:46-55.

Trentin, L., Marcer, G., Chilosi, M., Sci, M. C., Zambello, R., Agostini, C., Masciarelli, M., Bizzotto, R., Gemignani, C., Cipriani, A., Vittorio, G. D., and Semenzato, G. (1988). Longitudinal study of alveolitis in hypersensitivity pneumonitis patients: an immunologic evaluation. *J. Allergy Clin. Immunol.* **82**:577-585.

Warren, C. P. W. (1977). Extrinsic allergic alveolitis: a disease commoner in nonsmokers. *Thorax* **32**:567-569.

Yamasaki, H., Ando, M., Sakata, T., Araki, S., and Onoue, K. (1990). Importance of serotype-related antigen in the induction of experimental hypersensitivity pneumonitis by *Trichosporon cutaneum* in rabbits: correlation between granulomatous alveolitis and cellular and humoral immune responses to polysaccharide-rich antigen. *Am. Rev. Respir. Dis.* **141**:734-742.

Yoneda, R. (1983). Extrinsic allergic alveolitis and TBLB. *Pathol. Clin. Med.* (in Japanese) **1**:599-604.

Yoshida, K., Ando, M., Sakata, T., and Araki, S. (1988). Environmental mycological studies on the causative agent of summer-type hypersensitivity pneumonitis. *J. Allergy Clin. Immunol.* **81**:475-483.

Yoshida, K., Ando, M., Sakata, T., and Araki, S. (1989). Prevention of summer-type hypersensitivity pneumonitis: effect of elimination of *Trichosporon cutaneum* from the patients' homes. *Arch. Environ. Health* **44**:317-322.

Yung, C. W., Hanauer, S. B., Fretzin, D., Rippon, J. W., Shapiro, C., and Golzalez, M. (1981). Disseminated *Trichosporon beigelii* (*cutaneum*). *Cancer* **48**:2107-2111.

20

Diffuse Panbronchiolitis

MASANORI KITAICHI, KOICHI NISHIMURA, and TAKATERU IZUMI

Chest Disease Research Institute
Kyoto University
Kyoto, Japan

I. Introduction

Yamanaka and colleagues (1969) proposed the term *diffuse panbronchiolitis* (DPB) to define the disease entity characterized by chronic inflammation of respiratory bronchioles. Results of a Japanese nationwide survey on DPB were reported by Homma et al. (1983); a round table conference on DPB was held at the 11th World Congress on Sarcoidosis and Other Granulomatous Disorders in Milan in September, 1987.

Clinical features of DPB are chronic cough, sputum, and dyspnea particularly on exertion and associated chronic airflow limitation with or without restrictive pulmonary dysfunction and arterial hypoxemia. A chest roentgenogram reveals bilateral small nodular shadows often with hyperinflation of lungs. Patients with DPB usually do not have chronic inflammatory disorders except in the upper and lower respiratory system.

Although the clinical features of DPB are quite well known in Japan, very few cases have been reported from outside Japan.

This chapter reviews the current thoughts on diffuse panbronchiolitis. An illustrative case report is included to emphasize the clinical features and course of the disease.

II. Case Report

A 38-year-old Japanese man was examined in our hospital in July, 1987, because of chronic productive cough of 5 years' duration and diffuse abnormal shadows on a chest x-ray. He had worked as a medical technician in a hospital for many years. An exsmoker, he had smoked one to two packs of cigarettes daily for 7 years, before quitting 10 years earlier. He underwent an operation for chronic paranasal sinusitis at the age of 12. He was single; his parents and four siblings were alive and well. He had no history of exposure to industrial dusts or animals and was taking no medications. He denied any history of peripheral edema, orthopnea, dyspnea attacks, arthralgia, or alimentary problems.

At the time of admission in August, 1987, he appeared well except for an occasional cough and sputum production. His height was 177.7 cm and he weighed 60 kg. His body temperature was normal (35.6°C), his pulse rate was 100/min and his respiration rate was 28/min. His blood pressure was normal (118/60 mmHg). The accessory respiratory muscles were slightly prominent and clubbing of the fingers was suspected. Expirations were not prolonged. On auscultation of the chest, coarse crackles were heard over both lower lung areas.

Chest x-rays showed multiple small nodular shadows throughout the lung fields and a mild degree of hyperinflation of the lungs (Fig. 1). High resolution-computed tomographic scans of the lungs revealed small rounded and linear opacities (Fig. 2). Bronchographic examination of the right lung showed that small bronchi were mildly dilated (Fig. 3).

He expectorated approximately 10 ml of purulent sputum daily. Bacteriological culture revealed a few *Hemophilus influenzae*. No eosinophils were seen.

Urinalysis was normal. Mantoux's skin test was positive.

Blood examinations showed positive C-reactive protein and RA test, and elevated cold hemagglutination titer (x64), while antibody for *Mycoplasma pneumoniae* was negative. Otherwise, blood examinations were not remarkable: white blood cells 7200/mm^3 with 64% neutrophils, 28% lymphocytes, 4% eosinophils, and 4% monocytes. Serum protein was 7.8 g/dl with 16% gamma-globulins. The serum IgG level was 1564 mg/dl, IgA 425 mg/dl, and IgM 147 mg/dl; The IgE level was slightly elevated (425 IU/ml). Liver function test and serum electrolyte levels were normal in titer while antinuclear antibody and anti-DNA antibody were negative and alpha-1-anti-trypsin level was normal (262 mg/dl) (normal range, 148-317). Serum titers of CH_{50} and C_3 were almost normal (42.9 CH_{50}U/ml and 89 mg/dl, respectively; normal range, 30.0-40-0 and 59-120, respectively).

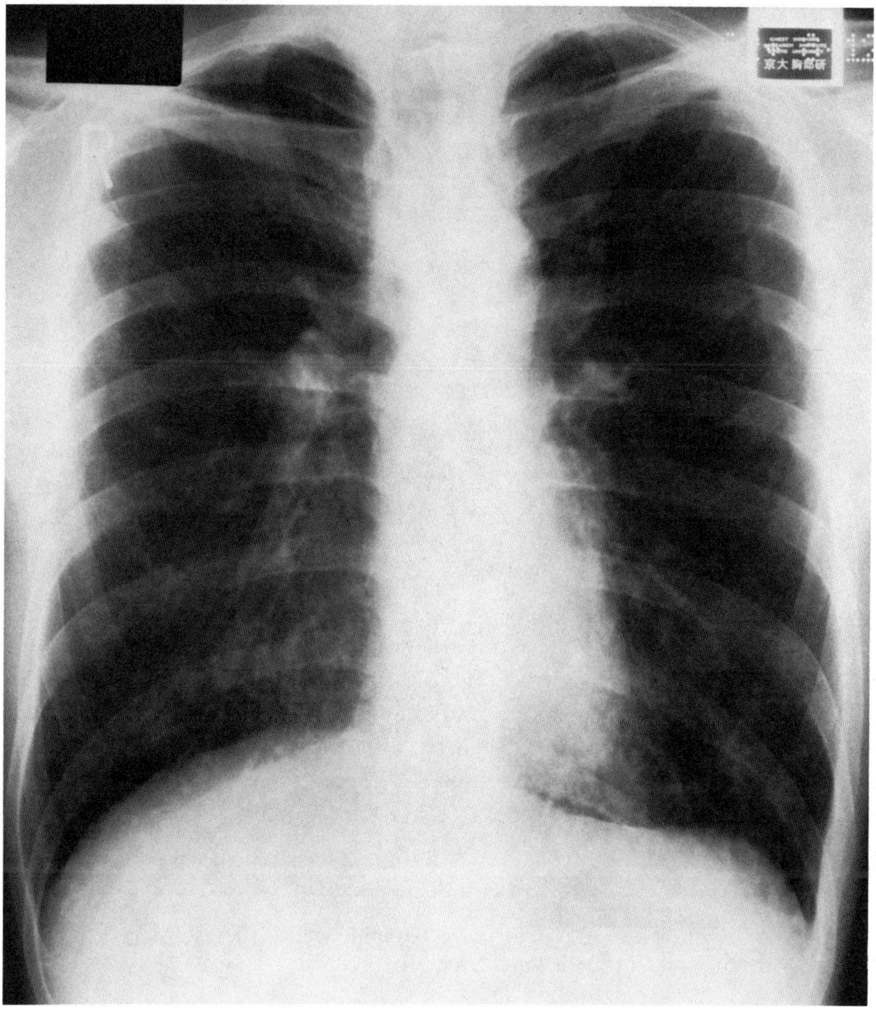

Figure 1 Chest x-ray on August 12, 1987, shows multiple small nodular shadows throughout bilateral lung fields and a mild degree of hyperinflation of the lungs.

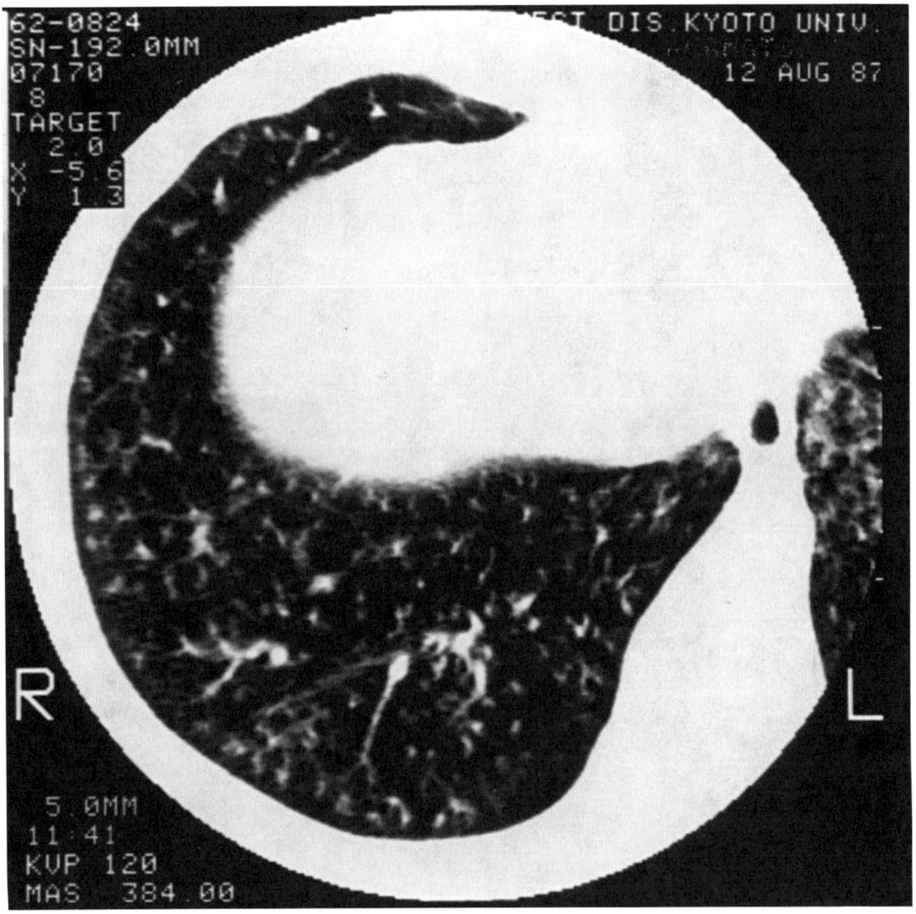

Figure 2 High-resolution computed tomographic scan of the right lung on August 12, 1987, shows small rounded and linear opacities.

Arterial blood gas analysis revealed hypoxemia during room air breathing: PaO_2 63.0 mmHg, $PaCO_2$ 41.3 mmHg, and pH 7.4 with widened A-a DO_2 (30.0 mmHg).

Pulmonary function test showed an irreversible obstructive dysfunction: vital capacity (VC) 3.40 L; 81.7% of the predicted value; forced vital capacity (FVC) 3.34 L; 73.4% predicted; forced expiratory volume in 1 s ($FEV_{1.0}$) 2.16 L; 55.8% of the predicted value and FEV_1/FVC 64.7%. There was no improvement after the inhalation of a beta-2 agonist. Methacholine challenge

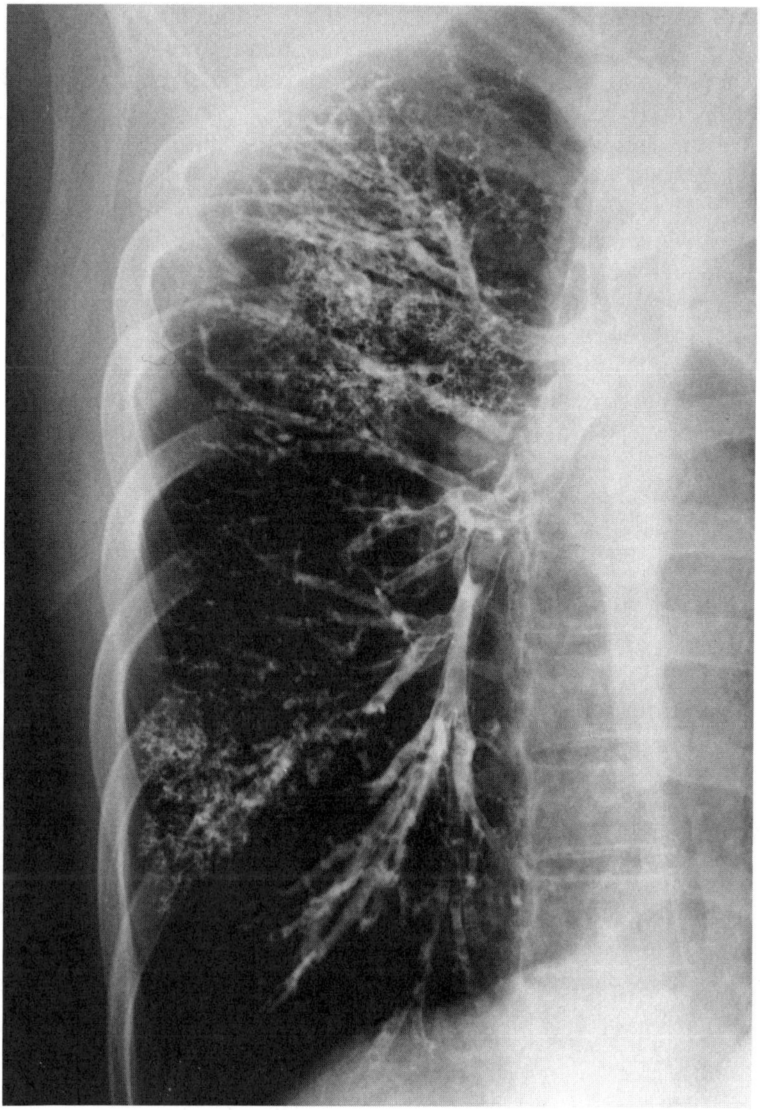

Figure 3 Bronchogram of the right lung on August 13, 1987, shows mild dilation of small bronchi.

test showed no airway reactivity even at the maximum methacholine concentration when PD_{20} was more than 225 cumulative units.

The diffusing capacity for carbon monoxide (DL_{CO}) using the single breath method was 29.4 ml/min/mmHg (95.5% of the predicted value). Body plethysmograph showed normal total lung capacity (TLC) with increased residual volume (RV): TLC 7.45 L; 107.5% of the predicted value and RV 4.12 L: 215.7% of the predicted value. The static compliance of the lung was increased: Cst 0.42 L/cmH_2O (normal range, 0.15-0.30).

He underwent an open lung biopsy to determine a definitive diagnosis on September 1, 1987. At the time of the left thoracotomy performed for lung biopsy, pleural adhesion or effusion was not noted. Biopsy samples were obtained from the upper and lower lobes of the left lung (segments 3 and 9). Both biopsy samples showed yellow nodular lesions measuring 2-6 mm in the lung parenchyma, although the degree of the lesions was milder in the upper lobe sample. Bacteriological examinations revealed few *Hemophilus influenzae* cultured from the fresh biopsy samples.

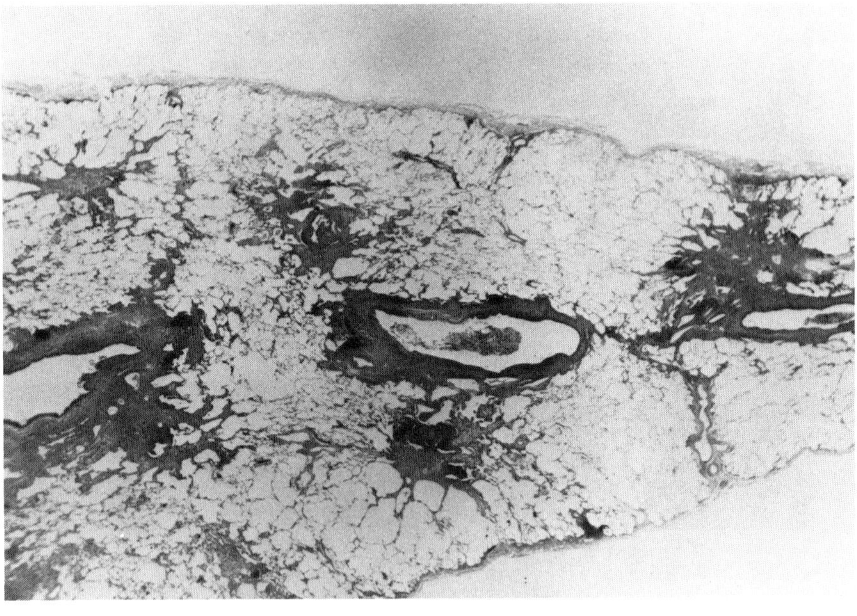

Figure 4 The lung biopsy sample from segment 9 of the left lower lobe shows several foci of centrilobular chronic inflammatory and fibrotic lesions and dilation of membranous bronchioles. The subpleural or peripheral zones of lobules were relatively free from lesions (Meyer's hematoxylin and eosin stain, ×5).

A biopsy sample of the lower lobe showed dilation of membranous bronchioles compared with the accompanying muscular pulmonary arteries. The bronchiolar lumen contained many PMN neutrophils and a few desquamated airway epithelial cells. The wall of membranous bronchioles showed focal desquamation of the epithelial layer and infiltration of many plasma cells, lymphocytes, and eosinophils. An elastic tissue stain showed inflammatory thickening of the lamina propria and partial disruption of elastic fibers of the airway wall. Regions of respiratory bronchioles and alveolar ducts showed chronic inflammatory lesions with fibrotic changes and interstitial accumulation of foamy cells, around which perifibrotic emphysematous changes were noted. Peripheral zones of lobules were often free from lesions (Figs. 4-6).

A biopsy sample from the upper lobe also showed predominantly centrilobular chronic inflammation with fibrotic changes and interstitial accu-

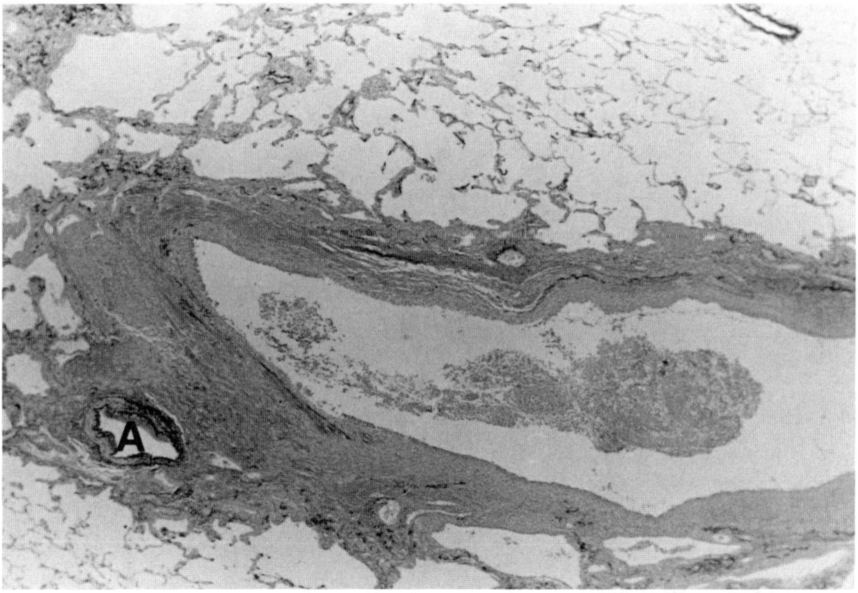

Figure 5 An elastic tissue stain of the lung sample in Figure 4. The membranous bronchiole showed dilation compared with the size of the accompanying muscular pulmonary artery (A). The bronchiolar lumen contained many PMN neutrophils, macrophages, desquamated airway epithelial cells, and basophilic exudates. The subepithelial layer of the bronchiole showed moderate infiltration of plasma cells, lymphocytes, and eosinophils with partial loss of the epithelial layer and partial disruption of elastic fibers of the wall (Weigert's elastic van Gieson stain, ×20).

mulation of foamy cells. A terminal portion of membranous bronchioles showed subepithelial infiltration of many plasma cells and a few eosinophils with fibrotic changes causing mild to moderate luminal stenosis. A few areas showed an accumulation of foamy cells with lymphoid cells in the wall of a respiratory bronchiole and adjacent alveolar ducts and alveoli; this is the unit lesion of panbronchiolitis described by Kitaichi (1988). PMN neutrophils and macrophages had infiltrated into the centrilobular terminal air spaces with basophilic exudates (Figs. 7-10).

After the lung biopsy, 2 g of ceftazidime (CAZ) was infused daily for 5 days and 2 g of latamoxef (LMOX) was infused daily for the next 16 days. Starting September 21, 1987, 600 mg of erythromycin orally was given daily. He was treated in the outpatient clinic for approximately 2 years and showed remarkable improvement (Fig. 11).

He visited our hospital on July 21, 1989, and claimed he expectorated less than five pieces of sputum daily and noted complete disappearance of exertional dyspnea. He had gained 5 kg to weigh 65 kg. No crackles were

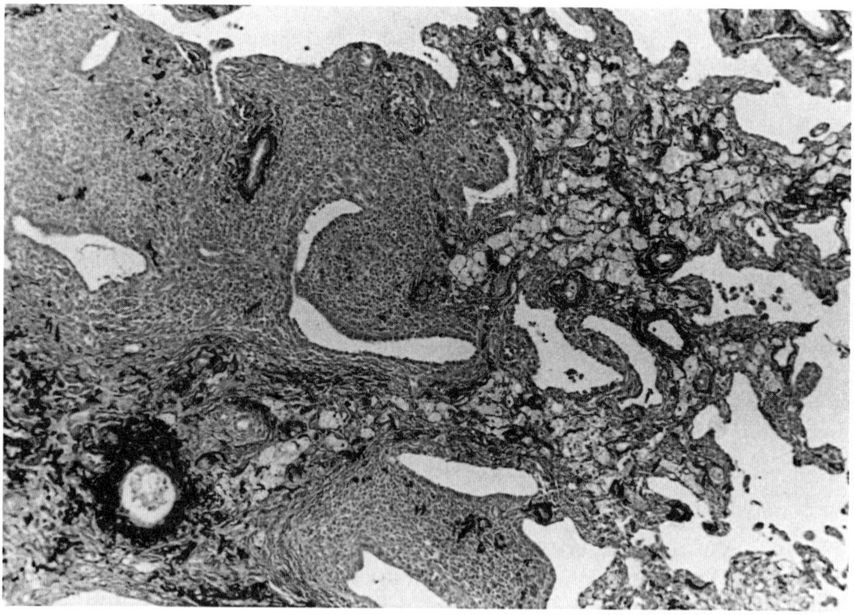

Figure 6 Another view of the same sample of the elastic tissue stain. One of the centrilobular chronic inflammatory lesions showed interstitial infiltration of lymphocytes and interstitial accumulation of foamy cells with fibrotic changes (Weigert's elastic van Gieson stein, ×50).

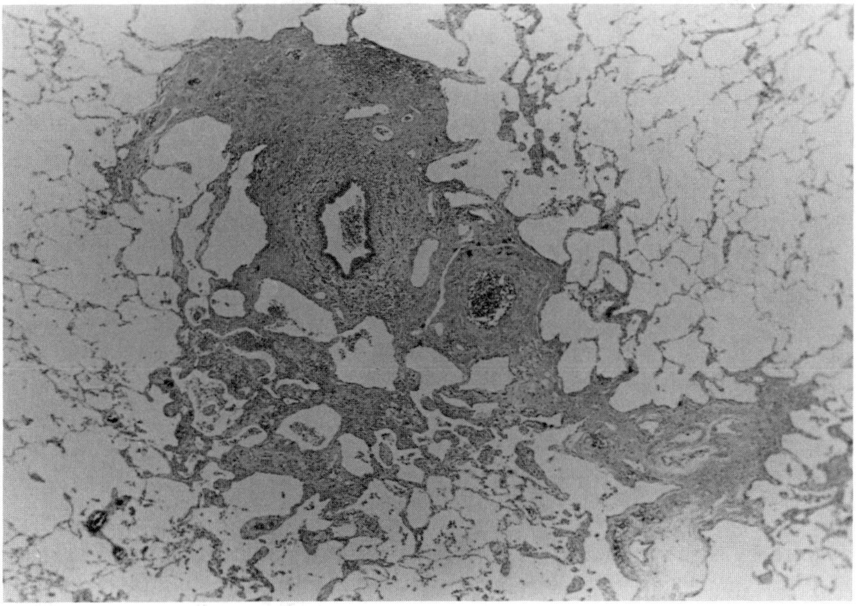

Figure 7 The biopsy sample from the segment 3 of the left upper lobe showed chronic inflammation and fibrotic lesions in and around the wall of a membranous bronchiole (Meyer's hematoxylin and eosin stain, ×20).

heard on the chest and the multiple small nodular shadows were reduced on a chest x-ray. The follow-up pulmonary function test showed a nadir on September 18, 1987, when FVC was 2.72 L: 59.6% of the predicted value; FEV_1 1.84 L: 47.7% predicted; and FEV_1/FVC 67.7%. In July 1989, a pulmonary function test showed better values: FVC 3.63 L: 83.5% predicted; FEV_1, 3.18 L: 87% predicted; and FEV_1/FVC: 87.8% (Fig. 11).

III. Epidemiological Aspects

A. Nationwide Surveys in Japan

The first nationwide survey of DPB was conducted in Japan from 1980 to 1982 under the sponsorship of the Ministry of Health and Welfare. Patients fulfilling the following criteria were admitted into the clinically diagnosed group:

1. Symptoms: chronic cough, sputum, and dyspnea on exertion
2. Physical signs: rales and rhonchi

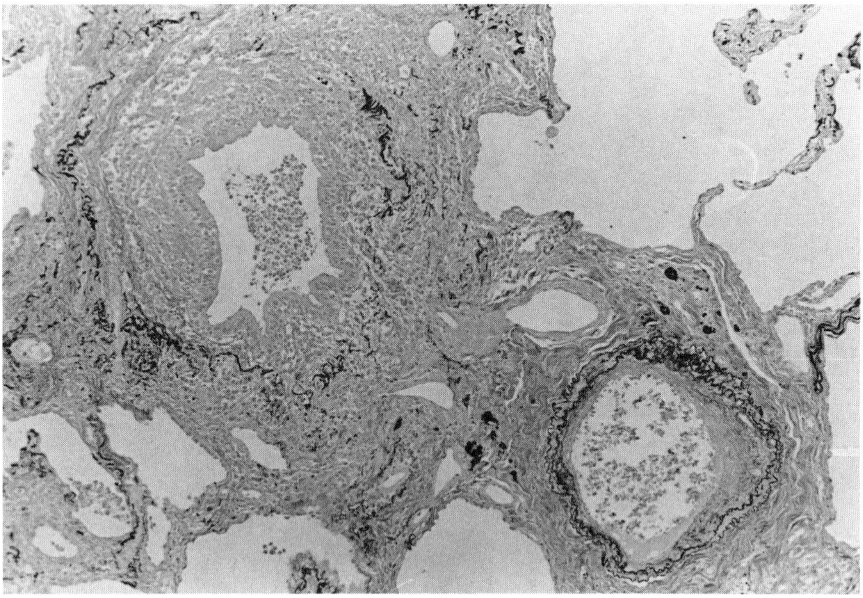

Figure 8 Higher magnification of an elastic tissue stain of the same region in Figure 7. The membranous bronchiole was stenosed, with subepithelial infiltration of many plasma cells and fibrotic changes. Elastic tissues in the bronchiolar wall showed partial disruption (Weigert's elastic van Gieson stain, ×50).

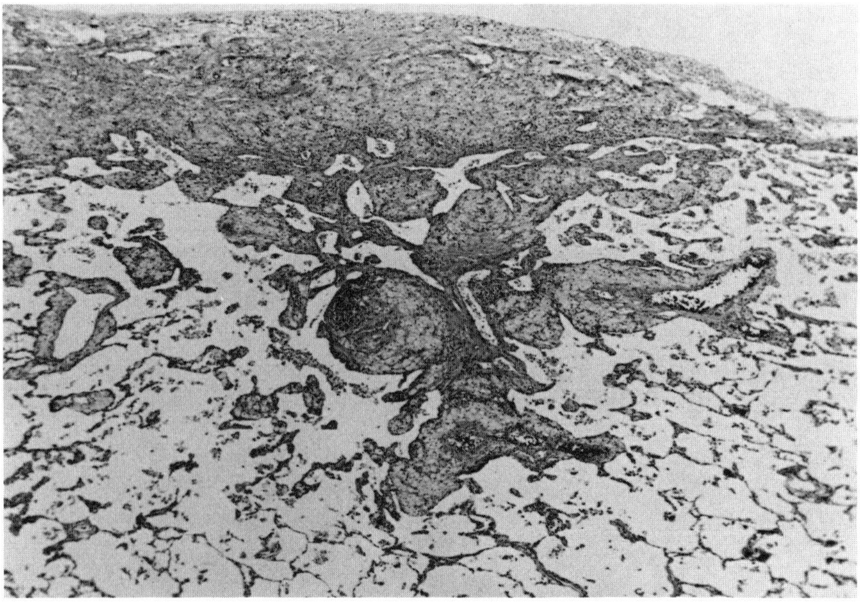

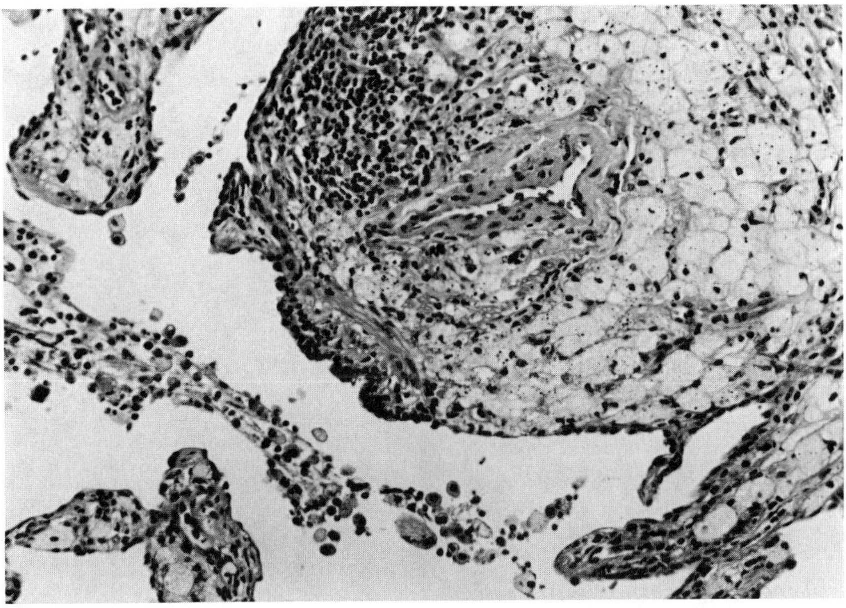

Figure 10 Higher-magnification view of Figure 9. The wall of a respiratory bronchiole showed accumulation of foamy cells with infiltration of lymphoid cells: the core portion of a unit lesion of panbronchiolitis. Accumulation of foamy cells was also seen in alveolar septae. Terminal airspace showed infiltration of macrophages and PMN neutrophils with basophilic exudates (Meyer's hematoxylin and eosin stain, ×200).

3. Chest x-ray findings: diffusely disseminated fine nodular shadows with hyperinflation of the lungs
4. Lung function studies (at least three conditions among the four abnormalities listed):
   a. $FEV_1/FVC < 70\%$
   b. $VC < 80\%$ of the predicted value
   c. $RV > 150\%$ of the predicted value or $RV/TLC > 45\%$
   d. $PaO_2 < 80$ mmHg

Figure 9 The lung biopsy sample from segment 3 of the left upper lobe showed an accumulation of foamy cells in the wall of respiratory bronchioles and adjacent alveolar ducts and alveoli. There was subpleural accumulation of foamy cells (Meyer's hematoxylin and eosin stain, ×20).

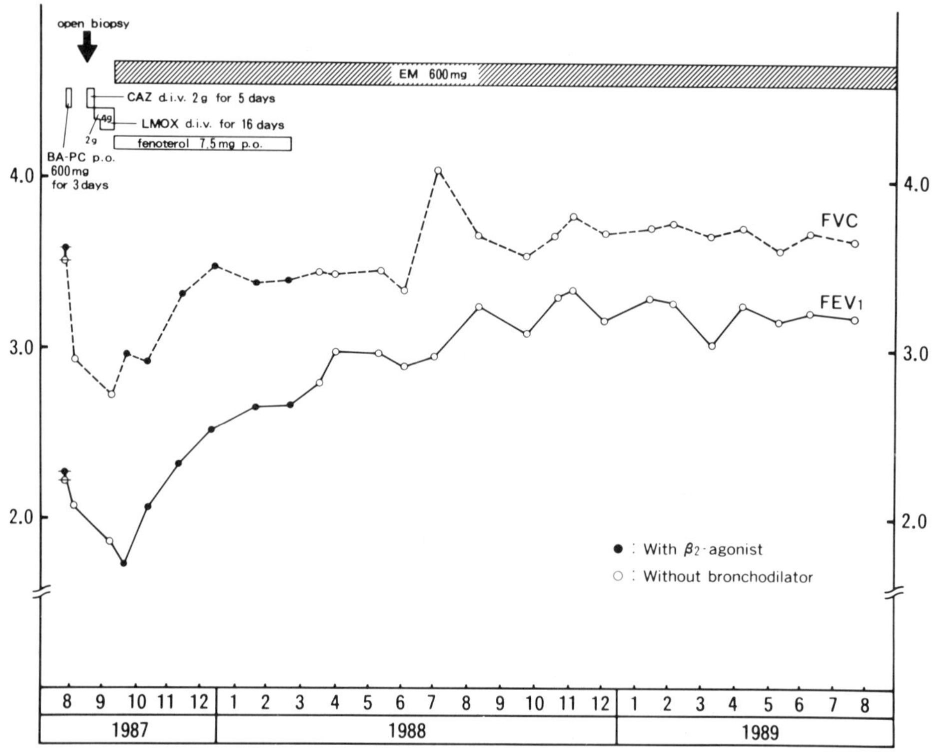

Figure 11 Patient's clinical course before and after the open lung biopsy done on September 1, 1987. The ordinate shows the value of FVC and FEV_1 in liters. BA-PC, bacampicillin; CAZ, ceftazidime; LMOX, latamoxef; EM, erythromycin.

The results have been summarized by Homma and co-workers (1983) and Izumi (1988). A total of 319 patients were diagnosed clinically as having DPB, including 48 patients with pathological findings. The 5 year survival of patients from the onset of dyspnea on exertion was 80.0%, and the 10 year survival was 53.9%.

The second nationwide survey of DPB was conducted in 26 major hospitals all over Japan in 1988 and 229 new cases (138 males and 91 females) were registered using the same diagnostic criteria of clinical DPB as in the first nationwide survey. The 26 hospitals participated in both nationwide surveys. After 1981, a tendency for the new patients to decline in frequency was observed, but a confirmation of the fact needs a longer term survey of DPB. The average survival years of 179 patients who died of DPB from the onset of exertional dyspnea was 14.1 ± 9.7 years. The survival time prior to

1980 for the 70 cases with DPB was 13.2 ± 10.1 years, while that after 1981 for 109 cases was 14.6 ± 9.5 years. These data shows no real advance in the treatment of DPB in the period studied.

B. Frequency in the Chest Disease Research Institute, Kyoto University

The frequency of DPB among patients with chronic airflow obstructive diseases in our Institute was reported by Izumi (1988) to be comparable to that of pulmonary emphysema, based upon clinical diagnostic criteria. Between June, 1982, and July, 1987, among cases of airflow obstructive diseases other than asthma, 47 cases were clinically diagnosed as having DPB while 53 cases were diagnosed as having pulmonary emphysema and 5 cases were suspected of having chronic bronchitis.

IV. Clinicopathological Correlation

A. Diffuse Panbronchiolitis

Five patients who underwent open lung biopsy and one patient who underwent lobectomy with a mean age of 35.2 years (range, 19-66) and 10 autopsy cases with a mean age of 58.5 years (range, 41-75) were studied.

Biopsy cases of DPB showed centrilobular inflammatory lesions with interstitial accumulation of foamy cells and fibrotic lesions. Accumulation of foamy cells was noted in the interstitium and alveolar spaces in the peripheral zones of lobules in several cases (Fig. 9).

In autopsy cases of DPB small bronchi and membranous bronchioles were usually dilated cylindrically throughout the lungs, as described by Nishimura and colleagues (1987). Many small yellow nodular lesions were noted in the lung parenchyma. The feature of PB unit lesions was recognized in all cases of DPB, as described by Kitaichi (1988), although the macroscopic yellow nodular lesions did not necessarily correspond to PB unit lesions.

Using serial section analysis, Maeda et al. (1987) studied the yellowish nodular lesions 2-4 mm in diameter in the lung parenchyma in 20 autopsy cases of DPB. They classified the centrilobular lesions into three types according to the presence or absence of intraluminal granulation tissue in the respiratory bronchioles, in addition to thickening of the walls of respiratory bronchioles. In their terminology, the granulation tissue varied considerably from fresh and active lesions abundant in proliferating fibroblasts and capillaries to those showing deposition of collagen fibers, hyalinization, and scarring. Contrary to the original theory that intramural bronchiolitis was an essential feature of DPB and bronchiolar obstruction was a type of modification due to secondary infection and occurred less commonly in DPB, they noted intraluminal granulation tissue in the respiratory bronchioles in 18 of the 20 autopsy cases and therefore concluded it to be an essential aspect of the DPB lesion. They discussed the differential diagnosis mainly in the context of bronchiolitis obliterans, as did King (1989).

Infertility in male cases of DPB is not observed, in contrast to cases of cystic fibrosis, Young's syndrome, and immotile cilia syndrome, which was reviewed by Davis et al. (1983). In 12 cases of DPB, sweat chloride concentration was reported to be reduced compared to that of healthy adults; none of the DPB cases showed a sweat chloride concentration over 60 mEq/L according to the study by Koshoubu et al. (1988). The bodies of patients with DPB did not show significant primary chronic lesions in the pancreas and gastrointestinal tracts, as seen in cases of cystic fibrosis and noted by Kitaichi (1988). Therefore DPB is a different entity from cystic fibrosis, although autopsy cases of both diseases showed bronchial dilation.

B. Comparative Clinicopathological Study of Inflammatory Airways Disorders

A total of 97 thoracotomy and 44 autopsy cases of inflammatory airways disorders in Japan, the United States, Canada, and the United Kingdom, including cases of DPB, chronic bronchitis, bronchiectasis, cystic fibrosis, *Mycoplasma pneumoniae* pneumonitis, hypersensitivity pneumonitis, bronchiolitis obliterans organizing pneumonia (BOOP), cryptogenic obliterative bronchiolitis, small airways disease, and follicular bronchitis/bronchiolitis, were studied pathologically by Kitaichi (1988) and Kitaichi et al. (1988) to clarify whether DPB is an independent clinical and pathological entity (Tables 1 and 2). We noticed that the most distinctive feature of DPB was an accumulation of foamy cells with lymphoid cells in the wall of a respiratory bronchiole and adjacent alveolar ducts and alveoli with a background of inflammatory airway lesions. This feature has been called the unit lesion of panbronchiolitis (PB unit lesion) by Kitaichi (1988) (Fig. 10). The frequency of the PB unit lesion in inflammatory airways disorders is shown in Table 3.

Chronic Bronchitis

Chronic bronchitis is basically diagnosed from clinical symptoms: expectoration of sputum for more than 3 months per year for more than 2 successive years. Pathological features have been described as increased Reid index or volume of glands, increased goblet cells in the bronchiolar epithelium, and mucin stasis in bronchiolar air spaces (Reid, 1954; Matsuba and Thurlbeck, 1973; Thurlbeck, 1976). It is rare to see cases of fatal chronic bronchitis in and around Kyoto and the authors noted only 1 case among some 300 adult autopsy cases. Five other fatal cases of chronic bronchitis were studied

Table 1 Cases of Inflammatory Airways Disorders

Disorder	Thoracotomy[a]	Autopsy	Total
DPB	6 (6)[b]	10 (10)[b]	16 (16)[b]
CB		6 (1)	6 (1)
BE	24 (21)	11 (11)	35 (32)
CF		13 (0)	13 (0)
Mycoplasma	7 (2)		7 (2)
HP	15 (11)		15 (11)
BOOP	29 (23)		29 (23)
Cryp OB	3 (2)	4 (0)	7 (2)
SAD	10 (0)		10 (0)
FB	3 (1)		3 (1)
Total	97 (66)	44 (22)	141 (88)

[a]Thoracotomy means an open lung biopsy except for a case of DPB with pulmonary adenocarcinoma and 24 cases of BE. The 25 cases underwent resection of pulmonary lobe(s).

[b]Numbers in parentheses show numbers of cases among Japanese.

Abbreviations: DPB: diffuse panbronchiolitis; CB: chronic bronchitis; BE: bronchiectasis; CF: cystic fibrosis; Mycoplasma: mycoplasma pneumonia; HP: hypersensitivity pneumonitis; BOOP: bronchiolitis obliterans organizing pneumonia (basically a type of interstitial pneumonia); Cryp OB: cryptogenic obliterative bronchiolitis; SAD: small airways disease (a generic term in North America for a disease showing features of bronchiolitis without any known entities); FB: follicular bronchitis/bronchiolitis.

at the University of Utah Medical Center in 1986. The six autopsy cases showed similar pulmonary lesions, as described above, and did not show accumulation of foamy cells in and around the walls of respiratory bronchioles (Fig. 12).

Bronchiectasis

Bronchiectasis was defined in the study as a long-standing pulmonary disorder excluding cystic fibrosis showing dilation of bronchi, which was attributed to clinical symptoms or required therapy. Among 11 autopsy cases, 4 cases showed dilation of bilateral bronchi including lower lobes. They did not show accumulation of foamy cells in and around the wall of respiratory bronchioles. Only 5 cases among 24 surgical cases of bronchiectasis showed interstitial accumulation of foamy cells (Figs. 13, 14). However, these cells had a tendency to spread out in the interstitium of peripheral lung tissues, and bronchiectasis was localized in these cases.

Table 2 A Summary of Histopathologic Features of Inflammatory Airways Disorders

	Bronchus	Membranous bronchiole	Respiratory bronchiole	Alveolar duct	Alveolus
DPB	Chronic mural inflammation Dilation in late stage		Mural and luminal inflammation with foamy cells in the wall		Interstitial accumulation of foamy cells
CB	Increase of glands and goblet cells	Increase of goblet cells with mucin stasis Mural bronchiolitis	Mucin stasis		
BE	Dilation with inflammation and hypervascularization in the wall Denudation of epithelial layer		Interstitial accumulation of foamy cells, rare.		
CF	Eosinophilic mucin stasis Dilation with mural hypervascularization and luminal acute inflammatory exudates Denudation of epithelial layer		Mural inflammation, mild		
Mycoplasma		Reparative epithelial metaplasia Mural bronchiolitis	Organizing exudates in air spaces		
HP			Organizing exudates in air spaces Cellular interstitial infiltrates and sarcoidlike granulomas		
BOOP			Granulation tissues in air spaces Cellular interstitial infiltrates		Septal fibrosis
Cryp OB	Mild mural inflammation	Granulation tissue formation in the lamina propria of the wall			
SAD		Muscular hypertrophy, chronic inflammation and subepithelial fibrosis in the wall; stenotic or dilated			
FB		Germinal centers and lymphoid follicles in and around the wall			

Table 3 Frequency of Unit Lesions of Panbronchiolitis

Disorder	Thoracotomy	Autopsy	Total
DPB	6/6 (100%)	10/10 (100%)	16/16 (100%)
CB		0/6	0/6
BE	5/24 (21%)	0/11	5/35 (14%)
CF		0/13	0/13
Myco	0/7		0/7
HP	0/15		0/15
BOOP	0/29		0/29
Cryp OB	0/3	0/4	0/7
SAD	0/10		0/10
FBB	0/3		0/3

Source: Kitaichi, M., Colby, T. V., et al. (abstract) *Am. Rev. Respir. Dis.* **137** (4): 155, 1988.

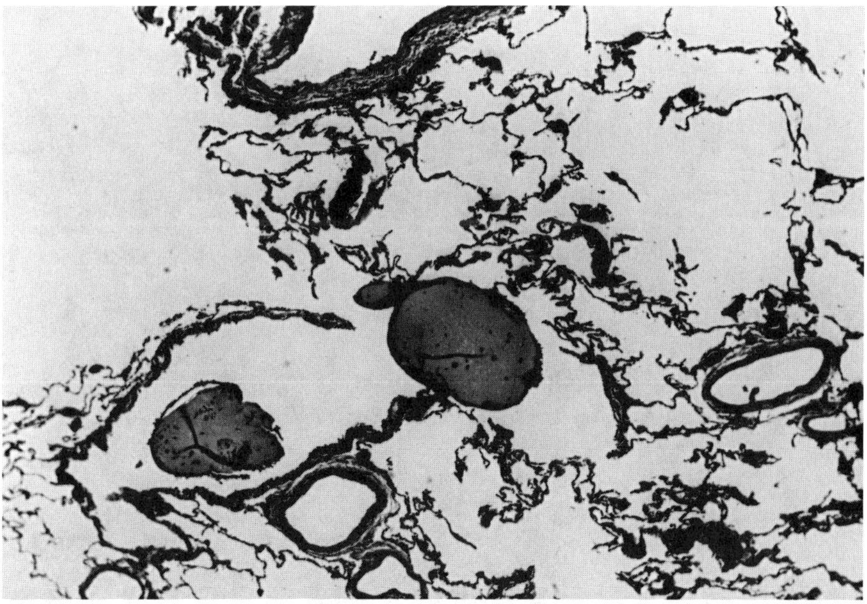

Figure 12 An autopsy case of chronic bronchitis. Mucin stasis was noted in the airspace of a respiratory bronchiole (Meyer's hematoxylin and eosin stain, ×20).

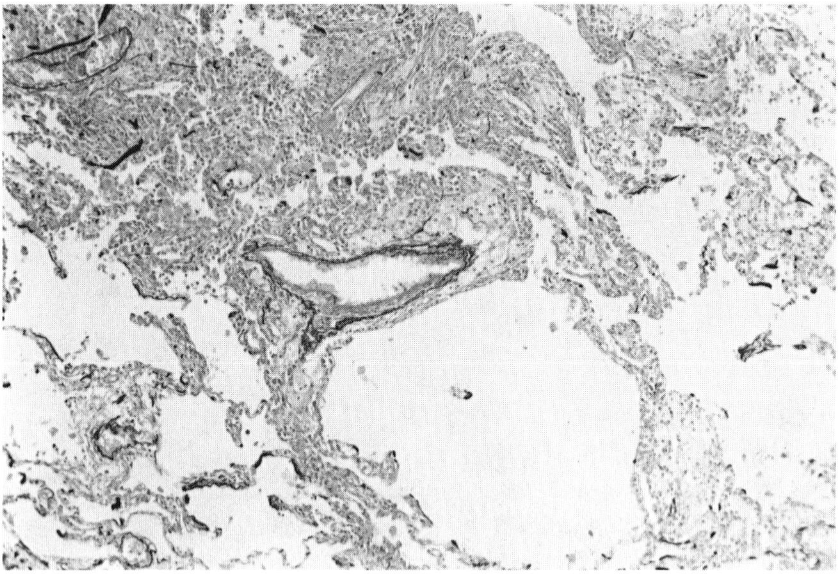

Figure 13 A surgical case of bronchiectasis. A 21-year-old Japanese woman underwent a right middle lobectomy after a 19 month symptomatic clinical course of localized bronchiectasis. A centrilobular inflammatory lesion showed accumulation of foamy cells around a muscular pulmonary artery (Meyer's hematoxylin and eosin stain, ×50).

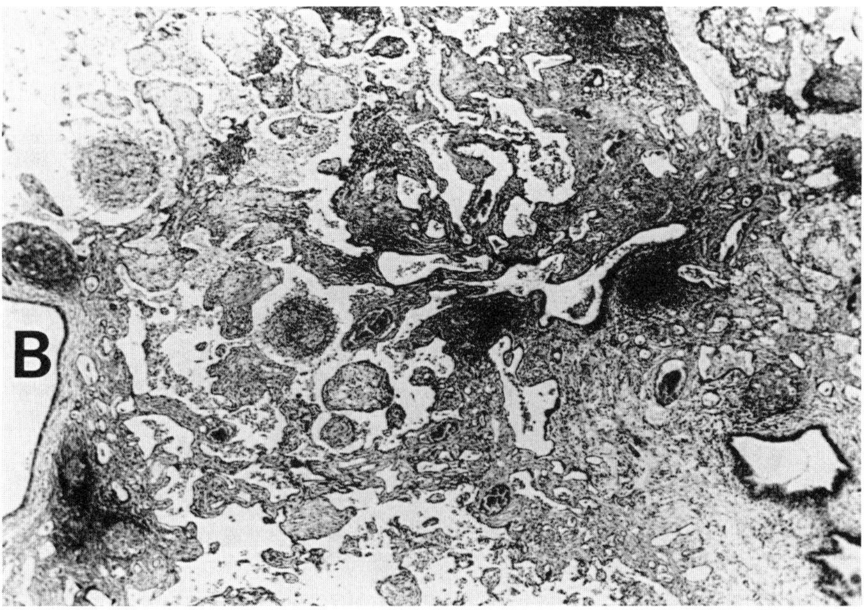

George and co-workers (1979) reported a 40 year experience of 3,133 cases of segmental bronchiectasis in their thoracic clinic since 1937, and noted that 1,067 of them underwent resection of the diseased bronchopulmonary segment and 99 (3.2%) underwent bilateral pulmonary resection.

Bronchiectasis was classified by Whitwell (1952) after a pathological study of 200 surgical specimens from 196 patients into follicular, saccular, and atelectatic bronchiectasis. Spencer (1985) cited this classification in his book. Gudbjerg (1955) reported that 6 among 112 cases of bronchiectasis showed involvement of the entire right and left lungs. Of these, four cases (3.6%) showed cylindrical-type bronchiectasis. Pathological studies of bronchiectasis were also done in 13 cases, including 11 autopsy cases, by Erb (1933); 35 lobectomy cases by Ogilvie (1941), who studied 31 histological specimens; 7 surgical cases by Moore et al. (1949); 45 surgical cases by Reid (1950); 2 autopsy cases by Cameron (1956); 3 surgical cases by Culiner (1963); and an autopsy case of diffuse bronchiectasis occurring after heroin intoxication by Warnock et al. (1972). Although Reid (1950) noted reduction of bronchial subdivision and Culiner (1963) noted obliterative changes of bronchi and bronchioles, none of these investigators noted interstitial accumulation of foamy cells such as the PB unit lesions in their histological studies of bronchiectasis. Nor did Rayl and colleagues (1961) note this kind of change, although they stated that cylindrical dilatation in chronic bronchitis usually had a generalized distribution.

Cystic Fibrosis

Cystic fibrosis is an inherited disease and often causes pulmonary complications in children, as summarized by Lloyd-Still (1983). Thirteen autopsy cases with a mean age of 13.9 years (range, 0.4-29) were studied. Pulmonary lesions showed marked dilation of multiple bronchi and membranous bronchioles with eosinophilic mucin stasis in their lumens. Areas of respiratory bronchioles did not show marked intramural changes or accumulation of foamy cells (Fig. 15).

Mycoplasma Pneumoniae *Pneumonia*

Approximately 90% of the DPB cases showed 64 times or higher cold agglutinin titers, but none showed elevation of serum antimycoplasma antibody titers, as reported by Izumi (1988).

Figure 14 Another surgical case of bronchiectasis. A 19-year-old Japanese man with Kartagener's syndrome underwent resection of the left middle lobe. The lung specimen showed marked dilation of bronchi and bronchioles (B) and formations of lymphoid follicles and germinal centers. There was extensive interstitial accumulation of foamy cells (Meyer's hematoxylin and eosin stain, ×20).

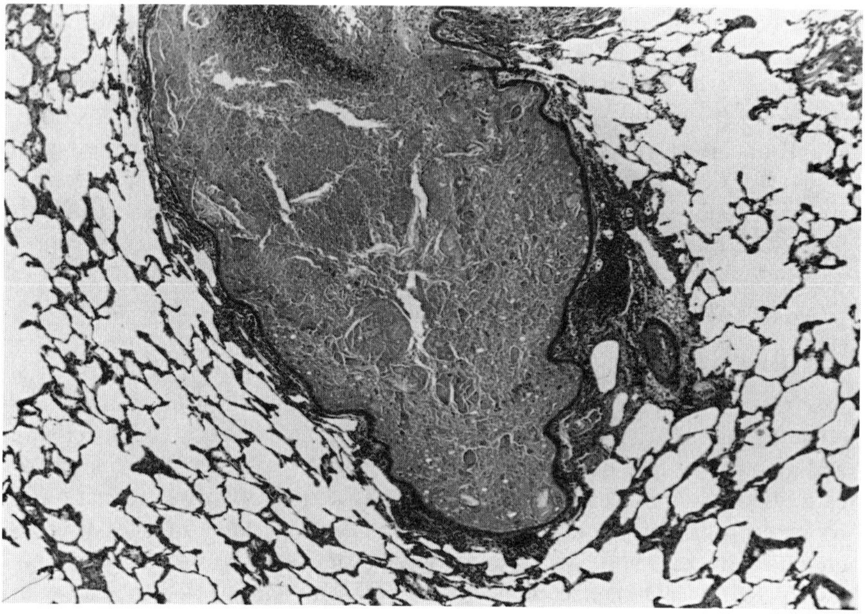

Figure 15 An autopsy case of cystic fibrosis. A membranous bronchiole showed marked dilation and was filled with eosinophilic mucin (Meyer's hematoxylin and eosin, ×50).

Seven biopsy cases with a mean age of 36.9 years who were proved microbiologically or serologically to have *Mycoplasma* infection showed a broad spectrum of inflammatory pulmonary lesions, including granulation tissues filling terminal and respiratory bronchioles (Fig. 16). A more distinct finding was reparative epithelial metaplasia of bronchioles, as reported by Rollins and co-workers (1986).

Hypersensitivity Pneumonitis

Fifteen biopsy cases with a mean age of 42.1 years were studied. They showed predominantly centrilobular lesions with bronchioloalveolitis, scattered small granulomas, and air-space accumulation of foamy cells, but none showed interstitial accumulation of foamy cells including PB unit lesions (Fig. 17). Histological features of these cases were summarized by Kitaichi (1986) and compared with those of pulmonary sarcoidosis.

Figure 17 A biopsy case of hypersensitivity pneumonitis. The respiratory bronchioles showed polypoid-type granulation tissues in the airspaces. Adjacent alveolar space showed foamy cells. Moderate number of lymphocytes had infiltrated into the interstitium (Meyer's hematoxylin and eosin stain, ×50).

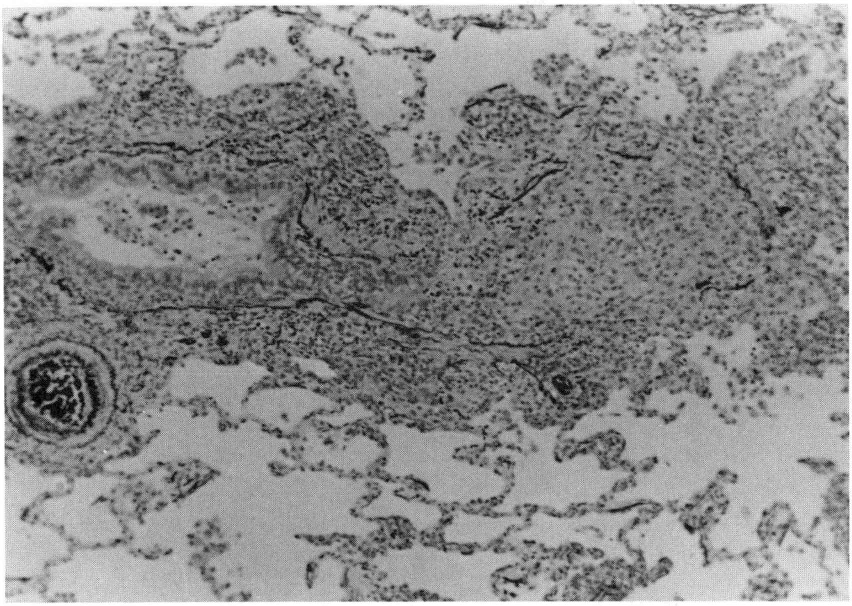

Figure 16 A biopsy case of *Mycoplasma pneumoniae* pneumonia. Terminal portion of the membranous bronchiole was obliterated with organizing and cellular exudate in the lumen (elastic Masson's stain, ×50).

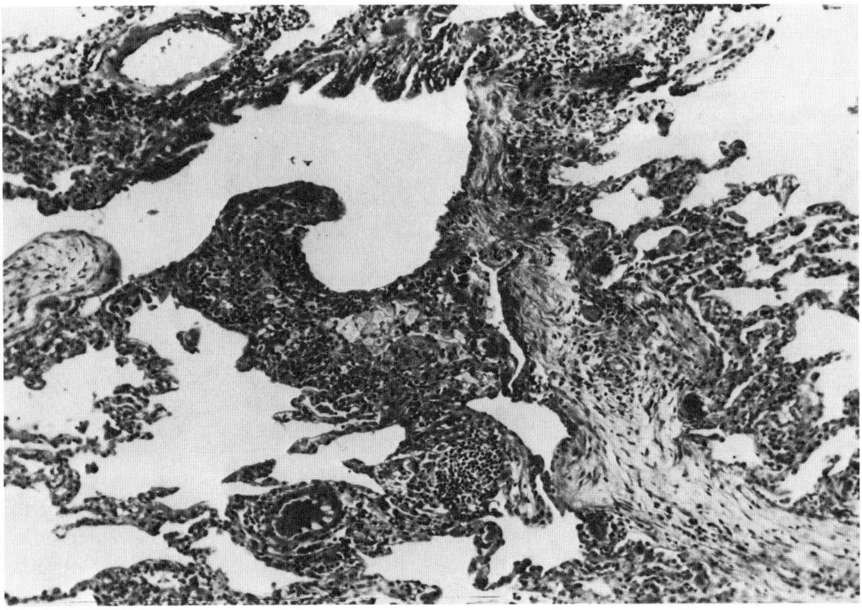

Bronchiolitis Obliterans Organizing Pneumonia

Because cases of idiopathic BOOP showed a polypoid type of bronchiolitis obliterans as reported by Epler et al. (1985), those cases were included in the study, although we consider that BOOP is basically a type of interstitial pneumonia of unknown cause. Six biopsy cases in the United States and 23 biopsy cases in Japan were studied. Accumulation of foamy cells was noted in some alveolar spaces but not in the wall of bronchioles. Histological features

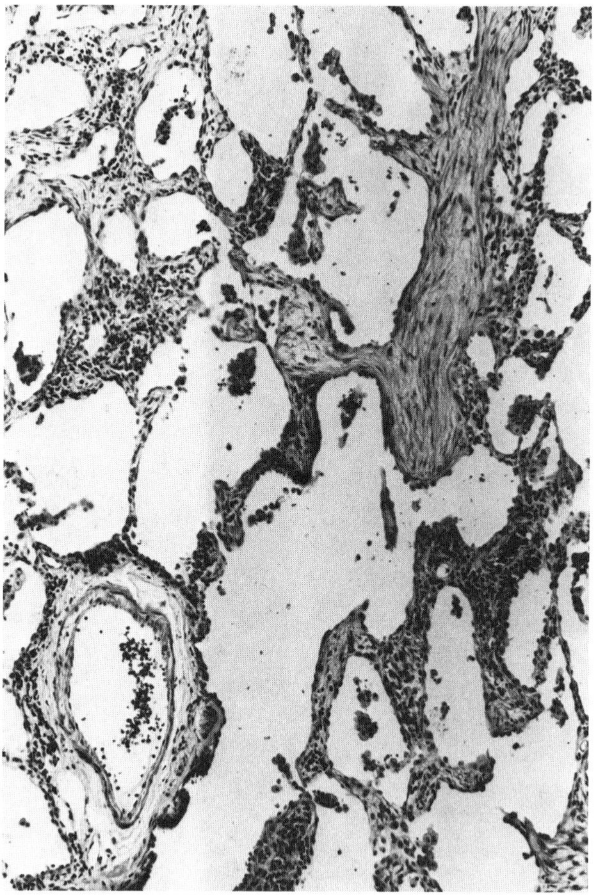

Figure 18 A biopsy case of BOOP. The lung sample showed diffuse alveolar septal thickening with fibrotic changes, infiltration of lymphocytes and plasma cells, and granulation tissue formed in a respiratory bronchiole and alveolar duct. The granulation tissue was continuous with the wall of the alveolar duct and alveoli (Meyer's hematoxylin and eosin stain, ×50).

of two of these Japanese cases were reported by Kitaichi and Izumi (1988) and by Imai and Kitaichi (1989) (Fig. 18).

Cryptogenic Obliterative Bronchiolitis

Three biopsy cases with a mean age of 51 years and 4 autopsy cases from the previous study reported by Geddes et al. (1977) were studied. The disorder was labeled *cryptogenic obliterative bronchiolitis* in adults by Turton and colleagues (1981). The most marked lesion showed granulation tissue formation in the lamina propria of membranous bronchioles, with infiltration of plasma cells (Fig. 19). Respiratory bronchioles showed much less marked lesions and were without PB unit lesions, although one case among them showed accumulation of foamy cells in the subepithelial layers of several membranous bronchioles.

Small Airways Disease

Small airways disease is a term introduced by Hogg et al. (1968) to encompass pathological changes observed in the peripheral conducting airways

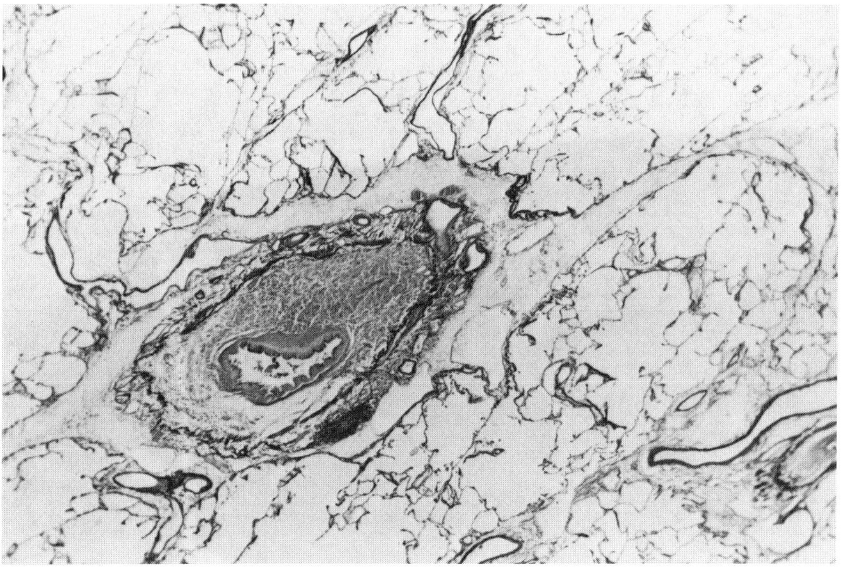

Figure 19 A biopsy case of cryptogenic obliterative bronchiolitis. The membranous bronchiole in the interlobular septum showed marked luminal stenosis with granulation tissue formation, hemorrhage, and infiltration of lymphoid cells in the subepithelial lamina propria (Weigert's elastic van Gieson's stain, ×20).

from cases of chronic obstructive pulmonary disease (COPD). These lesions included inflammation, fibrosis, smooth muscle hypertrophy, pigment deposition involving airways, and goblet cell metaplasia as summarized by Neiwoehner (1986). Changes of PB unit lesions were not noted in the pathological study of chronic bronchitis or COPD, as mentioned in the previous section.

Small airways disease is also used in North America as a generic term for a disease showing features of bronchiolitis without any known entities. Ten biopsy cases of small airways disease, as used in this sense, with a mean age of 45 were reviewed. They showed muscular hypertrophy, chronic inflammation, and subepithelial fibrosis in the wall of membranous and respiratory bronchioles, which were stenotic or dilated (Fig. 20).

Follicular Bronchitis/Bronchiolitis

Follicular bronchitis/bronchiolitis was described as a label for pulmonary disorder without COPD or bronchiectasis that shows formation of germinal

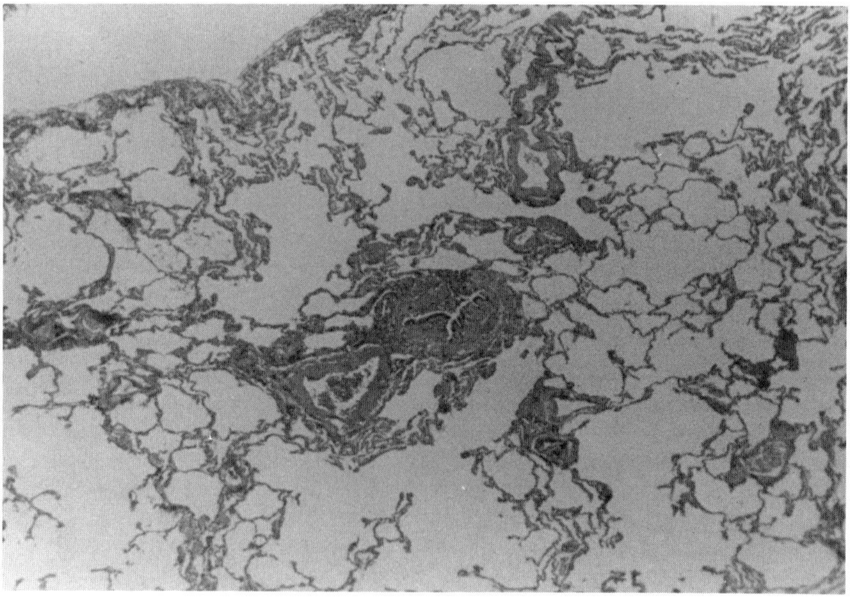

Figure 20 A biopsy case of small airways disease. The membranous bronchiole showed muscular hypertrophy, subepithelial chronic inflammation, and fibrotic changes causing luminal stenosis. The alveolar areas were free from lesions (Meyer's hematoxylin and eosin stain, ×25).

centers and lymphoid follicles around airways. This disorder was reported to be associated with autoimmune, immunodeficiency, or hypersensitivity disorders by Yousem et al. (1985a) and Fortoul et al. (1985).

Cases of DPB showed a positive serum rheumatoid factor with a frequency of 41% as reported by Izumi (1988), although they usually do not have joint symptoms or deformities as seen in cases of rheumatoid arthritis. Patients with rheumatoid arthritis developed several types of inflammatory airways disorders including obliterative bronchiolitis, follicular bronchitis/bronchiolitis, and BOOP as reported by Geddes et al. (1977) and Yousem et al. (1985a,b).

Three biopsy cases of follicular bronchitis/bronchiolitis associated with rheumatoid arthritis were studied. They showed germinal centers and/or lymphoid follicles in the wall of membranous and respiratory bronchioles, while alveolar areas were free from marked lesions (Fig. 21).

C. Summary of the Clinicopathological Studies

In our study, DPB stands as an independent disease only by the presence of PB unit lesions in the background of bilateral diffuse inflammatory airways disorder. However, cases showing exclusive or predominant distribution of

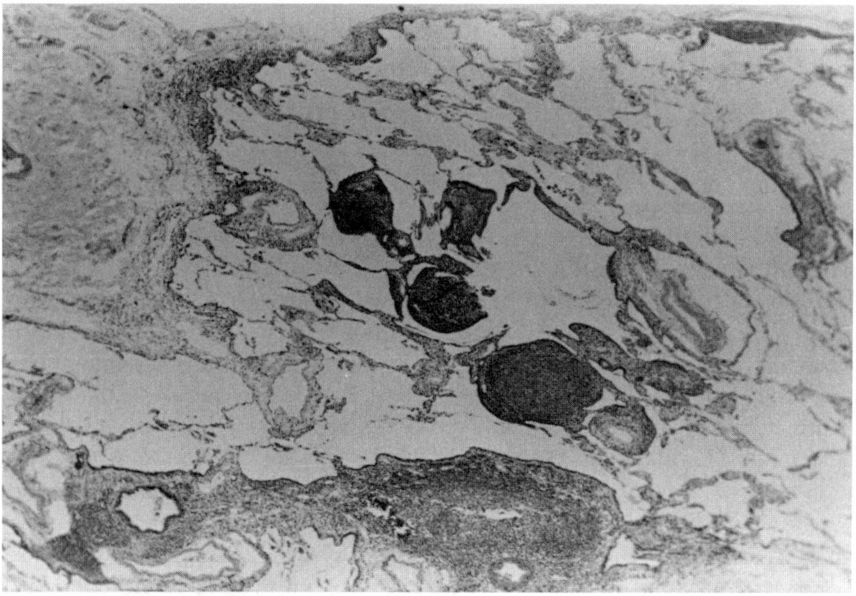

Figure 21 A biopsy case of follicular bronchiolitis. Lymphoid follicles and germinal centers were formed in the wall of respiratory bronchioles (Meyer's hematoxylin and eosin stain, ×20).

lesions in the region of respiratory bronchioles are infrequent, even among open lung biopsy cases, as seen in the case report (Figs. 4-10). In autopsy cases of DPB, cylindrical dilation of small bronchi and membranous bronchioles was usually noted throughout lungs as reported by Nishimura et al. (1987). Gudbjerg (1955) reported that among 112 cases of bronchiectasis, 4 (3.6%) showed cylindrical bronchiectasis with involvement throughout the entire right and left lungs. Among the surgical cases of bronchiectasis in our study, 5 (21%) among 24 cases showed interstitial accumulation of foamy cells. The five patients were all Japanese.

Bronchiectasis is an old disease, first described by Laennec in 1819, and has undergone great changes in its clinical features and prevalence, which were summarized by Lindskog (1986), and, recently, by Barker and Bardana (1988). Although previous studies of the pathology of bronchiectasis or chronic bronchitis, including a recent review by Reid (1986), did not describe similar lesions such as DPB with PB unit lesions, an international study of the pathology of these disorders will be required to establish the disease entity of DPB. The question is whether cases of DPB were described or included under a label of diffuse or bilateral bronchiectasis or fatal obstructive chronic bronchitis, as pointed out by Kitaichi (1988). Thurlbeck (1988) raised the possibility of an overlap between cases diagnosed as DPB in Japan and those diagnosed as bronchiectasis in North America.

V. Future of Diffuse Panbronchiolitis

A. Pathogenesis

The pathogenesis of DPB and that of the PB unit lesion is open to future study. Bronchiectasis was discussed by Davis et al. (1983) as having several theories of pathogenesis: pressure of secretion theory, atelectasis theory, traction theory, and infection theory. In DPB there was an inflammatory lesion causing disruption of elastic tissues in the wall of airways, as shown in Figures 5 and 8, which was similar to a process pointed out by Whitwell (1952) in cases of follicular bronchiectasis. Because cases of DPB have a frequent past history of chronic paranasal sinusitis (more than 80%), and a mean duration of 6-7 years of cough and sputum before development of dyspnea, as reported by Izumi (1988), many years of inflammatory changes in the airways are suspected of having been present before the full development of clinical features of DPB.

The socioeconomic environment of cases of DPB is also to be considered, because a major proportion of the DPB cases grew up soon after World War II, when Japan's environment was generally poor.

Bronchiectasis is the condition of dilation of the bronchi and bronchioles and has various causes, including primary ciliary dyskinesia (Editorial, 1975; Davis et al., 1983; and Barker and Bardana, 1988). However, cases of DPB did not reveal a particular cause as shown in the studies concerning airway cilia in three cases by Nagai (1983), and seven cases studied by Amitani et al. (1988).

B. Treatment and Prognosis

After the report by Kudoh et al. (1987) that showed a beneficial clinical effect of low-dose long-term erythromycin administration in 18 cases of DPB including an open lung biopsy case, a considerable number of cases of DPB have shown an amelioration and a better prognosis, as did the patient reported in this chapter. The mechanism of the beneficial effect of erythromycin is not always directly based upon its bacteriocidal or bacteriostatic effects. The mechanism remains open to the future study, although erythromycin was reported to decrease polymorphonuclear leukocyte directed migration in an animal experiment by Nelson et al. (1987). In any case erythromycin may change the overall prognosis of cases of DPB.

C. Diffuse Panbronchiolitis in Other Countries

Almost all cases of DPB have been recognized among Japanese, although one second-generation Korean-Japanese was recognized as having DPB clinically in Japan by Sugiyama et al. (1986) and a native Taiwanese adult who underwent an open lung biopsy was recognized as having DPB (Y. H. Tsai, 1989, personal communication). Population differences may be present in cases of DPB and these may be related to HLA-Bw54, as pointed out by Sugiyama et al. (1986), which is possessed by Japanese, Chinese, and Ashkenazi Jews with a frequency of 14.1%, 10.4%, and 0.8%, respectively, but is negative in Caucasians and other populations studied.

International communication regarding the pathology of cases of bronchiectasis and fatal obstructive chronic bronchitis is also to be requested to establish the independent diagnosis of DPB.

VI. Summary

We have discussed DPB to clarify the independence of the disease and determine that the PB unit lesion in the background of bilateral diffuse inflammatory airways disorder is the key to identifying DPB. However, the pathology of DPB, including open lung biopsy, rarely shows the exclusive or predominant distribution of changes in the region of respiratory bronchioles.

Analytical studies on DPB cited above were done primarily among the clinically diagnosed DPB cases. Therefore, DPB is open to further studies including pathogenesis and international communications in the general spectrum of inflammatory airways disorders.

Acknowledgments

The clinicopathological study in this article was done with Dr. T. V. Colby in 1986 and the results were briefly reported by Kitaichi (1988). The authors are grateful to many investigators in Japan, the United States, Canada, West Germany, and the United Kingdom who made the study possible.

References

Amitani, R., Tanaka, E., Suzuki, Y., Ishida, S., Takahasi, H., and Kuze, F. (1988). A study on ultrastructure and motility of tracheo-bronchial cilia in patients with diffuse panbronchiolitis. *Nihon Kyoubu Rinshou* (*Jpn. J. Chest Dis.*) **47**:483-490.

Barker, A. F., and Bardana, E. J. (1988). Bronchiectasis: update of an orphan disease. *Am. Rev. Respir. Dis.* **137**:969-978.

Cameron, A. H. (1956). Pulmonary hemosiderosis associated with bronchiectasis. *Thorax* **11**:105-112.

Culiner, M. M. (1963). Obliterative bronchitis and bronchiolitis with bronchiectasis. *Dis. Chest* **44**:351-361.

Davis, P. B., Hubbard, Y. S., McCoy, K., and Taussig, L. M. (1983). Familial bronchiectasis. *J. Pediatr.* **102**:177-185.

Editorial. (1975). Bronchiectasis today. *Br. Med. J.* **2**:605-606.

Epler, G. R., Colby, T. V., McLoud, T. C., Carrington, C. B., and Gaensler, E. A. (1985). Bronchiolitis obliterans organizing pneumonia. *N. Engl. J. Med.* **312**:152-158.

Erb, I. H. (1933). Pathology of bronchiectasis. *Arch. Pathol.* **15**:357-386.

Fortoul, T. I., Cano-Valle, F., Oliva, E., and Barrios, R. (1985). Follicular bronchiolitis in association with connective tissue diseases. *Lung* **163**: 305-314.

Geddes, D. M., Corrin, B., Brewerton, D. A., Davies, R. J., and Turner-Warwick, M. (1977). Progressive airway obliteration in adults and its association with rheumatoid disease. *Q. J. Med.* **46**:427-444.

George, S. A., Leonardi, H. K., and Overholt, R. H. (1979). Bilateral pulmonary resection for bronchiectasis: a 40-year experience. *Ann. Thorac. Surg.* **28**:48-53.

Gudbjerg, C. E. (1955). Roentgenologic diagnosis of bronchiectasis. An analysis of 112 cases. *Acta Radiol.* **43**:209-226.

Hogg, J. C., Macklem, P. T., and Thurlbeck, W. M. (1968). Site and nature of airway obstruction in chronic obstructive lung disease. *N. Engl. J. Med.* **278**:1355-1360.

Homma, H., Yamanaka, T., Tanimoto, S., Tamura, M., Chijimatsu, Y., Kira, S., and Izumi, T. (1983). Diffuse panbronchiolitis. A disease of the transitional zone of the lung. *Chest* **83**:63-69.

Imai, H., and Kitaichi, M. (1989). A case of bronchiolitis obliterans organizing pneumonia (BOOP) showing spontaneous regression after an open lung biopsy. *Nippon Kyoubu Shikkan Gakkai Zassi* (*Jpn. J. Thorac. Dis.*) **27**:829-836.

Izumi, T. (1988). A nation-wide survey of diffuse panbronchiolitis in Japan and the high incidence of diffuse panbronchiolitis seen in Japanese respiratory clinics. In *Sarcoidosis and Other Granulomatous Disorders*. Edited by C. Grassi, G. Rizzato, and E. Pozzi. Amsterdam, Elsevier Science Publishers B.V., pp. 753-757.

King, T. E. (1989). Review. Bronchiolitis obliterans. *Lung* **167**:69-93.

Kitaichi, M. (1986). Pathology of pulmonary sarcoidosis. *Clin. Dermatol.* **4**:108-115.

Kitaichi, M. (1988). Pathology of diffuse panbronchiolitis from the view point of differential diagnosis. In *Sarcoidosis and Other Granulomatous Disorders*. Edited by C. Grassi, G. Rizzato, and E. Pozzi. Amsterdam, Elsevier Science Publishers B.V., pp. 741-746.

Kitaichi, M., and Izumi, T. (1988). BOOP. *Kokyuu To Junkan* (*Respir. Circ.*) **36**:1075-1080.

Kitaichi, M., Colby, T. V., Izumi, T., Yamamoto, S., Kitatani, F., and Iwata, T. (1988). A comparative pathological study of inflammatory airways disorders (IAD): the significance of unit lesion of panbronchiolitis (PB) (abstract). *Am. Rev. Respir. Dis.* **137** (4):155.

Koshoubu, T., Hirai, H., Hikita, T., Kawasaki, Y., Burioka, N., and Sasaki, T. (1988). Sweat chloride concentration and pancreatic function diagnostant in patients with diffuse panbronchiolitis. *Nippon Kyoubu Shikkan Gakkai Zasshi* (*Jpn. J. Thorac. Dis.*) **26**:97-101.

Kudoh, S., Uetake, T., Hagiwara, K., Hirayama, M., Hus, L. H., Kimura, H., and Sugiyama, Y. (1987). Clinical effect of low-dose long-term erythromycin chemotherapy on diffuse panbronchiolitis. *Nippon Kyoubu Sikkan Gakkai Zassi* (*Jpn. J. Thorac. Dis.*) **25**:632-642.

Lindskog, G. E. (1986). Bronchiectasis revisited. *Yale J. Biol. Med.* **59**:41-53.

Lloyd-Still, J. D. (1983). Pathology. Pulmonary manifestations. In *Textbook of Cystic Fibrosis*. Edited by J. D. Lloyd-Still. Boston, John Wright/PSG Inc., pp. 19-31, 165-197.

Maeda, M., Saiki, S., and Yamanaka, A. (1987). Serial section analysis of the lesions in diffuse panbronchiolitis. *Acta Pathol. Jpn.* **37**:693-704.

Matsuba, K., and Thurlbeck, W. M. (1973). Disease of the small airways in chronic bronchitis. *Am. Rev. Respir. Dis.* **107**:552-558.

Moore, J. R., Kobernick, S. D., and Wigleworth, F. W. (1949). Bronchiectasis. A study of the segmental distribution of the pathologic lesions. *Surg. Gynecol. Obstet.* **89**:145-153.

Nagai, A. (1983). Ultrastructural characteristics of bronchial cilia in patients with respiratory infectious disease. *Nippon Kyoubu Sikkan Gakkai Zassi* (*Jpn. J. Thorac. Dis.*) **21**:564-573.

Nelson, S., Summer, W. R., Terry, P. B., Warr, G. A., and Jakab, G. J. (1987). Erythromycin-induced suppression of pulmonary antibacterial defenses. A potential mechanism of superinfection in the lung. *Am. Rev. Respir. Dis.* **136**:1207-1212.

Niewoehner, D. E. (1986). New messages from morphometric studies of chronic obstructive pulmonary disease. *Sem. Respir. Med.* **8**:140-146.

Nishimura, K., Furue, M., Kitaichi, M., Nagai, S., Kino, T., Izumi, T., Oshima, S., Suzuki, Y., Murata, K., and Itoh, H. (1987). A comparative study of computed tomography and pulmonary pathology in diffuse panbronchiolitis. *Hihon Kyoubu Rinshou* (*Jpn. J. Chest Dis.*) **46**: 481-486.

Oglivie, A. G. (1941). The natural history of bronchiectasis. A clinical, roentgenologic and pathologic study. *Arch. Intern. Med.* **68**:395-365.

Rayl, J. E., Peasley, E. D., and Joyner, J. T. (1961). Differential diagnosis of bronchiectasis and bronchitis. *Dis. Chest* **39**:591-600.

Reid, L. M. (1950). Reduction in bronchial subdivision in bronchiectasis. *Thorax* **5**:233-247.

Reid, L. M. (1954). Pathology of chronic bronchitis. *Lancet* **1**:275-278.

Reid, L. M. (1986). The pathology of obstructive and inflammatory airway diseases. *Eur. J. Respir. Dis.* **69**(Suppl 147):26-37.

Rollins, S., Colby, T. V., and Clayton, F. (1986). Open lung biopsy in *Mycoplasma pneumoniae* pneumonia. *Arch. Pathol. Lab. Med.* **110**:34-41.

Spencer, H. (1985). Diseases of the bronchial tree. In *Pathology of the Lung.* Oxford, Pergamon Press, pp. 131-165.

Sugiyama, Y., Takeuchi, K., Yotsumoto, H., Takaku, F., and Maeda, H. (1986). A case of diffuse panbronchiolitis in a second generation Korean male. *Nippon Kyoubu Shikkan Gakkai Zassi* (*Jpn. J. Thorac. Dis.*) **24**: 183-187.

Thurlbeck, W. M. (1976). The morphology of chronic bronchitis, asthma and bronchiectasis. In *Chronic Airflow Obstruction in Lung Disease.* Philadelphia, W. B. Saunders, pp. 31-95.

Thurlbeck, W. M. (1988). Chronic airflow obstruction. In *Pathology of the Lung.* Edited by W. M. Thurlbeck. Stuttgart, Thieme, pp. 519-575.

Turton, C. W., Williams, G., and Green, M. (1981). Cryptogenic obliterative bronchiolitis in adults. *Thorax* **36**:805-810.

Warnock, M. L., Ghahremani, C. G., Rattenborg, C., Ginsberg, M., and Valenzuela, J. (1972). Pulmonary complications of heroin intoxication. Aspiration pneumonia and diffuse bronchiectasis. *J.A.M.A.* **219**:1051-1053.

Whitwell, F. (1952). A study of the pathology and pathogenesis of bronchiectasis. *Thorax* **7**:213-239.

Yamanaka, A., Saiki, S., Tamura, S., and Saito, K. (1969). The problems of chronic obstructive pulmonary disease: especially concerning about diffuse panbronchiolitis. *Naika* (*Intern. Med.*) **23**:442-451.

Yousem, S. A., Colby, T. V., and Carrington, C. B. (1985a). Follicular bronchitis/bronchiolitis. *Hum. Pathol.* **16**:700-706.

Yousem, S. A., Colby, T. V., and Carrington, C. B. (1985b). Lung biopsy in rheumatoid arthritis. *Am. Rev. Respir. Dis.* **131**:770-777.

21

Pulmonary Complications of Drugs Commonly Used in Tropical Medicine

ADRIAN WILLIAMS

West Los Angeles Veterans Administration Hospital
and University of California School of Medicine
Los Angeles, California

Over the years we have become more aware of the importance of considering drug reactions in the differential diagnosis of lung diseases (Cooper et al., 1986; Demeter, 1979). The anatomical and physiological makeup of the organ reminds us that the lung is exposed to a host of potential insults. On the one hand, all of the cardiac output is delivered to the pulmonary capillaries, where metabolically active cells engage in the alteration and detoxification of materials presented to them (Pitt and Lister, 1989). On the other hand, all this occurs in an environment with the highest (i.e., atmospheric) concentration of oxygen available and where the potential for oxygen radical production is greatest (Brewis, 1981). In addition to this heightened potential for drug reactions, our recognition of such interactions is made more difficult by the limited nature of the lungs' response to insults (iatrogenic or not). This makes a questioning stance all the more appropriate.

It is well appreciated that the spectrum of disease in the tropics differs greatly from that in the "developed" world. Nutritional deficiencies and anemia constitute a large and important part and have not been considered here because drug therapy in the accepted sense of the word is not the pivotal element. The bulk of the remainder of "tropical" medicine is concerned with infestations (by helminths) and infections (by protozoae, bacteria, mycoses, rickettsiae, and viruses) and in the management of these by drug therapy the potential for pulmonary toxicity is ever present.

Table 1 provides an overview of those conditions most peculiar to the tropics and their recommended drug treatment. It draws attention to the pulmonary manifestations of the conditions themselves as well as the pulmonary complications of the agents used to treat them.

Although much recognition is given to drug reactions, currently available discussions do not address medicine peculiar to the tropics. This volume, devoted as it is to the pulmonary manifestations of tropical disease, would do the reader and practitioner a disservice by ignoring the potential impact on the lung of the exotic and unusual therapies used for exotic and unusual diseases. In this chapter we will address such concerns in relation to mechanisms of interaction and patterns of such interaction, together with the specific interactions themselves as they are known to date.

I. Mechanisms of Injury

The general mechanisms of drug interaction with the lung have been discussed in detail in recent reviews. (Cooper et al., 1986; Demeter et al., 1979). As with any adverse reaction to drugs, they may usefully be considered as toxic, idiosyncratic, or allergic.

Toxic effects are often direct, such as the cytotoxic effect on alveolar capillary endothelial cells of cytotoxic drugs (Ginsberg and Comis, 1982). In addition, although usually dose related (Van Barnerveld et al., 1987), such oxidant-mediated injury may be exaggerated by interaction with other factors, for example, the potentiation of nitrofurantoin lung disease by oxygen (Boyd et al., 1979).

Idiosyncratic reactions are best exemplified by those dependent on genetic susceptibility, such as in those with glucose-6-phosphate dehydrogenase deficiency and drug-induced hemolysis (Rollo, 1975), or acetylator status as in the case of hydralazine or isoniazid-related systemic lupus erythematosus (SLE), which occurs more frequently in slow acetylators of these drugs (Ginsberg, 1980).

Immune-mediated injury offers another mechanism for lung damage. This is best understood in terms of drug-induced SLE. There are two groups of drugs. In one, antinuclear antibody is prevalent in a large percentage of the individuals taking the drug (hydralazine, diphenylhydrantoin, penicillamine, and isoniazid). The second group is made up of numerous drugs whose use has been reported to induce SLE but that are not otherwise associated with positive antinuclear antibodies. Pulmonary infiltrates with eosinophils are an important subset that also represents a hypersensitivity response.

Table 1 Prevalent Tropical Diseases; Manifestations, and Complications of Therapy

Disease	Drug Treatment	Pulmonary Manifestations	Pulmonary Complications of Drug Therapy
Helminthic:		Asthma:	
Nematodes (Roundworms)		Pulmonary infiltrates with eosinophils (PIE), solitary pulmonary	
Filariasis	Diethylcarbamazine	nodule (*D. immitis*)	Asthma
Ascariasis (hookworms)	Piperazine	PIE, asthma, hemoptysis	Respiratory depression
Strongyloidiasis	Thiabendazole	PIE, Asthma, interstitial pneumonia	—
Trematodes: (Flukes)		PIE, pulmonary hypertension	
Schistosomiasis	Praziquantel	Cough, hemoptysis, "king cysts,"	—
Paragonomiasis	Praziquantel	effusion	—
Cestodes: (Tapeworms)			
Taeniasis	Praziquantel	None	—
Echinococcosis		Solitary pulmonary nodule mass	N/A
Protozoan:			
Malaria	Curative: Chlorquine	Cough, ARDS	—
	Quinine	("malarial lung")	Asthma
	Prophylactic: Primaquine		Methemoglobinemia, PIE
	Pyrimethamine-sulfadoxine Chloroquine		
African trypanosomiasis (sleeping sickness)	− CNS: Suramin	None	—
	Pentamidine		—
	+ CNS: Melarsoprol		—

(Table 1 continues)

Table 1 (continued)

Disease	Drug Treatment	Pulmonary Manifestations	Pulmonary Complications of Drug Therapy
American trypanosomiasis (Chagas' disease)	Nifurtimox	Congestive heart failure	—
Leishmaniasis	Pentamidine antimony (pentamidine)	None	—
Toxoplasmosis	Pyrimethamine-sulfadiazine Spiramycin (non-U.S.)	Interstitial pneumonia	Lupus
Pneumocystis	Trimethoprim-sulfamethoxazole	Pneumonia	Lupus syndrome and hypersensitivity pneumonia
Cryptosporidiosis	Spiramycin	Interstitial pneumonia	—
Amebiasis	Metronidazole	Effusion	—
Bacterial:			
Leprosy	Dapsone	None	Methemoglobinemia
	Clofazimine		—
	Rifampin		—
Tuberculosis	1st line: Isoniazid	Pulmonary TB	Lupus
	Rifampin		—
	Thiacetazone		—
	Pyrazinamide		—
	Streptomycin		—
	2nd line: Ethambutol		—
	P-aminosalicylic acid		H/S pneumonitis and pleural effusion
Plague	Tetracycline	Pneumonia	Lupus
Brucellosis	Tetracycline	Pneumonia	Lupus

Cholera	Tetracycline	None	Lupus
	Trimethoprim/sulfamethoxazole		Lupus and H/S pneumonitis
Shigellosis	Sulfonamides	Pneumonia	Lupus and H/S pneumonitis
	Chloramenicol	(typhoid)	—
Pseudomonas	Trimethoprim/sulphamethoxazole	Pneumonia	Lupus and H/S pneumonitis
(Melidiosis)	Chloramphenicol	Apical cavitation	—
Spirochetal:			
Syphilia	Penicillin	Gunmata	Lupus and H/S pneumonitis
Yaws	Penicillin	None	Lupus and H/S pneumonitis
Pinta	Penicillin	None	Lupus and H/S pneumonitis
Relapsing fever	Tetracycline	None	Lupus and H/S pneumonitis
Rickettsial:			
Typhus-like	Tetracycline or	Pneumonia	—
Chlamydial	Chloramphenicol	in all	—
Q-fever	For all		Lupus
Mycoses			
Actinomycosis	Penicillin	Empyema	Lupus and H/S pneumonitis
Nocardiosis	Sulfonamides	Bronchopneumonia	Lupus and H/S pneumonitis
Maduromycosis	Miconazole	Pneumonia	—
		Fungus ball	

II. Patterns of Presentation

The lung has a limited number of ways in which it responds to damage, whether due to disease or drugs (Tables 2, 3). As such it is important to remain vigilant for unexpected drug effects, the incidence of which may be greater than we believe. The symptoms and signs, clinical and radiological, that can occur with drug reactions can be considered in relation to the target tissues that make up the pulmonary system, specifically the airways, blood vessels, alveoli, chest wall (pleura and muscles) and neural connections to the central nervous system (CNS). Thus the clinical features that we might rationally expect will be those of asthma and bronchiolitis; pulmonary hypertension and hemorrhage; acute and subacute pulmonary fibrosis, and adult respira-

Table 2 Categories of Responses to Treatment

Asthma:
Quinine
Diethylcarbamazine
Methemoglobinemia:
Primaquine
Dapsone
Systemic Lupus Erythematosus:
Antibiotics
Sulfonamides
Antituberculous drugs
Tetracycline
Penicillin
Pleural Effusion:
P-aminosalicylic acid
Penicillin
Hypersensitivity Pneumonitis:
Antibiotics
Sulfonamides
P-aminosalicylic acid
Penicillin
Noncardiogenic Pulmonary Edema:
Aspirin
Narcotics
Amphotericin B

Table 3 Categories of Drugs and Associated Reactions

Antiprotozoals:
Asthma: quinine
Methemoglobinemia and cyanosis: primaquine

Antihelminthics:
Asthma: diethylcarbamazine

Antibiotics:
Systemic lupus erythematosus:
  Isoniazid, streptomycin, P-aminosalicylic acid
  Penicillin
  Sulfonamides
  Tetracycline

Hypersensitivity pneumonitis:
  Isoniazid, P-aminosalicylic acid
  Penicillin
  Sulfonamides

Pleural effusion:
  P-aminosalicylic acid
  Penicillin

Pulmonary infiltrates with eosinophils:
  Sulfonamides
  P-aminosalicylic acid

Analgesics:
Noncardiogenic pulmonary edema
  Aspirin, nonsteroidal anti-inflammatory agents
  Narcotics

Asthma
  Aspirin and other nonsteroidal anti-inflammatory agents

tory distress syndrome (ARDS); pleural effusions; and ventilatory failure. Discussion of these clinical features with specific examples will draw attention to the tropical drug interactions and highlight the broad possibilities. Where no "tropical" reaction is known, classic conventional drug examples are mentioned.

A. Asthma

Many drugs have been associated with the development of wheeze. The most common are those that interfere with the balance between bronchoconstricting and bronchodilating forces that determine airway caliber. In patients predisposed to reversible airways obstruction (those with hyperreactive airways) bronchospasm will be most easily induced. Classic examples given are the B-receptor blockers (Chester, 1981) as well as aspirin (Szczeklik, 1982). In this latter instance cyclooxygenase inhibition leads to increased lipooxygenase activity, with increased leukotriene production. However, asthma is also a typical feature of any anaphylactic reaction. This is most usually due to a penicillin (Reichlin et al., 1953), but in the tropics two other examples are to be found.

Quinine

Drug-resistant forms of *Falciparum malaria* should be treated with a regimen including quinine (often together with a dehydrofolate reductase inhibitor). When taken in overdosage, or by a hypersensitive individual, a typical cluster of symptoms occur called cinchonism. In this, asthma occurs together with disturbances of hearing and vision, nausea and vomiting, flushing, and pruritus (Rollo, 1975).

Diethylcarbamazine

Infection with the filarial worms *Wuchereria bancrofti* or *Brugia malayi* typically results in recurrent lymphangitis with fibrosis and lymphatic obstruction. Not infrequently this is associated with eosinophilia (generally greater than 3000/mm^3) cough (worse at night) with wheeze, and patchy mottling of the chest radiograph (so called tropical filarial eosinophilia). In the 1950s this syndrome was shown to respond to diethylcarbamazine. In addition to generalized untoward reactions, there are those from the filariacidal action (Rollo, 1975b). The drug sensitizes the microfilariae so that they become susceptible to phagocytosis by the fixed macrophages of the reticuloendothelial system. With this there is a release of filarial antigen, with resultant histamine release. In one case of bancroftian filariasis, this is associated with asthma. With onchocerciosis, there is intense pruritus.

B. Bronchiolitis

This is not likely to be of concern in the setting of tropical disease. A subtle condition, it is difficult to diagnose in the earlier stages but is characterized by increasing shortness of breath with an abnormal chest radiograph in some patients (localized acinonodular shadows [Epler et al., 1979]). To date, no drugs unique to tropical medicine have been implicated in its development.

C. Pulmonary Hypertension

The most common cause of pulmonary hypertension in the world is schistosomiasis (Barret-Conner, 1982). Over 200 million persons are thought to be infected by *Schistosoma* species worldwide and over 400,000 in the United States (Warren, 1984). Pulmonary disease may be seen as a late event in chronic hepatosplenic schistosomiasis when the hepatic injury of fibrosis fosters portosystemic collaterals, allowing eggs to bypass the liver and embolize the lungs. Eggs that lodge there incite an intense inflammatory response leading to pulmonary hypertension. Cor pulmonale occurs in 5% of infected individuals with hepatosplenomegaly (Barret-Conner, 1982). Pulmonary hypertension and/or vasculitis has rarely been linked to drug therapy (Demeter et al., 1979). The various case reports of angiitis have, for the most part, been discredited and the complication recognized as a part of an underlying disease.

D. Acute and Subacute Pulmonary Fibrosis

This grouping includes two types of reaction: hypersensitivity pneumonitis, and the pulmonary fibrosis of systemic lupus erythematosus (SLE). (Interstitial pneumonia and/or fibrosis occurs regularly as a direct cytotoxic effect of drugs such as bleomycin and nitrofurantoin but no "tropical" drug has been reported to induce such a reaction.) The distinction between the pulmonary manifestations of hypersensitivity pneumonitis and of SLE will often be difficult clinically. The symptomatic and radiographic features may be identical. However, the cause of the interstial pulmonary fibrosis may be revealed by transbronchial biopsy if granulomata are found. Drugs commonly used in the tropics that have been implicated are, of course, antibiotics, particularly sulfonamides (Weinstein, 1980), penicillin (Weinstein, 1980), and the antituberculous medicines (Rothfield et al., 1978). It is of particular note that part of the hypersensitivity response to a medication, sulfonamides being one (Schatz et al., 1981), may be a peripheral blood eosinophilia. In concert with diffuse peripheral pulmonary densities, this constitutes the syndrome of pulmonary infiltrates with eosinophils, which is itself a common tropical problem more usually due to parasitic infestations (i.e., Loeffler's syndrome) (Weingarten, 1943). In this latter instance, *Ascaris* infection is most often implicated. The characteristic features include cough, fever, eosinophilia, and roentgenographic parachymal infiltrates lasting 1-2 weeks. These are explained by eosinophilic pneumonitis due to the migration of larvae through the lung. Tropical filarial eosinophilia is another instance and has already been discussed. Pulmonary infiltrates with eosinophils may also, as noted, be produced by various drugs. Again, pulmonary infiltrates, fever, eosinophilia, and cough are characteristic with, in one series, most patients having rales on examination.

E. Noncardiogenic Pulmonary Edema

Overdose of sedative or narcotic medications produces the most frequent examples (Steinberg and Kaliner, 1968), but idiosyncratic reactions have been reported to several drugs that might be used routinely in the tropics, such as aspirin (Heffner and Sahn, 1981), hydrochlorothiazide (Bell and Lippman, 1977), and lidocaine (Howard et al., 1982). The characteristic response is acute, developing within minutes to days and is associated with dyspnea, cough, and typical radiographic changes. The mechanism believed to underly this phenomenon is one of increased permeability of the pulmonary capillary bed, perhaps due to endothelial cell damage.

F. Pleural Disease

The pleural space is often involved in the drug-induced lupus syndrome. Pleurisy has been reported in nearly half of the cases of lupus secondary to procainamide (Henningsen et al., 1975), while pleural effusions are a little less common. Isoniazide is an important cause of drug-induced lupus and, together with diphenylhydantoin, hydralazine and procainamide, account for 90% of the cases (Schoen and Trentham, 1981). In a prospective study of 102 patients receiving isoniazide for 1 year, 22% had antinuclear antibodies (Rothfield et al., 1978). Para-aminosalicylic acid has also been implicated as a cause of pleural effusion (Warring and Howlett, 1952). Since it is also known to cause hypersensitivity pneumonitis (Wold and Zahn, 1956) it may be another cause of drug-induced SLE.

G. Methemoglobinemia

Cyanosis may occur as a result of the use of primaquine for the treatment of malaria, as a consequence of the formation of abnormal amounts of methemoglobin. In this form of hemoglobin, the ferrous iron has been oxidized to ferric iron so that the hemoglobin molecule cannot combine with O_2 or CO_2. Methemoglobin is formed continuously in the normal red cell but the level is kept at or below 2% by intracellular reductive mechanisms facilitated by methemoglobin reductase. Primaquine increases the rate of oxidation beyond this reductive capacity, leading to methemoglobinemia. (Other mechanisms resulting in this are a congenital deficiency of methemoglobin reductase or the presence of hemoglobin M.) Clinical features vary with the blood levels. Concentrations of methemoglobin of 10-25% produce cyanosis. Levels above this are associated with fatigue and headache. Treatment is not usually necessary unless serious problems such as coma develop, in which case intravenous methylene blue (1-2 mg/kg of a 1% solution) is given slowly. Cyanosis usually disappears within 1 h (Szidon and Fishman, 1988).

IV. Conclusion

The clinician must retain a high index of suspicion that unexplained pulmonary disease may be caused by drugs. This particularily true given the similarity described here between the clinical features of the drug reaction itself and the primary pulmonary manifestation of the tropical disease. Much of the information presented here consists of case reports; a more complete understanding of the true incidence of these problems will only come with our continued vigilance.

References

Barret-Conner, E. (1982). Parasitic pulmonary disease. *Am. Rev. Respir. Dis.* **126**:558-563.

Bell, R. T., and Lippman, M. (1977). Hydrochlorothiazide-induced pulmonary edema. *Arch. Intern. Med.* **139**:817-819.

Boyd, M. R., Catignani, G. L., Sasame, H. A., Mitchell, J. R., and Stiko, A. W. (1979). Acute pulmonary injury in rats by nitrofurantoin and modification by vitamin E, dietary fat, and oxygen. *Am. Rev. Respir. Dis.* **120**:93-99.

Brewis, R. A. L. (1981). Respiratory disorders. In *Textbook of Adverse Drug Reactions*. Edited by D. M. Davies. Oxford, Oxford University Press. pp. 154-187.

Chester, E. H., Schwartz, H. J., and Fleming, G. M. (1981). Adverse effects of propranolol on airway function in non asthmatic chronic obstructive lung disease. *Chest* **79**:540-544.

Cooper, J. A. D., White, D. A., and Matthay, R. A. (1986). Drug-induced pulmonary disease. *Am. Rev. Respir. Dis.* **133**:321-340.

Dementer, S. L., Ahmad, M., and Tomashefski, J. F. (1979). Drug-induced pulmonary disease. *Clev. Clin. Quart.* **46**:89-124.

Epler, G. R., Snider, G. L., Gaensler, E. A., Cathicart, E. S., Fitzgerald, M. X., and Carrington, C. G. (1979). Bronchiolitis and bronchitis in connective tissue disease. A possible relationship to the use of penicillamine. *J.A.M.A.* **242**:528-532.

Ginsberg, S. J., and Comis, R. L. (1982). The pulmonary toxicity of antineoplastic agents. *Semin. Oncol.* **9**:34-51.

Ginsburg, W. W. (1980). Drug-induced systemic lupus erythematosus. *Semin. Respir. Med.* **2**:51-58.

Heffner, J. E., and Sahn, S. A. (1981). Salicylate-induced pulmonary edema: clinical features and prognosis. *Am. Intern. Med.* **95**:405-409.

Henningsen, N. C., Cederberg, A., and Hanson, A. (1975). Effects of long term treatment with procainamide. *Acta Med. Scand.* **198**:475-482.

Howard, J. J., Mohsenifar, Z., and Simmons, S. M. (1982). Adult respiratory distress syndrome following administration of lidocaine. *Chest* **81**:644-645.

Pitt, B. R., and Lister, G. (1989). Interpretation of metabolic function of the lung. In *Clinics in Chest Medicine* Vol. 10. Edited by S. G. Jenkinson. Philadelphia, W. B. Saunders, pp. 1-12.

Reichlin, S., Loveless, M. H., and Kane, E. G. (1953). Loeffler's syndrome following penicillin therapy. *Ann. Intern. Med.* **38**:113-120.

Rollo, I. M. (1975a). Drugs used in the chemotherapy of malaria. In *The Pharmacological Basis of Therapeutics.* Edited by A. G. Gilman, L. S. Goodman and A. Gilman. New York, MacMillan, pp. 1053.

Rollo, I. M. (1975b). Drugs used in the chemotherapy of helminthiasis. In *The Pharmacological Basis of Therapeutics.* Edited by A. G. Gilman, L. S. Goodman and A. Gilman. New York, Macmillan, pp. 1015-1016.

Rothfield, N. F., Bierer, W. F., and Garfield, J. W. (1978). Isoniazid induction of antinuclear antibodies: a prospective study. *Ann. Intern. Med.* **88**:650-652.

Schatz, M., Wasserman, S., and Patterson, R. (1981). Eosinophils and immunologic lung disease. *Med. Clin. North Am.* **65**:1055-1071.

Schoen, R. T., and Trentham, D. E. (1981). Drug-induced lupus: an adjuvant disease. *Am. J. Med.* **71**:5-8.

Steinberg, A. D., and Karliner, J. S. (1968). The clinical spectrum of heroin pulmonary edema. *Arch. Intern. Med.* **122**:122-127.

Szczeklik, A. (1982). Aspirin and asthma. *Eur. J. Respir. Dis.* **63**:376-379.

Szidon, J. P., and Fishman, A. P. (1988). Approach to the patient with respiratory signs and symptoms. In *Pulmonary Diseases and Disorders* (Second Edition) Vol. 1. Edited by A. P. Fishman. New York, MCGraw-Hill, pp. 351-352.

Van Barneveld, R. W. C., Sleifer, D. T., Vandermark, T. W., Mulder, H. H., Koops, H. S., Sluiter, H. J., and Peset, R. (1987). Fatal course of bleomycin-induced pneumonitis. *Am. Rev. Respir. Dis.* **135**:48-51.

Warring, F. C., and Howlett, K. S. (1952). Allergic reactions to para-aminosalicylic acid; report of seven cases, including one case of Loeffler's syndrome. *Am. Rev. Tuberc.* **65**:235-249.

Weingarten, R. J. (1943). Tropical eosinophilia. *Lancet* **1**:103-105.

Weinstein, A. (1980). Drug-induced systemic lupus erythematosus. *Prog. Clin. Immunol.* **4**:1-21.

Wold, D. E., and Zahn, D. W. (1956). Allergic (Loeffler's) pneumonitis occuring during antituberculous chemotherapy. Report of three cases. *Am. Rev. Tuberc.* **74**:445.

22

Pulmonary Function Laboratory in the Tropics

Needs, Problems, and Solutions

SURINDER K. JINDAL and P. L. WAHI

Postgraduate Institute of Medical Education and Research
Chandigarh, India

I. Introduction

The enormous burden of pulmonary tuberculosis (TB) has masked the equally staggering problem of nontuberculous pulmonary disease in most tropical countries. In India, the total burden of this problem was estimated at 21.76 million individuals, with an annual addition of 0.9 million (Sapru, 1983). Although 25-30% of total outpatient attendance at Indian hospitals was attributed to pulmonary diseases (Rao, 1971), around 65% of the patients attending the chest clinic of our hospital were diagnosed as having nontuberculous lung disease (Jindal et al., 1989). Unfortunately, the development of pulmonary medicine in this country, as in most other tropical countries, has not paralleled the enormity of the problem.

II. Existing Facilities

Information on testing facilities available in large hospitals with more than 500 beds and medical colleges, received from 60 Indian centers was revealing (Jindal, 1989). Although 20% of centers had no pulmonary function test

Table 1 Available Facilities in 60 PFT Labs of Indian Medical Colleges

Test	PFT Labs Using the Test No.	%	Tests per Week (Cumulative Average ± SD)
Spirometry	48	80	22 ± 15
Blood gas analysis	18	30	38 ± 28
Diffusion test	11	18.3	8 ± 3
Plethysmography	4	6.7	6
Exercise testing	3	5	<1

laboratory (PFT) at all, most others were ill equipped (Table 1). Frequently, the laboratory consisted of a spirometer, which was generally underutilized and often nonfunctional. The situation was similar in some of the neighboring countries, including Pakistan, Nepal, and Bangladesh, as revealed from the limited number of responses to our questionnaire (Jindal, 1989).

The need to develop a pulmonary service is now being realized (Malik, 1985; Jain, 1988). The American model can be considered as an example. In the late 1960s responsibility was assumed by the National Institutes of Health, and the National Heart, Lung and Blood Institute became the coordinating agency for programs for lung diseases (Cooper, 1970). Massive efforts were undertaken with partnership among the National Heart, Lung and Blood Institute, professional groups such as the American Thoracic Society and the National College of Chest Physicians, and individual pulmonary physicians and researchers to result in an overall improvement in staffing and pulmonary services (Schweizer and Lenfant, 1979). Raising staffing levels is the key to developing pulmonary centers. However, a real metamorphosis is required for internists and TB physicians dealing with lung diseases, who have generally lacked the initiative to enlighten themselves regarding advances in the field of pulmonary medicine to establish good, functional PFT laboratories.

III. Need for a PFT Laboratory

Although the need for a PFT laboratory may vary from center to center, the principal purpose of a clinical laboratory in a hospital is to assist the physician by providing a set of lung function tests to determine the presence of disease and to quantify the degree of respiratory disability. The tests may also provide objective assessment of type, degree, and progress of a disease and monitor therapy. A respiratory laboratory in an industrial or occupational setting has the more specific purpose of establishing the relationship between disease and to a particular exposure agent. Insurance companies are interested in the degree of disability for purposes of compensation. Research centers and those associated with training programs in pulmonary diseases need fully updated and research-oriented laboratories that reflect their specific area of research.

IV. Concept of a Laboratory in the Tropics

A small clinical PFT laboratory is required by any district level governmental or private hospital with 100 beds or more. A sturdy spirometer is the most basic requirement. Addition of a few peak flowmeters is useful. An arterial blood gas analyzer is optional for small laboratories, but mandatory for larger hospitals and laboratories at the level of state medical colleges (Malik, 1986a). These laboratories would also require facilities for measuring functional residual capacity and diffusion capacity, bronchoprovocation, and bronchoreversibility testing.

Referral laboratories established on a regional basis and for tertiary care centers need to be equipped with near-complete facilities, including whole body plethysmography, exercise testing, and mass spectrometry. It is useful to integrate facilities for cardiac catheterization and echocardiography to allow for an overall assessment of cardiopulmonary functions. Further additions can be made as needed, for example, assessment of respiratory regulation, polysomnography, and others, but a back up general-purpose computer is essential.

Respiratory laboratories play a vital role in hospitals that have intensive care units (ICU) because they help in monitoring hemodynamic and pulmonary mechanics. Lung mechanics can be assessed with volume, pressure, and flow measurements with the help of volume displacement (e.g., water-seal) spirometers and pneumotachographs. For the assessment of gas exchange, monitoring of inspired, expired, and arterial O_2 and CO_2 is required, necessitating O_2 and CO_2 monitors (preferably a mass spectrometer) and blood gas analyzers. Hemodynamic monitoring in the acute care setting occurs largely at the bedside, with central venous or right heart and pulmonary artery catheterization with flow-directed, double- or triple-lumen catheters. A thermodilution catheter with quadruple lumen has an additional line for computer connection to the thermister for measuring cardiac output.

A field unit is an important component as an "extended mobile laboratory", for epidemiological purposes, especially for obstructive lung diseases. The unit may be comprised of a trained team (including a physician, social worker, and a technician) and portable instruments (such as peak flowmeters) for the objective assessment of airway obstruction. The feasibility of field screening in a tropical country has been amply demonstrated in several studies from this center (Malik, 1986b).

Specialized laboratories such as those for industry, sports institutes, aviation, diving, and high-altitude science have more specific needs. The respiratory component is generally the same as expected for a referral laboratory, with added facilities for particular research interests. With increasing industrialization, developing countries are actively facing the issues of occupational exposures and compensation, and hence there is the need for these types of laboratories.

V. Specific Equipment Problems

Developing countries, including India, depend heavily on the importation of highly automated and sophisticated respiratory equipment. There are enormous financial and technical limitations in identifying, selecting, and procuring appropriate equipment. Both purchasing and maintaining the equipment pose problems. Lack of trained technologists, rapid changes in model designs, and nonavailability of spare parts add to the problems. It is not infrequent to find costly equipment remaining totally unused or rendered useless for want of minor repairs.

Financial considerations have a great bearing on establishing and running a laboratory. Heavy commissions charged by manufacturers and their dealers, export-import duties imposed by governments, and fluctuating foreign exchange rates often add heavily to the initial price of equipment. For example, in India it may cost between $30,000 and $50,000 to start an ordinary clinical laboratory. This excludes the costs for space and personnel. Establishment of a larger laboratory at the medical college level would require over $1,000,000.

As well as the initial investment, one must ensure the smooth running of equipment with adequate supplies of consumables and other spares. It is important not to go for the latest, exotic models, but for well-tested designs. Companies without adequate service facilities in the area should not even be considered. Reliability should be suitably checked through established laboratories of the region.

A strong case can be made for the indigenous development of technology, but accuracy must not be sacrificed. It may also do well for Western and Japanese manufacturers to "tropicalize" the equipment they are exporting. There is a greater need for sturdy and simple designs. Voltage fluctuations are wide and frequent in developing countries, necessitating built-in stabilizer designs. Hot and humid climates shorten the life of bags and tubing used for collecting and storing gas mixtures. There is also the minor problem of rats having a taste for polyvinyl-chloride-coated circuitry.

VI. Laboratory Management

As well as equipment and supplies, personnel are the anchor of a successful laboratory. The administrator in charge, equivalent to the Medical Director of an American laboratory, is usually the departmental head. It is difficult to prescribe definite qualifications, but they are expected to be similar to those recommended in an American hospital: a clinician with an M.D. degree who is authorized to practice medicine with certification (or eligibility for certification) by a subspeciality board of pulmonary diseases (Gardner et al., 1986a; Abramson and Van Kessel, 1982). A postdoctoral physician in pulmonary medicine is ideal to head a department and the laboratory. As an alternative, a postgraduate in medicine or in "tuberculosis and chest diseases" with at least 5 years of clinical and teaching experience on the faculty of a respiratory diseases department may be suitable to run the laboratory. The departmental head is responsible for the efficient working of the laboratory, accuracy of reports and their clinical interpretation, record keeping, and personnel management. He is directly accountable to the hospital administration.

The laboratory staff may include a technical supervisor and a few assistants, technicians, and laboratory attendants. The number depends upon the workload of the laboratory. It is difficult to specify qualifications for the technical staff since no regular teaching or training courses are available as yet. The American Thoracic Society recommends a high school background with strong mathematics training (Gardner et al., 1986a). In view of the huge technical inputs required for this country, it is advisable to create a pool of technical help by having a 2 year combined degree course in cardiopulmonary laboratory technology for graduates in science. Such courses can be started at two or three institutes equipped with the requisite resources. Until then, training is to be imparted on an inservice basis to individuals. The technician should be able not only to perform the test but also to understand the test, calculate the results, and assess its validity. He or she should be able to calibrate the equipment, perform periodic quality control procedures, and attend to minor troubleshooting.

Specific training is required for technicians for industrial laboratories. Several training manuals for this purpose are available (Make, 1979; Enright and Hyatt, 1987).

VII. Computer Requirements

Computer technology has invaded in a big way and has tremendous application in medicine in India (Jindal and Jindal, 1988). Most of the respiratory equipment, including spirometers, contains digital computers. These special-purpose systems are generally available as packages that include software and the test equipment. While the use of computers has increased the speed and accuracy of tests, it has posed problems of quality assurance and increased investment (Gardner et al., 1986b; Crapo et al., 1986). Moreover, most of the systems use Western values for predictive data. Software modifications may be essential to suit the needs of the local population. Since it may not be possible to alter the program of such a system, it may be useful to buy a general-purpose computer for a larger laboratory. This is expensive, but allows maximal flexibility. Software and programming for such a computer are most important and require trained personnel.

For routine use in a good laboratory, a 16 bit minicomputer with 64-256 K bytes of main memory and 1-5M bytes of disk storage is recommended (Larson, 1982). Smaller laboratories may continue to rely on special-purpose computer equipment, and manufacturing companies need to come to their help.

VII. Normal Lung Function Tests

There are significant variations in normal lung function values among different populations. These may relate to ethnic groups, environmental factors, altitude, level of habitual physical activity and habits of tobacco smoking (Woolcock et al., 1972). Variations on the order of 25% were found in different ethnic groups quantified on the basis of stature (Cotes, 1979). A difference of 13% for vital capacity (VC) and forced expiratory volume (FEV) has been reported between blacks and whites (Rossiter and Weil, 1974). Indian, Bantu, and Chinese have lower values than Europeans (Jain and Gupta, 1967; Jain and Ramiah, 1967, 1969; Johanssen and Erasmus, 1968; Woolcock et al., 1972; Da Costa, 1971). These differences are generally attributed to differences in body stature and lung size. True ethnic anthropometric variations may exist when age, body size, environmental, and nutritional status are standardized as far as possible (Miller et al., 1970).

A large number of reports on normal spirometric values have been produced in the last decade from several tropical countries of Asia and Africa, based on findings in both children and adults (Sliman et al., 1981, 1982; Udwadia et al., 1987; Kamat et al., 1982; Ayub et al., 1987; Lam et al., 1983; Malik and Jindal, 1985a; Malik et al., 1987a,b; Al Fayez et al., 1988; Sham-

Table 2 Minimal Recommendations for Spirometry Systems

Test	Range/Accuracy *BTPS*[a] (L)	Flow Range (L/s)	Time (s)	Resistance and Back Pressure	Test Signal
VC	7L ± 3% of reading or ± 0.050 L, whichever is greater	0-12	30		3 L Cal syringe
FVC	7 L ± 3% of reading or ± 0.050 L, whichever is greater	0-12	15		24 standard waveforms
FEV_1	7L ± 3% of reading or ± 0.050 L, whichever is greater	0-12	t	Less than 1.5 cm H_2O/L/s, from 0 to 12 L/s	
Time zero	The time point from which all FEV_t measurements are taken			Determined by extrapolation	
$FEF_{25-75\%}$	7.0 L ± 5% of reading or ± 0.200 L/s, whichever is greater	0-12	15	Same as FEV_t	24 standard waveforms
$\dot{V}$	± 12 L/s ± 5% of reading or ± 0.200 L/s, whichever is greater	0-12	15	Same as FEV_t	Manufacturer proof
MVV	Sine wave 250 L/min at TV of 2 L within ± 5% of reading	0-12 ± 5%	12-15 ±3%	Pressure less than ± 10 cmH_2O at 2 L TV at 2.0 Hz	Sine wave pump 0-4 Hz ± 10% at ± 12 L/s

Reproduced with permission of American Thoracic Society, 1987a.
[a]Body Temperature and Pressure, Saturated.

assain et al., 1988). Caution must be observed while deriving prediction formulae regarding standardization procedures. Guidelines published by American Thoracic Society including recommendations for spirometry systems (Table 2) are most useful (American Thoracic Society, 1987a). Volume and speed of spirometer should be regularly calibrated and leaks tested. Careful record ing of patients' age, height, and weight is important. Methodology should be precise and analysis accurate.

The criteria for an acceptable maneuver for expiratory flow include unhesitating start, apparent maximal effort, smooth continuous exhalation, and absence of cough, glottal closure, early termination, or leak. The FVC of best two of acceptable tracings should not vary by more than $\pm$ 5%. We use the "best test" FVC (i.e., the curve with largest sum of FVC and FEV_1) for all measurement, for convenience, rather than mixing computations from different tracings to obtain the "maximal data" (i.e., largest FEV_1 and largest FVC even if from different curves). This practice is largely followed in most of the laboratories and is supported by data on 1101 subjects in whom the difference between "maximal" and "best test" values was insignificant (Sorenson et al., 1980; Boushey and Dawson, 1982).

IX. Testing Lung Function in Children

Although the indications for lung function testing in children are similar to those in adults, the technical requirements and other specifications differ (Polgar and Promadhat, 1971; Taussig et al., 1980; Lemen, 1977). Several prediction equations available for white children are nearly identical (Polgar and Weng, 1979). These predictions may not be applicable to children of other racial groups (Binder et al., 1976). The earlier studies in children from India have reported volume and/or flow measurements for different age groups (Jain and Ramiah, 1968a,b; Bhattacharya and Banerjee, 1966). Recent studies from India and some other tropical countries including Libya and Jordan, have used prediction equations that incorporate coefficients for age and height (Malik and Jindal, 1985a; Sliman et al., 1982; Shamassain et al., 1988). These are likely to vary from place to place. It may not be feasible for each laboratory to have its own standards. However, each laboratory can test a group of normal subjects and compare these with the standards available for the particular racial group prevalent in the region.

Lungs are still growing in children, so no single value can be considered as normal for a particular age group and there is a broad range of normal values. Predictive values correlate significantly with selected physical characteristics such as age, height, weight, and body surface area (BSA). Although age is an index of lung maturity, BSA and height are determinants of body

Table 3 Regression Coefficients for Prediction Equations for Healthy Indian Children[a]

Function	K	Age (b_1)	Height (b_2)	S.D.
Boys				
VC(L)	− 0.4	0.02	0.0003	0.8
FEV_1 (L)	− 0.3	0.017	0.0003	0.7
$FEF_{25-75\%}$ (L/M)	11.0	1.08	0.04	54.8
Girls				
VC(L)	− 2.5	0.005	0.027	0.6
FEV_1 (L)	− 2.3	0.004	0.026	0.6
$FEF_{25-75\%}$	− 136.1	0.3	1.86	53.5

[a]Lung function = K + b_1 age (yrs) + b_2 height (cm).

size, and therefore, of lung size. Our predictions using age and height were similar to those using age and BSA (Malik and Jindal, 1985a). Because age and height are more reliable parameters in children, these are used for prediction (Table 3).

X. Testing Lung Function in Adults

Reports on lung function in adults from different places underline the importance of using local prediction equations. There is a general lowering of lung function as one moves towards the equator. While North African adults have values similar to those of Europeans and Americans, these values are lower in person living further south (Sliman et al., 1981; Johanssen and Erasmus, 1968; Woolcock et al., 1972; Miller et al., 1970; Cotes, 1979; Udwadia et al., 1987; Williams et al., 1978). On the Indian subcontinent, Pakistanis and North Indians have higher values than those of South Indians (Udwadia et al., 1987; Malik et al., 1987a,b; Ayub et al., 1987; Kamat et al., 1982). Highlanders are an exception, such as the natives of Nepal, Bhutan, Ladakh, New Guinea, and Peru, who have larger lung volumes (Cotes and Ward, 1966; Cotes, 1979; Woolcock et al., 1972; Boyce et al., 1974).

Most of the earlier studies used multiple linear equations relating the function to age, sex, and height, but the relationship with age is actually nonuniform (Knudson et al., 1976; Schoenberg et al., 1978). We derived equations using age and height as regression coefficients by the method of least squares, whereby the sum of squares of deviations of the observed from the predicted value is minimized and the "best fit" equation is chosen. To determine the final model, multiple coefficients including age, powers of age up to age to the third power, height, weight, and body surface area were included and the procedure of elimination was used. The "best fit" equations were those with height, age, and age squared as coefficients (Table 4). The predictions using these equations were compared for standardized height. The values are an improvement over those reported from the same region some 20 years ago (Jain and Ramiah, 1967b, 1969). It is interesting that our current values are similar to the Western values reported earlier (Goldman and Becklake, 1959; Ferris et al., 1965) (Fig. 1).

A. Lower Limit of Normal

The range of spirometric values in a normal population is rather broad and it is useful to define the "lower limit of normal" expressed as the lower 95th percentile, provided that the distribution of the data is Gaussian (Knudson and Lebowitz, 1978). This equals the mean minus 1.65 SD (Fig. 2). The lower 95th percentile is the value above which 95% of the normal subjects fall. The 5% of the population whose percentage predicted values fall below this normal 95th percentile are thus considered abnormal. This increases the sensitivity of prediction.

Table 4 Regression Coefficients for Prediction Equations for Healthy North Indian Adults

Function	K	Age (yrs) (b_1)	Age^2 (yrs) (b_2)	Ht. (cm) (b_3)	Lower Limit of Normal
Men					
FVC (L)	−3.44	−0.013	−0.00005	0.048	2.75
FEV_1 (L)	−1.9	0.025	0.00006	0.036	2.13
$FEF_{25\text{-}75\%}$ (L/M)	59	−2.6	0.007	1.5	87
Women					
FVC (L)	−2.05	−0.014	−0.00004	0.035	1.81
FEV_1 (L)	−1.07	−0.03	0.00013	0.027	1.53
$FEF_{25\text{-}75\%}$ (L/M)	23	−2.6	0.01	1.5	79

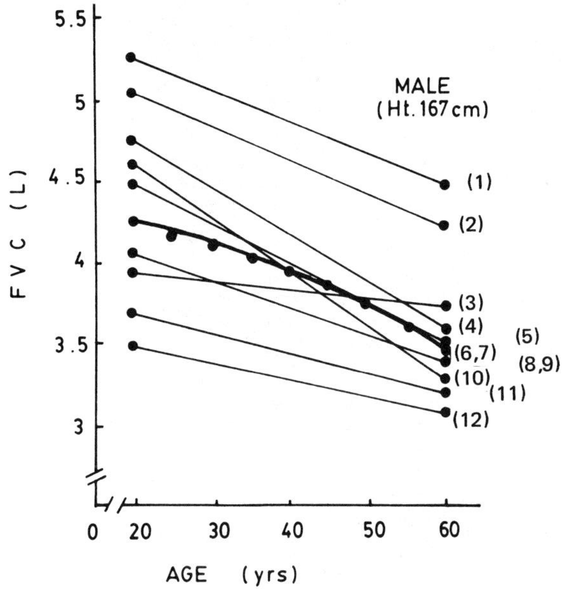

(a)

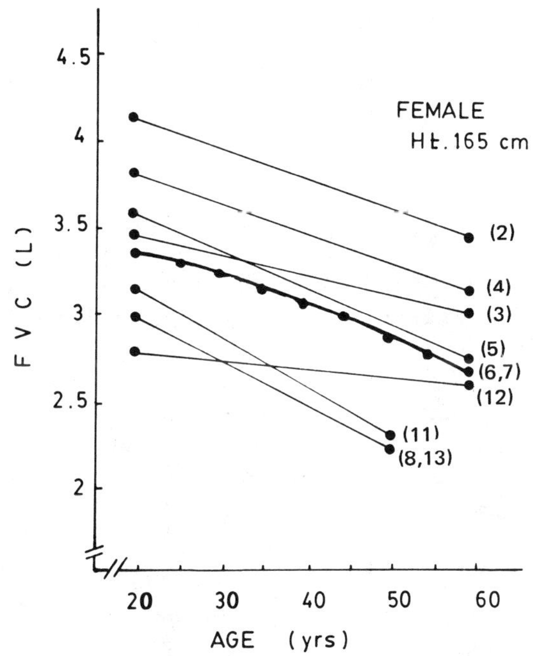

(b)

Figure 1 Regression lines for FVC derived from various prediction equations for healthy male (a) and female (b) subjects. 1. Cotes and Wand, 1966; 2, Sliman et al., 1987; 4, Ferris et al., 1965; 5, Goldman and Becklake, 1959; 6, 7, Malik et al., 1987a, b; 8, Jain and Gupta, 1967; 9, Jain and Ramiah 1969a; 10, Lam et al., 1983; 11, Kam et al., 1982; 12, Udwadia et al., 1987; 13, Jain and Ramiah, 1967b.

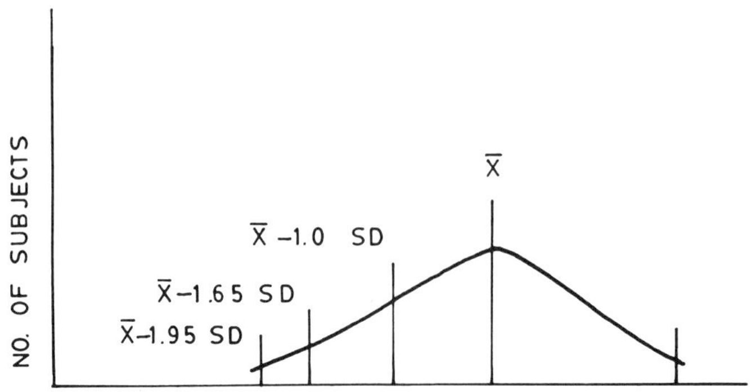

A	% OF POPULATION >A
$\bar{X}$ −1.95 SD	97.5
$\bar{X}$ −1.65 SD	95.0
$\bar{X}$ −1.0 SD	84.0
$\bar{X}$	50.0

Figure 2 Proportion of a population above various limits of normal (reproduced with permission from Clausen, 1982).

B. Variation in Measurements

Lung function may change due to factors other than disease, which are often dismissed as "noise" by clinicians (Hruby and Butler, 1975). The measurements may differ in the same subject at different times. The different technical and biological sources of variation were recently reviewed (Becklake, 1986). Although the technical factors may relate to the instrument and the procedure, the biological factors may vary with the subject and the environment. A well-judged and balanced measurement is therefore essential while interpreting these tests.

C. Peak Expiratory Flow Rate

Peak expiratory flow rate (PEFR) remains an important test for both epidemiological and clinical purposes (Prime, 1973; Gregg and Nunn, 1973). This is especially true for tropical countries because it is cheaper and easier to perform. The values are closely correlated with estimates of FEV_1 and of airway resistance (Wright and McKerrow, 1959; Zamel et al., 1963).

Since sensitive electronic instruments such as FEV_1-FVC-meters or minispirometers are not suitable in the field because of problems due to weather conditions and quality control, a peak flowmeter is preferable. Moreover, for epidemiological studies such great sensitivity is not required. The PEFR is therefore quite satisfactory. On the other hand, high sensitivity of electronic meters may introduce too many false-positve results.

Similar criteria apply to PEFR as to spirometry. Curvilinear equations based on height and age are most suitable (Gregg and Nunn, 1973; Jindal et al., 1974; Malik and Jindal, 1985b).

D. Blood Gases

Determination of arterial gas pressures and pH has a great significance in patient management. This facility is generally required around the clock for most of the clinical departments of a large hospital. Therefore, it is better managed as a centralized facility than locating it in a PFT laboratory. It is difficult to specify absolute quality control requirements because of the differences in analyzers and quality control procedures. Accuracy and precision are the minimum requirements.

E. Pulmonary Diffusion Capacity

The clinical usefulness of diffusion capacity is doubtful, but the applications include diagnosis of diffuse interstitial pulmonary diseases and suspected emphysema. Several factors, such as blood hemoglobin levels, pulmonary vascular blood volume, exercise, and other metabolic activities, influence normal values. Standard technique should be followed to minimize the variation (American Thoracic Society, 1987b). With the recent availability of computerized, electronic equipment, it has become easier to measure diffusion capacity. Reports on normal subjects from India have been scanty (Guleria et al., 1971; Pande et al., 1975). In a recent study on normal subjects from Bombay, diffusion capacity was found to be lower among Indians (Udwadia et al., 1987).

XI. Clinical Applications of Laboratory Data

A. Diagnostic

Caution is necessary regarding diagnosis by overinterpretation of lung function test results (Butler, 1981; Becklake, 1986). Abnormal lung function indicates respiratory defect. The defect may relate to ventilation (obstructive or restrictive), perfusion, or gas exchange. Obstructive diseases such as bronchial asthma, chronic bronchitis, and emphysema are the common diseases that require PFT laboratory assistance for diagnosis. Pulmonary parenchymal involvement, both primary and secondary to systemic diseases, also shows characteristic findings on lung function assessment. Some of these problems, such as tropical eosinophilia and schistosomiasis, are characteristically seen in tropical countries. A 6 year analysis from this Institute gives a general trend of diagnostic applications (Table 5).

Around 50% of pulmonary function tests are done for preoperative assessment, which is very similar to the Western experience (Malik and Jindal, 1988; Woolf, 1968; Hughes and Empey, 1972). In the field, PFT is used to document airway obstruction, which is a forerunner of respiratory disability (Fletcher and Peto, 1977).

Table 5 Disease-Related Distribution of Indications for Pulmonary Function Tests[a] at the Postgraduate Institute, Chandigarh, for a 6 Year Period

			Total	
Disease	Males	Females	No.	%
Pulmonary				
COPD	891	179	1070	20.1
Asthma	292	239	531	10.0
Interstitial	122	129	251	4.7
Collagen vascular	58	106	164	3.1
Bronchiectasis	72	49	121	2.3
Tuberculosis	37	11	48	0.9
Lung cancer	77	11	88	1.7
Others	174	74	248	4.7
Cardiac				
Congenital	236	165	401	7.6
Rheumatic	194	140	334	6.3
Others	33	17	50	0.9
Miscellaneous, Medical				
Neurological	47	25	72	1.4
General	153	79	232	4.4
Preoperative assessment				
Thoracic[b]	14	5	19	0.4
Urological	1094	113	1207	22.7
Gynecological	—	96	96	1.8
Neurosurgical	83	50	133	2.5
General, surgical	178	69	247	4.6
Total	3755 (70.7%)	1557 (29.3%)	5312	100.0

[a]Multiple follow up tests for one patient are considered only once.
[b]Excluding cardiac and pulmonary.

B. Therapeutic

The role of lung function assessment in both determining treatment and following the response to therapy for diseases of airways, as well as those of lung parenchyma, is well established. In tropical countries, most clinicians have generally relied on clinical judgement. This was because of both the magnitude of disease and the limited availability of resources. This is no longer true. With the routine availability of peak flowmeters and cheaper office spirometers, ventilatory monitoring has become easier and more practical. This is especially important for asthma, in which fluctuations in airway obstruction are wide and clinical assessment can be misleading.

Deciding on treatment and monitoring the progress of parenchymal and interstitial diseases are more problematic on the basis of simple lung function tests, especially spirometry. A battery of tests, done repeatedly, is often required. However, these diseases are relatively uncommon and are generally diagnosed and treated in a referral hospital, where a better-equipped laboratory is often available. Abnormal spirometry may serve as a screening tool only. With the help of PFT laboratories diseases such as fibrosing alveolitis, sarcoidosis, and others, hitherto considered "extremely rare" in these countries, have been recognized and treated with increasing frequency (Jindal et al., 1979; Sharma et al., 1984; Bambery et al., 1987).

References

Abramson, J. F., and Van Kessel, A. L. (1982). Laboratory management; qualifications of personnel. In *Pulmonary Function Testing Guidelines and Controversies.* Edited by J. L. Clausen. New York, Academic Press.

Al Fayez, S. F., Salieh, M., Ardawf, M., and Zahran, F. M. (1988). Effect of sheesha and cigarette smoking on pulmonary function of Saudi males and females. *Trop. Geogr. Med.* **40**:115-123.

American Thoracic Society. (1987a). Standardization of spirometry—1987 update *Am. Rev. Respir. Dis.* **136**:1285-1298.

American Thoracic Society. (1987b). Statement. Single breath carbon monoxide diffusing capacity (transfer factor). *Am. Rev. Respir. Dis.* **136**: 1299-1307.

Ayub, M., Zaidi, S. H., and Burki, N. K. (1987). Spirometry and flow-volume curves in healthy normal Pakistanis. *Br. J. Dis. Chest* **81**:35-44.

Bambery, P., Behera, D., Gupta, A. K., Kaur, U., Jindal, S. K., Deodhar, S. D., and Malik, S. K. (1987). Sarcoidosis in North India: clinical profile of 40 patients. *Sarcoidosis* **4**:155-158.

Becklake, M. R. (1986). Concepts of normality applied to the measurement of lung function. *Am. J. Med.* **80**:1158-1164.

Bhattacharya, A. K., and Banerjee, S. (1966). Vital capacity in children and young adults of India. *Indian J. Med. Res.* **54**:62-71.

Binder, R. E., Mitchell, C. A., Schoenberg, J. B., and Bouhuys, A. (1976). Lung function among black and white children. *Am. Rev. Respir. Dis.* **114**:955-959.

Boushey, H. A., and Dawson, A. (1982). Spirometry and flow-volume curves. In *Pulmonary Function Testing Guidelines and Controversies*. Edited by J. L. Clausen. New York, Academic Press.

Boyce, A. J., Haight, J. S., Rimmer, D. B., and Harrison, G. A. (1974). Respiratory function in Peruvian Quechua Indians. *Ann. Hum. Biol.* **1**:137-148.

Butler, J. (1981). The pulmonary function test—cautious overinterpretation. *Chest* **79**:498-500.

Clausen, J. L. (Ed.). (1982). Predictors of normal values. In *Pulmonary Function Testing: Guidelines and Controversies*. New York, Academic Press.

Cooper, T. (1970). National Heart and Lung Institute. *Am. Rev. Respir. Dis.* **101**:631.

Cotes, J. E. (1979). *Lung Function*. Oxford, Blackwell Scientific Publishers, pp. 329-387.

Cotes, J. E., and Ward, M. P. (1966). Ventilatory capacity in normal Bhutanese. *J. Physiol.* **186**:88.

Crapo, R. O., Gardner, R. M., Berlin, S. L., and Morris, A. H. (1986). Automation of pulmonary function equipment—user beware! *Chest* **90**:1-2.

Da Costa, J. L. (1971). Pulmonary function studies in healthy Chinese adults in Singapore. *Am. Rev. Respir. Dis.* **104**:128-131.

Enright, R. L., and Hyatt, R. D. (1987). *Office Spirometry*. Philadelphia, Lea & Febiger.

Ferris, B. G., Jr., Anderson, D. O., and Zickmantel, R. (1965). Prediction values for screening tests of pulmonary function. *Am. Rev. Respir. Dis.* **91**:252-261.

Fletcher, C. M., and Peto, R. (1977). The natural history of chronic airflow obstruction. *Br. Med. J.* **1**:1645-1648.

Gardner, R. M., Clausen, J. L., Epler, G., Hankinson, J. L., Permutt, S., and Plummer, A. L. (1986a). Pulmonary function laboratory personnel qualifications. *Am. Rev. Respir. Dis.* **134**:623-624.

Gardner, R. M., Clausen, J. L., Cotton, D. J., Crapo, R. O., Epler, G., Hankinson, J. L., and Johnson, R. L., Jr. (1986b). Computer guidelines for pulmonary laboratories. *Am. Rev. Respir. Dis.* **134**:628-629.

Goldman, H. I., Becklake, M. R. (1959). Respiratory function tests. Normal values at median altitudes and the prediction of normal results. *Am. Rev. Tuberc.* **79**:457-467.

Gregg, I., and Nunn, A. J. (1973). Peak expiratory flow in normal subjects. *Br. Med. J.* **3**:282-284.

Guleria, J. S., Pande, J. N., Sethi, P. K., and Roy, S. B. (1971). Pulmonary diffusing capacity and high altitudes. *J. Appl. Physiol.* **31**:536-543.

Hruby, J., and Butler, J. (1975). Variability of routine pulmonary function tests. *Thorax* **30**:548-553.

Hughes, D. T. D., and Empey, D. W. (1972). Ten years experience in running a pulmonary function laboratory. *Br. Med. J.* **4**:470-473.

Jain, S. K. (1988). Is teaching and respiratory medicine keeping pace with the clinical needs? *Ind. J. Chest Dis. Allied Sci.* **30**:1-4.

Jain, S. K., and Gupta, C. K. (1967). Lung function studies in healthy men and women over forty. *Indian J. Med. Res.* **55**:612-691.

Jain, S. K., and Ramiah, T. J. (1967). Spirometric studies in healthy women 15-40 years age. *Indian J. Chest Dis.* **9**:1-12.

Jain, S. K., and Ramiah, T. J. (1968a). Lung volumes and mechanics of breathing in healthy boys 7-14 years old. *Indian J. Chest Dis.* **10**:63-68.

Jain, S. K., and Ramiah, T. J. (1968b). Prediction of ventilatory 'norms' in healthy boys 7-14 years of age. *Indian J. Chest. Dis.* **10**:69-79.

Jain, S. K., and Ramiah, T. J. (1969). Normal standards of pulmonary function tests for healthy men 15-40 years old. Comparison of different regression equations (prediction formulae). *Indian J. Med. Res.* **57**:1453-1466.

Jindal, S. K. (1989). Pulmonary training facilities in medical colleges in India *Indian J. Chest Dis. Allied Sci.* **31**:295-298.

Jindal, S. K., and Jindal, U. N. (1988). Computer use in medical field. In *Hospital Administration and Management,* Vol. I. Edited by S. L. Goel and R. Kumar. New Delhi, Deep and Deep Publ., pp. 213-229.

Jindal, S. K., Bansal, S. K., and Malik, S. K. (1974). Peak expiratory flow rate in healthy North Indian adults. *Bull. Postgrad. Inst.* (*Chadigarh*) **8**:92-96.

Jindal, S. K., Malik, S. K., Deodhar, S. D., and Sharma, B. K. (1979). Fibrosing alveolitis: a report of 61 cases seen over the past five years. *Indian J. Chest. Dis. Allied Sci.* **21**:174-179.

Jindal, S. K., Bhaskar, B. V., and Behera, D. (1989). Respiratory disease pattern in a large referral hospital in India. *Lung India* **7**:119-121.

Johannsen, Z. M., and Erasmus, L. D. (1968). Clinical spirometry in normal Bantu. *Am. Rev. Respir. Dis.* **97**:585-597.

Kamat, S. R., Tyagi, N. K., and Rashid, S. S. A. (1982). Lung function in Indian adult subjects. *Lung India* **1**:1-11.

Knudson, R. J., and Lebowitz, M. D. (1978). Maximal mid expiratory flow: normal limits and assessment of sensitivity. *Am. Rev. Respir. Dis.* **117**: 609-610.

Knudson, R. J., Slatin, R. C., Lebowitz, M. D., and Burrows, B. (1976). The maximal expiratory flow-volume curve: normal standards, variability and effects of age. *Am. Rev. Respir. Dis.* **113**:587-600.

Lam, K. K., Pang, S. C., Allan, W. G. L., Hill, L. E., Snell, N. J. C., Fayers, P. M., Nunn, A. J., and Prime, F. J. (1983). Predictive nomograms for forced expiratory volume, forced vital capacity, and peak expiratory flow rate in Chinese adults and children. *Br. J. Dis. Chest* **77**:391-396.

Larson, J. K. (1982). Selection of a computer for the pulmonary laboratory. In *Pulmonary Function Testing Guidelines and Controversies.* Edited by J. L. Clausen. New York, Academic Press.

Lemen, J. R. (1977). Pulmonary function testing in the office and clinic. In *Disorders of the Respiratory Tract in Children.* Edited by E. L. Kendig and L. C. Chernick. Philadelphia, W. B. Saunders.

Make, B. (1979). Minimum criteria for training in spirometric testing in industry. *Bull. Am. Coll. Chest Physicians* **18**:24-26.

Malik, S. K. (1985). Developing pulmonary medicine (pulmonology) in India—a view point. *Indian J. Chest Dis. Allied Sci.* **27**:254-256.

Malik, S. K. (1986a). Setting up pulmonary laboratories in India. *Indian J. Chest Dis. Allied Sci.* **28**:257-262.

Malik, S. K. (1986b). Profile of chronic bronchitis in North India—the PGI experience (1972-1985). *Lung India* **4**:89-100.

Malik, S. K., and Jindal, S. K. (1985a). Pulmonary function tests in healthy children. *Indian Pediatr.* **22**:677-681.

Malik, S. K., and Jindal, S. K. (1985b). Normal values of PEFR in healthy North Indian adults.—revision of prediction formulae. *Indian J. Chest Dis. Allied Sci.* **27**:50-51.

Malik, S. K., and Jindal, S. K. (1988). Clinical pulmonary function laboratory, fifteen years on—an assessment. *Lung India* **6**:59-60.

Malik, S. K., Jindal, S. K., and Jindal, V. K. (1987a). Vital capacity and forced expiratory volume, one second (FEV_1) in normal, healthy North Indian adults (I). *Bull. Postgrad. Inst. (Chadigarh)* **21**:179-186.

Malik, S. K., Jindal, S. K., and Jindal, V. K. (1987b). Forced expiratory flows in normal, healthy, North Indian adults (II). *Bull. Postgrad. Inst. (Chandigarh)* **21**:187-210.

Miller, G. J., Ashcroft, M. T., Swan, A. V., and Beadnell, H. M. G. S. (1970). Ethnic variation in forced expiratory volume and forced vital capacity of African and Indian adults in Guyana. *Am. Rev. Respir. Dis.* **102**:979-981.

Pande, J. N., Gupta, S. P., and Guleria, J. S. (1975). Clinical significance of the measurement of membrane diffusing capacity and pulmonary capillary blood volume. *Respiration* **32**:317-324.

Polgar, G., and Promadhat, V. (1971). *Pulmonary Function Testing in Children: Techniques and Standards.* Philadelphia, W. B. Saunders.

Polgar, G., and Weng, T. R. (1979). The functional development of the respiratory system. *Am. Rev. Respir. Dis.* **120**:625-695.

Prime, F. J. (1973). Respiratory function tests for a clinician. *Br. Thorac. Tuberc. Assoc. Rev.* **3**:1-12.

Rao, K. N. (1971). Epidemiology of chest diseases. *Indian J. Chest Dis.* **13**: 17-24.

Rossiter, C. E., and Weil, H. (1974). Ethnic difference in lung function: evidence for proportional differences. *Int. J. Epidemiol.* **3**:55-66.

Sapru, R. P. (1983). Cardiovascular and nontuberculous chest diseases—an estimate of the size of the problem in India. *Ann. Natl. Acad. Sci. (India)* **19**:179-193.

Schoenberg, J. B., Beck, G. J., and Bouhuys, A. (1978). Growth and decay of pulmonary function in healthy blacks and whites. *Respir. Physiol.* **33**:367-393.

Schweizer, M., and Lenfant, C. (1979). Report on a decade: the lung program of the National Heart, Lung and Blood Institute. *Am. Rev. Respir. Dis.* **120**:1-4.

Shamassain, M. H., Thompson, J., and Ogston, S. A. (1988). Forced expiratory indices in normal Libyan children aged 6-19 years. *Thorax* **43**: 467-470.

Sharma, S. K., Pande, J. N., and Guleria, J. S. (1984). Diffuse interstitial pulmonary fibrosis. *Indian J. Chest Dis. Allied Sci.* **26**:214-219.

Sliman, N. A., Dajani, B. M., and Dajani, H. M. (1981). Ventilatory function test values of healthy adult Jordanians. *Thorax* **36**:546-549.

Sliman, N. A., Dajani, B. M., and Shubair, K. S. (1982). Pulmonary function in normal Jordanian children. *Thorax* **37**:854-857.

Sorensen, J. B., Morris, A. H., Crapo, R.O., and Gardner, R. M. (1980). Selection of the best spirometric values for interpretation. *Am. Rev. Respir. Dis.* **122**:802-805.

Taussig, L. M., Chernick, V., Wood, R., Farrel, P., and Mellins, R. B. (1980). Standardization of lung function testing in children. *J. Pediatr.* **97**:668-678.

Udwadia, F. E., Sunavala, J. D., and Shetye, V. M. (1987). Lung function studies in healthy Indian subjects. *J. Assoc. Physicians India* **36**:491-496.

Williams, D. E., Miller, R. D., and Taylor, W. F. (1978). Pulmonary function studies in healthy Pakistani adults. *Thorax* **33**:243-249.

Woolcock, A. M., Colman, M. H., and Blackburn, C. R. B. (1972). Factors affecting normal values for ventilatory lung function. *Am. Rev. Respir. Dis.* **106**:692-709.

Woolf, C. R. (1968). Organization of a hospital routine pulmonary function laboratory. *Can. Med. Assoc. J.* **98**:542-549.

Wright, B., McKerrow, C. G. (1959). Maximum forced expiratory flow rate as a measure of ventilatory capacity. *Br. Med. J.* **2**:1041-1047.
Zamel, N., Youssef, H. H., and Prime, F. J. (1963). Airway resistance and peak expiratory flow rates in smokers and non-smokers. *Lancet* **1**:1237-1238.

23

Tropical Pulmonary Eosinophilia

C. N. DEIVANAYAGAM

Tamilnadu Arasu Medical Science and Research Institute
Madras, India

I. Introduction

Tropical pulmonary eosinophilia is a component of the spectrum of filariasis. Filariasis is endemic in many coastal and subcoastal areas of the tropics. Filariasis is the result of infestation with many filarial parasites, the majority being due to the two species, *Wucheria bancrofti* and *Brugia malayi* (Spry and Kumaraswamy, 1982). Filariasis is a systemic disease and is the result of repeated transmissions of microfilariae to humans by biting mosquitoes—mainly the *Aedes* species.

The other names for tropical pulmonary eosinophilia are eosinophilic lung, tropical eosinophilia, and occult filariasis (Lie Khan, 1962).

II. Geographical Distribution

Most reported cases of tropical pulmonary eosinophilia originate from India, Malaysia, Indonesia, Pakistan, Bangladesh, Srilanka, Singapore, and the South Pacific Islands. In all these areas chronic filariasis is endemic, with visible deformities of filarial elephantiasis being the marker for this spectrum. Africa and South Africa have less number of patients (Manson-Bahr, 1987).

III. Clinical Features

Nothing prevents filariasis from coexisting with other disorders and diseases in the same individual. It has been reported that tropical pulmonary eosinophilia is distinct from chronic filariasis. This is no longer valid (Spry and Kumaraswamy, 1982). In order to clarify the clinical features, I report those subjects who are suffering only from tropical pulmonary eosinophilia. The cohort of 102 patients was seen by the author at Madras between the years 1971 and 1989. There were 62 males with a mean age of 23.7 years and 40 females with a mean age of 22.5 years. The sex ratio (3:2) is at variance with previous reports (Manson-Bahr, 1987).

The youngest and oldest males were 2 and 83 years of age, respectively. The female counterparts were 3 and 60 years, respectively. Clearly this is a disorder of young adults, with no age being exempt. One can speculate that infants below 2 years of age are generally protected in the tropics from mosquito bites and hence escape.

The criteria for diagnosis must be strictly defined. Short history of illness with predominant respiratory component, residence in endemic areas (sojournees usually escape), and a peripheral absolute blood count of more than 2000 cells/mm^3 (Vijayan et al., 1988a). Other authors have used counts of 3000 cells/mm^3 as the floor value (Spry and Kumaraswamy, 1982; Danaraj-etal, 1959.)

In this series, the mean absolute count was 3995 cells/mm^3. The highest being 19,120 and the lowest 1980. The threshold of 2000 is no magic dividing line; spontaneous drops in counts (without specific therapy) have been reported (Ray, 1986). The range of 1500-2000 cells/mm^3 is the grey area of overlap between allergic bronchial asthmatic syndromes (including allergic bronchopulmonary aspergillosis) and tropical eosinophilia. Clinical judgement and follow up are required for identification. Symptoms in the order of frequency are shown in Table 1.

Some patients present with no symptoms and others have only general systemic symptoms such as tiredness, anorexia, and weight loss. Rare reports include limb pain, acute giddiness, and testicular pain (Danaraj, 1958). The general systemic symptoms (in the absence of proven toxin production by the micro and adult filarial parasites), as well as the pain or giddiness referred to above point to the systemic nature of the illness. This is not surprising in view of the microfilaremia which occurs in every individual with filarial infection.

Table 1

Symptom	Percent
Cough	72.5
Expectoration	63.7
Wheezing and Stridor	41.2
Breathlessness and tightness of chest	33.3
Fever/rigor	31.4
Chest pain	28.4

Earlier workers emphasized the absence of microfilaria in the peripheral blood of tropical pulmonary eosinophilia (Danaraj, 1958), in both the day smear and night smear. In the author's series, two young men have had all the classical features of tropical pulmonary eosinophilia and persistant microfilariae in the peripheral blood for six months, despite specific therapy. It has been suggested that, in tropical pulmonary eosinophilia, the microfilariae are sequestrated in the pulmonary circulation (clearance from the circulation) and hence very few of them are available in the peripheral circulation (Ottesen et al., 1979).

On examination, these subjects exhibit features of some anxiety, are warm and tachypneic. The chest wall is usually resonant (occasionally tender) and vesicular breath sounds are accompanied by inspiratory and expiratory rhonchi and scattered crepitations. These rhonchi do diminish partially with forced coughing and chest wall percussion. Prolongation of expiration is uncommon and inconstant. Sputum had shown an increase in eosinophils and an intense eosinophilic alveolitis has been described in bronchoalveolar lavage studies (Pinkiston et al., 1987).

IV. Radiological Features

These are highly suggestive but not diagnostic. The most common features are (in the order of frequency)

Increased irregular and linear markings

Irregular hilar shadow

Fine to medium sized nodules (2-4 mm)

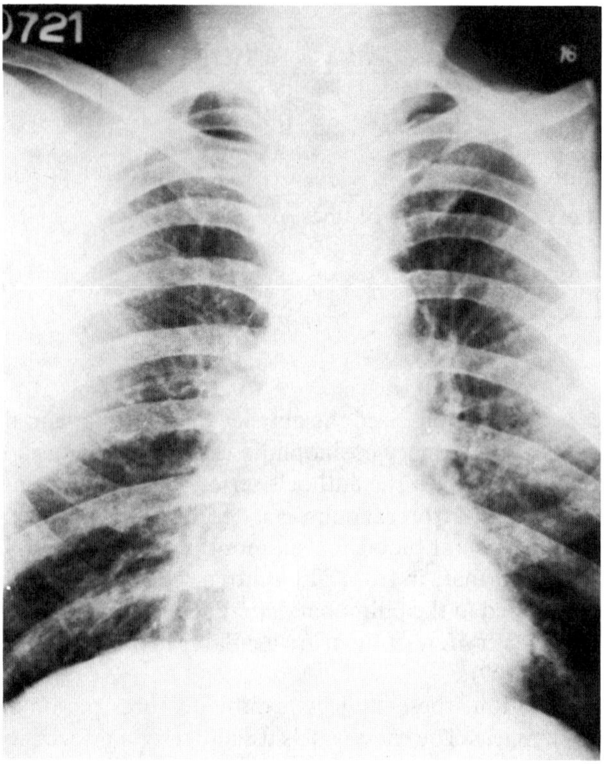

Figure 1 Skiagram chest PA view of adult male (48 years) with short history and absolute eosinophil count of $9000/mm^3$. Reticulations, striations, fine nodules and right hilar density are seen.

Air bronchogram especially in the right lower zone

Reticular shadows

Hilar density

Also described, but uncommon are pleural thickening, pleural effusions, pneumonic patches, and abscesslike opacities.

The erythrocyte sedimentation rate is usually raised.

V. Pulmonary Function Impairment

These are usually reductions in forced vital capacity (FVC) readings. There may be elements of obstruction or restriction of airflow and sometimes both elements may coexist. In subjects with obstruction as the major feature, the response to bronchodilator is only mild or moderate; the post bronchodilator FVC enhancement is usually less than 10% above the baseline reading. However, Ray has reported a higher response to isoprenaline in relapsing tropical pulmonary eosinophilia (1986). Diffusing capacity levels are low as are arterial oxygen tension levels (Vijayan et al., 1988b).

VI. Serological Tests

Complement fixation test using 1% alcoholic extract of dried Dirofilaria Immites has been found in the high liters in 95.3% patients and falling to low levels after therapy (Danavaj et al., 1959). Filarial fluorescent antibody levels are also high.

VII. Histopathological Features

Well-defined nodules 1-5 mm in diameter in the lung, lymph nodes, liver, and spleen have been described by Lie Kian Joe (1962). The cells are predominantly eosinophilic and in the center are seen microfilaria or its remnants. Surrounding these, are histiocytes and giant cells. Some fibrosis may be seen at the periphery. It is difficult to discern the microfilaria especially if they are sectioned across. The microfilaria can be made out easily if they are cut longitudinally. In the lymph nodes, the increase in size is due to proliferation of endothelial cells and germinal follicles infiltration with eosinophils and increased vascularity. Special and diligent search is required in the lungs to locate and identify these tubercles (Webb et al., 1960). In the lungs some of these nodules can mimic microabscesses.

VIII. Diagnosis

Diagnosis is readily made in the endemic areas by the classical symptomatology and absolute eosinophilia. Clinicians in these areas have long used response to diethylcarbamazine as a supplemental confirmatory diagnostic test.

The problem group represents patients who have other diseases and have additionally been subject to tropical pulmonary eosinophilia. In the author's experience, the coexistence has been noted with pulmonary tuberculosis, bronchial asthma, interstitial lung fibrosis and bronchiectasis. It would be necessary to keep this association in mind in considering atypical presentation.

IX. Natural History

The natural course of tropical pulmonary eosinophilia is of short duration and has been known to remit spontaneously. Relapses have been recorded in up to 20% of treated cases (Ray, 1986). These relapsing forms of the diseases may represent true relapses (i.e., no fresh injection of microfilaria by mosquito) or reinfection due to the ubiquitous mosquitoes, parasites, and man chain being available in endemic areas. Even these relapses rarely persist for more than 6 to 9 months. Lung fibrosis is rare in the experience of the author. The response to diethyl carbamazine is so good that persistance and fibrosis are rare consequences.

X. Treatment

Diethylcarbamazine in a dose to 8-10 mg/kg body weight for 21 days is the accepted treatment in many endemic areas. A few subjects complain of dizziness or unsteadiness and may require 4-5 mg/kg body weight dose for a few weeks. The response is often dramatic, clinical symptoms remit in 2 to 7 days, pulmonary function and radiological features improve more slowly. By 14 days the response is complete in the majority of patients.

A few patients may require a second or third course. Fewer than 5% may show resistance to diethylcarbamazine and may require steroids (prednisolone 0.25 mg/kg) upto 3-6 weeks for full recovery. It is good practice to continue diethylcarbamazine along with prednisolone. Prognosis is excellent. Morbidity is low and mortality is unreported. Relapses have to be diligently managed.

Prevention is intimately related to improved sanitation, removal of breeding areas, survey of the area for mosquito density, antimosquito measures (biological and chemical), as well as early identification of microfilariae in night smear. Wire/nylon mesh protection of houses, closing the windows and doors from 4-6 p.m. (the peak entry of mosquitoes into human dwellings in South India occurs at this hours) and the use of mosquito repellents (pyrethrum) are all necessary. Effective treatment of endemic filariasis will reduce the availability of microfilaria for transmission by mosquitoes. Endemicity reduces with improved socioeconomic prosperity of the population.

Widespread community treatment with diethylcarbamazine has been tried in Southeast Asia and may be tried elsewhere as part of a package of measures along with the foregoing public health measures.

References

Danaraj, T. J. (1958). The treatment of eosinophilic lung (tropical eosinophilia) with diethylcarbamazine. *Quart. J. Med.* **27**:243-263.

Danaraj, T. J., Da Silva, L. S., and Schacher, J. F. (1959). The serological diagnosis of eosinophilic lung (tropical eosinophilia) and its etiological implications. *Am. J. Trop. Med. Hyg.* **8**:151-159.

Lie Kian Joe. (1962). Occult filariasis: its relationship with tropical pulmonary eosinophilia. *Am. J. Trop. Med. Hyg.* **II**, 646-652.

Manson-Bahr, P. (1987). Tropical pulmonary eosinophilia (occult filariasis). In *Manson's Tropical Diseases*, 19th Ed. London, Balliere Tindal, pp. 371-373.

Ottesen, E. A., Neva, F. A., Paranjape, R. S., Tripathy, S. P., Thirvengadam, K. V., and Beaven, M. A. (1979). Specific allergic sensitization to filarial antigens in tropical eosinophilia syndrome. *Lancet* **1**:1158-1161.

Pinkiston, P., Vijayan, V. K., Nutman, T. B., et al. (1987). Acute tropical pulmonary eosinophilia—characterization of the lower respiratory tract inflammation and its response to therapy. *J. Clin. Invest.* **80**:216-225.

Ray, D. (1986). Bronchial response to inhaled isoprenaline in tropical pulmonary eosinophilia. *Lung India* **4**:25-28.

Spry, C. J. F., and Kumaraswamy, V. (1982). Tropical eosinophilia. *Sem. Hematol.* **19**:107-115.

Vijayan, V. K., Kuppurao, K. V., Sankaran, K., Venkatram, P., and Prabhakar, R. (1988a). Diffusing capacity in acute untreated tropical eosinophilia. *Ind. J. Chest Dis. All. Sci.* **30**:71-77.

Vijayan, V. K., Kuppurao, K. V., Venkataram, P., and Prabhakar, R. (1988b). Arterial hypoxaema in acute tropical pulmonary eosinophilia. *Lung India* **6**:183-185.

Webb, J. K. G., Job, C. K., and Gault, E. W. (1960). Tropical eosinophilia, demonstration of microfilaria in lung, liver and lymph nodes. *Lancet* **1**:835-845.

AUTHOR INDEX

Italic numbers give the page on which the complete reference is listed.

B

C

D

E

F

H

I

L

M

O

Q

R

S

T

X

Y

Z

SUBJECT INDEX

A